CHALLENGES IN CLINICAL PRACTICE

Pharmacologic and Psychosocial Strategies

Edited by

**MARK H. POLLACK
MICHAEL W. OTTO
JERROLD F. ROSENBAUM**

THE GUILFORD PRESS
New York London

©1996 The Guilford Press
A Division of Guilford Publications, Inc.
72 Spring Street, New York, NY 10012

Printed in the United States of America

This book is printed on acid-free paper.

Last digit is print number: 9   8   7   6   5   4   3   2   1

Library of Congress cataloging-in-publication data
is available from the Publisher.

ISBN 1-57230-067-1

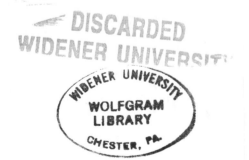

CHALLENGES IN CLINICAL PRACTICE

Contributors

J. Stuart Ablon, B.A., Pediatric Psychopharmacology Unit, Department of Psychiatry, Massachusetts General Hospital, Boston, MA

Lee Baer, Ph.D., Obsessive–Compulsive Disorder Unit, Department of Psychiatry, Massachusetts General Hospital East, Charlestown, MA

Claudia F. Baldassano, M.D., Bipolar Research Program, Clinical Psychopharmacology Unit, Department of Psychiatry, Massachusetts General Hospital, Boston, MA

Joseph Biederman, M.D., Pediatric Psychopharmacology Unit, Department of Psychiatry, Massachusetts General Hospital, Boston, MA

Carol Birnbaum, M.D., Perinatal and Reproductive Psychiatry, Clinical Psychopharmacology Unit, Department of Psychiatry, Massachusetts General Hospital, Boston, MA

Andrew Brotman, M.D., Department of Psychiatry, New England Deaconess Hospital, Boston, MA

Lee Cohen, M.D., Perinatal and Reproductive Psychiatry, Clinical Psychopharmacology Unit, Department of Psychiatry, Massachusetts General Hospital, Boston, MA

Katharine Davidson, B.A., Depression Research Program, Department of Psychiatry, Massachusetts General Hospital, Boston, MA

Scott E. Ewing, M.D., Consolidated Department of Psychiatry, McLean Hospital, Belmont, MA

William E. Falk, M.D., Geriatric Neurobehavioral Clinic, Clinical Psychopharmacology Unit, Department of Psychiatry, Massachusetts General Hospital, Boston, MA

Stephen Faraone, Ph.D., Pediatric Psychopharmacology Unit, Department of Psychiatry, Massachusetts General Hospital, Boston, MA

Maurizio Fava, M.D., Depression Research Program, Clinical Psychopharmacology Unit, Department of Psychiatry, Massachusetts General Hospital, Boston, MA

David R. Gastfriend, M.D., Addiction Services, Department of Psychiatry, Massachusetts General Hospital, Boston, MA

Alan J. Gelenberg, M.D., Department of Psychiatry, University of Arizona Health Sciences Center, Tucson, AZ

S. Nassir Ghaemi, M.D., Affective Disorders Unit, Department of Psychiatry, Medical College of Virginia, Richmond, VA

Donald C. Goff, M.D., Freedom Trail Clinic, E. Lindemann Mental Health Center, Boston, MA

Robert A. Gould, Ph.D., Cognitive-Behavior Therapy Program, Department of Psychiatry, Massachusetts General Hospital, Boston, MA

Paul Hamburg, M.D., Eating Disorders Unit, Department of Psychiatry, Massachusetts General Hospital, Boston, MA

David C. Henderson, M.D., Freedom Trail Clinic, E. Lindemann Mental Health Center, Boston, MA

David B. Herzog, M.D., Eating Disorders Unit, Department of Psychiatry, Massachusetts General Hospital, Boston, MA

Michael A. Jenike, M.D., Obsessive–Compulsive Unit, Department of Psychiatry, Massachusetts General Hospital East, Charlestown, MA

Junko Kaji, B.A., Depression Research Program, Department of Psychiatry, Massachusetts General Hospital, Boston, MA

Kathleen Kiely, B.A., Pediatric Psychopharmacology Unit, Department of Psychiatry, Massachusetts General Hospital, Boston, MA

Eric Mick, B.A., Pediatric Psychopharmacology Unit, Department of Psychiatry, Massachusetts General Hospital, Boston, MA

Michael W. Otto, Ph.D., Cognitive-Behavior Therapy Program, Department of Psychiatry, Massachusetts General Hospital, Boston, MA

Joel A. Pava, Ph.D., Depression Research Program, Department of Psychiatry, Massachusetts General Hospital, Boston, MA

Susan J. Penava, Ph.D., Cognitive-Behavior Therapy Program, Department of Psychiatry, Massachusetts General Hospital, Boston, MA

Mark H. Pollack, M.D., Anxiety Disorders Program, Department of Psychiatry, Massachusetts General Hospital, Boston, MA

Rachel A. Pollack, B.A., Clinical Psychopharmacology Unit, Department of Psychiatry, Massachusetts General Hospital, Boston, MA

Scott L. Rauch, M.D., Obsessive–Compulsive Disorder Unit, Department of Psychiatry, Massachusetts General Hospital East, Charlestown, MA

Jerrold F. Rosenbaum, M.D., Outpatient Psychiatry Department, Massachusetts General Hospital, Boston, MA

Gary S. Sachs, M.D., Bipolar Research Program, Clinical Psychopharmacology Unit, Department of Psychiatry, Massachusetts General Hospital, Boston, MA

Jordan W. Smoller, M.D., Anxiety Disorders Program, Department of Psychiatry, Massachusetts General Hospital, Boston, MA

Thomas J. Spencer, M.D., Pediatric Psychopharmacology Unit, Department of Psychiatry, Massachusetts General Hospital, Boston, MA

Susan Sprich-Buckminster, M.A., Cognitive-Behavior Therapy Program, Department of Psychiatry, Massachusetts General Hospital, Boston, MA

Jeffrey B. Weilburg, M.D., Neuropsychiatry Section, Clinical Psychopharmacology Unit, Department of Psychiatry, Massachusetts General Hospital, Boston, MA

Maureen L. Whittal, Ph.D., Cognitive-Behavior Therapy Program, Department of Psychiatry, Massachusetts General Hospital, Boston, MA

Timothy E. Wilens, M.D., Pediatric Psychopharmacology Unit, Department of Psychiatry, Massachusetts General Hospital, Boston, MA

Ari Zaretsky, M.D., General Psychiatry Service, Department of Psychiatry, Massachusetts General Hospital, Boston, MA

Preface

Clinicians have available a powerful armamentarium of interventions to bring to bear in the treatment of psychiatric disorders. Research on the phenomenology, etiology, and treatment of psychiatric disorders holds the promise of additional progress in our ability to understand and treat complex and challenging conditions. Despite recent advances, however, systematic inquiry confirms what experienced clinicians have long known: Although the majority of patients with psychiatric disorders improve with treatment, a substantial number remain symptomatic and impaired.

The impact of untreated and inadequately treated psychiatric disorders on the physical, social, and economic functioning of individuals is marked and rivals that of chronic medical disorders. Yet, despite its pressing clinical importance, the question of "what to do next" for a patient who has failed to respond to initial interventions has only recently been the focus of systematic study. Consequently, clinicians and researchers must rely on their experience and creativity to expand empirically based treatments to patients who fail to achieve a satisfactory outcome with standard treatments. This volume brings together experts in pharmacologic and psychosocial treatments to address the challenges presented by psychiatric disorders, with special attention to strategies for treatment-refractory patients.

Each chapter targets a serious psychiatric condition encountered in clinical practice. The treatment of major depression is discussed from both pharmacologic and cognitive-behavioral perspectives, with attention to clinical strategies appropriate to various stages of the disorder and treatment response. The management of bipolar disorder is reviewed primarily from a pharmacologic perspective, but includes discussion of important psychosocial influences. Initial treatment strategies and alternatives for nonresponders are detailed in separate chapters devoted to the anxiety disorders, including pharmacologic and cognitive-behavioral perspectives on panic disorder, social phobia, generalized anxiety disorder, obsessive–

compulsive disorder, and posttraumatic stress disorder. Subsequent chapters address the difficult task of treating eating disorders, with review of treatment strategies from psychodynamic, pharmacologic, and cognitive-behavioral perspectives. The chapter on treatment-resistant psychotic disorders emphasizes newer pharmacologic strategies. The complex issues presented by individuals with substance use disorders are discussed, along with relevant clinical strategies for their treatment. Additional chapters are devoted to the management of patients with personality disorders, adult attention-deficit/hyperactivity disorder, premenstrual dysphoric disorder, and refractory insomnia. Treatment-emergent side effects are major causes of noncompliance and poor outcome with pharmacotherapy; two chapters are devoted to issues and strategies in the management of antidepressant- and neuroleptic-induced side effects.

Throughout this volume, emphasis is placed on empirically supported treatments. Nonetheless, like all clinicians who struggle with patients who remain ill despite treatment, the authors range beyond systematically collected data to address the spectrum of management issues and strategies pertinent to clinical practice. By offering theoretical perspectives and clinical interventions from both pharmacologic and psychosocial domains, they provide the reader with a range of clinical strategies and guidelines for deciding how and when to consider alternative or combined treatment modalities.

The approach to patient care presented throughout this book reflects the accumulated wisdom and experience of the many clinicians, clinical researchers, and trainees at our center over the years at the Massachusetts General Hospital—caregivers who have created a high standard of dedication to patients, indefatigability and persistence in the face of chronic disorders, and commitment to the alleviation of suffering. We would especially like to thank our mentors and teachers, the late Thomas P. Hackett, M.D., and Ned Cassem, M.D. (former and current chairmen of the Department of Psychiatry), and George Murray, M.D. (its limbic system).

Contents

III. EATING DISORDERS

IV. OTHER DISORDERS

V. TREATMENT-EMERGENT SIDE EFFECTS

CHALLENGES IN CLINICAL PRACTICE

I

MOOD DISORDERS

1

Pharmacologic Strategies for Treatment-Resistant Major Depression

MAURIZIO FAVA
JUNKO KAJI
KATHARINE DAVIDSON

Depressed patients who fail to achieve and sustain euthymia with adequate antidepressant treatment can be considered treatment-resistant. However, no universally accepted definition of "treatment-resistant depression" exists, in part because of continually evolving standards of adequate antidepressant dose and treatment duration in psychiatric practice (Nierenberg & Amsterdam, 1990). Most clinicians tend to treat patients for 4–6 weeks with standard doses of antidepressants before presuming that treatment resistance exists. There are different levels of resistance: Some patients show little or no response ("nonresponders"), whereas others improve but retain significant symptomatology ("partial responders").

The issue of treatment resistance is a major concern in the clinical management of depressed patients, as many fail to achieve full remission of their symptoms after one or more adequate trials with antidepressants. It is therefore crucial that clinicians understand the factors underlying partial response and nonresponse, and that they be aware of therapeutic strategies to improve outcome. Unfortunately, the literature on this topic is scanty, and the clinician must rely on recommendations derived from a mixture of clinical reports, case series, open trials, and very few, small controlled studies. For now, familiarity with the issues and options for treatment-resistant depression is the best foundation for clinical practice.

PREVALENCE OF TREATMENT RESISTANCE

Between 15% and 30% of depressed patients do not reach a state of well-being and functioning following an initial adequate trial of antidepressant medication. The proportion of treatment-resistant patients is even larger if one includes patients who experience improvement with antidepressant treatment but suffer from residual symptoms that affect functioning in a wide range of social and occupational roles. Furthermore, researchers estimate that a substantial proportion of responders will have a relapse or a recurrence within 1 year while continuing on antidepressants (Fava & Kaji, 1994). However, it is debatable whether one should classify a return of depressive symptoms in someone who initially responded to the original antidepressant dose as a form of treatment resistance.

Other possible forms of treatment resistance include inconsistent types of responses (i.e., placebo-like) and intermittent depressive symptoms during continued antidepressant treatment following an initial robust response.

CONTRIBUTING ROLE OF DEPRESSIVE SUBTYPES

There is some evidence of an association between resistance to treatment and specific depressive subtypes. Some clinicians believe that "endogenous" or "melancholic" depression, characterized by symptoms such as non-reactivity of mood, pervasive anhedonia, and psychomotor retardation, is less likely to respond to selective serotonin reuptake inhibitors (SSRIs) than to tricyclic antidepressants (TCAs). However, this view has recently been challenged by results from a large multicenter study, which found nonsignificantly higher rates of response to fluoxetine in subjects with melancholic depression than in those without melancholia (Rosenbaum et al., 1993). Another subtype traditionally viewed as relatively resistant to treatment with certain types of antidepressants is "atypical" depression, commonly defined by mood reactivity plus associated features such as overeating, oversleeping, leaden paralysis, and/or chronic oversensitivity to rejection (Liebowitz et al., 1988). Depressed patients with atypical depression appear to respond less favorably to TCAs than to monoamine oxidase inhibitors (MAOIs) (Liebowitz et al., 1988; Thase, Carpenter, Kupfer, & Frank, 1991) or SSRIs (Pande, Haskett, & Greden, 1992).

A common source of partial response is "double depression" (Keller & Shapiro, 1982), a major depressive episode superimposed upon a dysthymic disorder. In fact, patients with double depression may recover quickly with treatment from a major depressive episode, but may take much longer to recover from the dysthymia (Keller, Lavori, Endicott, Coryell, & Klerman, 1983). These data suggest that patients with major depression superimposed upon chronic dysthymia are likely to display at least some level of treatment resistance, maintaining residual symptoms long after the acute depression has remitted.

Treatment resistance may also stem from the presence of certain comorbid conditions that require specific treatments. For example, comorbid depression and obsessive–compulsive disorder (OCD) may be less responsive to a TCA alone, as this class of antidepressants is known to have little efficacy in OCD treatment, than to any of the SSRIs, whose efficacy in this disorder is supported by numerous studies (Jenike et al., 1990). In addition, resistance to TCA treatment alone is relatively common in psychotic or delusional depression (Chan et al., 1987), especially in those subjects with a late-onset form (Aronson, Shukla, Hoff, & Cook, 1988). Overall, patients with psychotic depression seem to be relatively resistant to treatment with antidepressants alone, with the possible exception of amoxapine, which is in part metabolized to a neuroleptic (Anton & Burch, 1990). It appears that the combination of antidepressants with antipsychotics is significantly more effective than antidepressant treatment alone in this population (Spiker et al., 1985). Since the efficacy of antidepressants in the treatment of other psychiatric disorders differs across classes, resistance in a depressed patient with a comorbid condition may reflect failure of the selected antidepressant to treat the concurrent disorder. When no class of antidepressant is known to reduce symptoms of the comorbid condition, the use of other psychotropic drugs (i.e., antianxiety and antipsychotic drugs) with specific efficacy in the treatment of the concurrent disorder is indicated. Of course, comorbid medical conditions can also contribute to treatment resistance. In a study on outcome of psychiatric treatment in the medically ill, only 40% of patients with medical comorbidity responded to antidepressant treatment (Popkin, Callies, & Mackenzie, 1985). For these reasons, clinicians should always consider the possibility of medical comorbidity contributing to resistance in depressed patients, and should gather a complete medical history before initiating further treatment.

Depressed patients with high anxiety levels may show less response to antidepressants and have a poorer long-term prognosis than nonanxious depressed patients (Fawcett & Kravitz, 1983; Clayton et al., 1991), although a recent study failed to support this view (Joffe, Bagby, & Levitt, 1993a). It is unclear whether or not the presence of comorbid panic disorder contributes to resistance to antidepressant treatment in depression, in spite of reports that depressed patients with panic attacks have a poorer outcome than those without panic attacks (van Valkenburg, Akiskal, Puzantian, & Rosenthal, 1984). On the other hand, anger attacks (explosive outbursts of anger accompanied by symptoms of autonomic arousal in patients with marked irritability) may contribute to treatment resistance. In fact, there is some anecdotal evidence that TCAs may be less effective than SSRIs in the treatment of depressed patients with anger attacks (Fava, Anderson, & Rosenbaum, 1993). Depressed patients frequently have comorbid personality disorders (Fava et al., 1994a); these may contribute to resistance, depending on the type of antidepressant drug selected as well as on the severity and number of comorbid personality disorders

(Rosenbaum, Fava, Nierenberg, & Sachs, 1995). Finally, clinical studies show that ongoing substance abuse tends to be present in a high proportion of partial responders and nonresponders to antidepressant treatment (MacEwan & Remick, 1988), and it is possible that the concomitant mild or moderate use (not abuse) of psychoactive substances such as alcohol may have a negative effect on outcome (Worthington et al., 1994).

COMMONLY USED CLINICAL STRATEGIES

When a depressed patient fails to respond to an antidepressant after an optimized medication trial, four pharmacologic treatment strategies are available: augmentation of the failed antidepressant, increasing the dose of the failed antidepressant, combining two classes of antidepressants, or switching to another antidepressant. The choice among these four strategies is affected by a number of different factors. If the initial drug trial has resulted in partial remission without adverse drug reactions, then either augmentation or a higher dose may be advisable. If, however, a partial remission is accompanied by significant side effects, then switching may be a better strategy. If the failed drug has caused no improvement whatsoever, many physicians favor switching, even though no data are available to show that switching is superior to augmentation or combination.

The following subsections review the studies on augmentation strategies, higher doses of antidepressants, combination strategies, and switching. The results of these studies are summarized below in Tables 1.1 through 1.4.

Augmentation Strategies

Over the past 30 years, clinicians have been adding a number of different drugs to antidepressants in treatment-resistant patients (see Table 1.1). The most common augmenting agents are probably lithium and thyroid hormone, although the popularity of adding stimulants or dopaminergic agents is increasing. The strategy of augmentation offers the basic advantage of maintaining continuity of treatment, since patients can be kept on the same antidepressant without changes in dosing or switching to different antidepressants. Patients who tolerate their initial antidepressant well but fail to achieve adequate response are good candidates for this approach.

Lithium Augmentation

Lithium augmentation is a popular strategy in the management of treatment-resistant depression (Nierenberg & Cole, 1991). Although isolated case reports on the efficacy of lithium augmentation of antidepressants were published in the 1970s, wider clinical use followed a report by

TABLE 1.1. Clinical Trials of Augmentation Strategies

Augmenting agent	Initial drug	Investigators	n	Design[a]	Dose range	% Responders	Significantly more effective than placebo?
Lithium	TCA & mianserin	Heninger et al. (1983)	15	RCT	900–1200 mg	5 of 8 (63%)	Yes
	TCA	Courneyer et al. (1984)	12	RCT; c/o	900 mg	?	Yes
	TCA	Kantor et al. (1986)	7	RCT	900 mg	1 of 4 (25%)	No
	TCA & MAOI	Zusky et al. (1988)	16	RCT	≥300 mg	3 of 5 (60%)	No
	TCA, SSRI, etc.	Schopf et al. (1989)	27	RCT	≥800 mg	7 of 7 (100%)	Yes
	TCA	Stein & Bernadt (1993)	34	RCT	250 mg / 750 mg	6 of 34 (18%) / 15 of 34 (44%)	No / Yes
	TCA	Joffe et al. (1993c)	50	RCT	900 mg	9 of 17 (53%)	Yes
	Fluoxetine	Fava et al. (1994b)	41	RCT	300–600 mg	4 of 14 (29%)	–
Thyroid hormone (T$_3$)	TCA	Targum et al. (1984)	21	Open	25 µg	7 of 21 (33%)	–
	Imipramine	Gitlin et al. (1987)	16	RCT; c/o	25 µg	–	No
	Imipramine	Thase et al. (1989b)	20	Open	25 µg	5 of 20 (25%)	–
	TCA	Joffe et al. (1993c)	50	RCT	37.5 µg	10 of 17 (59%)	Yes
Dopaminergic agents	SSRI, TCA, MAOI, etc.	Bouckoms & Mangini (1992)	20	Open	? mg pergolide	11 of 20 (55%)	–
Stimulants	MAOI	Fawcett et al. (1991)	32	Open	18.75–112.5 mg pemoline, 5–40 mg D-amphetamine	25 of 32 (78%)	–
	Fluoxetine	Metz & Shader (1991)	21	Open	9.375–37.5 mg pemoline	16 of 21 (76%)	–

[a]In this and subsequent tables, RCT, randomized controlled trial; c/o, crossover.

de Montigny, Grunberg, and Mayer (1981) in which antidepressant non-responders showed dramatic improvement within 48 hours after the addition of lithium to at least 3 weeks of treatment with tricyclic antidepressants. Johnson (1991) reviewed all case reports, case series, and controlled studies published over the subsequent 10 years concerning lithium augmentation of TCAs, MAOIs, SSRIs, trazodone, bupropion, and carbamazepine, and concluded that the bulk of the studies supported the efficacy of this strategy, particularly with TCAs. The quality and time course of response tended to vary from study to study. A meta-analysis of all available data up to 1991 (Austin, Souza, & Goodwin, 1991) concluded that the addition of lithium to an ongoing but failed antidepressant trial reduced the odds of patients' remaining ill by between 56% and 95%. Price (1990) set the probability of complete response to lithium augmentation at 30%, with another 25% to 35% of patients gaining substantial improvement but not returning fully to euthymia. As yet, however, only a few controlled reports have focused on lithium augmentation of SSRIs. One group found that although lithium appeared to be equally effective when added to either desipramine or fluoxetine, 33% of lithium augmentation responders who had failed to respond to fluoxetine alone had a relapse within 14 weeks, whereas none of the patients who had been taking desipramine relapsed (Ontiveros, Fontaine, & Elie, 1991). We have recently found that lithium augmentation of fluoxetine in patients failing to respond to 8 weeks of treatment with a standard dose of fluoxetine was less effective than raising the dose among partial responders, but as effective as raising the fluoxetine dose and more effective than adding desipramine among nonresponders (Fava et al., 1994b).

Traditionally, clinicians tend to aim at therapeutic (0.5–1.2 mEq/liter) blood levels of lithium when treating patients with mood disorders. However, researchers have used a very broad range of lithium doses for augmentation of antidepressants. In fact, as noted in the review by Johnson (1991), several studies and case series reported successful outcome with low doses and low lithium blood levels, as well as with blood levels within the traditional therapeutic range. A double-blind, placebo-controlled study in 34 depressed patients failing to respond to antidepressants showed that the addition of lithium at a dose of 250 mg/day was not significantly better than placebo, but that the addition of lithium at 750 mg/day was superior to both 250 mg of lithium and placebo (Stein & Bernadt, 1993). In contrast, Thase, Kupfer, Frank, and Jarrett (1989a) found that no relationship existed between lithium dose or blood levels and augmentation response in their series of 20 patients. It is apparent that the relevance of lithium dose and blood levels for response to lithium augmentation merits further study.

Adverse effects associated with the addition of lithium are those typical of this drug; they may include nausea, vomiting, diarrhea, sedation, tremors, polyuria, renal toxicity, hypothyroidism, and exacerbation of myoclonus or orthostatic hypotension (Baldessarini, 1985; Johnson, 1991).

Clinicians should routinely monitor lithium blood levels, as well as renal and thyroid function.

Clinicians often disagree on the timing for the addition of lithium to the ongoing failed antidepressant trial. Some investigators have added lithium to an antidepressant after 12 weeks of antidepressant nonresponse (Austin, Arana, & Ballenger, 1990; Thase et al., 1989a), but in actual clinical practice, most physicians would choose to intervene at 4 weeks or earlier for patients who show no sign of improvement. Although some patients will respond within a few days, others will experience a delay of onset for up to 6 weeks, making it advisable for clinicians to continue at least 4 weeks before abandoning this strategy.

Very little is known about the long-term course of patients who respond to lithium augmentation, including how many patients will maintain response or suffer a recurrence over time. It is also unclear whether it is best to discontinue lithium first or the antidepressant, to minimize the risk for relapses or recurrences. The most conservative approach would be to continue to prescribe both the antidepressant and lithium for continuation or maintenance therapy; alternatively, the adjunctive lithium could be discontinued first and restored if symptoms recur (Rosenbaum et al., 1995). Although Joffe, Levitt, Bagby, Macdonald, and Singer (1993b) found that nonresponders to lithium augmentation were more severely depressed and had more insomnia and weight loss than responders, it has not been established whether particular depressive subtypes may be more likely to respond to this strategy.

In sum, although many patients can benefit from lithium augmentation, there is no evidence for a clear dose–response relationship. However, it seems reasonable to use at least 600 mg/day of lithium for at least 4 weeks before assuming lack of efficacy.

Thyroid Augmentation

The addition of thyroid hormone to antidepressants for nonresponders has been reported since the late 1960s. When prescribed in addition to an antidepressant, thyroid hormone yielded a faster response in depressed women than an antidepressant alone did (Prange, Wilson, & Robon, 1969; Wilson, Prange, & McClaine, 1970). Later case reports and series extended these results, suggesting that a broader spectrum of patients benefited from adding thyroid to a failed antidepressant trial (Earle, 1970; Ogura et al., 1974; Banki, 1975; Tsutsui, Yamazaki, Namba, & Tsushima, 1979). A study by Joffe, Singer, Levitt, and MacDonald (1993c) found a response rate of 59% for triiodothyronine (T_3), significantly greater than the 19% rate for placebo, even though a much smaller previous study (Gitlin, Weiner, & Fairbanks, 1987) had failed to show a difference between T_3 (25 µg/day) and placebo added to an unsuccessful 4-week trial of imipramine (mean dose, 206 mg/day; mean imipramine plus desipramine blood levels, 200 ng/dl).

Adverse effects associated with the addition of thyroid are typically absent or mild, but may include increased anxiety, jitteriness, tachycardia, insomnia, and sweating, with very infrequent occurrence of atrial irritability or high-output cardiac failure (Rosenbaum et al., 1995). For these reasons, clinicians should be cautious when giving thyroid to patients with cardiac insufficiency or to elderly patients.

Most reports have involved dosing ranges of 25 to 50 μg of T_3, in the form of liothyronine, with lower doses in the elderly and higher (e.g., 75 μg) in some younger patients. Usual thyroid replacement doses of thyroxine (T_4) (e.g., 150 μg) have been used for the treatment of refractory depressed patients. Higher doses of both T_3 and T_4 may be considered for selected patients as long as side effects are monitored carefully. No guidelines exist as to the duration of an adequate acute trial of thyroid augmentation, but most patients who respond appear to do so within 2–3 weeks. The longest reported duration of a thyroid augmentation study is 4 weeks (Thase, Kupfer, & Jarrett, 1989b). As in the case of lithium augmentation, the literature is not a particularly helpful guide to clinical practice, since few longitudinal studies and no double-blind discontinuation studies of thyroid augmentation responders have been completed. A reasonable strategy would be to test whether the adjunct remains necessary for maintaining a response by gradually discontinuing thyroid hormone 6 months after a response to T_3 or T_4 augmentation. If the patient experiences a relapse during the discontinuation trial, the thyroid adjunct can be reinstated. No significant predictors of response to T_3 augmentation have been found (Joffe et al., 1993b).

In sum, the evidence for thyroid augmentation of antidepressants in euthyroid unipolar depressed patients suggests that some patients may benefit from this strategy. One controlled study suggests that thyroid augmentation is superior to placebo and equal to lithium augmentation in its effects (Joffe et al., 1993c). Further research is needed to clarify treatment decisions with regard to duration of an adequate acute trial and maintenance therapy with this adjunct.

Augmentation with Dopaminergic Agents

There is some evidence that dopaminergic agents, such as bromocriptine, amantadine, and pergolide, may be useful as adjuncts for some depressed patients. Bromocriptine and piribedil are dopamine agonists used for Parkinson's disease that also appear to have antidepressant properties, as suggested by four open trials (Agnoli, Ruggieri, & Casacchia, 1978; Colonna, Petit, & Lepine, 1979; Nordin, Siwers, & Bertilsson, 1981; Silverstone, 1984) and three double-blind trials comparing bromocriptine to imipramine and amitriptyline (Bouras & Bridges, 1982; Theohar, Fischer-Cornelssen, Brosch, Fischer, & Petrovic, 1982; Waehrens & Gerlach, 1981). According to some anecdotal reports, dopaminergic agents seem to be effective within days when added to antidepressants in the treatment of refractory patients. Pergolide, a dopamine agonist 20 to 30 times more potent than bromocriptine, was an effective adjunct in 55% of 4 bipolar and 16 unipolar depressed patients who had failed to respond to either fluoxetine, TCAs, MAOIs, or trazodone (Bouckoms & Mangini, 1992). Adverse drug reactions with the use of dopaminergic agents have included nausea, headache, dizziness, fatigue, lightheadedness, vomiting, nervousness, insomnia, ataxia, and mania. At higher doses, the use of these drugs has been associated with confusion, delusions, hallucinations, and dyskinesias. Although some clinicians currently employ dopamine agonists as adjuncts to antidepressants, no controlled studies on these agents are yet available.

Guidelines for the prescription of dopaminergic agents are based on clinical experience rather than controlled trials. These drugs can be started in low doses and increased to the maximum dose recommended for use in Parkinson's disease (American Medical Association, 1993). Pergolide is usually started at 0.05 mg daily, with increases of 0.1 to 0.15 mg every 2–3 days to a maximum of 5 mg daily in divided doses; bromocriptine is started at 1.25 mg daily or twice daily and increased every 2 weeks by 1.25-mg increments up to 20 mg daily, although some patients may require up to 100 mg. Amantadine can be started at 25 to 50 mg daily (when given in syrup form) and increased up to 200 mg in divided doses.

Stimulant Augmentation

Although stimulants such as amphetamine, methylphenidate, and pemoline have abuse potential in populations of patients with a history of substance abuse, depressed patients have taken these drugs responsibly in stable doses for up to 20 or 30 years (Chiarello & Cole, 1987). There are no controlled trials on the use of stimulants as depressive adjuncts. Evidence from case reports and series suggests that stimulants are effective in augmenting fluoxetine (Linet, 1989; Metz & Shader, 1991), MAOIs alone, and MAOIs in combination with TCAs (Feighner, Herbstein, & Damlouji, 1985; Fawcett, Kravitz, Zajecka, & Schaff, 1991). Feighner et al. (1985) and Fawcett et al. (1991) reported their experience with D-amphetamine (dose range, 5–40 mg daily), methylphenidate (dose range, 10–15 mg daily), and pemoline (dose range, 18.75–112.5 mg daily) as adjuncts for a total of 45 severely treatment-resistant patients. Of this group, 57% responded to D-amphetamine, 50% responded to pemoline, and 60% responded to methylphenidate when these drugs were added to failed aggressive trials of MAOIs alone and in combination with other psychotropic classes of medications. The response to the addition of stimulants may be transient, as suggested by a study showing that only 32% of 25 responding patients maintained their improvement (Fawcett et al., 1991).

Adverse events with the use of stimulants may include nervousness, anorexia, nausea, weight loss, insomnia, impotence, dizziness, orthostatic hypotension, elevated blood pressure, tachycardia, shakiness, memory difficulties, parkinsonian symptoms, mania, and fatigue. Stimulants may also increase blood levels of other drugs. Extreme caution should be used when stimulants are combined with MAOIs; patients should be instructed about the risk and symptoms of a hypertensive crisis, and stimulants should be added at very low doses with gradual increases.

Stimulants are often prescribed on the basis of clinical experience rather than controlled trials. D-Amphetamine and methylphenidate are usually started at low doses (e.g., 2.5 to 5.0 mg daily, respectively), with gradual increases up to 40–60 mg/day in divided doses. Pemoline can be started at 18.75 mg daily and increased up to 112.5 mg daily. The use of stimulants as adjuncts is best avoided in patients who have a recent history of substance abuse or are perceived to be at risk for developing drug dependence. Patients should be informed that stimulants are a controlled substance and that they should be taken only as prescribed.

High Doses of Antidepressants

An alternative approach to augmentation is the use of relatively high doses of antidepressant monotherapy (see Table 1.2). In an open-label study of higher doses of tranylcypromine (doses ranging from 90 to 170 mg/day), four (57%) of seven treatment-resistant subjects responded (Amsterdam & Berwish, 1989). Similarly, one retrospective study asserted the relative safety and efficacy of high-dose TCAs in treatment-resistant depression (Schuckit & Feighner, 1972), and another found that 64% of 22 treatment-resistant depressed patients responded to an open trial with trazodone up to 800 mg/day (Cole, Schatzberg, Sniffin, Zolner, & Cole, 1981). In addition, an open study of 15 patients who had failed to respond after 8–12 weeks of treatment with a standard 20-mg dose of the SSRI fluoxetine showed a significant improvement in depressive symptoms following a dose increase up to 80 mg/day (Fava et al., 1992). The only controlled study of high-dose antidepressants found that patients treated with high-dose fluoxetine did significantly better than patients treated with fluoxetine plus lithium and those treated with fluoxetine plus desipramine (Fava et al., 1994b). Although further controlled studies are necessary to confirm the potential usefulness of this approach, high-dose SSRIs (which are safer than high-dose TCAs) may be helpful in managing patients who are resistant to standard doses.

In clinical practice, some patients who fail to respond to treatment with a standard dose of a TCA will improve when the dose of the TCA is titrated up to 400 or 500 mg/day, if this can be tolerated (Rosenbaum et al., 1995). When using TCAs, clinicians should carefully monitor electrocardiograms (EKGs) and blood levels to minimize the risk of toxicity. In addition, some patients not responding to a standard dose of an SSRI have been treated with doses up to 80 to 100 mg/day of fluoxetine or paroxetine, up to 300 mg/day of sertraline, and up to 450 mg/day of venlafaxine. No guidelines exist as to the adequate duration of a higher-dose

TABLE 1.2. Clinical Studies of High-Dose Strategies

Antidepressant (class)	Investigators	Number of failed trials	n	Design	Dose range	% Responders
Tranylcypromine (MAOI)	Amsterdam & Berwish (1989)	3 to 14	7	Open-label	90–170 mg/day	4 of 7 (57%)
Amitriptyline, imipramine, doxepin (TCAs)	Schuckit & Feighner (1972)	?	40	Retrospective	100–500 mg amitriptyline, 150–600 mg imipramine, 250–350 mg doxepin	None discontinued due to side effects
Trazodone	Cole et al. (1981)	≥1	22	Retrospective	Up to 800 mg/day	14 of 22 (64%)
Fluoxetine (SSRI)	Fava et al. (1992)	1	15	Open	Up to 80 mg/day	15 of 15 (100%)
Fluoxetine (SSRI)	Fava et al. (1994b)	1	41	RCT	40–60 mg/day	8 of 15 (53%)

antidepressant therapy trial, but 6 weeks is likely to be a sufficient duration. If the higher dose is tolerated, treatment following response can be maintained for 6–9 months, followed by a decrease through tapering.

Combined Antidepressant Treatments

Combination of antidepressants is often useful when depressive symptoms do not improve after treatment with a single antidepressant (see Table 1.3). For example, when patients do not respond to a TCA alone, the dose of the TCA may be reduced and a standard dosage of an SSRI added. On the other hand, when patients fail to respond to treatment with an SSRI alone, clinicians may initially add TCAs in low doses from 10 to 25 mg/day without changing the SSRI dose, and can raise the TCA dose while monitoring the blood levels. MAOIs have also been combined with TCAs, often by initiating both drugs simultaneously and gradually raising their doses to standard antidepressant levels. For safety, neither SSRIs nor clomipramine should be combined with MAOIs. When buspirone or high-potency benzodiazepines are added to an antidepressant, the dose of the antidepressant may usually remain unchanged.

No guidelines exist as to the duration of an adequate trial of a combination strategy. Patients who respond have shown initial improvement in a range from 24 hours to several weeks. There are no reports of longitudinal studies or double-blind discontinuation studies of responders to combination strategies. To test whether the added antidepressant remains necessary for maintaining a response, a trial discontinuation may be used 6 months or more after a response. If relapse occurs during the discontinuation trial, the combination agent may be reinstated.

Combined MAOIs and TCAs

Combined antidepressant therapy with MAOIs and TCAs was common in the 1960s (Tyrer & Murphy, 1990), until rising concern over the safety of this combination led to decreased clinical use (Sheperd, Lader, & Rodnight, 1968). However, the combination of MAOIs and TCAs appears safe if the agents are simultaneously initiated in low doses and increased gradually (Spiker & Pugh, 1976; White & Simpson, 1981). The combination of MAOIs with imipramine or clomipramine should be avoided, however, as the risk of toxicity is greater (Lader, 1983).

Some uncontrolled reports and studies on combined MAOI and TCA treatment reported efficacy in treatment-refractory depression (Sethna, 1974; Goldberg & Thornton, 1978; Lippmann, Baldwin, & Manshadi, 1982; Manshadi & Lippmann, 1984; Feighner et al., 1985; Tyrer & Murphy, 1990). In a retrospective study, 68% of 94 inpatients with treatment-resistant depression responded to combinations of MAOIs with TCAs and tetracyclic antidepressants (Schmauss, Kapfhammer, Meyr, & Hoff,

TABLE 1.3. Clinical Studies of Combination Strategies

Drug combination	Investigators	n	Design	Failed trial	Dose ranges	% Response
MAOI + TCA	Sethna (1974)	12	Open	TCA, MAOI	75 mg amitriptyline, 45 mg phenelzine	83% response to comb.
	Davidson et al. (1978)	17	RCT	Adequate trial w/ conventional treatment	20–100 mg amitriptyline, 15–45 mg phenelzine	Less effective than ECT
	Riise & Holm (1984)	27	Open	MAOI or TCA alone	0.5 mg/kg isocarboxazid, 30–90 mg mianserin	74% response to comb.
	Feighner et al. (1985)	11	Retrospective	2-yr history of treatment resistance	5–15 mg MAOI, 15–400 mg TCA	64% response to comb.
	Schmauss et al. (1988)	94	Retrospective	≥2 TCAs or tetracyclics	10–30 mg tranylcypromine, 50–300 mg TCA	68% response to comb.
SSRI + TCA	Weilburg et al. (1989)	30	Retrospective	Non-MAOI	20–60 mg fluoxetine, 37.5–400 mg TCA	87% response to comb.
	Weilburg et al. (1991)	20	Retrospective	Fluoxetine alone	20–40 mg fluoxetine, 10–100 mg TCA	65% response to comb.
	Fava et al. (1994b)	41	RCT	Fluoxetine alone	20 mg fluoxetine, 25–50 mg desipramine	25% response to comb.
Buspirone + SSRI	Jacobsen (1991)	7	Open	Fluoxetine alone	30 mg buspirone, 20–40 mg fluoxetine	86% full or partial response
	Joffe & Schuller (1993)	25	Open	TCA, MAOI, SSRI alone, or lithium	20–50 mg buspirone, 20–60 mg fluoxetine, 100–200 mg fluvoxamine,	68% response to comb.

1988). Furthermore, in a survey of 27 treatment-resistant patients treated with a combination of the MAOI isocarboxazid and mianserin, 20 (74%) patients responded (Riise & Holm, 1984). A controlled study on the efficacy of MAOI and TCA combinations in treatment refractory patients had different results: Electroconvulsive therapy (ECT) proved to be more effective than combined amitriptyline and phenelzine (n = 17) (Davidson, McLeod, Law-Yone, & Linnoila, 1978). The negative results may be explained by the small sample size, the presence of psychotic depression in some of the patients, and the use of a relatively low average dosage of amitriptyline and phenelzine. Overall, it appears that the combination of MAOIs and TCAs may be relatively safe and effective in treatment-resistant patients. In contrast, the combination of MAOIs and SSRIs (or clomipramine) can cause potentially fatal reactions and is contraindicated (Feighner, Boyer, Tyler, & Neborsky, 1990).

Combined SSRIs and TCAs

Combining fluoxetine or other SSRIs with a TCA in refractory patients has become increasingly popular. Some case reports suggested efficacy in treatment-resistant depression of adding a TCA to SSRIs such as fluoxetine and sertraline (Eisen, 1989; Seth, Jennings, Bindman, Phillips, & Bergmann, 1992), and of adding fluoxetine or citalopram to TCAs (Seth et al., 1992; Baettig, Bondolfi, Montaldi, & Amey, 1993). Weilburg et al. (1989) conducted a retrospective study on 30 depressed nonresponders and found that 26 (87%) improved when fluoxetine was added to a non-MAOI antidepressant. When the non-MAOI antidepressant treatment was withdrawn for 12 of the responders, 8 relapsed on fluoxetine treatment alone and recovered after readminstration of the discontinued agent (Weilburg et al., 1989). In another retrospective study, the addition of a TCA to fluoxetine led to significant improvement in 13 of 20 (65%) depressed patients failing to respond adequately to fluoxetine alone (Weilburg, Rosenbaum, Meltzer-Brody, & Shustari, 1991). However, the only prospective, controlled study showed that fluoxetine plus desipramine was less effective than fluoxetine plus lithium in nonresponders to fluoxetine alone, and was also less efficacious than high-dose fluoxetine in both nonresponders and partial responders (Fava et al., 1994b).

Like all SSRIs, fluoxetine inhibits the metabolism of drugs metabolized by cytochrome P450IID6, and cases of toxicity resulting from elevations in TCA blood levels have been reported when a TCA was coadministered with fluoxetine (Ciraulo & Shader, 1990). However, it is possible to administer fluoxetine with TCAs safely if a low dosage of the latter (25–50 mg/day) is used and plasma levels are monitored (Fava et al., 1994b). Although most reports of SSRI–TCA combinations feature fluoxetine, it is likely that other SSRIs could be used.

Combined Buspirone and SSRIs

Buspirone is an azospirodecanedione anxiolytic and a partial serotonin (5-HT$_{1A}$) agonist that may increase the efficacy of SSRIs. In one report, three nonresponders to fluoxetine alone showed marked improvement when buspirone was added (Bakish, 1991). In an open trial with seven fluoxetine nonresponders, partial or full response was observed in six (86%) when buspirone (10 mg three times daily) was added to the regimen (Jacobsen, 1991). A larger open study on 25 depressed patients who had had several previous unsuccessful treatments and had not responded to treatment with either fluoxetine or fluvoxamine found that 17 (68%) had marked or complete response when they received buspirone for 3 weeks in addition to their SSRI (Joffe & Schuller, 1993). These uncontrolled reports suggest that the addition of buspirone may be helpful in patients failing to respond to monotherapy with an SSRI (Rosenbaum et al., 1995).

Combined Bupropion and Other Antidepressants

Although no studies have been conducted on the efficacy of the combination of SSRIs and bupropion, one case report described rapid response when this combination was given to a depressed patient who had failed several previous trials (Novac, 1992). When this strategy is used clinically, the most common procedure is to add bupropion in twice-daily doses of either 75 or 100 mg to the original SSRI. The reason for using low doses of bupropion is that SSRIs may inhibit the metabolism of bupropion and elevate its plasma levels, leading to an increased risk of seizure (Callahan, Fava, & Rosenbaum, 1993). There are currently no reports in the literature on the safety or efficacy of the combination of MAOIs and bupropion.

Combined Antidepressants and Anticonvulsants or Benzodiazepines

Marked improvement in patients with treatment-resistant depression was observed when the anticonvulsant carbamazepine (300 mg/day) was added to desipramine (Cullen et al., 1991). Similarly, the addition of sodium valproate to fluoxetine in a nonresponder and to fluvoxamine in a partial responder was followed by marked improvement in both patients (Corrigan, 1992). The combination of benzodiazepine anxiolytics and antidepressants is very commonly prescribed. In some cases, the benzodiazepine is added to the antidepressant to manage such side effects as insomnia and nervousness; in other instances, this combination is used to treat patients with anxious depression or comorbid anxiety disorders. Case reports have found the combination of MAOIs and high-potency benzodiazepines such as alprazolam to be efficacious in treating resistant depression with panic attacks (Ries & Wittkowsky, 1986; Deicken, 1987). The potential useful-

ness of the combination of antidepressants and anticonvulsants or benzodiazepines requires further study.

Switching Strategies

When patients fail to respond to treatment with one antidepressant, a
common clinical strategy is to switch antidepressants (see Table 1.4). Most
clinicians believe that a switch from one antidepressant class to another
yields a greater chance of benefit than switching within the same class
(Nierenberg & Amsterdam, 1990). When patients fail to respond to treatment with an antidepressant alone, switching from a TCA to an SSRI
or vice versa does not typically require washout, but rather a tapering of
the first antidepressant and initiation of the second one (Rosenbaum et
al., 1995). To avoid a lapse in treatment, clinicians can start the new drug
while tapering the failed agent, although the period of overlap may create
drug interaction side effects. When switching to an MAOI, clinicians
should wait at least 1 week after discontinuing TCAs (with the exception
of protriptyline, which requires 3 weeks of washout) and at least 2 weeks
after discontinuing SSRIs (with the exception of fluoxetine, which requires
at least 5 weeks of washout) (Rosenbaum et al., 1995). Clinicians switching from an MAOI to an SSRI or a TCA should wait at least 2 weeks
before starting the new antidepressant. When clinicians switch to an antidepressant of the same class, no washout is necessary, except for the change
from phenelzine to tranylcypromine. For patients responding to a switch,
the antidepressant may be continued for at least 6 months following
response and then gradually discontinued.

Switching to MAOIs

Several studies have examined the efficacy of MAOIs in the treatment
of patients failing to respond to TCAs. In an open-label study, 23 of 40
(58%) depressed patients who had been unsuccessful in sustained, adequate
treatment with imipramine and interpersonal psychotherapy responded
to treatment with either tranylcypromine or phenelzine (Thase, Frank,
Hamer, & Kupfer, 1992). The response rate in this study was greater in
the anergic/atypical subgroup of patients (67%) than in the typical subgroup (31%), consistent with reports of greater efficacy of MAOIs than
of TCAs in atypical depression (Liebowitz et al., 1988). Similarly, in a
crossover study of atypical depressives, 4 (29%) of 14 nonresponders to
phenelzine responded to imipramine, but 17 (65%) of 26 nonresponders
to imipramine responded to phenelzine (McGrath, Stewart, Harrison, &
Quitkin, 1987). Of 47 patients with major depression who had failed to
respond to treatment with at least two antidepressants, 1 (5%) of 22 patients treated with either L-5-hydroxytryptophan (L-5-HTP) or nomifensine responded, while 13 (52%) of 25 patients responded to tranylcypromine
(Nolen et al., 1988b). In addition, 8 (67%) of 12 nonresponders to L-5-HTP

TABLE 1.4. Clinical Trials of Switching Strategies

Agent class	Investigators	Failed agent	Antidepressant switch	n	Design	Dose ranges	% Response
MAOIs	McGrath et al. (1987)	Imipramine or phenelzine	Imipramine or phenelzine	101	Double-blind, c/o	60–90 mg phenelzine, 200–300 mg imipramine	4 of 14 (29%) imipramine, 17 of 26 (65%) phenelzine
	Nolen et al. (1988b)	TCA	Tranylcypromine	47	Controlled, partial c/o	20–100 mg	13 of 25 (52%)
	Thase et al. (1992)	Imipramine	Tranylcypromine, phenelzine	42	Open	20–60 mg tranylcypromine, 30–90 mg phenelzine	23 of 40 (58%) MAOI
SSRIs	Delgado et al. (1988)	TCA	Fluvoxamine	28	Open	100–300 mg	8 of 28 (29%)
	Nolen et al. (1988a)	TCA	Fluvoxamine, oxaprotiline	71	Double-blind, partial c/o	100–300 mg fluvoxamine, 100–300 mg oxaprotiline	10% fluvoxamine, 39% oxaprotiline
	Beasley et al. (1990)	TCA	Fluoxetine	132	Open	Up to 300 mg TCA, up to 80 mg fluoxetine	51.4–62.1% (varied by definition of treatment response)
	White et al. (1990)	Desipramine	Fluvoxamine	11	Open	50–300 mg	9 of 11 (82%)
	Nierenberg et al. (1993)	≥3 adequate trials	Venlafaxine	70	Open	150–450 mg	33% response
Bupropion	Stern et al. (1983)	TCA	Bupropion	33	Open	150–600 mg	62% of nonresponders

(continued)

TABLE 1.4. cont.

Agent class	Investigators	Failed agent	Antidepressant switch	n	Design	Dose ranges	% Response
Naturally occurring compounds	Takahashi et al. (1975)	TCA	L-5-HTP	16	Open	300 mg/day	6 of 16 (38%)
	Nolen et al. (1988b)	TCA	L-5-HTP	47	Controlled, partial c/o	20–200 mg/day	0 of 12 (0%)
	Rosenbaum et al. (1990)	>1 prior adequate trial	SAMe	9	Open	400–1600 mg/day	2 of 9 (22%)
Anticonvulsants and steroid-suppressing agents	Prasad (1985)	Standard antidepressants	Carbamazepine	12	Open	400–600 mg/day	11 of 12 (92%)
	Post et al. (1986)	Unspecified antidepressants	Carbamazepine	11	RCT	400–2000 mg /day	5 of 11 (45%)
	Pearson Murphy et al. (1991)	Standard antidepressants	Steroid suppressors (aminoglutethimide, metyrapone, & ketoconazole)	8	Open	500–1000 mg aminoglutethimide, 500–2000 mg metyrapone, 600–1200 mg ketoconazole	6 of 8 (75%)

and 5 (62%) of 8 nonresponders to nomifensine eventually responded to tranylcypromine in the crossover phase of the study. Thus, the switch from a TCA to an MAOI is a very efficacious alternative to augmentation for treatment-resistant depressed patients.

Switching to SSRIs

The switch to an SSRI from a TCA appears to be effective clinically, although this method lacks support from controlled trials. An open-label study on 132 patients who had failed to respond to or to tolerate TCAs observed a response rate to fluoxetine between 51.4% and 62.1%, depending on the definition of "response" employed (Beasley, Sayler, Cunningham, Weiss, & Masica, 1990). Thus, patients who have failed to respond to TCAs may show a favorable response after switch to an SSRI. In an open study with another SSRI, 8 (29%) of 28 depressed patients refractory to TCAs responded to treatment with fluvoxamine alone (Delgado, Price, Charney, & Heninger, 1988). A double-blind, partial-crossover study of 71 patients who failed to respond to earlier treatment with TCAs reported response in 10% of patients treated with fluvoxamine, but in 39% of patients treated with the selective norepinephrine reuptake inhibitor oxaprotiline (Nolen et al., 1988a). In an open study, 9 (82%) of 11 patients who had failed to respond to desipramine responded to treatment with fluvoxamine (White, Wykoff, Tynes, Schneider, & Zemansky, 1990). A study on 70 depressed patients with a history of failure to at least two different antidepressant classes showed a 33% response to open treatment with venlafaxine (Nierenberg, Feighner, Rudolf, Cole, & Sullivan, 1994), which can be considered an SSRI on the basis of its pharmacologic properties *in vitro* (Fava & Rosenbaum, 1995). Overall, the switch from a TCA to an SSRI is a promising alternative to augmentation for treatment-resistant depressed patients, although controlled studies need to be done.

Switching to Bupropion

A study by Stern, Harto-Truax, and Bauer (1983) in 33 outpatients with a history of nonresponse or nonresponse plus intolerance to TCAs found that these patients markedly improved with open treatment on the atypical antidepressant bupropion. These results are at best suggestive, given the lack of a controlled design.

Switching to Naturally Occurring Compounds or Steroid-Suppressing Agents

The efficacy of L-5-HTP, a serotonin precursor, in the treatment of nonresponders was initially suggested by an open trial (Takahashi, Kondo, & Kato, 1975). However, another report indicates that none (0%) of 12 patients with major depression who had failed to respond to treatment with at least two antidepressants responded to treatment with L-5-HTP (Nolen et al., 1988b). Finally, S-adenosyl-L-methionine (SAMe), a naturally occurring methyl donor observed to increase serotonergic turnover, was found in an open study to induce remission in 2 (22%) of 9 treatment-resistant patients (Rosenbaum et al., 1990). Although L-5-HTP and SAMe may be helpful in some refractory patients, their efficacy in this population has not yet been adequately investigated.

Similarly, there is some suggestion that steroid-suppressing agents may be helpful in refractory depression. One study found that six (75%) of eight treatment-resistant depressed patients who completed 2 months of treatment with one or more steroid-suppressing agents (aminoglutethimide, ketoconazole, and/or metyrapone) showed full response (Pearson Murphy, Dhar, Ghadirian, Chouinard, & Keller, 1991). The efficacy of this type of treatment may derive from hypercortisolism in depression, but the data are clearly very preliminary.

Switching to Anticonvulsants

Of nine treatment-resistant depressed patients, four (44%) showed moderate or marked response following treatment with the anticonvulsant carbamazepine alone (Cullen et al., 1991). In an open study, 11 (92%) of 12 cases of chronic depression resistant to treatment with TCAs and MAOIs showed a definite improvement after treatment with carbamazepine alone at doses of 400 to 600 mg/day (Prasad, 1985). In a double-blind, placebo-controlled study, 5 (45%) of 11 unipolar depressed patients responded to carbamazepine after having been unsuccessfully treated with other antidepressant treatments (Post, Uhde, Roy-Byrne, & Joffe, 1986). There are no controlled, published data yet on the efficacy of valproic acid, another anticonvulsant used in mood disorders, in the treatment of refractory patients. Overall, the switch to anticonvulsant drugs such as carbamazepine may be helpful in refractory patients, particularly in those with highly recurrent depression.

ELECTROCONVULSIVE THERAPY

Although ECT is generally regarded as the most potent treatment for depression, limited patient acceptance and concerns about cost often result in its underutilization. In view of its safety and efficacy, ECT is a particularly attractive option for any depressed treatment-resistant patient, and should be considered as such rather than as treatment of last resort. For some patient groups, including patients who are acutely suicidal, are psychotic, have medical complications, or are pregnant, ECT may be the treatment of choice (Rosenbaum et al., 1995).

A course of ECT for acute depression typically consists of 4 to 12 seizures induced electrically while the patient is under anesthesia. Within the range of common clinical practice, the intensity of electrical stimulus and the waveform (sine wave, brief pulse) seem to contribute to differential adverse effects, whereas the format of stimulus placement (bilateral vs. unilateral) appears to affect both adverse events and efficacy. Some investigators (Mukherjee, Sackeim, & Schnur, 1994) and many clinicians find better response to bilateral treatment, but unilateral nondominant ECT is associated with less memory impairment than is bilateral ECT. Therefore, many clinicians will start treatment with unilateral ECT and switch to bilateral ECT only if the patient fails to respond.

A study by Prudic, Sackeim, and Devanand (1990) found that patients who had previously failed to respond to adequate antidepressant pharmacotherapies had a poorer response rate and also a higher relapse rate after ECT treatment than patients who had responded to a trial of adequate prior antidepressant medication. This was supported by the findings of a study by the British Medical Research Council showing a 71% response rate to ECT in treatment-naive patients, with response rates of only 50% in phenelzine nonresponders and 55% in imipramine nonresponders (Medical Research Council, 1965).

PSYCHOTHERAPY

Various forms of psychotherapy are currently used in the treatment of depression. In particular, numerous studies support the antidepressant efficacy of interpersonal psychotherapy and cognitive-behavioral therapy in both the short and the long term (Fava & Kaji, 1994), and their strategies are discussed in detail by Otto, Pava, and Sprich-Buckminster in Chapter 2 of this volume. Of course, psychotherapy is often used in combination with pharmacotherapy in patients with partial response, to address residual symptoms that are not improved by drug treatment alone; the efficacy of this strategy remains to be demonstrated, however. Psychotherapy alone or in combination with pharmacotherapy is also used in refractory depression, but again there is only limited empirical support for this clinical strategy (see Otto et al., Chapter 2). Our field needs to conduct systematic studies to evaluate the role of various forms of psychotherapy in populations of depressed patients resistant to treatment.

CONCLUSION

Treatment-resistant major depression is clearly not a simple phenomenon, but reflects issues of diagnostic subtypes, comorbidity, treatment adequacy, augmentation, and alternatives. The clinician must establish and address possible factors contributing to each patient's relative resistance to treatment, in order to maximize the patient's chances of recovery. Persistence of nonresponse or partial response in the face of adequate treatment and comprehensive evaluation of possible contributing factors may be addressed by a wide range of clinical strategies, which vary across practitioners and patients according to the needs of each individual case. In general, initial choices for treating resistant depression are best drawn from options with the most support from clinical research and reports. From our review of the literature, it appears that lithium or thyroid augmentation, high-dose SSRIs, and combinations of TCAs with either MAOIs or SSRIs may be the most promising first approaches. However, even if these three strategies fail, clinicians can draw on ample additional resources, including other psychotropic agents, psychotherapy alone or in combination with pharmacotherapy, and ECT. Even though the literature has not yet provided empirical evidence for the efficacy of many of these strategies, it is certainly suggestive of their potential usefulness.

REFERENCES

Agnoli, A., Ruggieri, S., & Casacchia, M. (1978). Restatement and perspectives of ergot alkaloids in clinical neurology and psychiatry. *Pharmacology, 16*(Suppl. 1), 174–188.

American Medical Association. (1993). *AMA drug evaluations.* Chicago: Author.

Amsterdam, J. D., & Berwish, N. J. (1989). High dose tranylcypromine therapy for refractory depression. *Pharmacopsychiatry, 22,* 21–25.

Anton, R. F., Jr., & Burch, E. A., Jr. (1990). A comparison study of amoxapine vs. amitriptyline plus perphenazine in the treatment of psychotic depression. *American Journal of Psychiatry, 147,* 1203–1208.

Aronson, T. A., Shukla, S., Hoff, A., & Cook, B. (1988). Proposed delusional depression subtypes: Preliminary evidence from a retrospective study of phenomenology and treatment course. *Journal of Affective Disorders, 14,* 69–74.

Austin, L. S., Arana, G. W., & Ballenger, J. C. (1990). Rapid response of patients simultaneously treated with lithium and nortriptyline. *Journal of Clinical Psychiatry, 51,* 124–125.

Austin, M.-P., Souza, F. G. M., & Goodwin, G. M. (1991). Lithium augmentation in antidepressant-resistant patients: A quantitative analysis. *British Journal of Psychiatry, 159,* 510–514.

Baettig, D., Bondolfi, G., Montaldi, S., & Amey, M. (1993). Tricyclic antidepressant plasma levels after augmentation with citalopram: A case study. *European Journal of Clinical Pharmacology, 44,* 403–405.

Bakish, D. (1991). Fluoxetine potentiation by buspirone: Three case histories. *Canadian Journal of Psychiatry, 36,* 749–750.

Baldessarini, R. J. (1985). *Chemotherapy in psychiatry: Principles and practice.* Cambridge, MA: Harvard University Press.

Banki, C. M. (1975). Triiodothyronine in the treatment of depression. *Orvosi Hetilap, 116,* 2543–2547.

Beasley, C. M., Sayler, M. E., Cunningham, G. E., Weiss, A. M., & Masica, D. N. (1990). Fluoxetine in tricyclic refractory major depressive disorder. *Journal of Affective Disorders, 20,* 193–200.

Bouckoms, A., & Mangini, L. (1992). *Pergolide: An antidepressant adjuvant for mood disorders?* Paper presented at the meeting of the New Clinical Drug Evaluation Unit, Boca Raton, FL.

Bouras, N., & Bridges, P. K. (1982). Bromocriptine and depression. *Current Medical Research and Opinion, 8,* 150–153.

Callahan, A. M., Fava, M., & Rosenbaum, J. F. (1993). Drug interactions in psychopharmacology. *Psychiatric Clinics of North America, 16,* 647–671.

Chan, C. H., Janicak, P. G., Davis, J. M., Altman, E., Andriukaitis, S., & Hedeker, D. (1987). Response of psychotic and nonpsychotic depressed patients to tricyclic antidepressants. *Journal of Clinical Psychiatry, 48,* 197–200.

Chiarello, R. J., & Cole, J. O. (1987). The use of psychostimulants in psychiatry. *Archives of General Psychiatry, 44,* 286–295.

Ciraulo, D. A., & Shader, R. I. (1990). Fluoxetine drug–drug interactions: I. Antidepressants and antipsychotics. *Journal of Clinical Psychopharmacology, 10,* 48–50.

Clayton, P. J., Grove, W. M., Coryell, W., Keller, M., Hirschfeld, R., & Fawcett, J. (1991). Follow-up and family study of anxious depression. *American Journal of Psychiatry, 148,* 1512–1517.

Cole, J. O., Schatzberg, A. F., Sniffin, C., Zolner, J., & Cole, J. P. (1981). Trazodone in treatment-resistant depression: An open study. *Journal of Clinical Psychopharmacology, 1*(6, Suppl.), 49S–54S.

Colonna, L., Petit, M., & Lepine, J. P. (1979). Bromocriptine in affective disorders. *Journal of Affective Disorders, 1,* 173–177.

Corrigan, F. M. (1992). Sodium valproate augmentation of fluoxetine or fluvoxamine effects [Letter]. *Biological Psychiatry, 31,* 1178–1179.

Courneyer, G., de Montigny, C., Oullette, J., Leblanc, G., Langlois, R., & Elie, R. (1984). Lithium addition in tricyclic-resistant unipolar depression: A placebo-controlled study. *Abstracts Collegium Internationale Neuropsychopharmacologicum,* 179.

Cullen, M., Mitchell, P., Brodaty, H., Boyce, P., Parker, G., Hickie, I., & Wilhelm, K. (1991). Carbamazepine for treatment-resistant melancholia. *Journal of Clinical Psychiatry, 52,* 472–476.

Davidson, J., McLeod, M., Law-Yone, B., & Linnoila, M. (1978). A comparison of electroconvulsive therapy and combined phenelzine–amitriptyline in refractory depression. *Archives of General Psychiatry, 35,* 639–642.

de Montigny, C., Grunberg, F., & Mayer, A. (1981). Lithium induces rapid relief of depression in tricyclic antidepressant drug non-responders. *British Journal of Psychiatry, 138,* 252–256.

Deicken, R. F. (1987). Combined alprazolam and phenelzine treatment of refractory depression with panic attacks. *Biological Psychiatry, 22,* 762–766.

Delgado, P. L., Price, L. H., Charney, D. S., & Heninger, G. R. (1988). Efficacy of fluvoxamine in treatment-refractory depression. *Journal of Affective Disorders, 15,* 55–60.

Earle, B. V. (1970). Thyroid hormone and tricyclic antidepressants in resistant depressions. *American Journal of Psychiatry, 126,* 1667–1669.

Eisen, A. (1989). Fluoxetine and desipramine: A strategy for augmenting antidepressant response. *Pharmacopsychiatry, 22,* 272–273.

Fava, M., Anderson, K., & Rosenbaum, J. F. (1993). Are thymoleptic-responsive "anger attacks" a discrete clinical syndrome? *Psychosomatics, 34,* 350–355.

Fava, M., Bouffides, E., Pava, J. A., McCarthy, M. K., Steingard, R. J., & Rosenbaum, J. F. (1994a). Personality disorder comorbidity with major depression and response to fluoxetine treatment. *Psychotherapy and Psychosomatics, 62*, 160–167.

Fava, M., & Kaji, J. (1994). Continuation and maintenance treatments of major depressive disorder. *Psychiatric Annals, 24*, 281–290.

Fava, M., & Rosenbaum, J. F. (1995). Pharmacotherapy and somatic therapies. In E. E. Beckham & W. R. Leber (Eds.), *Handbook of depression* (2nd ed., pp. 280–281). New York: Guilford Press.

Fava, M., Rosenbaum, J. F., Cohen, L., Reiter, S., McKarthy, M., Steingard, R., & Clancy, K. (1992). High-dose fluoxetine in the treatment of depressed patients not responsive to a standard dose of fluoxetine. *Journal of Affective Disorders, 25*, 229–234.

Fava, M., Rosenbaum, J. F., McGrath, P. J., Stewart, J. W., Amsterdam, J. D., & Quitkin, F. M. (1994b). Lithium and tricyclic augmentation of fluoxetine treatment for resistant major depression: A double-blind, controlled study. *American Journal of Psychiatry, 151*, 1372–1374.

Fawcett, J., & Kravitz, H. M. (1983). Anxiety syndromes and their relationship to depressive illness. *Journal of Clinical Psychiatry, 44*, 8–11.

Fawcett, J., Kravitz, H. M., Zajecka, J. M., & Schaff, M. R. (1991). CNS stimulant potentiation of monoamine oxidase inhibitors in treatment-refractory depression. *Journal of Clinical Psychopharmacology, 11*, 127–132.

Feighner, J. P., Boyer, W. F., Tyler, D. L., & Neborsky, R. J. (1990). Adverse consequences of fluoxetine–MAOI combination therapy. *Journal of Clinical Psychiatry, 51*, 222–225.

Feighner, J. P., Herbstein, J., & Damlouji, N. (1985). Combined MAOI, TCA, and direct stimulant therapy of treatment-resistant depression. *Journal of Clinical Psychiatry, 46*, 206–209.

Gitlin, M. J., Weiner, H., & Fairbanks, L. (1987). Failure of T_3 to potentiate tricyclic antidepressant response. *Journal of Affective Disorders, 13*, 267–272.

Goldberg, R. S., & Thornton, W. E. (1978). Combined tricyclic–MAOI therapy for refractory depression: A review, with guidelines for appropriate usage. *Journal of Clinical Pharmacology, 18*, 143–147.

Heninger, G. R., Charney, D. S., & Sternberg, D. E. (1983). Lithium carbonate augmentation of antidepressant treatment. *Archives of General Psychiatry, 40*, 1335–1342.

Jacobsen, F. M. (1991). Possible augmentation of antidepressant response by buspirone. *Journal of Clinical Psychiatry, 52*(5), 217–220.

Jenike, M. A., Hyman, S., Baer, L., Holland, A., Minichello, W. E., Buttolph, L., Summergrad, P., Seymour, R., & Ricciardi, J. (1990). A controlled trial of fluvoxamine in obsessive–compulsive disorder: Implications for a serotonergic theory. *American Journal of Psychiatry, 147*, 1209–1215.

Joffe, R. T., Bagby, M., & Levitt, A. (1993a). Anxious and nonanxious depression. *American Journal of Psychiatry, 150*, 1257–1258.

Joffe, R. T., Levitt, A. T., Bagby, R. M., Macdonald, C., & Singer, W. (1993b). Predictors of response to lithium and triiodothyronine augmentation of antidepressants in tricyclic non-responders. *British Journal of Psychiatry, 163*, 574–578.

Joffe, R. T., & Schuller, D. R. (1993). An open study of buspirone augmentation of serotonin reuptake inhibitors in refractory depression. *Journal of Clinical Psychiatry, 54*, 269–271.

Joffe, R. T., Singer, W., Levitt, A. J., & MacDonald, C. (1993c). A placebo-controlled comparison of lithium and triiodothyronine augmentation of tricyclic antidepressants in unipolar refractory depression. *Archives of General Psychiatry, 50*, 387–393.

Johnson, F. N. (1991). Lithium augmentation therapy. *Review of Contemporary Pharmacotherapy, 2*, 1–52.

Kantor, D., McNeuen, S., Leichner, P., Harper, D., & Krenn, M. (1986). The benefit of lithium carbonate adjunct in refractory depression—fact or fiction? *Canadian Journal of Psychiatry, 31*, 416–418.

Keller, M. B., Lavori, P. W., Endicott, J., Coryell, W., & Klerman, G. L. (1983). "Double depression": Two-year follow-up. *American Journal of Psychiatry, 140*, 689–694.

Keller, M. B., & Shapiro, R. W. (1982). "Double depression": Superimposition of acute depressive episodes on chronic depressive disorders. *American Journal of Psychiatry, 139*, 438–442.

Lader, M. (1983). Combined use of tricyclic antidepressants and monoamine oxidase inhibitors. *Journal of Clinical Psychiatry, 44*, 20–24.

Liebowitz, M. R., Quitkin, F. M., Stewart, J. W., McGrath, P. J., Harrison, W. M., Markowitz, J. S., Rabkin, J. G., Tricamo, E., Goetz, D. M., & Klein, D. F. (1988). Antidepressant specificity in atypical depression. *Archives of General Psychiatry, 45*, 129–137.

Linet, L. S. (1989). Treatment of a refractory depression with a combination of fluoxetine and D-amphetamine [Letter]. *American Journal of Psychiatry, 146*, 803–804.

Lippman, S., Baldwin, H., & Manshadi, M. (1982). Combined trimipramine/phenelzine treatment of depression: Case report. *Journal of Clinical Psychiatry, 43*, 430–431.

MacEwan, W. G., & Remick, R. A. (1988). Treatment-resistant depression: A clinical perspective. *Canadian Journal of Psychiatry, 33*, 788–792.

Manshadi, M. S., & Lippmann, S. B. (1984). Combined treatment of refractory depression with an MAO inhibitor and a tricyclic. *Psychosomatics, 25*, 929–931.

McGrath, P. J., Stewart, J. W., Harrison, W., & Quitkin, F. M. (1987). Treatment of tricyclic refractory depression with a monoamine oxidase inhibitor antidepressant. *Psychopharmacology Bulletin, 23*, 169–172.

Medical Research Council. (1965). Clinical trial of treatment of depressive illness. *British Medical Journal, i*, 881–886.

Metz, A., & Shader, R. I. (1991). Combination of fluoxetine with pemoline in the treatment of major depressive disorder. *International Journal of Clinical Psychopharmacology, 6*, 93–96.

Mukherjee, S., Sackeim, H. A., & Schnur, D. B. (1994). Electroconvulsive therapy of acute manic episodes: A review of 50 years' experience. *American Journal of Psychiatry, 151*(2), 169–176.

Nierenberg, A. A., & Amsterdam, J. D. (1990). Treatment-resistant depression: Definition and treatment approaches. *Journal of Clinical Psychiatry, 51*(Suppl.), 39–47.

Nierenberg, A. A., & Cole, J. O. (1991). One antidepressant fails: What next? A survey of Northeastern psychiatrists. *Journal of Clinical Psychiatry, 52*, 383–385.

Nierenberg, A. A., Feighner, J. P., Rudolph, R., Cole, J. O., & Sullivan, J. (1994). Venlafaxine for treatment-resistant unipolar depression. *Journal of Clinical Psychopharmacology, 14*, 419–423.

Nolen, W. A., van de Putte, J. J., Dijken, W. A., Kamp, J. S., Blansjaar, B. A., Kramer, H. J., & Haffmans, J. (1988a). Treatment strategy in depression: I. Non-tricyclic and selective reuptake inhibitors in resistant depression. A double-blind partial crossover study on the effects of oxaprotiline and fluvoxamine. *Acta Psychiatrica Scandinavica, 78,* 668–675.

Nolen, W. A., van de Putte, J. J., Dijken, W. A., Kamp, J. S., Blansjaar, B. A., Kramer, H. J., & Haffmans, J. (1988b). Treatment strategy in depression: II. MAO inhibitors in depression resistant to cyclic antidepressants: Two controlled crossover studies with tranylcypromine versus L-5-hydroxytryptophan and nomifensine. *Acta Psychiatrica Scandinavica, 78,* 676–683.

Nordin, C., Siwers, B., & Bertilsson, L. (1981). Bromocriptine of depressive disorders: Clinical and biochemical effects. *Acta Psychiatrica Scandinavica, 64,* 25–33.

Novac, A. (1992). Fluoxetine and bupropion treatment of bipolar disorder, type II, associated with GAD. *Journal of Clinical Psychiatry, 52,* 67.

Ogura, C., Okuma, T., Uchida, Y., Imai, S., Yogi, H., & Sumami, Y. (1974). Combined thyroid (triiodothyronine)–tricyclic antidepressant treatment in depressive states. *Folia Psychiatrica et Neurologica Japonica, 28,* 179–186.

Ontiveros, A., Fontaine, R., & Elie, R. (1991). Refractory depression: The addition of lithium to fluoxetine or desipramine. *Acta Psychiatrica Scandinavica, 83,* 188–192.

Pande, A. C., Haskett, R. F., & Greden, J. F. (1992). *Fluoxetine treatment of atypical depression.* Paper presented at the 145th Annual Meeting of the American Psychiatric Association, Washington, DC.

Pearson Murphy, B. E., Dhar, V., Ghadirian, A. M., Chouinard, G., & Keller, R. (1991). Response to steroid suppression in major depression resistant to antidepressant therapy. *Journal of Clinical Psychopharmacology, 11,* 121–126.

Popkin, M. K., Callies, A. L., & Mackenzie, T. B. (1985). The outcome of antidepressant use in the medically ill. *Archives of General Psychiatry, 42,* 1160–1163.

Post, R. M., Uhde, T. W., Roy-Byrne, P. P., & Joffe, R. T. (1986). Antidepressant effects of carbamazepine. *American Journal of Psychiatry, 143,* 29–34.

Prange, A. J., Wilson, I. C., & Robon, A. M. (1969). Enhancement of imipramine antidepressant activity by thyroid hormone. *American Journal of Psychiatry, 126,* 457–469.

Prasad, A. J. (1985). Efficacy of carbamazepine as an antidepressant in chronic resistant depressives. *Journal of the Indian Medical Association, 83,* 235–237.

Price, L. H. (1990). Pharmacological strategies in refractory depression. In A. Tasman, S. M. Goldfinger, & C. A. Kaufman (Eds.), *American Psychiatric Press review of psychiatry* (Vol. 9, pp. 116–131). Washington, DC: American Psychiatric Press.

Prudic, J., Sackeim, H. A., & Devanand, D. P. (1990). Medication resistance and clinical response to electroconvulsive therapy. *Psychiatry Research, 31,* 287–296.

Ries, R. K., & Wittkowsky, A. K. (1986). Synergistic action of alprazolam with tranylcypromine in drug-resistant atypical depression with panic attacks. *Biological Psychiatry, 21,* 519–521.

Riise, I. S., & Holm, P. (1984). Concomitant isocarboxazid/mianserin treatment of major depressive disorder. *Journal of Affective Disorders, 6,* 175–179.

Rosenbaum, J. R., Fava, M., Nierenberg, A. A., & Sachs, G. (1995). Treatment-resistant mood disorders. In G. O. Gabbard (Ed.), *Treatments of psychiatric disorders* (2nd ed., pp. 1275–1328). Washington, DC: American Psychiatric Association.

Rosenbaum, J. F., Fava, M., Falk, W. E., Pollack, M. H., Cohen, L. S., Cohen, B. M., & Zubenko, G. S. (1990). The antidepressant potential of oral S-adenosyl-l-methionine. *Acta Psychiatrica Scandinavica, 81,* 432–436.

Rosenbaum, J. F., Quitkin, F. M., Fava, M., Amsterdam, J., Fawcett, J., Zajecka, J., Lebegue, B. J., Reimherr, F. W., & Beasley, C. M. (1993). *Fluoxetine vs. placebo: Long-term treatment of MDD.* Paper presented at the 32nd Annual Meeting of the American College of Neuropsychopharmacology, Maui, HI.

Schmauss, M., Kapfhammer, H. P., Meyr, P., & Hoff, P. (1988). Combined MAO-inhibitor and tri- (tetra-)cyclic antidepressant treatment in therapy-resistant depression. *Progress in Neuropsychopharmacology and Biological Psychiatry, 12,* 523–532.

Schopf, J., Baumann, P., Lemarchand, T., & Rey, M. (1989). Treatment of endogenous depressions resistant to tricyclic antidepressants or related drugs by lithium addition. *Pharmacopsychiatry, 22,* 183–187.

Schuckit, M. A., & Feighner, J. P. (1972). Safety of high-dose tricyclic antidepressant therapy. *American Journal of Psychiatry, 128,* 140–143.

Seth, R., Jennings, A. L., Bindman, J., Phillips, J., & Bergmann, K. (1992). Combination treatment with noradrenalin and serotonin reuptake inhibitors in resistant depression. *British Journal of Psychiatry, 161,* 562–565.

Sethna, E. R. (1974). A study of refractory cases of depressive illnesses and their response to combined antidepressant treatment. *British Journal of Psychiatry, 124,* 265–271.

Sheperd, M., Lader, M., & Rodnight, R. (1968). *Clinical psychopharmacology.* London: English Universities Press.

Silverstone, T. (1984). Response to bromocriptine distinguishes bipolar from unipolar depressions. *Lancet, i,* 903–904.

Spiker, D. G., & Pugh, D. D. (1976). Combining tricyclic and monoamine oxidase inhibitor antidepressants. *Archives of General Psychiatry, 33,* 828–830.

Spiker, D. G., Weiss, J. C., Dealy, R. S., Griffin, S. J., Hanin, I., Neil, J. F., Perel, J. M., Rossi, A. J., & Soloff, P. H. (1985). The pharmacological treatment of delusional depression. *American Journal of Psychiatry, 142,* 430–436.

Stein, G., & Bernadt, M. (1993). Lithium augmentation therapy in tricyclic-resistant depression: A controlled trial using lithium in low and normal doses. *British Journal of Psychiatry, 162,* 634–640.

Stern, W. C., Harto-Truax, N., & Bauer, N. (1983). Efficacy of bupropion in tricyclic-resistant or intolerant patients. *Journal of Clinical Psychiatry, 44,* 148–152.

Takahashi, S., Kondo, H., & Kato, N. (1975). Effect of L-5-hydroxytryptophan on brain monoamine metabolism and evaluation of its clinical effect in depressed patients. *Journal of Psychiatric Research, 12,* 177–187.

Targum, S. D., Greenberg, R. D., Harmon, R. L., Kessler, K., Salerian, A. J., & Fram, D. H. (1984). Thyroid hormone and the TRH simulation test in refractory depression. *Journal of Clinical Psychiatry, 45,* 345–346.

Thase, M. E., Carpenter, L., Kupfer, D. J., & Frank, E. (1991). Clinical significance of reversed vegetative subtypes of recurrent major depression. *Psychopharmacology Bulletin, 27,* 17–22.

Thase, M. E., Frank, E., Hamer, T., & Kupfer, D. J. (1992). Treatment of imipramine-resistant recurrent depression: III. Efficacy of monoamine oxidase inhibitors. *Journal of Clinical Psychiatry, 53,* 5–11.

Thase, M. E., Kupfer, D. J., Frank, E., & Jarrett, D. B. (1989a). Treatment of imipramine-resistant recurrent depression: II. An open clinical trial of lithium augmentation. *Journal of Clinical Psychiatry, 50,* 413–417.

Thase, M. E., Kupfer, D. J., & Jarrett, D. B. (1989b). Treatment of imipramine-resistant recurrent depression: I. An open clinical trial of adjunctive L-triidothyronine. *Journal of Clinical Psychiatry, 50,* 385–388.

Theohar, C., Fischer-Cornelssen, K., Brosch, H., Fischer, E. K., & Petrovic, D. (1982). A comparative, multicenter trial between bromocriptine and amitriptyline in the treatment of endogenous depression. *Arzneimittelforschung, 32,* 783–787.

Tsutsui, S., Yamazaki, Y., Namba, T., & Tsushima, M. (1979). Combined therapy of T_3 and antidepressants in depression. *Journal of International Medical Research, 7,* 138–146.

Tyrer, P., & Murphy, S. (1990). Effect of combined antidepressant therapy in resistant neurotic disorder. *British Journal of Psychiatry, 156,* 115–118.

van Valkenburg, C., Akiskal, H. S., Puzantian, V., & Rosenthal, T. (1984). Anxious depression: Clinical, family history and naturalistic outcome. Comparison with panic and major depressive disorders. *Journal of Affective Disorders, 6,* 67–82.

Waehrens, J., & Gerlach, J. (1981). Bromocriptine and imipramine in endogenous depression: A double-blind controlled trial in out-patients. *Journal of Affective Disorders, 3,* 193–202.

Weilburg, J. B., Rosenbaum, J. F., Biederman, M. D., Sachs, G. S., Pollack, M. H., & Kelly, K. (1989). Fluoxetine added to non-MAOI antidepressants converts non-responders to responders: A preliminary report. *Journal of Clinical Psychiatry, 50,* 447–449.

Weilburg, J. B., Rosenbaum, J. F., Meltzer-Brody, S., & Shustari, J. (1991). Tricyclic augmentation of fluoxetine. *Annals of Clinical Psychiatry, 3,* 209–213.

White, K., & Simpson, G. (1981). Combined MAOI–tricyclic antidepressant treatment: A reevaluation. *Journal of Clinical Psychopharmacology, 1,* 264–282.

White, K., Wykoff, W., Tynes, L. L., Schneider, L., & Zemansky, M. (1990). Fluvoxamine in the treatment of tricyclic-resistant depression. *Psychiatric Journal of the University of Ottawa, 15,* 156–158.

Wilson, I. C., Prange, A. J., & McClaine, T. K. (1970). Thyroid hormone enhancement of imipramine in non-related depressions. *New England Journal of Medicine, 282,* 1063–1067.

Worthington, J. J., Fava, M., Agustin, C. M., Alpert, J. E., Nierenberg, A. A., Pava, J. A., & Rosenbaum, J. F. (1994). *Consumption of alcohol, nicotine, and caffeine among depressed outpatients: Relationship with response to treatment.* Paper presented at the 41st Annual Meeting of the Academy of Psychosomatic Medicine, Phoenix, AZ.

Zusky, P. M., Biederman, J., Rosenbaum, J. F., Manschreck, T. C., Grass, C. C., Weilburg, J. B., & Gastfriend, D. R. (1988). Adjunct low dose lithium carbonate in treatment-resistant depression: A placebo-controlled study. *Journal of Clinical Psychopharmacology, 8,* 120–124.

2

Treatment of Major Depression: Applications and Efficacy of Cognitive-Behavioral Therapy

MICHAEL W. OTTO
JOEL A. PAVA
SUSAN SPRICH-BUCKMINSTER

Research to date provides a wealth of evidence for both pharmacologic and psychosocial approaches to the treatment of major depression. Of psychosocial treatments, cognitive-behavioral therapy (CBT) and interpersonal psychotherapy (IPT) have received the most empirical support. Because of the relatively larger research base for CBT, this chapter focuses primarily on CBT and discusses the role of this treatment as an alternative to pharmacotherapy, as an adjunct to ongoing pharmacologic treatment, and as a relapse prevention strategy for patients maintaining or discontinuing their pharmacologic regimen. In all applications, emphasis is placed on the role of CBT in maximizing short-term treatment outcome and lessening the likelihood of relapse and recurrence over the long term. An algorithm of interventions for treatment-resistant patients is also presented.

Beck's cognitive model of depression (Beck, 1983; Beck, Rush, Shaw, & Emery, 1979) has been especially influential in characterizing the interplay of cognitive, affective, and behavioral dimensions of depression. In this model, a number of developmental, hereditary, and learning factors are thought to predispose individuals to depression. Among learning

factors, the model posits that individuals may develop negative or dysfunctional belief systems about themselves, the world, and the future as
the result of their experiences. Upon exposure to negative life events, negative schemas and dysfunctional attitudes are activated, and negative automatic thoughts may result. These thoughts are typically irrational,
unproductive statements about events in the past, present, or future; by
their nature, they act to disrupt adaptive behavior, decrease motivation,
and worsen mood, thereby contributing to the occurrence and maintenance
of depression.

CBT for depression is an active, structured approach that typically
consists of a variety of cognitive restructuring, problem-solving, and activity-
planning interventions (Beck et al., 1979; Fennell, 1989; Lewinsohn,
Biglan, & Zeiss, 1976). Cognitive restructuring is a central component
of treatment and is designed to help patients learn to identify, question,
and modify their negative automatic thoughts. Cognitive restructuring is
achieved through a combination of informational interventions, careful
monitoring and logical examination of thoughts, and the use of behavioral
assignments and monitoring to challenge the veracity of dysfunctional beliefs. In addition to these cognitive restructuring components, patients are
often asked to monitor their daily activities and schedule events that are
pleasurable and that lead them to feel competent. Training in problem-
solving skills may also be included. Typically, these treatment components
are provided within a collaborative, problem-oriented approach, with special
emphasis on helping patients identify their underlying negative assumptions
and learn the skills of cognitive restructuring and activity management.

Like CBT, IPT (Klerman, Weissman, Rounsaville, & Chevron, 1984)
is an active, collaborative, problem-oriented treatment approach that focuses on the acquisition of skills for more adaptive interactions. The focus of treatment is on the identification of problem areas such as grief,
role transitions, role disputes, and interpersonal deficits, and the development of appropriate interpersonal skills for altering these difficulties.

THE EFFICACY OF CBT FOR DEPRESSION

Evaluation of the effectiveness of CBT for depression is aided by two meta-
analyses of the depression treatment literature. In the first, Dobson (1989)
examined 28 studies that (1) compared Beck's cognitive therapy to other
treatment modalities, and (2) used the Beck Depression Inventory (Beck,
Ward, Mendelson, Mock, & Erbaugh, 1961) as an outcome measure. These
studies were conducted between 1976 and 1987. Dobson found that when
cognitive therapy was compared with a no-treatment or a waiting-list control
group, the mean effect size was 2.15. This effect size indicates that the
average cognitive therapy patient did better than 98% of the control patients. Similarly, when cognitive therapy was compared with treatments
emphasizing only behavioral strategies, the mean effect size was 0.46, in-

dicating that the average cognitive therapy patient did better than 67% of patients receiving behavioral interventions alone. Finally, in studies that compared cognitive therapy to pharmacotherapy, the average effect size was 0.53, showing that the average CBT patient did better than 70% of the pharmacotherapy patients.

A second meta-analysis was conducted by Robinson, Berman, and Neimeyer (1990). These authors included 58 studies of psychotherapy for the treatment of depression published between 1976 and 1986. They included studies of depressed adult patients which compared a psychological treatment to either a no-treatment control, a placebo control, or another treatment. Of the psychological treatments examined, forms of CBT were identified as significantly more effective than general psychotherapies. In addition, the psychosocial treatments were found to be significantly more effective than antidepressant treatments. However, these significant differences were reduced to the level of trends when the influence of investigator allegiance was examined. That is, studies carried out by investigators with allegiance to a particular type of treatment—CBT, general psychotherapy, or pharmacotherapy—generally found stronger effect sizes for their own treatment under study. A similar effect was reported by Greenberg, Bornstein, Greenberg, and Fisher (1992) for pharmacologic treatments. They found that the efficacy of medication treatments, as assessed by effect size, appeared to be inflated under conditions where clinical researchers were more likely to be aware that a patient was receiving an active agent.

These issues make it hard to draw firm conclusions about the relative efficacy of CBT and pharmacologic interventions, at least for diverse samples of depressed patients. It is possible, however, that differences in efficacy between these treatments are more pronounced within specific subgroups of patients. Crossover studies support the idea that nonresponders to one treatment approach will respond to an alternative treatment (Stewart, Mercier, Agosti, Guardin, & Quitkin, 1993). This finding encourages the search for predictors of differential response to pharmacologic treatment and CBT.

BIOLOGIC MARKERS OF TREATMENT RESPONSE

It is a common clinical opinion that patients with endogenous features will require pharmacotherapy rather than psychotherapy. This opinion has intuitive appeal; it rests on the assumption that a condition marked by physiologic disturbances will require physiologic interventions. Endogenous depression is characterized by severe neurovegetative and affective symptoms that include weight loss, early morning awakening, psychomotor disturbances, anhedonia, loss of mood reactivity, and diurnal mood variation. It is also frequently marked by disruption of neuroendocrine regulation or sleep neurophysiology. In particular, nonsuppression of plasma cortisol following adminstration of the dexamethasone suppression test (DST) and decreased latency to rapid-eye-movement (REM) sleep are associated with endogenous depression, and have been suggested to be markers of conditions requiring pharmacologic treatment (Thase, Simons, Cahalane, & McGeary, 1991b). However, recent studies provide evidence against a necessary matching of biologic interventions to conditions involving biologic disruptions.

To address this issue empirically, Thase et al. (1991b) examined the effects of a 16-week, 20-session program of CBT in patients who met Research Diagnostic Criteria for probable or definite endogenous depression. Treatment was associated with marked reduction in depressive symptoms, and approximately 75% of patients met criteria for treatment response by the end of the protocol. Response was defined as at least a 50% reduction in the 17-item Hamilton Rating Scale for Depression (HRSD; Hamilton, 1960) score from pretreatment and an HRSD score of 10 or less for at least the last 2 consecutive weeks of treatment. Approximately half of these patients had the biologic marker of reduced REM sleep latency. These patients did not respond poorly to CBT; rather, they demonstrated more rapid response on several measures. This finding does not support the hypothesis that reduced REM latency should be used to identify patients who will require pharmacotherapy rather than CBT.

Like reduced REM latency, nonsuppression to the DST test has also been identified as a marker for depression requiring pharmacologic treatment. This notion was effectively challenged by a study by McKnight, Nelson-Gray, and Barnhill (1992). McKnight et al. examined the differential effectiveness of 8 weeks of CBT versus 8 weeks of tricyclic medications for the treatment of depression in women classified as abnormal or normal DST responders. Tricyclic treatment consisted of amitriptyline or desipramine treatment; the dose of these medications was titrated upward until all patients achieved a plasma level of 125–150 ng/ml. McKnight et al. (1992) found that the DST was not a useful predictor of differential response to the CBT and antidepressant medication treatments. Both treatments significantly decreased depressive symptomatology, with patients with normal DST improving more in both the CBT and antidepressant treatment conditions. As anticipated, a high association was obtained between DST nonsuppression and melancholic status. When patients were reclassified according to the presence or absence of melancholia, there again was no evidence of differential effectiveness between the CBT and antidepressant treatment conditions.

This study also examined posttreatment DST status. It is noteworthy that effective treatment with CBT, like that with antidepressant medications, was associated with normalization of posttreatment DST status. It is equally important to note that successful treatment with either CBT or antidepressant medication resulted in significant decreases in dysfunctional thoughts associated with depression, although this reduction was greater in the CBT condition. These findings challenge the specificity of classic physiologic and psychologic markers of depression; both are correlates of depression, and both may change with effective treatment, whether this is behavioral or pharmacologic. As Thase et al. (1991b) discuss, the finding that reduced REM latency predicted a more rapid response to treatment, coupled with findings that reduced REM latency is associated with a favorable response to tricyclic medications, may indicate that this biologic marker may be a general predictor of treatment response per se rather than an indicator of a need for pharmacologic interventions. In summary, these studies and others (Simons & Thase, 1992; Thase, Bowler, & Harden, 1991a) challenge the notion that depression marked by biologic disruption requires a biologic intervention; support the efficacy of short-term CBT for patients with endogenous depression; and encourage clinicians to consider CBT as well as pharmacologic interventions for patients with depression, regardless of the presence of endogenous features or neurophysiologic markers.

MOOD REACTIVITY

In 1984, Liebowitz and associates described a subtype of depression ("atypical depression") characterized by mood reactivity, hyperphagia, hypersomnia, rejection sensitivity, and leaden paralysis (see also Quitkin et al., 1989). Patients with atypical depression tend to be in the moderate range of severity, but often have a chronic or recurrent course. This subtype has been hypothesized to show preferential response to monoamine oxidase inhibitors (Quitkin et al., 1989), although recent research suggests that it also responds to fluoxetine treatment (Pande, Haskett, & Greden, 1992) as well as a brief course of CBT (Mercier, Stewart, & Quitkin, 1992).

THE INFLUENCE OF DEPRESSION SEVERITY

Although biologic subtype of depression and atypical depression may not differentiate the effects of pharmacologic treatment versus CBT, there is limited evidence for differential effects of depression severity. For example, in the recent National Institute of Mental Health (NIMH) Treatment of Depression Collaborative Research Program (Elkin et al., 1989), endogenicity was not associated with differential response to pharmacologic and psychosocial treatments, but severity of depression was. In this study, 250 depressed patients were randomly assigned to CBT, IPT, imipramine plus clinical management, or placebo plus clinical management. After 16 weeks of treatment, all four groups showed significant improvement. Although there were no significant differences among the three active treatments, imipramine plus clinical management resulted in the best outcome on many measures; placebo plus clinical management resulted in the worst outcome; and the outcomes of the two psychosocial treatments were in between, usually closer to that of imipramine than to that of placebo. When the patients were stratified by initial depression severity, imipramine emerged as the preferable treatment for severely depressed patients, with some evidence for IPT for this group. However, as Munoz, Hollon, McGrath, Rehm, and Vanden Bos (1994) point out, this finding was not robust across sites, and several other studies support the efficacy of CBT with more severely depressed patients (Hollon et al., 1992a; Thase et al., 1991b; Thase, Simons, Cahalane, McGeary, & Harden, 1991c).

In summary, research to date supports the efficacy of CBT as an alternative to pharmacologic treatment, particularly for patients with mild to moderate levels of depression. Select studies have suggested that pharmacotherapy may offer greater efficacy for severely depressed patients than CBT alone, although contradictory evidence exists.

THE ROLE OF COMBINED TREATMENTS

Support for the individual effectiveness of CBT and pharmacologic treatments has raised hopes that the combination of these treatments may be more effective than either treatment alone. Studies to date have provided mixed support for this proposition. Although several studies have reported trends toward greater acute efficacy for combination treatment, these trends generally do not reach significance (Blackburn, Bishop, Glen, Whalley, & Christie, 1981; Hollon, DeRubeis, & Seligman, 1992b; Simons, Murphy, Levine, & Wetzel, 1986; Weissman, 1979). In addition, a number of studies have found that the addition of pharmacotherapy to a course of CBT appears to do little to improve outcome, either in the short term or at longer-term follow-up (Beck, Hollon, Young, Bedrosian, & Budenz, 1985; Murphy, Simons, Wetzel, & Lustman, 1984). However, in a recent "mega-analysis" that pooled subjects from several independent studies (n = 600), Thase et al. (1995) found that combined pharmacologic and psychosocial treatments (CBT or IPT) were better than psychosocial treatment alone for patients with severe depression. There was no evidence for additive effects for the combined treatment for less severe patients. Notably, the patients studied in this mega-analysis were often characterized by numerous previous episodes; hence, the advantage of combined treatments over CBT alone for severe depression may be most applicable to patients with recurrent depression.

There is more consistent evidence that the addition of CBT to a pharmacologic regimen may benefit the maintenance of treatment gains. For example, Simons et al. (1986) studied 70 depressed patients who were randomly assigned to one of four treatment groups: cognitive therapy alone, cognitive therapy plus nortriptyline, cognitive therapy plus active placebo, or nortriptyline alone. The treatment took place over a 12-week period. All four treatment groups demonstrated significant improvement in depression severity, and the amount of improvement did not differ as a function of treatment group. Study medications were tapered at the end of this study period. At the end of a 1-year follow-up phase, 52% of the responders in the medication conditions had relapsed, compared with 19% of patients in the other two conditions. Patients who received cognitive therapy and responded were much less likely to relapse (28% relapse rate) than responders to medication who had no exposure to cognitive therapy (66% relapse rate).

The important role of CBT in maintaining outcome is also reflected in studies comparing CBT and antidepressant treatments. A number of studies of treatment responders provide evidence for a lower relapse rate for CBT than for pharmacotherapy following treatment discontinuation (Blackburn, Eunson, & Bishop, 1986; Kovacs, Rush, Beck, & Hollon, 1981; McLean & Hakstian, 1990; Simons et al., 1986). For example, McLean and Hakstian (1990) examined the outcome for 121 patients treated over 10 weeks with CBT, nondirective (psychodynamic) psychotherapy, relaxation training, or pharmacotherapy (amitriptyline) and followed for over 2 years. Over this follow-up period, patients who received CBT were significantly improved on a number of mood, social activity, and productivity variables. The nondirective psychotherapy and pharmacotherapy conditions were not significantly different from the relaxation control group on these measures. In contrast, at follow-up approximately twice as many patients in the CBT condition (63%) as in the other treatment conditions were within one standard deviation of a normal, nondepressed control group on measures of depressed mood.

USE OF CBT FOR RELAPSE PREVENTION

CBT appears to offer a useful alternative to maintenance pharmacotherapy. Relative to a brief regimen of antidepressant treatment, maintenance pharmacotherapy is associated with reduced relapse rates (see Fava, Kaji, & Davidson, Chapter 1, this volume). Short-term CBT appears to offer a similar level of protection for these patients. For example, Evans et al. (1992) examined the effect of prior cognitive therapy relative to continuation imipramine treatment in a sample of 44 depressed men and women who had responded to an initial course of treatment. They found that prior cognitive therapy was as effective as continued pharmacotherapy for maintaining treatment response at a 1-year follow-up evaluation, with 18% and 20% relapse rates, respectively. Likewise, across studies, the degree of relapse risk reduction afforded by maintenance pharmacotherapy and CBT appears to be equal (58% and 59% respectively; Hollon et al., 1992b). In addition, CBT programs (Miller, Norman, & Keitner, 1989) integrated into standard inpatient treatment have been associated with lower relapse rates, at least as defined by rates of rehospitalization. CBT protocols for short-stay inpatient treatment for depression are also available (Thase & Wright, 1991). Some of the unique advantages of CBT relative to pharmacologic treatment are as follows:

- Consistent evidence for equal efficacy in patients with mild to moderate depression and in both endogenous and nonendogenous subtypes of depression, without exposure to medication risks or side effects.
- Evidence for lower relapse rates than pharmacotherapy when treatment is discontinued.
- Evidence for long-term effectiveness equal to that of maintenance pharmacotherapy.
- Greater tolerability than many pharmacologic agents.
- Avoidance of long-term medication effects, including potential effects on chronicity, as well as pregnancy-related health concerns.

An emphasis on the role of CBT for relapse prevention introduces a novel strategy for combined pharmacologic treatment and CBT. Clinical researchers in depression (Pava, Fava, & Levenson, 1994b; Thase, 1990) have suggested that for severe depression, treatment may be initiated with pharmacotherapy and then followed by psychotherapy for treatment of residual symptoms and consolidation of improvement. Pava et al. (1994a) further recommend that the course of treatment be adapted to the patient's profile of depression. They suggest that a standard course of CBT (20 sessions in 16 weeks) may be sufficient for patients with nonchronic, nonrecurrent depression. Longer treatment with booster sessions is recommended for patients with chronic and recurrent patterns of depression.

Therapeutic attention to a patient's conceptualization of his or her disorder is often important if CBT is initiated after an initial response to pharmacotherapy. Some of these patients may conceptualize their disorder as "biologic" because they responded to a biologic intervention. Hence, they may not be fully engaged in a psychosocial treatment and may not be motivated to apply CBT strategies if relapse symptoms arise. For these patients we provide information on the nature of treatment effects, predictors of treatment response, and the effects of relapse prevention treatment relative to maintenance pharmacotherapy. This discussion may be aided by reviewing other findings documenting that psychosocial interventions also have biologic effects (e.g., imaging studies of obsessive–compulsive disorder patients treated with CBT; Baxter et al., 1992). Altogether, this discussion is targeted at the patient's belief systems surrounding treatment, with the goal of eliminating logical errors that may preclude full involvement in CBT.

The core elements of CBT extend naturally to the goal of relapse prevention, largely because CBT is conceptualized as a treatment that operates by skill acquisition. First, treatment emphasizes the development of skills to observe and modify dysfunctional cognitions associated with depression; second, high-risk situations are identified, and homework exercises are used to encourage independent application of skills; and, third, this process is reinforced by a collaborative treatment approach, which attends to and underscores procedures that were especially helpful during the course of treatment. As discussed by Hollon et al. (1992b):

Therapy is therefore most likely to produce long-lasting gains if it is approached from a skills-training perspective; that is, the goal in treatment should not only be to produce change, but in the process, to teach the client how those changes were achieved. Rather than simply working to modify a client's existing beliefs, we try to teach the client a methodology for identifying and exploring the validity of his or her own inferences. Our goal is not so much to produce a cure as to teach a strategy that can be applied broadly across time and contexts. (p. 93)

This process can be aided by more explicit "therapist training" interventions that instruct a patient in the problem-solving format used by the therapist in selecting specific thoughts and behaviors for intervention. As part of this training, the course of treatment is reviewed to illustrate how these procedures were applied to the patient's specific patterns of difficulties. The patient is provided with the expectation that difficulties may arise in the future, and the emergence of these difficulties is a signal for the full application of the skills learned in CBT.

Patients may also benefit from the addition of specific self-help procedures for relapse prevention. For example, for the behavioral treatment of agoraphobia, Öst (1989) described the use of mail-in, self-monitoring forms to help patients apply behavioral skills when problems were encountered. Use of these procedures was associated with continued improvement, lower numbers of patients requiring further treatment, and fewer relapses during follow-up monitoring. Similar procedures may be helpful in depression, particularly as restriction of mental health care visits becomes the norm. Research supports the efficacy of bibliotherapy for mildly and moderately depressed patients (Scogin, Jamison, & Gochneaur, 1989), and hence such materials may offer promise as a strategy for relapse prevention following the conclusion of short-term treatment.

Because of the evidence supporting the role of CBT in preventing relapse (for similar findings for IPT, see Frank, Kupfer, Wagner, McEachran, & Cornes, 1991), CBT may have an especially important role for patients requiring medication discontinuation. For example, we currently offer a brief program of CBT (12–16 sessions) to women with recurrent depression who wish to discontinue their antidepressant treatment because of pregnancy or the desire to become pregnant. Patients receive four to six sessions before a medication taper is initiated, and continue with weekly sessions through the period of medication discontinuation and acute adjustment. Initial sessions provide an overview of the cognitive-behavioral model of depression, with particular attention to depressogenic reactions to initial symptoms (see Fennell & Teasdale, 1987) and chronic explanatory styles (Hollon et al., 1992b; Nolen-Hoeksema, 1991). Homework assignments focus on self-monitoring, cognitive restructuring, and activity monitoring/scheduling. Few subjects have completed this pilot program, but the outcome of treatment to date provides encouraging evidence for the efficacy of CBT in preventing relapse among these patients.

Programs such as this are also encouraged by the application of CBT as a primary prevention strategy. A number of studies are now underway to examine the usefulness of a cognitive therapy approach for preventing the emergence of major depression in samples of euthymic individuals at risk for such episodes. For example, Hollon et al. (1992b) describe a program of eight 2-hour sessions that is modeled on cognitive therapy and designed to identify and modify depressotypic, negative belief systems. This program deemphasizes some of the behavioral activation strategies included in CBT, and instead focuses on negative beliefs and explanatory styles, such as the tendency to explain negative outcomes in terms of stable personal deficiencies (e.g., "It happened because I am unlovable"). Reports of full trials are pending, but data from pilot projects suggest that such programs hold promise for reducing the risk for onset of depression (see Hollon et al., 1992b).

CONTINUATION TREATMENT WITH CBT

Although maintenance of treatment effects tends to be higher for CBT than for brief pharmacologic treatments, relapse rates among patients treated with CBT are still causes for concern. Thase and Simons (1992) found a 32% rate of relapse into depression over a 1-year prospective follow-up period following either a 16- or a 20-week trial of CBT. Patients who relapsed tended to have had higher pretreatment depression severity and higher residual symptoms at the end of the acute treatment trial. Only 9% of patients who met the criteria for full recovery by the end of acute treatment relapsed, compared to 52% of patients achieving only partial recovery. These data underscore the importance of full treatment of patients in the original episode of treatment, and/or the provision of occasional booster sessions to insure continued remission.

Thase and Simons (1992) suggest that maintenance treatment with CBT may parallel that for pharmacotherapy; extended treatment may offer specific benefit to patients with residual depression symptoms who are at a higher risk for relapse. As conceptualized by Pava et al. (1994a), the role of continuation treatment is as follows:

(1) to reduce residual symptomatology (i.e., subsyndromal depressive symptoms per se, comorbid psychiatric disorders, and/or psychological sequelae of having suffered from major depressive episodes);
(2) to focus directly on relapse prevention strategies; and
(3) to impact positively on the overall quality of life in recovered depressed patients. (p. 216)

One goal of this treatment is to identify and modify long-standing maladaptive patterns of thinking and behaving that leave patients vulnerable to relapse. This work often centers on the identification of core beliefs that influence thoughts, behaviors, and emotions in a wide range of situations. Two types of core beliefs are especially prominent: beliefs that one is personally incompetent, and beliefs that one is unlovable. Risk for recurrence of depression from these dysfunctional attitudes appears to depend on an interaction between these beliefs and belief-relevant stressful life events. For example, Segal, Shaw, Vella, and Katz (1992) found that the congruence between negative life events and cognitive schemas predicted relapse in a longitudinal study. Patients were identified at baseline as being sensitive to affiliation issues (need for approval) or achievement issues (self-criticism centering around performance demands). Patients identified as being more achievement-oriented relapsed more often after exposure to achievement-related stressful events than to noncongruent stressors. The congruency effect was less strong for patients sensitive to affiliation issues, but was evident at a select assessment point. Similar findings have been reported by other investigators (Hammen, Ellicott, & Gitlin, 1989). Accordingly, Segal et al. (1992) emphasize that the identification of core concerns and the rehearsal of proactive strategies may help prepare patients to cope with future stressful life events that are likely to be especially depressogenic.

This approach underscores the importance of therapeutic attention to residual levels of dysfunctional attitudes. Successful treatment of depression with pharmacologic or psychosocial treatments results in marked reductions in negative thoughts and dysfunctional attitudes (Dohr, Rush, & Bernstein, 1989; Fava, Bless, Otto, Pava, & Rosenbaum, 1994; Peselow, Robins, Block, Barouche, & Fieve, 1990), although high residual levels of dysfunctional attitudes and negative responses to symptoms remain in some patients (Pava, Nierenberg, Carey, Rosenbaum, & Fava, 1994b; see also Eaves & Rush, 1984; Nolen-Hoeksema, Girgus, & Seligman, 1992). These residual cognitive symptoms predict depression relapse (e.g., Simons et al., 1986; Thase et al., 1992).

Nolen-Hoeksema et al. (1992) found in a longitudinal study of children that a period of depression appeared to lead to the development of a more pessimistic explanatory style. This style is itself linked with both risk and length of future depressive episodes (Nolen-Hoeksema et al., 1992; Nolen-Hoeksema, Morrow, & Fredrickson, 1993). Chronic depression may also bring with it problems in self-definition. Markowitz (1994) suggests that patients with dysthymia tend to attribute their difficulties to a personality defect, rather than to the effects of a chronic mood disorder. In our experience, a central task in the early stages of CBT for chronic depression is to help the patient attribute their difficulties to the effects of the mood disorder, rather than to global and negative personal traits (e.g., "I'm defective," "I'm weak," or "If I was any kind of person, I could pull myself out of this depression"). At times, these negative attributions have been reinforced by family members and/or by cultural biases. Also, these negative beliefs may be unwittingly reinforced by experiences in insight-oriented treatments, in which therapists in good faith have confused the depressive disorder with personality characteristics, and may " 'blame the victim' by assigning the patient responsibility for his or her mood disorder" (Markowitz, 1994, p. 1116). This typically results in increased guilt and depressed mood and is counterproductive. For these patients, CBT may be especially important for helping suppress self-critical responses to symptoms (Fennell & Teasdale, 1987), as well as for introducing the step-by-step skill acquisition and activity assignments that will be required in treatment.

ADHERENCE AND COMPLIANCE ISSUES IN CBT

A number of therapy variables have been linked with CBT outcome. For example, in the NIMH multicenter study (Elkin et al., 1989), one explanation for the site differences in the efficacy of CBT is poor *therapist* adherence to core CBT interventions (Hollon, Shelton, & Loosen, 1991). In addition, the therapist's empathy and experience have been found to have nonredundant influences on the response to CBT for depression (Burns & Nolen-Hoeksema, 1992). Accordingly, nonresponse to the CBT offered by a particular therapist can not be equated with nonresponse to CBT itself. Therapist behavior in the sessions needs to be evaluated for drift from the active, skill-oriented focus of traditional CBT. Consultation with an experienced cognitive-behavioral therapist, and/or efforts to maximize empathy, may also be helpful for therapists faced with nonresponse to initial CBT sessions.

Given the emphasis in CBT on the acquisition and rehearsal of cognitive and behavioral skills, it is not surprising that low homework compliance also adversely influences therapy outcome (Burns & Nolen-Hoeksema, 1992). Strategies for addressing compliance issues in CBT have been discussed by Newman (1994). In general, these strategies include conducting a functional analysis of the noncompliant or resistant behaviors, and intervening with a variety of informational, motivational, self-monitoring, and cognitive restructuring interventions when appropriate.

In addition to general compliance issues, CBT for depression faces specific issues concerning the willingness and ability of patients to identify negative automatic thoughts. In the standard course of treatment, patients are educated about the cognitive model of depression and are asked to monitor thoughts. Some patients, however, have marked difficulty with this task. Rather than identifying the direct content of their thoughts, they tend to report edited or intellectualized versions of their cognitions. Beck, Freeman, and Associates (1990) have described this subgroup of patients as appearing to be "cognitive avoiders"—individuals who, "despite their hyperawareness of painful feelings, . . . shy away from identifying unpleasant thoughts" (p. 44). The cost of this strategy to effective treatment is the restriction of access to some of the "hot" cognitions that are hypothesized to affect mood. The consequence is that these cognitions are not modified and continue to pose a risk for affective disturbances.

Clinically, we have discriminated two subtypes of patients within this broader category of cognitive avoiders. One subtype appears to avoid difficult cognitions as a consequence of past experiences with intense and painful affect. Individuals who have suffered through previous episodes of depression (or other aversive mood states) may believe that negative affective experiences are by their nature unmanageable. Depressed feelings are equated with the emergence of depression and accompanying disability. Accordingly, patients are motivated to avoid these feelings and the thoughts that herald them. The unfortunate long-term consequence of this strategy is restriction of the opportunity to learn adaptive skills for subtle mood changes; this restriction helps insure that emotional issues are left unsolved, and increases the likelihood of additional problems.

A second subtype of cognitive avoiders consists of individuals who employ narcissistic strategies for avoiding a focus on negative core beliefs. Because of their concern that schemas of inadequacy or unlovability may be accurate, these patients avoid acknowledging thoughts related to these schemas. Acknowledgment of these negative thoughts is sufficiently threatening that when the thoughts are identified, patients may rush into global repudiation of them (e.g., "I should not worry about their comments on my work, because I am much smarter"). Unfortunately, these global repudiations may be just as inaccurate as the global negative thoughts. These "empty" coping responses engender competition between inaccurate global cognitions, rather than the development of realistic self-views based on evidence and behavioral experiments in specific situations. The global repudiations of negative thoughts may also inhibit therapeutic action toward modest, stepwise completion of tasks that are useful for decreasing depression.

Our general approach to treating patients who display high levels of cognitive avoidance employs two strategies. First, emphasis is placed on informational interventions that demonstrate the longer-term consequences of cognitive avoidance strategies in terms of a cost–benefit analysis of the strategies' mood and behavioral effects. Second, because the cognitive avoidance restricts access to "hot" cognitions, emphasis is placed on the cognitive-behavioral patterns that emerge directly in the therapy session. That is, self-monitoring and cognitive restructuring assignments are brought into the therapy session by devoting attention to (1) naturally occurring changes in mood in the session, or (2) changes in mood and behavior that arise from specific role-playing assignments or behavioral tests conducted in session. Subsequently, cognitive restructuring and more adaptive interpersonal behaviors can be practiced in the context of these in-session emotional events. Exposure to a range of emotional experiences in session also allows therapists to help patients reduce their avoidance of emotional experience and increase their tolerance of negative emotions

(Cordova & Kohlenberg, 1994). Emphasis on the evocation of issues and emotions in session allows for the development of self-monitoring skills in a safe environment, where patients can be introduced to an increasing hierarchy of emotional intensity.

MARITAL ISSUES AND THE TREATMENT OF DEPRESSION

Almost half of patients presenting for treatment of depression have significant marital issues, and the degree of marital problems has been linked with treatment outcome (for a review, see Beach, Whisman, & O'Leary, 1994). Accordingly, it appears that among distressed couples, cognitive-behavioral marital therapy may be an effective treatment for depression. For example, Beach and O'Leary (1992) found that individual CBT and cognitive-behavioral marital therapy were of equal efficacy for the treatment of depressed women (women with major depression, dysthymia, or both) in discordant marital relationships. After treatment, 47% of patients in each treatment scored in the nondepressed range (9 or less) on the Beck Depression Inventory. Fully 87% of patients in marital therapy, relative to 25% of patients in individual CBT, reported a distinctly improved marital environment. Cognitive-behavioral marital therapy, like individual CBT, is also associated with good maintenance of treatment outcome for depression (Beach et al., 1994).

The degree of marital discord appears to be an important predictor of the efficacy of marital therapy for depression. Jacobson, Dobson, Fruzzetti, Schmaling, and Salusky (1991) found that cognitive-behavioral marital therapy was not helpful for treating depression in patients with low marital discord, but was as effective as individual CBT in patients with marital issues. Among patients with the most extreme marital discord, marital therapy tended to be more effective than individual CBT. These findings encourage consideration of cognitive-behavioral marital therapy for depressed patients with significant marital issues, particularly those that do not fully respond to individual CBT.

COMORBID CONDITIONS INFLUENCING THE COURSE OF TREATMENT

Numerous studies suggest that the presence of a personality disorder and pathologic personality traits is associated with poorer treatment outcome for depression (Shea, Widiger, & Klein, 1992). This is true for both pharmacologic and psychosocial interventions, although the influence of Axis II disorders appears to be less strong for CBT for depression. Nonetheless, specific Axis II disorders (e.g., borderline personality disorder) have been found to have negative effects on the outcome of CBT for depression (Burns

& Nolen-Hoeksema, 1992). Although low homework compliance is linked with poorer outcome for CBT, and poorer compliance may well be associated with Axis II pathology, the influence of a borderline personality disorder diagnosis appears to be independent of compliance issues.

CBT methods for Axis II conditions have emerged in the last decade (Beck et al., 1990; Katz & Levendusky, 1990; Linehan, 1993). Many of these methods emphasize the provision of emotional regulation and interpersonal skills to replace existing skill deficits and reliance on maladaptive strategies (Farrell & Shaw, 1994; Linehan, 1993). Accordingly, these interventions may provide important adjuncts for patients with both major depression and Axis II pathology. In addition to these adjuncts, CBT for depression in patients with Axis II pathology will probably necessitate a number of other important changes. Beck et al. (1990) emphasize that cognitive therapy for patients with personality disorders requires the establishment of a closer and warmer therapeutic relationship than may be required by the treatment of an acute disorder alone. Accordingly, greater emphasis is placed on the therapeutic relationship relative to other techniques early in treatment, and treatment is expected to proceed at a slower pace. Emphasis is also placed on gaining control of dichotomous thinking, and a greater range of techniques may be required to achieve changes in dominant schemas in these patients (Mercier & Leahy, 1992; Young, 1990). Additional emphasis may be placed on the core negative beliefs and underlying assumptions that give rise to maladaptive strategies and negative automatic thoughts (Beck et al., 1990).

Comorbid Axis I conditions are also common in depressed patients. For example, of 197 patients presenting for treatment of major depression at the Center for Cognitive Therapy at the University of Pennsylvania School of Medicine, 59% received at least one additional Axis I diagnosis (Sanderson, Beck, & Beck, 1990). Anxiety and substance use disorders were the most common, with 12% with comorbid panic disorder or agoraphobia, 15% with comorbid social phobia, 20% with comorbid generalized anxiety disorder, 4% with obsessive–compulsive disorder, and 15% with substance abuse or dependence. In most cases, the onset of the depressive disorder preceded the onset of the comorbid condition.

Because distress from comorbid conditions may contribute significantly to depression severity and/or treatment nonresponse (Grunhaus, 1988; see Hirschfeld, Hasin, Keller, Endicott, & Wunder, 1990, for the absence of such evidence for comorbid alcoholism), treatment of the depressive disorder must often address the comorbid disorder. Self-monitoring assignments provide an excellent source of material on the nature of current distress, and provide the clinician with a means to examine the role of dysfunctional cognitions associated with comorbid conditions. The need for a flexible approach to address the heterogeneity of problems that may be encountered in these patients is reflected by the use of a module approach that targets the cognitive-behavioral patterns in specific problem areas, while maintaining an overall focus on the management of depression with traditional CBT methods (Pava & McDermott, 1994).

AN ALGORITHM FOR
THE TREATMENT OF DEPRESSION

Figure 2.1 illustrates the range of applications of CBT to patients with major depression. The potential advantages of CBT alone over pharmacotherapy are best documented for patients with mild to moderate depression. For these patients, CBT has the advantages of effectiveness equivalent to that of medication alone or of combination treatments; freedom from drug-related side effects; and maintenance of treatment effects over time. Despite these advantages, it is clear that a large number of patients will continue to receive pharmacotherapy as an initial intervention for depression, in part because antidepressant treatment may be initiated by primary care physicians long before referral is considered. For patients receiving pharmacotherapy, Pava et al. (1994a) have suggested a specific role for CBT in relapse prevention and treating residual symptoms: Patients demonstrating at least a partial response to medications continue their pharmacotherapy and receive adjunctive CBT. This treatment is designed to

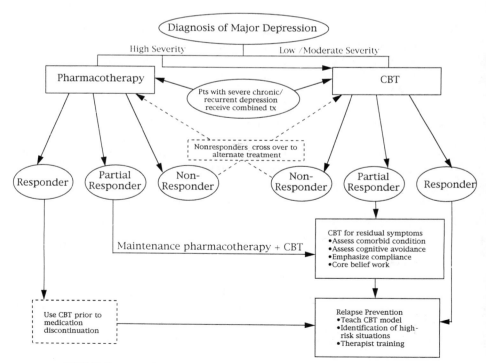

FIGURE 2.1. Algorithm of treatment options for depressed patients.

emphasize the core component of the cognitive-behavioral approach, but also devotes attention to comorbid conditions and core beliefs that may pose a risk for relapse over time.

Although there is some evidence suggesting that pharmacotherapy has advantages over CBT in the treatment of more severe cases of depression, this finding is far from robust. Consequently, severity of depression should not be considered a clear stratification variable for treatment assignment. Because patients failing to respond to one modality may respond well to the other, patients failing to respond to initial pharmacologic treatment or CBT should be considered for the opposite intervention. However, given the difficulties in successfully treating chronic and treatment-resistant cases of depression, we believe that it makes practical sense (especially given the modest effects reported for either form of therapy alone with chronic depression) to adopt a more aggressive treatment approach, combining CBT and pharmacologic strategies. To conserve mental health benefits, one strategy is to initiate treatment with pharmacotherapy, conserving CBT sessions for continuation treatment that emphasizes the elimination of residual symptoms and relapse prevention training. This treatment should proceed with an understanding on the part of all clinicians involved of the goals of each modality, and with a strong attempt on the part of both psychopharmacologists and psychotherapists to collaborate on integrating the two treatments.

As an attempt to reduce the relapse rates for all patients, the introduction of specific relapse prevention training at the conclusion of the course of CBT is recommended. Patients with an early and robust response to pharmacotherapy may also benefit from relapse prevention treatment that is initiated when medication tapering begins.

SUMMARY

In summary, research to date supports the efficacy of both pharmacologic treatment and CBT for major depression. Although many patients respond to short-term interventions, additional clinical strategies are often necessary to guard against relapse and help nonresponders to short-term treatment. Clinical programs and research suggest that CBT offers a range of successful applications for depressed patients who are medication-free, are receiving maintenance pharmacotherapy, or are considering medication discontinuation.

REFERENCES

Baxter, L. R., Schwartz, J. M., Guze, B. H., Bergman, K. S., Szuba, M. P., Guze, B. H., Mazziotta, J. C., Alazraki, A., Selin, C. E., Ferng, H.-K., Munford, P., & Phelps, M. E. (1992). Caudate glucose metabolic rate changes with both drug and behavior therapy for obsessive–compulsive disorder. *Archives of General Psychiatry, 49,* 681–689.

Beach, S. R. H., & O'Leary, K. D. (1992). Treating depression in the context of marital discord: Outcome and predictors of response for marital therapy vs. cognitive therapy. *Behavior Therapy, 23,* 507–528.

Beach, S. R. H., Whisman, M. A., & O'Leary, K. D. (1994). Marital therapy for depression: Theoretical foundation, current status, and future directions. *Behavior Therapy, 25,* 345–371.

Beck, A. T. (1983). Cognitive therapy of depression: New perspectives. In P. J. Clayton & J. E. Barrett (Eds.), *Treatment of depression: Old controversies and new approaches* (pp. 265–284). New York: Raven Press.

Beck, A. T., Freeman, A., & Associates. (1990). *Cognitive therapy of personality disorders.* New York: Guilford Press.

Beck, A. T., Hollon, S. D., Young, J. E., Bedrosian, R. C., & Budenz, D. (1985). Treatment of depression with cognitive therapy and amitriptyline. *Archives of General Psychiatry, 42,* 142–148.

Beck, A. T., Rush, A. J., Shaw, B. F., & Emery, G. (1979). *Cognitive therapy of depression.* New York: Guilford Press.

Beck, A. T., Ward, C. H., Mendelson, M., Mock, J., & Erbaugh, J. (1961). An inventory for measuring depression. *Archives of General Psychiatry, 4,* 561–567.

Blackburn, I. M., Bishop, S., Glen, A., Whalley, L., & Christie, J. (1981). The efficacy of cognitive therapy in depression: A treatment trial using cognitive therapy and pharmacotherapy, each alone and in combination. *British Journal of Psychiatry, 139,* 181–189.

Blackburn, I. M., Eunson, K. M., & Bishop, S. (1986). A two-year naturalistic follow-up of depressed patients treated with cognitive therapy, pharmacotherapy and a combination of both. *Journal of Affective Disorders, 10,* 67–75.

Burns, D. D., & Nolen-Hoeksema, S. (1992). Therapeutic empathy and recovery from depression in cognitive-behavioral therapy: A structural equation model. *Journal of Consulting and Clinical Psychology, 60,* 441–449.

Cordova, J. V., & Kohlenberg, R. J. (1994). Acceptance and the therapeutic relationship. In S. C. Hayes, N. S. Jacobson, V. M. Follette, & M. J. Dougher (Eds.), *Acceptance and change: Content and context in psychotherapy* (pp. 125–142). Reno, NV: Context Press.

Dobson, K. S. (1989). A meta-analysis of the efficacy of cognitive therapy for depression. *Journal of Consulting and Clinical Psychology, 57,* 414–419.

Dohr, K. B., Rush, A. J., & Bernstein, I. H. (1989). Cognitive biases and depression. *Journal of Abnormal Psychology, 98,* 263–267.

Eaves, G. G., & Rush, A. J. (1984). Cognitive patterns in symptomatic and remitted unipolar major depression. *Journal of Abnormal Psychology, 93,* 31–40.

Elkin, I., Shea, T., Watkins, J. T., Imber, S. D., Sotsky, S. M., Collins, J. F., Glass, D. R., Pilkonis, P. A., Leber, W. R., Docherty, J. P., Fiester, S. J., & Parloff, M. B. (1989). National Institute of Mental Health Treatment of Depression Collaborative Research Program: General effectiveness of treatments. *Archives of General Psychiatry, 46,* 971–982.

Evans, M., Hollon, S., DeRubeis, R., Piasecki, J., Grove, W., Garvey, M., & Tuason, V. (1992). Differential relapse following cognitive therapy and pharmacotherapy for depression. *Archives of General Psychiatry, 49,* 802–808.

Farrell, J. M., & Shaw, I. A. (1994). Emotional awareness training: A prerequisite to effective cognitive-behavioral treatment of borderline personality disorder. *Cognitive and Behavioral Practice, 1,* 71–91.

Fava, M., Bless, E., Otto, M. W., Pava, J. A., & Rosenbaum, J. F. (1994). Dysfunctional attitudes in major depression: Changes with pharmacotherapy. *Journal of Nervous and Mental Disease, 182,* 45–49.

Fennell, M. J. V. (1989). Depression. In K. Hawton, P. Salkovskis, J. Kirk, & D. M. Clark (Eds.), *Cognitive behaviour therapy for psychiatric problems: A practical guide* (pp. 169–234). New York: Oxford University Press.

Fennell, M. J. V., & Teasdale, J. D. (1987). Cognitive therapy for depression: Individual differences and the process of change. *Cognitive Therapy and Research, 11,* 253–271.

Frank, E., Kupfer, D. J., Wagner, E. F., McEachran, A. B., & Cornes, C. (1991). Efficacy of interpersonal psychotherapy as a maintenance treatment of recurrent depression: Contributing factors. *Archives of General Psychiatry, 48,* 1053–1059.

Greenberg, R. P., Bornstein, R. F., Greenberg, M. D., & Fisher, S. (1992). A meta-analysis of antidepressant outcome under "blinder" conditions. *Journal of Consulting and Clinical Psychology, 60,* 664–669.

Grunhaus, L. (1988). Clinical and psychobiological characteristics of simultaneous panic disorder and major depression. *American Journal of Psychiatry, 145,* 1214–1221.

Hamilton, M. (1960). A rating scale for depression. *Journal of Neurology, Neurosurgery and Psychiatry, 23,* 56–62.

Hammen, C., Ellicott, A., & Gitlin, M. (1989). Vulnerability to specific life events and prediction of course of disorder in unipolar depressed patients. *Canadian Journal of Behavioural Science, 21,* 377–388.

Hirschfeld, R. M. A., Hasin, D., Keller, M. B., Endicott, J., & Wunder, J. (1990). Depression and alcoholism: Comorbidity in a longitudinal study. In J. D. Maser & C. R. Cloninger (Eds.), *Comorbidity of mood and anxiety disorders* (pp. 293–303). Washington, DC: American Psychiatric Press.

Hollon, S. D., DeRubeis, R. J., Evans, M. D., Wiemer, M. J., Garvey, M. J., Grove, W. M., & Tuason, V. B. (1992a). Cognitive therapy and pharmacotherapy for depression: Singly and in combination. *Archives of General Psychiatry, 49,* 774–781.

Hollon, S. D., DeRubeis, R. J., & Seligman, M. E. P. (1992b). Cognitive therapy and the prevention of depression. *Applied and Preventive Psychology, 1,* 89–95.

Hollon, S. D., Shelton, R. C., & Loosen, P. T. (1991). Cognitive therapy and pharmacotherapy for depression. *Journal of Consulting and Clinical Psychology, 59,* 88–99.

Jacobson, N. S., Dobson, K., Fruzzetti, A. E., Schmaling, D. B., & Salusky, S. (1991). Marital therapy as a treatment for depression. *Journal of Consulting and Clinical Psychology, 59,* 547–557.

Katz, S. E., & Levendusky, P. G. (1990). Cognitive-behavioral approaches to treating borderline and self-mutilating patients. *Bulletin of the Menninger Clinic, 54*(3), 398–408.

Klerman, G. L., Weissman, M. M., Rounsaville, B. J., & Chevron, E. S. (1984). *Interpersonal psychotherapy of depression.* New York: Basic Books.

Kovacs, M., Rush, A. T., Beck, A. T., & Hollon, S. D. (1981). Depressed outpatients treated with cognitive therapy or pharmacotherapy: A one-year follow-up. *Archives of General Psychiatry, 38,* 33–39.

Lewinsohn, P. M., Biglan, A., & Zeiss, A. M. (1976). Behavioral treatment of depression. In P. O. Davidson (Ed.), *The behavioral management of anxiety, depression, and pain* (pp. 91–146). New York: Brunner/Mazel.

Liebowitz, M. R., Quitkin, F. M., Stewart, J. W., McGrath, P. J., Harrison, W., Rabkin, J., Tricamo, E., Markowitz, J. S., & Klein, D. F. (1984). Phenelzine vs. imipramine in atypical depression: A preliminary report. *Archives of General Psychiatry, 41*, 669–677.

Linehan, M. M. (1993). *Cognitive-behavioral treatment of borderline personality disorder.* New York: Guilford Press.

Markowitz, J. C. (1994). Psychotherapy of dysthymia. *American Journal of Psychiatry, 151*, 1114–1121.

McLean, P. D., & Hakstian, A. R. (1990). Relative endurance of unipolar depression treatment effects: Longitudinal follow-up. *Journal of Consulting and Clinical Psychology, 58*, 482–488.

McKnight, D. L., Nelson-Gray, R. O., & Barnhill, J. (1992). Dexamethasone suppression test and response to cognitive therapy and antidepressant medication. *Behavior Therapy, 23*, 99–111.

Mercier, M. A., & Leahy, R. L. (1992). *Cognitive therapy of dysthymia: A treatment manual.* Unpublished manuscript, Columbia–Presbyterian Hospital, New York.

Mercier, M. A., Stewart, J. W., & Quitkin, F. M. (1992). A pilot sequential study of cognitive therapy and pharmacotherapy of atypical depression. *Journal of Clinical Psychiatry, 53*, 166–170.

Miller, I., Norman, W., & Keitner, G. (1989). Cognitive-behavioral treatment of depressed inpatients: Six- and twelve-month follow-up. *American Journal of Psychiatry, 146*, 1272–1279.

Munoz, R. F., Hollon, S. D., McGrath, E., Rehm, L. P., & Vanden Bos, G. R. (1994). On the AHCPR Depression in Primary Care guidelines: Further considerations for practitioners. *American Psychologist, 49*, 42–61.

Murphy, G., Simons, A., Wetzel, R., & Lustman, P. (1984). Cognitive therapy and pharmacotherapy, singly and together in the treatment of depression. *Archives of General Psychiatry, 41*, 33–41.

Newman, C. F. (1994). Understanding client resistance: Methods for enhancing motivation to change. *Cognitive and Behavioral Practice, 1*, 47–69.

Nolen-Hoeksema, S. (1991). Responses to depression and their effects on the duration of depressive episodes. *Journal of Abnormal Psychology, 100*, 569–582.

Nolen-Hoeksema, S., Girgus, J. S., & Seligman, M. E. P. (1992). Predictors and consequences of childhood depressive symptoms: A 5-year longitudinal study. *Journal of Abnormal Psychology, 101*, 403–422.

Nolen-Hoeksema, S., Morrow, J., & Fredrickson, B. L. (1993). Response styles and the duration of episodes of depressed mood. *Journal of Abnormal Psychology, 102*, 20–28.

Öst, L. G. (1989). A maintenance program for behavioural treatment of anxiety disorders. *Behaviour Research and Therapy, 27*, 123–130.

Pande, A. C., Haskett, R. F., & Greden, J. F. (1992). *Fluoxetine treatment of atypical depression.* Paper presented at the 145th Annual Meeting of the American Psychiatric Association, Washington, DC.

Pava, J. A., Fava, M., & Levenson, J. A. (1994a). Integrating cognitive therapy and pharmacotherapy in the treatment and prophylaxis of depression: A novel approach. *Psychotherapy and Psychosomatics, 61*, 211–219.

Pava, J. A., & McDermott, S. P. (1994). *Cognitive therapy for remitted depressives at relatively high risk for relapse/recurrence.* Unpublished manuscript, Massachusetts General Hospital, Boston.

Pava, J. A., Nierenberg, A. A., Carey, M., Rosenbaum, J. F., & Fava, M. (1994b). *Residual symptoms in major depressive disorder: I. A comparison with normal controls.* Paper presented at the 147th Annual Meeting of the American Psychiatric Association, Philadelphia.

Peselow, E. D., Robins, C., Block, P., Barouche, F., & Fieve, R. R. (1990). Dysfunctional attitudes in depressed patients before and after clinical treatment and in normal control subjects. *American Journal of Psychiatry, 147,* 439–444.

Quitkin, F. M., McGrath, P. J., Stewart, J. W., Harrison, W., Wager, S. G., Nunes, E., Rabkin, J. G., Tricamo, E., Markowitz, J., & Klein, D. F. (1989). Phenelzine and imipramine in mood reactive depressives: Further delineation of the syndrome of atypical depression. *Archives of General Psychiatry, 46,* 787–793.

Robinson, L. A., Berman, J. S., & Neimeyer, R. A. (1990). Psychotherapy for the treatment of depression: A comprehensive review of controlled outcome research. *Psychological Bulletin, 108,* 30–49.

Sanderson, W. C., Beck, A. T., & Beck, J. (1990). Syndrome comorbidity in patients with major depression or dysthymia: Prevalence and temporal relationship. *American Journal of Psychiatry, 147,* 1025–1028.

Scogin, F., Jamison, C., & Gochneaur, K. (1989). Comparative efficacy of cognitive and behavioral bibliotherapy for mildly and moderately depressed older adults. *Journal of Consulting and Clinical Psychology, 57,* 403–407.

Segal, Z. V., Shaw, B. F., Vella, D. D., & Katz, R. (1992). Cognitive and life stress predictors of relapse in remitted unipolar depressed patients: Test of the congruency hypothesis. *Journal of Abnormal Psychology, 101,* 26–36.

Shea, M. T., Widiger, T. A., & Klein, M. H. (1992). Comorbidity of personality disorders and depression: Implications for treatment. *Journal of Consulting and Clinical Psychology, 60,* 857–868.

Simons, A. D., Murphy, G. E., Levine, J. L., & Wetzel, R. D. (1986). Cognitive therapy and pharmacotherapy for depression: Sustained improvement over one year. *Archives of General Psychiatry, 43,* 43–48.

Simons, A. D., & Thase, M. E. (1992). Biological markers, treatment outcome, and 1-year follow-up in endogenous depression: Electroencephalographic sleep studies and response to cognitive therapy. *Journal of Consulting and Clinical Psychology, 60,* 392–401.

Stewart, J. W., Mercier, M. A., Agosti, V., Guardin, M., & Quitkin, F. M. (1993). Imipramine is effective after unsuccessful cognitive therapy: Sequential use of cognitive therapy and imipramine in depressed outpatients. *Journal of Clinical Psychopharmacology, 13,* 114–119.

Thase, M. E. (1990). Relapse and recurrence in unipolar major depression: Short-term and long-term approaches. *Journal of Clinical Psychiatry, 51,* 51–57.

Thase, M. E., Bowler, K., & Harden, T. (1991a). Cognitive behavior therapy of endogenous depression: Part 2. Preliminary findings in 16 unmedicated inpatients. *Behavior Therapy, 22,* 469–477.

Thase, M. E., Greenhouse, J. B., Frank, E., Reynolds, C. F., Pilkonis, P. A., Hurley, K., Grochocinski, V., & Kupfer, D. J. (1995). *Correlates of remission of major depression during standardized trials of psychotherapy, pharmacotherapy, or their combination: Results from the Pittsburgh 600.* Manuscript submitted for publication.

Thase, M. E., & Simons, A. D. (1992). Cognitive behavior therapy and relapse of nonbipolar depression: Parallels with pharmacotherapy. *Psychopharmacology, 28,* 117–122.

Thase, M. E., Simons, A. D., Cahalane, J. F., & McGeary, J. (1991b). Cognitive behavior therapy of endogenous depression: Part 1. An outpatient clinical replication series. *Behavior Therapy, 22,* 457–467.

Thase, M. E., Simons, A. D., Cahalane, J. F., McGeary, J., & Harden, T. (1991c). Severity of depression and response to cognitive behavior therapy. *American Journal of Psychiatry, 148,* 784–789.

Thase, M. E., Simons, A. D., McGeary, J., Cahalane, J., Hughes, C., Harden, T., & Friedman, E. (1992). Relapse after cognitive behavior therapy of depression: Potential implications for longer courses of treatment. *American Journal of Psychiatry, 149,* 1046–1052.

Thase, M. E., & Wright, J. H. (1991). Cognitive behavior therapy manual for depressed inpatients: A treatment protocol outline. *Behavior Therapy, 22,* 579–595.

Weissman, M. M. (1979). The psychological treatment of depression: Evidence for the efficacy of psychotherapy alone, in comparison with, and in combination with pharmacotherapy. *Archives of General Psychiatry, 36,* 1261–1269.

Young, J. E. (1990). *Cognitive therapy for personality disorders: A schema-focused approach.* Sarasota, FL: Professional Resource Exchange.

3

Treatment-Resistant Bipolar Disorder: Clinical Aspects and Management

S. NASSIR GHAEMI
GARY S. SACHS
CLAUDIA F. BALDASSANO

Kraepelin (1921) conceptualized "manic–depressive insanity" as an illness characterized by discrete episodes with prominent affective symptoms and by complete recovery between episodes. Since the introduction of the *Diagnostic and Statistical Manual of Mental Disorders,* third edition (DSM-III, American Psychological Association, 1980), bipolar disorder has been defined primarily on the basis of the occurrence of a manic or hypomanic episode. As a result, the population meeting criteria for bipolar disorder overlaps with the population exhibition Kraepelin's manic–depressive insanity, but excludes those patients with only depressive episodes and includes many more severely ill patients, such as those with prominent psychotic symptoms and patients who may never have enjoyed a complete remission. Although many Kraepelinian concepts can still be applied, bipolar disorder, as defined by the fourth edition of DSM (DSM-IV; American Psychological Association, 1994) should be recognized as including a broader array of patients. Specifically, experience with bipolar disorder since the introduction of DSM-III shows it to be a complicated condition in which complete recovery is relatively uncommon and in which treatment resistance is often a prominent feature.

TABLE 3.1 Efficacy of Lithium

Condition	Degree of efficacy
Acute mania	Strong
Acute depression	Weak/moderate
Prevention of mania	Strong
Prevention of depression	Moderate

The concept of treatment resistance is often applied to bipolar disorder when an episode of mood elevation or depression persists or recurs
despite adequate treatment with lithium (or another appropriate medication). As noted in Table 3.1, lithium possesses varying efficacy in the treatment and prophylaxis of bipolar disorder. In the first part of this chapter,
we review clinical aspects of treatment-resistant bipolar disorder; in the
second, we describe psychopharmacologic strategies for treatment-resistant
patients.

CLINICAL ASPECTS OF
TREATMENT-RESISTANT BIPOLAR DISORDER

Estimated Prevalence

The clinical complexity of the illness hampers the process of estimating
the prevalence of treatment-resistant bipolar disorder. Whereas research
on unipolar depression has been aided by relatively straightforward definitions for recovery, relapse, and recurrence, bipolar disorder often demon-
strates an irregular episodic course, in which the potential exists to mislabel
a switch in polarity as recovery from a preceding phase.

The median duration of acute episodes provides one context for defining treatment resistance. For example, in 155 patients with bipolar disorder followed during open naturalistic treatment, Keller et al. (1986)
reported that the median duration of acute episodes was 10 weeks for pure
mania, 19 weeks for pure depression, and 36 weeks for mixed episodes.
Recurrence rates can also be used to define treatment resistance; for instance, it has been suggested that patients diagnosed in adolescence with
bipolar disorder may experience 10 or more acute episodes in a lifetime
(Deister & Mameros, 1993; Lish et al., 1994; Sachs, 1995a). However,
the variation among individuals in duration of episodes and cycle frequency
limits the usefulness of defining treatment resistance in these ways.

Defining Treatment-Resistant Bipolar Disorder

Despite the difficulties in formulating a comprehensive definition for
treatment-resistant bipolar disorder, it may be possible to advance our un-

derstanding of it by formulating definitions that capture differences between extremes of response and resistance at the outer range of clinical experience. We offer the following working clinical definitions:

"Treatment-refractory mania": Mania without remission despite 6 weeks of adequate therapy with at least two antimanic agents (lithium, a neuroleptic, an anticonvulsant, etc.), in the absence of antidepressants or other mood-elevating agents.

"Treatment-refractory bipolar depression": Depression without remission despite two adequate trials of standard antidepressant agents (6 weeks each), with or without augmentation strategies.

"Treatment-refractory mood cycling": Continued cycling despite maximal tolerated lithium in combination with valproate and/or carbamazepine for a period three times the average cycle length, or 6 months (whichever is longer), in the absence of antidepressants or other cycle-promoting agents.

Diagnostic Subtypes Associated with Treatment Resistance

Treatment resistance thus defined can be associated with any class of bipolar disorder, but it has been particularly closely linked with a number of specific diagnostic subtypes, such as mixed bipolar disorder, rapid-cycling bipolar disorder, and bipolar disorder associated with comorbid psychiatric or medical conditions.

Bipolar Disorder with Mixed Episodes

Several investigators report poorer outcome with lithium therapy in patients with mixed episodes (dysphoric mania, depressive mania) than in patients with pure affective episodes (Dilsaver, Swann, Shoaib, Bowers, & Halle, 1993; Himmelhoch & Garfinkel, 1986; Himmelhoch, Mulla, Neil, Detre, & Kupfer, 1976; Keller et al., 1986; Secunda et al., 1987). Although such patients may respond better to anticonvulsants than to lithium (Calabrese, Woyshville, Kimmel, & Rapport, 1993; Post & Uhde, 1987; Post et al., 1989), the outcome of anticonvulsant therapy for mixed mania may be less robust than the response of patients with pure manic episodes. Mixed episodes may arise spontaneously (simple mixed episodes), or may result from the co-occurrence of a primary mood disorder and a secondary neuropsychiatric condition. In a sample of patients treated at our clinic, mixed episodes were most often complicated by abuse of alcohol or other substances, migraine headaches, nonparoxysmal electroencephalographic abnormalities, attention-deficit/hyperactivity disorder, bulimia nervosa, thyroid disorders, and autoimmune disorders (systemic lupus erythematosus, multiple sclerosis). Himmelhoch et al. (1976), who noted that 46% of patients with mixed bipolar disorder met criteria for substance abuse, compared to 20% of patients with pure bipolar disorder,

reported that treatment of such secondary neuropsychiatric conditions improved treatment responsiveness of the mixed state.

Rapid-Cycling Bipolar Disorder

Rapid-cycling bipolar disorder, defined as at least four affective episodes
in a given year, has been described as less responsive to treatment with
lithium (Calabrese et al., 1993; Kukopulos et al., 1980). Some reports
(Calabrese et al., 1993; Schaff, Fawcett, & Zajecka, 1993) suggest that
rapid-cycling patients are more likely to respond to the anticonvulsants
carbamazepine or valproate. However, even these reports found that a substantial percentage of rapid-cycling patients failed to respond to a trial
of anticonvulsant medication. One report (Levy, Drake, & Shy, 1988) suggested that mood swings in some rapid-cycling patients may be the
manifestation of a subclinical seizure disorder, thus accounting for anticonvulsant responsiveness. Rapid cycling has also been associated with antidepressant use, as noted below (Kukopulos et al., 1980; Wehr & Goodwin,
1979).

Bipolar Disorder with Comorbid Medical and Psychiatric Conditions

Another significant correlate of treatment resistance in bipolar disorder
is the presence of comorbid medical or psychiatric conditions. Anxiety
disorders and attention-deficit/hyperactivity disorder (Wozniak et al., 1995)
are associated with patients whose bipolar disorder began early in childhood or young adulthood; this early-onset cohort tends to be more
treatment-resistant than patients whose bipolar disorder begins later in
adulthood. In addition, past substance abuse has been associated with poor
outcome in bipolar patients followed after a first psychotic episode (Tohen, Waternaux, & Tsuang, 1990). Furthermore, thyroid hormone abnormalities (Cowdry, Wehr, Zis, & Goodwin, 1983; Joyce, 1991) and temporal
lobe epileptiform abnormalities (Levy et al., 1988) have been associated
with rapid-cycling bipolar disorder, which (as noted above) has been
described as refractory to lithium.

The Relationship of Clinical Phenomenology
to Treatment Resistance

In a review of five studies that included data on sequence of affective episodes in bipolar disorder (combined $n = 576$), Faedda, Baldessarini, Tohen, Strakowski, and Waternaux (1991) noted decreased responsiveness
to lithium treatment among those whose illness began with a depressive
episode, compared with those whose illness began with a manic or hypomanic episode. Since patients presenting with an initial depressive episode are usually not yet diagnosed as bipolar and thus are likely to receive
antidepressant medication, Faedda et al.'s finding may be confounded, because treatment with antidepressants alone may have a role in the induc-

tion of treatment resistance (as discussed below). Also, the occurrence of psychotic features has been associated with poor outcome (Tohen et al., 1990). On the other hand, lack of insight into illness and need for treatment following recovery from an acute manic episode have not been associated with poor outcome (Ghaemi, Pope, & Stoll, 1995a).

The Antidepressant Problem

Patients with bipolar disorder are more often aware of depression and its concomitant symptoms than they are aware of mood elevation. Hence, even in the midst of an episode of mood elevation (often but not exclusively dysphoric), they may present requesting antidepressant treatment and often refuse mood stabilizers. Regardless of whether these patients are simply less concerned about the consequences of mood elevation or are relatively insensitive in perceiving mood elevation, the demand for antidepressant treatment presents a clinical dilemma. Considerable evidence suggests a relationship between chronic antidepressant treatment, especially without concurrent mood-stabilizing treatment, and development of treatment resistance in patients with bipolar disorder. Goodwin and Jamison (1990) have reviewed this matter and marshaled much of the relevant data. Briefly, in three double-blind outcome studies, the rate of manic episodes in patients with bipolar disorder treated with antidepressants and lithium was roughly twice the rate of such episodes in patients treated with lithium alone (Prien et al., 1984; Prien, Klett, & Caffey, 1974; Quitkin, Kane, Rifkin, Ramos-Lorenzi, & Nayak, 1981a). In two studies of patients with rapid cycling, antidepressants were thought to be the likely causes of rapid cycling in 26–35% of cases (n = 85) (Goodwin, 1994; Kukopulos et al., 1980). Using mood charting, Wehr and Goodwin (1979) also documented increased frequency of affective cycles in patients treated with desipramine and lithium compared to lithium alone. The absence of systematic or objective measures for cycling may account for the general underrecognition of this phenomenon. Simple reliance on a patient's subjective self-report is often insufficient. The limitations of self-report can be decreased by systematically collecting information from other sources, such as mood charting and family report.

Although some clinicians describe generally good results when prescribing antidepressants to patients with bipolar disorder, it is difficult to completely ignore the apparent risks. Until better data are available, it seems prudent to limit exposure of bipolar patients to antidepressants to the periods of their acute depressive episodes, and to provide concurrent mood-stabilizing treatment.

Sudden Discontinuation of Lithium: Another Possible Factor in Treatment Resistance

Recent evidence suggests that sudden discontinuation of lithium increases the risk of subsequent mania significantly beyond the risk attributable to the natural history of the illness. In a review of data culled from previous studies, Suppes, Baldessarini, Faedda, and Tohen (1991) reported in a sample of 257 patients that the average time to an affective episode after sudden lithium discontinuation was 5 months. In a subgroup for whom information about subsequent course of illness while untreated was available (*n* = 16), the time to relapse was only 1.7 months, far shorter than the pretreatment cycle length of 11.6 months. When lithium was tapered over a few weeks, however, relapse rates were no more rapid than before treatment. Rosenbaum, Sachs, Kane, Keller, and Gelenberg (1992) confirmed these findings in a reanalysis of data from Gelenberg et al. (1989). The reanalysis demonstrated that patients with sudden decreases in lithium dose suffered a threefold increased risk of relapse, compared to patients maintained at stable lithium levels in the range of either 0.8–1.0 mmol/liter or 0.4–0.6 mmol/liter. In addition, Post, Leverich, Altshuler, and Mikalauskas (1992) reported that sudden discontinuation was associated with later nonresponse to resumption of lithium treatment in 14% of a population of 66 patients with refractory bipolar disorder. Although this finding has not been confirmed, the accumulating evidence on the deleterious effects of sudden discontinuation of lithium suggests that lithium should be tapered as slowly as is consistent with the patient's clinical needs; a decrease in dose by 300 mg/day each month may be a reasonable pace, to avoid any excess risk of relapse.

MANAGEMENT OPTIONS IN TREATMENT-RESISTANT BIPOLAR DISORDER

In managing a patient with treatment-resistant bipolar disorder, one must be vigilant about the possibility of a switch in affect, as well as the current symptomatology. Self-report may be the only available means of evaluating the patient's illness, yet this subjective database is itself colored by the pathological mood state. In addition, bipolar patients often present with comorbid medical and psychiatric conditions that challenge the treatment process. Clinicians can better meet the clinical needs of these patients by drawing together an array of clinical tools, which should include a systematic approach to evaluation and the use of treatment algorithms.

General Treatment Approach for Bipolar Patients

The Therapeutic Alliance and Mood Charting

After the diagnosis of bipolar disorder is made, the single most important element in any treatment is the therapeutic alliance between patient and psychiatrist. The psychiatrist should provide explicit detailed instructions and education about the illness and its treatment, and should discuss anticipated problems in management. It should be made clear that the patient and psychiatrist are entering into a partnership for the purpose of treating the mood disorder. The goals of this alliance are to insure the patient's safety, treat acute episodes, attempt to prevent recurrence, and maximize the patient's quality of life between episodes. In most cases, these primary goals can be made explicit in an individualized treatment contract written by the patient, with input from care providers, family, and friends. The contract sets out the parameters by which normal mood, depression, and mood elevation will be assessed, as well as the treatment plan for each phase of the illness.

Mood charting (Figure 3.1) is also frequently an indispensable aid to successful treatment. All patients should be encouraged to chart their moods, sleep patterns, and treatment on a daily basis. At follow-up, a clinician can review a patient's chart and incorporate this information into a monthly mood chart. The data accumulated over time in the mood charts provide a record of typical precipitants, frequency, possible seasonality, and duration of episodes. Knowledge of the individual patient's mood cycles often enables the clinician to be a better judge of the impact of treatments and to determine the most appropriate duration for the continuation of treatment.

Medical Workup

Since treatment resistance may be secondary to other medical problems, a patient's prior neuropsychiatric workup should be reviewed, and additional studies should be ordered as indicated. Appropriate physical examination and laboratory workup should be carried out if necessary to rule out general medical and neuroendocrine disease. In particular, thyroid disease appears to be common among bipolar patients, both as a preexisting condition and as a consequence of treatment (lithium, carbamazepine). Given the association between thyroid disease and treatment-refractory conditions such as rapid cycling and mixed states, evaluation and optimization of thyroid status may be a key to improving treatment response. Unfortunately, practical management guidelines for such cases are complicated and remain controversial, because laboratory values for thyroid function may vary widely and still be in the normal range. In light of this, use of a thyroid preparation for optimization of thyroid function could be indicated in two situations: (1) To achieve a normalization of thyroxine (T_4), free T_4, or thyroid-stimulating hormone if these values are outside the normal range; or (2) to reestablish baseline thyroid function, if on repeated measurement one of these values has changed by 50% or more during the course of treatment (even if all thyroid functions remain within normal limits).

The Antidepressant Factor and Other Drugs

The treating clinician should eliminate cycle-promoting agents, particularly antidepressants. This appears to be the single most successful inter-

NAME ____________

MOOD CHART

Month / Yr: ________

TREATMENTS (Enter number of tablets taken each day)

MOOD (Rate with 2 marks each day to indicate best and worst)

___mg	Neuroleptic ___mg	___mg	Antidepressant ___mg	Anticonvulsant ___mg	Benzodiazepine ___mg	Lithium ___mg	Verbal therapy	Daily notes	Irritability (0 = none, 1 = mild, 2 = moderate, 3 = severe)	Anxiety (0 = none, 1 = mild, 2 = moderate, 3 = severe)	Hours slept last night	Depressed: Severe — Significant impairment, Not able to work	Depressed: Mod. — Significant impairment, Able to work	Depressed: Mild — Without significant impairment	WNL: Mood not definitely elevated or depressed, no symptoms. Circle date to indicated menses	Elevated: Mild — Without significant impairment	Elevated: Mod. — Significant impairment, Able to work	Elevated: Severe — Significant impairment, Not able to work	Psychotic sxs, Strange ideas, hallucinations
															1				
															2				
															3				
															4				
															5				
															6				
															7				
															8				
															9				
															10				
															11				
															12				
															13				
															14				
															15				
															16				
															17				
															18				
															19				
															20				
															21				
															22				
															23				
															24				
															25				
															26				
															27				
															28				
								Weight							29				
															30				
															31				

FIGURE 3.1. Mood chart. Created by Gary S. Sachs.

vention for reducing rapid cycling (Kukopulos et al., 1980; Wehr, Sack, Rosenthal, & Cowdry, 1988). Neuroleptics can be cycle-promoting, and some patients improve when they discontinue these agents. In addition, reduction of stimulants (including caffeine) and bronchodilators (albuterol, theophylline) may be beneficial.

Psychoeducation

Improvement in treatment outcome can be achieved in some cases by providing the family and patient with education about the nature of bipolar disorder and principles of good mood hygiene. Although studies associating onset of episodes with environmental events find little correlation beyond the earliest episodes, many patients are able to learn and benefit from simple strategies to lessen conflict or avoid precipitants. Encouragement to maintain a stable sleep–wake schedule, to eat and exercise regularly, and to avoid extremes in workload and travel across time zones often have salutary effects. Although (as for many of the somatic therapies described below) there are no empirical data showing the effectiveness of these strategies in treatment-refractory bipolar patients, clinical experience and their low cost and low risk justify their recommendation.

Psychotherapeutic Aspects of Psychopharmacologic Management

Although no verbal therapy has demonstrated conclusive benefit in treatment of acute mania, and few (with the exception of cognitive-behavioral therapy) have established benefit in acute depression, empirical studies suggest that psychotherapies of all types help to prevent recurrence when they are added to pharmacologic treatment in the prophylaxis of bipolar disorder (Kanas, 1993; Lesser, 1983; Mayo, O'Connell, & O'Brien, 1979; Miklowitz, Goldstein, Nuechterlein, Snyder, & Mintz, 1988; Van Gent, Vida, & Zwart, 1988; Vasile et al., 1987). The active elements of psychotherapy remain unclear; however, the prophylactic efficacy of verbal therapies, like that of lithium treatment, appears to require continued treatment. Negative expressed emotion especially appears to be associated with increased relapse rates in patients with bipolar disorder maintained on lithium for more than 3 years (Priebe, Wildgrube, & Müller-Oerlinghausen, 1989).

In general, treaters also need to be flexible and to adjust the content, frequency, and duration of therapy sessions according to patients' mood states. For instance, as patients become acutely ill, sessions should become more frequent but shorter, with focus on acute signs and symptoms and on maintaining the patients' safety. Many patients also report benefit from self-help groups such as the National Depressive and Manic Depressive Association.

Management of Mood Elevation or Failure of Prophylaxis

Figure 3.2 summarizes an algorithm for the management of mood elevation or rapid cycling in patients with bipolar disorder. The rationale for the steps of the algorithm is reflected in the literature for each of the treatment options, as discussed below.

The Limits of Lithium

Lithium is widely regarded as the treatment of choice for bipolar disorder. Placebo-controlled data from studies conducted in the 1960s and 1970s (Baastrup, Poulsen, Schou, Thomsen, & Amdisen, 1970; Coppen et al., 1971; Cundall, Brooks, & Murray, 1972; Dunner, Stallone, & Fieve, 1976; Fieve, Kumbaraci, & Dunner, 1976; Melia, 1970; Prien et al., 1974) led to the conclusion that "the response rate of acute mania to lithium is roughly 70 to 80 percent" (Prien & Potter, 1990, p. 410). Widely accepted and widely cited, this myth led many clinicians to expect that 70–80% of lithium-treated bipolar patients would achieve full remission.

Unfortunately, data accumulated over the last 20 years suggest that this expectation is often unfulfilled. After lithium use became widespread in Great Britain, Symonds and Williams (1981) observed an increase in readmission rates for bipolar patients. Retrospective studies of bipolar patients given lithium or other treatments in open practice often failed to find much significant prophylactic benefit from lithium (Harrow, Goldberg, Grossman, & Meltzer, 1990; Mander, 1986; Markar & Mander, 1989). For instance, Mander (1986) reported that manic inpatients who were prescribed lithium at the time of discharge had the same rate (30%) of early relapse—less than 3 months from hospital discharge—as those patients receiving no lithium (28%). Among 41 bipolar outpatients started on lithium prophylaxis compared with a group treated without lithium, Markar and Mander (1989) failed to detect a significant difference in relapse rate. Over a 1.7-year naturalistic follow-up period in patients with bipolar disorder, Harrow et al. (1990) found a 40% recurrence rate of mania in those receiving lithium prophylaxis, as opposed to a 42% recurrence rate in those receiving other treatments. Regardless of whether or not lithium was administered, "a considerable percentage show[ed] at least moderately impaired functioning at follow-up" compared with unipolar depressed patients (Harrow et al., 1990, p. 669). Consistent with this finding, Gillberg, Hellgren, and Gillberg (1993) reported that 89% of a sample diagnosed bipolar with illness during adolescence received full disability benefits by age 30, despite adequate treatment with lithium.

Although these were open retrospective studies, in which less intensive management and noncompliance may have diminished the protective benefit of lithium maintenance, rigorous double-blind maintenance studies have also had disappointing results. Gelenberg et al. (1989) reported that response to lithium did not differ much regardless of whether or not

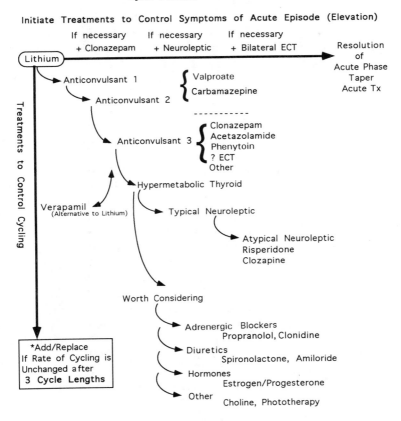

Cycle Duration < 4 Weeks

Initiate Treatments to Control Symptoms of Acute Episode (Elevation)

FIGURE 3.2. Rapid-cycling treatment algorithm. Copyright 1994 by Gary S. Sachs. Reprinted by permission.

lithium levels were therapeutic or low in bipolar patients with three or more prior episodes; in contrast, higher lithium doses resulting in therapeutic levels definitely produced more improvement in symptoms than did low-dose lithium treatment in bipolar patients with fewer than three prior episodes. This finding is consistent with the observations that lithium is less effective for rapid-cycling bipolar patients (Dunner & Fieve, 1974; Kukopulos et al., 1980).

In open clinical practice, the detectable benefit of lithium monotherapy is modest. Only 4% of the patients in a sample (total $n = 100$) in our bipolar program were episode-free when treated with lithium alone (Sachs et al., 1994a). This may reflect, in part, the treatment-resistant characteristics of patients referred to a hospital-affiliated specialty clinic;

however, many of these patients were initially referred for treatment of their first episode. The percentage of bipolar patients achieving sustained full remission was quite low, regardless of treatment. If treatment success was defined as sustained remission during at least 3 years of treatment with therapeutic levels of lithium, carbamazepine, or valproate, nearly all (more than 75%) bipolar patients in that sample could have been considered treatment-resistant. Most required treatments in addition to lithium.

Anticonvulsants: Their Role in Prophylaxis

Numerous controlled studies support the use of carbamazepine and valproate in bipolar disorder. Both anticonvulsants have been shown to be at least equal in efficacy to lithium in double-blind studies (Bowden et al., 1994; Coxhead, Silverstone, & Cookson, 1992; Freeman, Clothier, Pazzaglia, Lesem, & Swann, 1992; Small et al., 1991).

The claim of acute antimanic efficacy of carbamazepine is based on at least 12 studies with a total n of 327 (Ballenger & Post, 1978; Cookson, 1987; Emrich, Dose, Gunther, & Von Zerssen, 1985; Grossi et al., 1984; Klein, Bental, Lerer, & Belmaker, 1984; Lerer, Moore, Meyendorff, Cho, & Gershon, 1987; Lusznat, Murphy, & Nunn, 1988; Okuma et al., 1979, 1981, 1989; Placidi, Lenzi, Lazzerini, Cassano, & Akiskal, 1986; Watkins, Callender, Thomas, Tidmarsh, & Shaw, 1987). Four additional studies found antimanic efficacy when carbamazepine was given in combination with lithium or neuroleptics (Klein et al., 1984; Kramlinger & Post, 1989; Moller et al., 1989; Muller & Stoll, 1984). With respect to prophylaxis, five studies show an overall response rate of 72% in 81 bipolar and schizoaffective patients (Ballenger & Post, 1978; Lusznat et al., 1988; Okuma et al., 1981; Placidi et al., 1986; Watkins et al., 1987).

Acute antimanic efficacy of valproic acid has been established by eight controlled studies (six double-blind) with a total n of 506 (Brennan, Sandyk, & Borsook, 1984; Brown, 1989; Calabrese et al., 1993; Emrich, Okuma, & Muller, 1984; Emrich, Von Zerssen, Kissling, Moller, & Windorfer, 1980; McElroy, Keck, & Hudson, 1988; Pope, McElroy, Keck, & Hudson, 1991; Prasad, 1984). This includes the two largest placebo-controlled double-blind trials conducted in the past 25 years on bipolar patients. Although less rigorously controlled, 10 studies of valproate maintenance report a 54% response to valproate prophylaxis among 375 bipolar and schizoaffective patients (Brennan et al., 1984; Calabrese et al., 1993; Emrich et al., 1984; Hayes, 1989; Lambert, 1984; Lambert et al., 1975; McElroy et al., 1988; Post & Uhde, 1987; Semadeni, 1976; Sovner, 1989).

Combining Lithium and Anticonvulsants

Most of the literature on combination treatments of mood stabilizers is uncontrolled (Post, 1990). However, these studies seem to provide increasing evidence for the utility of combining lithium with valproate, carbamazepine, or both. In Post's (1990) review of this literature, there were 15 uncontrolled studies of valproate augmentation of lithium in bipolar disorder; when combined, these yielded a 62% (246/400) success rate in acute treatment, and a 48% (183/380) success rate in prophylaxis. In another recent study, 75% (47/63) of patients with refractory affective disorders (mostly bipolar disorder) responded when valproate was added to either lithium or carbamazepine (Schaff et al., 1993). A number of recent reports have noted the efficacy and relative safety of combining valproate and carbamazepine in the treatment of refractory bipolar disorder (Keck, McElroy, Vuckovic, & Friedman, 1992; Ketter, Pazzaglia, & Post, 1992; Tohen, Castillo, Pope, & Herbstein, 1994a).

Combining mood stabilizers requires attention to the pharmacokinetic effects of the medications. In particular, carbamazepine should be cautiously introduced when a patient is using other medications that are metabolized by hepatic cytochrome P450 enzymes, since carbamazepine strongly induces these enzymes and thus lowers the level of medications metabolized by them (such as neuroleptics and antidepressants). Valproate, on the other hand, tends to inhibit these hepatic enzymes, thus potentially raising the levels of medications metabolized by this system. In rare circumstances severe consequences of enzyme induction may follow, as when a toxic metabolite is produced in significant quantities because of the induction of the P450 system. An interaction of this type can occur when valproate and carbamazepine are given concurrently. Under most circumstances in adults, valproate is metabolized mostly in the mitochondria by beta-oxidation, and a relatively small amount is metabolized by the P450 metabolic pathway in the smooth endoplasmic reticulum. The latter pathway produces a potentially toxic metabolite, (Kesterson, Granneman, & Machinist, 1984; Patsalos et al., 1985), but since the amount metabolized by this pathway is typically small, this effect is usually not clinically significant. If a valproate-treated patient is treated with carbamazepine as well, or with another drug that induces the P450 pathway, the resulting increase in the toxic metabolite may reach potentially lethal levels. Although recent case reports suggest that patients often tolerate concurrent use of valproate and carbamazepine (Keck et al., 1992; Tohen et al., 1994a) the use of this combination warrants caution and careful monitoring.

Benzodiazepines

Several case reports suggest that benzodiazepines can be effective treatments for acute mania. In the only double-blind study of clonazepam, Chouinard, Young, and Annable (1983) used a crossover design to compare the acute antimanic efficacy of clonazepam and lithium in 12 patients over a 10-day period. The main finding reported from this study was a statistically significant advantage for clonazepam in controlling one of five of the manic symptoms rated. This finding is often criticized, however, because the efficacy of lithium is not usually apparent during the first 10 days of treatment.

Two studies in which clonazepam was given in place of a neuroleptic during maintenance treatment obtained contrasting results. In an open study reported by Aronson, Shukla, and Hirschowitz (1989), five of five bipolar patients who were refractory to lithium alone, and who had improved only with the addition of neuroleptic agents to lithium, suffered relapse of psychotic mania within 15 weeks of switching from the neuroleptics to clonazepam. This study is often cited as evidence of the non-efficacy of clonazepam, but no treatment has been shown to be effective in a population of neuroleptic-refractory bipolar patients.

Using a similar open design for the treatment of bipolar patients not refractory to neuroleptic treatment and maintained on lithium and neuroleptic agents, Sachs (1990) found that within the limitations of the design, patients could be safely switched from neuroleptic maintenance to clonazepam maintenance. Furthermore, over a 12-month follow-up period there was a trend (not reaching statistical significance) showing a lower incidence of relapse into depression in clonazepam-treated patients and no difference in the rate of recurrence of mania/hypomania. On the other hand, Bradwejn, Shriqui, Koszycki, and Meterissian (1990) reported a blind comparison of clonazepam and lorazepam in acute mania that found lorazepam to be superior. It is difficult to interpret the results from this study, given the other reports, since this study detected almost no response to clonazepam. At this time, the relative advantages of various benzodiapines are unclear.

Neuroleptics and Atypical Antipsychotic Agents

Patients with bipolar disorder often receive neuroleptic maintenance treatment, despite the well-known risks associated with chronic neuroleptic use (Sachs, 1990). Given the frequency of this practice, it is surprising that there are no studies reporting an advantage for neuroleptic maintenance in bipolar patients. However, recurrence of mania or psychotic symptoms after tapering of neuroleptics may provide a clinical rationale for this treatment. The high frequency of maintenance neuroleptic use may reflect an underutilization of other treatments for acute mania or the existence of a significant subgroup requiring chronic neuroleptic treatment.

The only studies of neuroleptic maintenance in bipolar patients suggest little benefit. A 2-year double-blind crossover study compared the neuroleptic flupenthixol to a placebo as an adjunct to lithium maintenance. Patients receiving flupenthixol experienced more episodes of depression than did placebo-treated patients (Esparon et al., 1986). No significant difference was observed in outcome between bipolar patients continuing lithium and a neuroleptic and patients openly switched to lithium and clonazepam, but a trend indicating higher incidence of depressive relapse was observed in the neuroleptic-treated patients (Sachs, 1990).

The atypical antipsychotic agents risperidone and clozapine may offer better results than older agents, but the literature available on the use of these agents with bipolar patients is limited to case reports and open series. The reports are encouraging, however: Bipolar patients refractory to neuroleptics, anticonvulsants, and lithium are reported to derive substantial acute improvement from atypical antipsychotic agents, and this improvement persists in the maintenance phase.

Clozapine was reported to be beneficial for seven of seven bipolar patients with mixed episodes (Suppes, McElroy, Gilbert, Dessain, & Cole, 1992). Treatment was continued for 3–5 years, during which the patients' psychosocial functioning improved substantially. Case reports also describe positive response during maintenance treatment in bipolar patients previously refractory to lithium, anticonvulsants, and typical neuroleptic drugs (Frankenburg, 1993). In an open retrospective review that included 52 patients with bipolar disorder, the outcome of treatment with clozapine was noted to be better for the patients with bipolar disorder than for patients with schizoaffective disorder, schizophrenia, or unipolar depression (Banov et al., 1994). Daily dosage of clozapine for treatment of bipolar patients ranges from 50 to 600 mg. It should be noted that the risk of seizures increases with increasing clozapine dose, being 1–2% with doses of less than 300 mg/day, 3–4% with doses of 300–600 mg/day, and 5% with doses of 600–900 mg/day. Thus, when a patient is being treated with more than 400–500 mg/day, prophylactic anticonvulsant treatment is indicated. Carbamazepine is not commonly used with clozapine because of a possibly greater combined risk of agranulocytosis. Phenytoin does not suppress bone marrow activity, but, like carbamazepine, induces hepatic P450 enzymes and thus will lower clozapine levels. Valproate tends to raise clozapine levels somewhat and is thus a preferable anticonvulsant to combine with clozapine. Also, one report has suggested that the addition of valproate may enhance the clinical mood-stabilizing effect of clozapine (Kando, Tohen, Castillo, & Centorrino, 1994).

Two case series have reported improvement in bipolar patients treated openly with risperidone (Tohen et al., 1994b; Ghaemi, Sachs, Baldassano, & Truman, 1995b). Doses typically were lower (1–3 mg/day) than the 6-mg daily dose recommended for treatment of schizophrenia. In contrast with these two case series in which no patient worsened during risperidone treatment, Dwight, Keck, Stanton, Strakowski, and McElroy (1994) have described worsening of symptoms of mania in seven schizoaffective inpatients treated with risperidone. These patients were followed every other day with depression and mania ratings (Hamilton Depression Rating Scale, Hamilton, 1960; Young Mania Rating Scale, Young, 1978), and their depression scores fell while their mania scores rose. The interpretability of this report is hampered by the small sample, its open design, the use of the most extreme score for statistical analysis, and the use of rating scales designed for use at weekly intervals but administered every other day. Each of these factors may have contributed toward biased positive results.

Although in need of replication in controlled double-blind studies, these suggestive results may justify the use of risperidone and clozapine for treatment-refractory bipolar patients. Clozapine should be used with caution because of the risk of agranulocytosis (which requires weekly monitoring of white blood cell count), a substantial risk of seizures, drug interactions, and its high cost. It is reasonable to reserve clozapine for patients who are unresponsive to other therapies; risperidone may serve as a safer initial alternative.

Electroconvulsive Therapy: Its Role in Prophylaxis

Electroconvulsive therapy (ECT) appears to be a potent and beneficial treatment for bipolar disorder. Use of ECT may be appropriate at any time during the course of either unipolar depression or bipolar disorder. Although it is generally regarded as the most potent treatment for depression, limited patient acceptance and administrative barriers result in underuse of ECT. Because of its effectiveness and safety, ECT is a particularly attractive option for any affectively ill treatment-resistant patient, and should always be offered as a treatment option rather than held as a treatment of last resort. Indeed, for some patient groups ECT may be the treatment of choice, as Fava, Kaji, and Davidson have noted in Chapter 1 of this volume.

A course of ECT for acute depression or mania typically consists of 4–12 seizures induced electrically while the patient is under anesthesia. Seizure induction takes place two or three times per week. Within the range of common clinical practice, the intensity of the electrical stimulus and the waveform (sine wave, brief pulse) seem to contribute more to differential adverse effects than to differences in efficacy.

ECT, like all effective antidepressant therapies, has been reported to induce mania in some depressed patients. However, ECT is also an effective treatment for mania, with a remission rate of approximately 80% (Mukherjee, Sackeim, & Schnur, 1994). In a large open case series, acute antimanic ECT treatment appeared to be superior to lithium or to the combination of lithium and neuroleptic (Black, Winokur, & Nasrallah, 1987; Thomas & Reddy, 1982). Three studies have reported that for the treatment of mania, the efficacy of ECT is equal to or greater than that of neuroleptics or lithium (Black et al., 1987; McCabe & Norris, 1977; Thomas & Reddy, 1982). In another study of patients with refractory mania, ECT nonresponse was associated with irritability and suspiciousness, but not with severity of mania (Schnur, Mukherjee, Sackheim, Lee, & Roth, 1992). Most of these studies found unilateral ECT to be effective for mania. However, Small, Milstein, Kellams, and Klapper (1985) reported that unilateral nondominant ECT resulted in worsening of mania in six of six patients, but that all six improved when treatment was changed to bilateral ECT. Since unilateral nondominant ECT is associated with less memory impairment than is bilateral ECT, many clinicians will start treatment with unilateral ECT and switch to bilateral ECT only if a patient fails to respond. However, patients should not be considered nonresponsive to ECT unless they have had an adequate course of bilateral ECT.

A high relapse rate may be expected if successful treatment with ECT in the acute phase is not followed by continuation and/or maintenance antidepressant or antimanic prophylaxis. Case reports have described successful continuation and maintenance treatment with ECT, but no controlled study has been published (Monroe, 1991).

Hypermetabolic Thyroid Hormone

The relationship between rapid cycling and hypothyroidism remains the subject of some debate. A number of studies (Bauer et al., 1993; Cho, Bone, Dunner, Colt, & Fieve, 1979; Cowdry et al., 1983) have found that hypothyroidism is present in 31–50% of patients with rapid cycling, as opposed to 0–2% of non-rapid-cycling bipolar patients. Wehr et al. (1988), however, found hypothyroidism in about 40% of non-rapid-cycling as well as rapid-cycling patients.

There are no double-blind studies reporting the therapeutic use of thyroid hormone in bipolar patients. Stancer and Persad (1982) reported that administration of 300–500 μg of T_4 abolished rapid cycling in 5 of 10 patients. In another open trial, Bauer and Whybrow (1990) added high-dose levothyroxine to the mood-stabilizing treatment regimen of 11 rapid-cycling bipolar patients. They reported that 10 of the 11 experienced "clear-cut" improvement in the depressive phase; among the seven with mania at baseline, five responded. Interestingly, response in these patients was independent of initial thyroid status. At the time of clinical response, however, T_4 and free T_4 were found to be above the upper limit of normal in nearly all subjects. Bauer et al. (1993) observed loss of benefit when patients' doses of thyroid hormone were tapered below supernormal levels, including some under blind conditions.

Candidates for hypermetabolic thyroid hormone treatment should be screened for medical contraindications (such as cardiac conduction defects, hypertension or past stroke, and osteoporosis) and started with levothyroxine at 0.1 mg per day. Dosage is gradually titrated upward by increasing the daily dosage 0.05–0.1 mg every 1–2 weeks as tolerated until the free T_4 is about 150% of the laboratory upper limit or the patient experiences intolerable side effects (anxiety, agitation, tremor, sweating, palpitations). Use of hypermetabolic thyroid treatment is carried out as an adjunct to a standard mood-stabilizing regimen. Considerations in long-term use of this treatment include the possibility of demineralization of bone, loss of calcium from teeth, loss of muscle mass, and paroxysmal atrial fibrillation.

Calcium Channel Blockers

The reasoning for use of calcium channel blockers in bipolar disorder comes from studies finding abnormalities of calcium metabolism in affective ill-

ness (Dubovsky, Lee, Christiano, & Murphy, 1991; Meltzer, 1986). Calcium concentration in the cerebrospinal fluid of bipolar patients has been
found in some studies to correlate with mood state (Carman, Post, Runkle, Bunney, & Wyatt, 1979). During the 1980s, trials carried out with
bipolar patients suggested that calcium channel blockers might be effective alternatives or adjuncts to lithium treatment of acute mania. On the
basis of two small double-blind studies, verapamil appears to have antimanic effects (Dubovsky, Franks, Allen, & Murphy, 1986; Giannini, Houser, Loiselle, Giannini, & Price, 1984). Unfortunately, verapamil does not
appear to be particularly effective for treatment-refractory patients. Kennedy, Ozevsky, and Robillard (1986) described two patients refractory to lithium and carbamazepine who failed to benefit from verapamil. Furthermore,
none of the five verapamil responders reported by Dubovsky et al. (1986)
had failed a previous trial of lithium. Dosage of verapamil is 160–480 mg
given on a split twice-daily or three-times-daily basis. In the treatment
algorithm for mood cycling (Figure 3.2), verapamil is placed on a branch
off the sequence of other anticycling treatments as an alternative rather
than an adjunct to these treatments, largely because of drug interactions
with lithium (lithium toxicity is perhaps attributable to rising intracellular levels despite lower serum levels) and carbamazepine (leading to neu-
rotoxicity). The currently available data suggest that verapamil's main use
will be in patients who are intolerant of lithium or anticonvulsants. Other
calcium channel blockers are structurally different and exert effects on
intracellular calcium through different mechanisms. It remains to be seen
whether these other agents, such as diltiazem, nifedipine, or nimodipine,
have therapeutic value for treatment-refractory bipolar patients.

Adrenergic Agents

Adrenergic agents, such as clonidine, may be another possible treatment
for the nonresponsive patient with bipolar disorder. Open data (Hardy,
Lecrubier, & Witlocher, 1986; Jouvent, Lecrubier, Puech, Simon, & Witlocher, 1980; Zubenko, Cohen, Lipinski, & Jonas, 1984) suggest that clonidine is an effective alternative or adjunctive treatment for acute mania,
in which antimanic response appears within days of reaching an effective
dose (0.2–0.6 mg twice a day). Two double-blind studies obtained less positive results. In one, clonidine was found to be inferior to verapamil in
lithium-nonresponsive acute mania (Giannini, Luiselle, Price, & Giannini, 1985); in another, clonidine was inferior to lithium in treating acute
mania (Zubenko et al., 1984). The meaning of this last finding is unclear,
since the sample was comprised of lithium-responsive patients, and there
was no placebo control group for comparison. Although no maintenance
studies have been reported, clonidine may be a useful adjunct to other
mood-stabilizing agents. Treatment with clonidine is often limited by sedation and hypotension, however.

Alternative Approaches

It is preferable to base clinical practice on empirical data, but in many areas of medicine this preference is recognized as a wish for a state of knowledge more advanced than current reality. Clinicians treating bipolar patients, however, frequently confront a more acute dilemma: They are often compelled to treat the severe symptoms of patients who have proven refractory to the few empirically grounded therapies discussed above. In order to further the rational treatment of these severely ill patients, it is useful to consider the limited knowledge available on alternative treatments. The reader must exercise caution, since the nature of these reports (open data, anecdotal, or theoretical) does not permit confident conclusions as to the true benefit of most of the following therapies.

Cholinergic drugs have been reported to have antimanic effects (Janowsky, El-Yousef, Davis, & Sekereke, 1972). Cohen, Lipinski, and Altesman (1982) presented a controlled study supporting the use of lecithin, a precursor of choline for the treatment of manic patients. Stoll, Sachs, Cohen, Lafer, and Renshaw (1994) have demonstrated that oral administration of choline bitartrate raises brain choline levels. An open trial of choline bitartrate as an adjunct to lithium produced promising results in five of six rapid-cycling patients; the only patient who failed to respond was also the only patient who failed to demonstrate an increase in brain choline level during choline treatment. Typical choline doses used are 4–10 mg/day, and the few side effects that have been noted include occasional diarrhea, abdominal discomfort, fishy breath, and a few reports of worsened depression. There have been reports that vanadium-lowering agents (such as ascorbic acid, 4 mg/day; ethylenediaminetetraacetic acid [EDTA], 4 mg/day; and methylene blue, 300 mg/day) produce improvement in bipolar depression comparable to that produced by treatment with traditional antidepressants, although the antimanic benefits of these agents seem weaker than those of lithium (Kay, Naylor, Smith, & Greenwood, 1984; Naylor, Martin, Hopwood, & Watson, 1986). Side effects reported with methylene blue included nausea, dysuria, increased urination, and diarrhea; few side effects were reported with EDTA or ascorbic acid. Reduction of sleep time and the use of light have been reported to improve depression, but may cause abnormal mood elevation (Sachs, 1989). Subcaudate stereotactic tractomy reportedly helped a small group of patients with intractable bipolar symptoms in an uncontrolled study (Poynton, Bridges, & Bartlett, 1988). Some patients with bipolar disorder have also been reported to respond to acetazolamide, adinazolam, estrogen–progesterone, reserpine, and spironolactone (Sachs, 1989).

Management of Treatment-Resistant Bipolar Depression

The algorithm presented (in Figure 3.3) for treatment-resistant bipolar depression attempts to balance the need for antidepressant treatment and

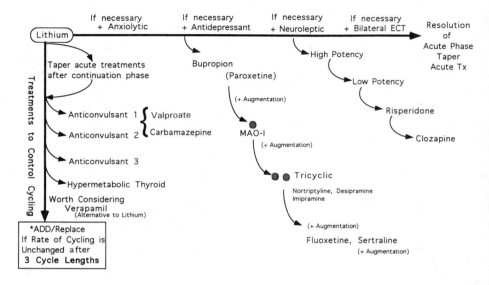

FIGURE 3.3. Bipolar depression treatment algorithm. Copyright 1994 by Gary S. Sachs. Reprinted by permission.

the risk of treatment-induced mania or rapid cycling. The treatment algorithm is divided into two dimensions. Along the horizontal dimension are treatments that target symptoms of the acute episode. These treatments are started at the time of diagnosis (acute phase).

Each individual treatment trial is carried out to one of three end points: (1) discontinuation because the patient is unable to tolerate adverse effects of treatment; (2) discontinuation because the patient has failed to respond to a maximal trial of the treatment (including, if warranted, augmentation strategies); or (3) improvement.

In the case of treatment success, the therapy should be continued for a period of time (often 2–4 months may be sufficient) to prevent relapse (continuation phase), and then should be tapered gradually. Relapse during the taper period should be managed by resumption of acute-phase strategies. Antidepressant doses should be raised to effective levels and another taper attempted following another continuation phase. As a rule, for the majority of bipolar patients, maintenance treatment with antidepressants should be avoided. Those patients who suffer multiple relapses during attempts to discontinue their antidepressant treatment may be candidates for a prophylactic regimen that includes an antidepressant as well as a mood stabilizer. Even in such cases, it is prudent to find the lowest effective dose of antidepressant medication. After resolution of the acute episode, patients continue treatment directed at preventing recurrence (the vertical dimension of Figure 3.3). During this phase, symptoms are treated and plotted on a mood chart (see Figure 3.1) to allow determination of the rate of cycling of episodes.

The Limits of Lithium

The bipolar depression treatment algorithm starts with lithium, because among untreated bipolar depressed patients in open practice, lithium monotherapy appears to be sufficient treatment for about one-third of these patients (Sachs, 1995b). If effectively treated by lithium, patients are spared the risk of antidepressant-induced mania. Since lithium does not carry the risk of inducing mania and appears to reduce the risk of affective switch during treatment with standard antidepressant agents, initiating treatment with lithium is an appealing first step in the management of episodes of depressive disorder in bipolar patients. In cases where depression occurs despite ongoing adequate lithium maintenance, it is often suggested that raising lithium levels will optimize antidepressive efficacy. No controlled data are available to support this, and many clinicians describe cases refractory to high therapeutic lithium levels. If lithium is not sufficient treatment for the acute depression, the combination of lithium and a standard antidepressant appears to carry less risk of affective switch than does treatment with antidepressant alone (Prien et al., 1984; Prien, Klett, & Caffey, 1973; Quitkin et al., 1981a).

Standard Antidepressant Medications

Few clinicians doubt that the antidepressants found to be effective for unipolar depressed patients are also effective for bipolar patients. Unfortunately, because bipolar patients are routinely excluded from most antidepressant treatment trials, empirical data with eight or more bipolar patients are limited to only seven studies. These relatively few studies—and, as reviewed by Zornberg and Pope (1993), additional reports with very small samples—do appear to confirm the clinical impression that standard antidepressant agents also effectively treat the depressed phase of bipolar disorder.

Quitkin, McGrath, Liebowitz, Stewart, and Howard (1993) reported that up to two-thirds of bipolar patients responded to a tricyclic antidepressant. Among the tricyclic nonresponders, two-thirds responded to a monoamine oxidase inhibitor (MAOI). Consistent with this, Himmelhoch, Thase, Mallinger, and Houck (1991) found a higher response rate among bipolar patients treated with tranylcypromine than among those receiving imipramine. Baumhackl et al. (1989) reported that treatment with imipramine as effective as treatment with the MAOI moclobemide for bipolar depression. Fluoxetine and perhaps other selective serotonin reuptake inhibitors (SSRIs) appear to be very potent treatments for bipolar depression.

Cohn, Collins, Ashbrook, and Wernicke (1989) found fluoxetine superi-
or to imipramine in a study of bipolar depressed patients. Sachs et al. (1994a)
reported that desipramine and bupropion possessed equivalent antidepressant properties in patients with bipolar depression. Although sparse, the
available data suggest little difference in antidepressant efficacy among
standard agents.

As reviewed by Goodwin and Jamison (1990), rates of treatment-
emergent mania in bipolar I patients treated with tricyclic antidepressants
alone range from 31% to 70%. All effective standard antidepressant agents
have been associated with treatment-emergent mania. It is possible, however, that the various antidepressants differ in their propensity to induce
mania. Among the few studies comparing antidepressant treatment in bipolar patients, even fewer report rates of treatment-emergent hypomania/ma-
nia. Cohn et al. (1989) reported that the incidence of hypomania/mania
during 3–6 weeks of treatment for depressed bipolar patients receiving fluoxetine, imipramine, and placebo was 19%, 9.5%, and 7.7%, respectively.
However, since the rate of lithium use differed among the three groups
as well (33.3% in the fluoxetine group, 16.6% in the imipramine group,
and 20.7% in the placebo group), the findings may not represent equivalent comparison conditions. Nonetheless, the trend toward increased mood
elevation with fluoxetine is suggestive; interestingly, the authors also noted
a 16% switch rate into hypomania or mania with open fluoxetine treatment
for those who failed to respond to imipramine or placebo treatment (n
= 25). Over a year of double-blind treatment, Sachs et al. (1994a) found
that 50% of desipramine-treated patients versus 11% of bupropion-treated
patients experienced hypomania/mania. Fogelson, Bystritsky, and Pasnau
(1992), however, reported an uncontrolled open case series in which 6 of
11 bipolar patients experienced hypomania or mania during treatment with
bupropion. Design differences may account for the disparity between these
results. Fogelson et al.'s sample probably included patients at higher risk for
affective switch. In this study, 10 of the 11 subjects had experienced mania
during prior antidepressant treatment, and the dose of bupropion was rapidly
escalated (the maximum dose of 450 mg/day was usually reached by day 6).
Sachs et al. (1994a) excluded patients with a history of treatment-emergent
mania and used a more gradual titration of dosage (all subjects had 2 weeks
or more of treatment at 300 mg/day before further dosage increase).

Replication of the findings by Sachs et al. (1994a) is necessary to as-
sure the validity of the findings. Nonetheless based on the available data
it appears that bupropion is less likely to induce hypomania/mania than
reuptake-inhibitor-type antidepressants. The SSRIs, on the other hand,
may be particularly potent mood elevators.

Anticonvulsants

There are six reports with results for eight or more bipolar patients who
received a trial of an anticonvulsant alone for acute treatment of depres-

sion; only two of these were double-blind (see Table 3.2). The results are quite modest if judged by the very low frequency of marked improvement in double-blind trials. Given that the samples in these studies included many treatment-resistant patients, the moderate improvement rate may justify including the anticonvulsants as options for the acute treatment phase. Perhaps the main advantage of using anticonvulsants in the acute phase is avoiding the risk of antidepressant-induced mood elevation.

Treatment of Anxiety during Depressive Episodes

Anxiety is a very common feature of acute depressive episodes; it may intensify dysphoria and, particularly when it causes insomnia, may interfere with treatment response or lead to affective switch. Therefore, use of an anxiolytic agent is often warranted, both to ameliorate the anxiety itself and to facilitate response to antidepressant treatment. Use of high-potency benzodiazepines (lorazepam, alprazolam, clonazepam) appears to produce rapid benefit by significantly relieving dysphoria in some bipolar depressed patients. It remains unclear whether this represents a true antidepressant effect in these patients or is simply the result of diminished anxiety.

For those patients with prominent anxiety who fail to benefit from a benzodiazepine, or for whom this class of medication may be contraindicated, clonidine and propranolol may be useful adjuncts. These adrenergic blockers must be used with caution, since they may act as depressogens and interfere with the antidepressant activity of standard antidepressant medications.

TABLE 3.2. Acute Trials of Anticonvulsants for Bipolar Depression (Reporting Results of at Least Eight Bipolar Subjects)

Drug; investigators; n	Design	Improvement		
		Marked	Moderate	None
Carbamazepine; Ballenger & Post (1978); n = 9	Double-blind, crossover	0%	44%	56%
Carbamazepine; Okuma (1983); n = 9	Open	22%	–	78%
Carbamazepine; Post et al. (1984); n = 25	Double-blind (placebo, drug, placebo, drug)	–	48%	52%
Valproate; Lambert & Venaud (1984); n = 103[a]	Open	2%	22%	76%
Valproate; Calabrese & Delucchi (1990); n = 11	Open	57%	6%	37%
Clonazepam; Kishimoto et al. (1988) n = 9	Open	44%	33%	23%

[a]It is not clear what percentage of these patients would actually meet DSM-IV criteria for bipolar disorder.

For many bipolar patients, tapering of anxiolytic drugs is indicated following the successful resolution of the acute phase of the affective episode and stabilization during the continuation phase of the affective episode. Other bipolar patients appear to benefit from maintenance anxiolytic therapy. Bipolar patients may be maintained on lithium and a benzodiazepine with prophylactic efficacy at least as great as that achieved by lithium and a neuroleptic (Sachs, Lafer, Truman, Noeth, & Thibault, 1994b) or lithium and an antidepressant (Thibault, Sachs, Lafer, Kokoletsky, & Rosenbaum, 1993).

Treatment of Psychosis during Depressive Episodes

The presence of psychotic features in bipolar disorder appears to increase the likelihood of poor outcome (Tohen et al., 1990). Because of the increased severity of their illness, psychotic depressed bipolar patients are typically treated with three or more medications (lithium, an antidepressant, and a neuroleptic). In the absence of data specific to treatment of bipolar depression with psychotic features, the approach to treatment may be guided by experience with unipolar psychotic depression.

SUMMARY

Bipolar disorder is often a refractory illness. Treatment resistance is particularly prominent in particular diagnostic subtypes of bipolar disorder, such as those involving mixed episodes or rapid cycling, and it also appears to be associated with chronic antidepressant treatment. Clinical correlates of treatment resistance include onset of illness with a major depressive episode, substance abuse, mood-incongruent psychotic features, and psychiatric and medical comorbidities.

Management involves replacing or combining lithium treatment with anticonvulsants or atypical antipsychotic agents. Other adjuncts include benzodiazepines, thyroid hormone, verapamil, clonidine, and ECT. Antidepressants should be used cautiously, mainly in the acute depressive episode, and always with concomitant mood stabilizers. Above all, the treatment of bipolar disorder, whether refractory or not, is complex, and requires careful attention to the therapeutic alliance.

REFERENCES

American Psychological Association. (1980). *Diagnostic and statistical manual of mental disorders* (3rd ed.). Washington, DC: Author.

American Psychological Association. (1994). *Diagnostic and statistical manual of mental disorders* (4th ed.). Washington, DC: Author.

Aronson, T. A., Shukla, S., & Hirschowitz, J. (1989). Clonazepam treatment of five lithium-refractory patients with bipolar disorder. *American Journal of Psychiatry, 146*, 77–80.

Baastrup, P. C., Poulsen, J. C., Schou, M., Thomsen, K., & Amdisen, A. (1970). Prophylactic lithium: Double blind discontinuation in manic-depressive and recurrent-depressive disorders. *Lancet, 7668,* 326–330.

Ballenger, J. C., & Post, R. M. (1978). Therapeutic effects of carbamazepine in affective illness: A preliminary report. *Community Psychopharmacology, 2,* 159–175.

Banov, M. D., Zarate, C. A., Jr., Tohen, M., Scialabba, D., Wines, J. D., Jr., Kolbrener, M., Kim, J., & Cole, J. O. (1994). Clozapine therapy in refractory affective disorders: Polarity predicts response in long-term follow-up. *Journal of Clinical Psychiatry, 55*(7), 295–300.

Bauer, M. S., Kurtz, J., Winokur, A., Phillips, J., Rubin, L. B., & Marcus, J. G. (1993). Thyroid function before and after four-week light treatment in winter depressives and controls. *Psychoneuroendocrinology, 18*(5–6), 437–443.

Bauer, M. S., & Whybrow, P. (1990). Rapid cycling bipolar affective disorder: II. Treatment of refractory rapid cycling with high-dose levothyroxine: A preliminary study. *Archives of General Psychiatry, 47,* 435–440.

Baumhackl, U., Biziere, K., Fischbach, M., Geretstegger, C. H., Hebenstreit, G., Radmayr, E., & Stabl, M. (1989). Efficacy and tolerability of meclobemide compared with imipramine in depressive disorder (DSM III): An Austrian double-blind, multicentre study. *British Journal of Psychiatry, 155*(Suppl.), 78–83.

Black, D. W., Winokur, G., & Nasrallah, A. (1987). Treatment of mania: A naturalistic study of electroconvulsive therapy versus lithium in 438 patients. *Journal of Clinical Psychiatry, 48,* 132–139.

Bowden, C., Brugger, A., Swann, A., Calabrese, J., Janicak, R., Petty, F., Dilsaver, S., Davis, J., Rush, A., Small, J., Garza-Tevino, E., Risch, C., Goodnick, P., & Morris, D. (1994). Efficacy of divalproex vs. lithium and placebo in the treatment of mania. *Journal of the American Medical Association, 271,* 918–924.

Bradwejn, J., Shriqui, C., Koszycki, D., & Meterissian, G. (1990). Double-blind comparison of the effects of clonazepam and lorazepam in mania. *Journal of Clinical Psychopharmacology, 10,* 403–408.

Brennan, M., Sandyk, R., & Borsook, D. (1984). Use of sodium valproate in the management of affective disorders: Basic and clinical aspects. In H. M. Emrich, T. Okuma, & A. A. Muller (Eds.), *Anticonvulsants in affective disorders* (pp. 56–65). Amsterdam: Elsevier.

Brown, R. (1989). U.S. experience with valproate in manic depressive illness: A multicenter trial. *Journal of Clinical Psychopharmacology, 50*(Suppl.), 13–16.

Calabrese, J. R., & Delucchi, G. A. (1990). Spectrum of efficacy of valproate in 55 patients with rapid-cycling bipolar disorder. *American Journal of Psychiatry, 147*(4), 431–434.

Calabrese, J. R., Woyshville, M. J., Kimmel, S. E., & Rapport, D. J. (1993). Predictors of valproate response in bipolar rapid cycling. *Journal of Clinical Psychopharmacology, 13*(4), 280–283.

Carman, J. S., Post, R. M., Runkle, D. C., Bunney, W. E., & Wyatt, R. J. (1979). Increased serum calcium and phosphorus with the 'switch' into manic or excited psychotic states. *British Journal of Psychiatry, 135,* 55–61.

Cho, J. T., Bone, S., Dunner, D. L., Colt, E., & Fieve, R. R. (1979). The effect of lithium treatment on thyroid function in patients with primary affective disorder. *American Journal of Psychiatry, 136,* 115–116.

Chouinard, G., Young, S. N., & Annable, L. (1983). Antimanic effect of clonazepam. *Biological Psychiatry, 18,* 451–466.

Cohen, B. M., Lipinski, J. F., & Altesman, R. I. (1982). Lecithin in the treatment of mania: Double blind, placebo-controlled trials. *American Journal of Psychiatry, 139*(9), 1162–1164.

Cohn, J. B., Collins, G., Ashbrook, E., & Wernicke, J. F. (1989). A comparison of fluoxetine, imipramine and placebo in patients with bipolar depressive disorder. *International Clinical Psychopharmacology, 4,* 313–322.

Cookson, J. C. (1987). Carbamazepine in acute mania: A practical view. *International Clinical Psychopharmacology, 2,* 11–22.

Coppen, A., Noguera, R., Bailey, J., Burns, B., Swani, M., Hare, E., Gardner, R., & Maggs, R. (1971). Prophylactic lithium in affective disorders. *Lancet, 7719,* 275–279.

Cowdry, R., Wehr, T., Zis, A., & Goodwin, F. (1983). Thyroid abnormalities associated with rapid-cycling bipolar illness. *Archives of General Psychiatry, 40,* 414–420.

Coxhead, N., Silverstone, T., & Cookson, J. (1992). Carbamazepine versus lithium in the prophylaxis of bipolar affective disorder. *Acta Psychiatrica Scandinavica, 85,* 114–118.

Cundall, R. L., Brooks, P. W., & Murray, L. G. (1972). A controlled evaluation of lithium prophylaxis in affective disorders. *Psychological Medicine, 2,* 308–311.

Deister, A., & Mameros, A. (1993). Predicting the long-term outcome of affective disorders. *Acta Psychiatrica Scandinavica, 88,* 174–177.

Dilsaver, S. C., Swann, A. C., Shoaib, A. M., Bowers, T. C., & Halle, M. T. (1993). Depressive mania associated with nonresponse to antimanic agents. *American Journal of Psychiatry, 150*(10), 1548–1551.

Dubovsky, S., Franks, R., Allen, S., & Murphy, J. (1986). Calcium antagonists in mania: A double-blind study of verapamil. *Psychiatry Research, 18,* 309–320.

Dubovsky, S., Lee, C., Christiano, J., & Murphy, J. (1991). Elevated platelet intracellular calcium concentration in bipolar depression. *Biological Psychiatry, 29,* 441–450.

Dunner, D. L., & Fieve, R. (1974). Clinical factors in lithium carbonate prophylaxis failure. *Archives of General Psychiatry, 30,* 229–233.

Dunner, D. L., Stallone, F., & Fieve, R. R. (1976). Lithium carbonate and affective disorders. *Archives of General Psychiatry, 33,* 117.

Dwight, M. M., Keck, P. E., Jr., Stanton, S. P., Strakowski, S. M., & McElroy, S. L. (1994). Antidepressant activity and mania associated with risperidone treatment of schizoaffective disorder. *Lancet, 344,* 554–555.

Emrich, H. M., Dose, M., Gunther, R., & Von Zerssen, D. (1985). The use of valproate and oxcarbazepine in affective disorders. In P. Pichot, P. Berner, R. Wolf, & K. Thau (Eds.), *Psychiatry: The state of the art* (pp. 455–458). New York: Plenum Press.

Emrich, H. M., Okuma, T., & Muller, A. A. (Eds.). (1984). *Anticonvulsants in affective disorders.* Amsterdam: Elsevier.

Emrich, H. M., Von Zerssen, D., Kissling, W., Moller, H. J., & Windorfer, A. (1980). Effect of sodium valproate on mania: The GABA-hypothesis of affective disorder. *Archiv für Psychiatrie und Nervenkrankheiten, 229,* 1–16.

Esparon, J., Kolloori, J., Naylor, G. J., McHarg, A. M., Smith, A. H. W., & Hopwood, S. E. (1986). Comparison of the prophylactic action of flupenthixol with placebo in lithium treated manic–depressive patients. *British Journal of Psychiatry, 148,* 723–725.

Faedda, G. L., Baldessarini, R. J., Tohen, M., Strakowski, S. M., & Waternaux, C. (1991). Episode sequence in bipolar disorder and response to lithium treatment. *American Journal of Psychiatry, 148*, 1237–1239.

Fieve, R. R., Kumbaraci, T., & Dunner, D. L. (1976). Lithium prophylaxis of depression in bipolar I, bipolar II, and unipolar patients. *American Journal of Psychiatry, 133*(8), 925–929.

Fogelson, D., Bystritsky, A., & Pasnau, R. (1992). Bupropion in the treatment of bipolar disorders: The same old story. *Journal of Clinical Psychiatry, 53*(12), 443.

Frankenburg, F. R. (1993). Clozapine and bipolar disorder. *Journal of Clinical Psychopharmocology, 13*(4), 289–290.

Freeman, T. W., Clothier, J. L., Pazzaglia, P., Lesem, M. D., & Swann, A. C. (1992). A double-blind comparison of valproate and lithium in the treatment of acute mania. *American Journal of Psychiatry, 149*, 108–111.

Gelenberg, A. J., Kane, J. M., Keller, M. B., Lavori, P., Rosenbaum, J. F., Cole, K., & Lavelle, J. (1989). Comparison of standard and low serum levels of lithium for maintenance treatment of bipolar depression. *New England Journal of Medicine, 321*(22), 1489–1493.

Ghaemi, S. N., Pope, H. G., & Stoll, A. L. (1995). Lack of insight in bipolar disorder. *Journal of Nervous and Mental Disease, 183*, 464–467.

Ghaemi, S. N., Sachs, G. S., Baldassano, C. F., & Truman, C. J. (1995b). *Management of bipolar disorder with adjunctive risperidone.* Abstract presented at the 148th Annual Meeting of the American Psychiatric Association, Miami, FL.

Giannini, A. J., Houser, W. L., Loiselle, R. H., Giannini, M. C., & Price, W. A. (1984). Antimanic effects of verapamil. *American Journal of Psychiatry, 141*, 1602–1603.

Giannini, A. J., Luiselle, R. H., Price, W. A., & Giannini, M. C. (1985). Comparison of antimanic efficacy of clonidine and verapamil. *Journal of Clinical Pharmacology, 25*, 307–308.

Gillberg, I. C., Hellgren, L., & Gillberg, C. (1993). Psychotic disorders diagnosed in adolescence: Outcome at age 30 years. *Journal of Child Psychology and Psychiatry, 34*(7), 1173–1185.

Goodwin, F. K., & Jamison, K. R. (1990). *Manic depressive illness.* New York: Oxford University Press.

Goodwin, G. M. (1994). Recurrence of mania after lithium withdrawal: Implications for the use of lithium in the treatment of bipolar affective disorder. *British Journal of Psychiatry, 164*, 149–152.

Grossi, E., Sacchetti, E., Vita, A., Conte, G., Faravelli, C., Hautman, G., Zerbi, D., Mesina, A. M., Drago, F., & Motta, A. (1984). Carbamazepine vs. chlorpromamazine in mania: A double-blind trial. In H. M. Emrich, T. Okuma, & A. A. Muller (Eds.), *Anticonvulsants in affective ddisorders* (pp. 177–187). Amsterdam: Elsevier.

Hamilton, M. (1960). A rating scale for depression. *Journal of Neurology, Neurosurgery and Psychiatry, 23*, 56–62.

Hardy, M., Lecrubier, Y., & Witlocher, D. (1986). Efficacy of clonidine in 24 patients with acute mania. *American Journal of Psychiatry, 143*(11), 1450–1453.

Harrow, M., Goldberg, J. F., Grossman, L. S., & Meltzer, H. Y. (1990). Outcome in manic disorders. *Archives of General Psychiatry, 47*, 665–671.

Hayes, S. G. (1989). Long-term use of valproate in primary psychiatric disorders. *Journal of Clinical Psychiatry, 50*(Suppl.), 35–39.

Himmelhoch, J. M., & Garfinkel, M. E. (1986). Sources of lithium resistance in mixed mania. *Psychopharmacology Bulletin, 22*(3), 613–620.

Himmelhoch, J. M., Mulla, D., Neil, J. F., Detre, T. P., & Kupfer, D. J. (1976). Incidence and significance of mixed affective states in a bipolar population. *Archives of General Psychiatry, 33,* 1062–1066.

Himmelhoch, J. M., Thase, M. E., Mallinger, A. G., & Houck, P. (1991). Tranylcypromine versus imipramine in anergic bipolar depression. *American Journal of Psychiatry, 148*(7), 910–916.

Janowsky, D. S., El-Yousef, M. K., Davis, J. M., & Sekereke, H. J. (1972). A cholinergic–adrenergic hypothesis of mania and depression. *Lancet, 7778,* 632–635.

Jouvent, R., Lecrubier, Y., Puech, A. J., Simon, P., & Witlocher, D. (1980). Antimanic effect of clonidine. *American Journal of Psychiatry, 137*(10), 1275–1276.

Joyce, P. R. (1991). The prognostic significance of thyroid function in mania. *Journal of Psychiatric Research, 25,* 1–6.

Kanas, N. (1993). Group psychotherapy with bipolar patients: A review and synthesis. *International Journal of Group Psychotherapy, 43*(3), 321–333.

Kando, J. C., Tohen, M., Castillo, J., & Centorrino, F. (1994). Concurrent use of clozapine and valproate in affective and psychotic disorders. *Journal of Clinical Psychiatry, 55,* 255–257.

Kay, D. S. G., Naylor, G. J., Smith, A. H., & Greenwood, C. (1984). The therapeutic effect of ascorbic acid and EDTA in manic–depressive psychosis: Double-blind comparisons with standard treatments. *Psychological Medicine, 14,* 533–539.

Keck, P. E., McElroy, S. L., Vuckovic, A., & Friedman, L. M. (1992). Combined valproate and carbamazepine treatment of bipolar disorder. *Journal of Neuropsychiatry and Clinical Neurosciences, 4,* 319–322.

Keller, M., Lavori, P., Coryell, W., Andreasen, N., Endicott, J., Clayton, P., Klerman, G., & Hirschfeld, R. (1986). Differential outcome of pure manic, mixed/cycling, and pure depressive episodes in patients with bipolar illness. *Journal of the American Medical Association, 255,* 3138–3142.

Kennedy, S., Ozevsky, S., & Robillard, M. (1986). Refractory bipolar illness may not repond to verapamil [Letter]. *Journal of Clinical Psychopharmacology, 6*(5), 316–317.

Kesterson, J. W., Granneman, G. R., & Machinist, J. M. (1984). The hepatotoxicity of valproic acid and its metabolites in rats. *Hepatology, 4,* 1143–1152.

Ketter, T. A., Pazzaglia, P. J., & Post, R. M. (1992). Synergy of carbamazepine and valproic acid in affective illness: Case report and review of the literature. *Journal of Clinical Psychopharmacology, 12*(4), 276–281.

Kishimoto, A., Kamata, K., Sughira, T., Ishiguro, S., Hazama, K., Mizukawa, R., & Kunimoto, N. (1988). Treatment of depression with clonazepam. *Acta Psychiatrica Scandinavica, 77,* 81–86.

Klein, E., Bental, E., Lerer, B., & Belmaker, R. H. (1984). Carbamazepine and haloperidol versus placebo and haloperidol in excited psychoses: A controlled study. *Archives of General Psychiatry, 41,* 165–170.

Kraepelin, E. (1921). *Manic–depressive insanity and paranoia* (R. M. Barclay, Trans.). Edinburgh: E & S Livingstone.

Kramlinger, K. G., & Post, R. M. (1989). The addition of lithium carbonate to carbamazepine: Antimanic efficacy in treatment-resistant mania. *Archives of General Psychiatry, 35,* 794–800.

Kukopulos, A., Reginaldi, P., Laddomada, G., Floris, G., Serra, G., & Tondo, L. (1980). Course of the manic–depressive cycle and changes caused by treatments. *Pharmakopsychiatria, 13,* 156–167.

Lambert, P. A. (1984). Acute and prophylactic therapies of patients with affective disorders using valproate. In H. M. Emrich, T. Okuma, & A. A. Muller (Eds.), *Anticonvulsants in affective disorders* (pp. 33–44). Amsterdam: Elsevier.

Lambert, P. A., Carraz, G., Borselli, S., & Bouchardy, M. (1975). Dipropylacetamide in the treatment of manic–depressive psychosis. *Encephale, 1,* 25–31.

Lambert, P. A., & Venand, G. (1987). The use of valpromide in psychiatry. *L'Encephale, 13,* 367–373.

Lerer, B., Moore, N., Meyendorff, E., Cho, S. R., & Gershon, S. (1987). Carbamazepine versus lithium in mania: A double-blind study. *Journal of Clinical Psychiatry, 48,* 88–93.

Lesser, A. L. (1983). Hypomania and marital conflict. *Canadian Journal of Psychiatry, 28,* 362–366.

Levy, A. B., Drake, M. E., & Shy, K. E. (1988). EEG evidence of epileptiform paroxysms in rapid-cycling bipolar patients. *Journal of Clinical Psychiatry, 49,* 802–803.

Lish, J. D., Dime-Meenan, S., Whybrow, P. C., Price, R. A., & Hirschfeld, R. M. (1994). The national depressive and manic-depressive association (DMDA) survey of bipolar members. *Journal of Affective Disorders, 31,* 281–294.

Lusznat, R. M., Murphy, D. P., & Nunn, C. M. H. (1988). Carbamazepine vs. lithium in the treatment and prophylaxis of mania. *British Journal of Psychiatry, 153,* 198–204.

Mander, A. J. (1986). Clinical prediction of outcome and lithium response in bipolar affective disorder. *Journal of Affective Disorders, 11,* 35–41.

Markar, H. R., & Mander, A. J. (1989). Efficacy of lithium prophylaxis in clinical practice. *British Journal of Psychiatry, 155,* 496–500.

Mayo, J. A., O'Connell, R. A., & O'Brien, J. D. (1979). Families of manic–depressive patients: Effect of treatment. *American Journal of Psychiatry, 136*(12), 1525–1529.

McCabe, M. S., & Norris, B. (1977). ECT versus chlorpromazine in mania. *Biological Psychiatry, 12,* 245–254.

McElroy, S. L., Keck, P. E. J., & Hudson, J. I. (1988). Valproate in the treatment of rapid cycling bipolar disorder. *Journal of Clinical Psychopharmacology, 8,* 275–279.

Melia, P. I. (1970). Prophylactic lithium: A double-blind trial in recurrent affective disorders. *British Journal of Psychiatry, 116,* 621–624.

Meltzer, H. L. (1986). Lithium mechanisms in bipolar illness and altered intracellular calcium functions. *Biological Psychiatry, 21,* 492–510.

Miklowitz, D., Goldstein, M., Nuechterlein, K., Snyder, K., & Mintz, J. (1988). Family factors and the course of bipolar affective disorder. *Archives of General Psychiatry, 45,* 225–231.

Moller, M. J., Kissling, W., Riehl, T., Bauml, J., Binz, U., & Wendt, G. (1989). Double-blind evaluation of the antimanic properties of carbamazepine as a comedication to haloperidol. *Progress in Neuropsychopharmacological and Biological Psychiatry, 13,* 127–136.

Monroe, R. R. (1991). Maintenance electroconvulsive therapy. *Electroconvulsive Therapy, 14,* 947–960.

Mukherjee, S., Sackeim, H. A., & Schnur, D. B. (1994). Electroconvulsive therapy of acute manic episodes: A review of 50 years' experience. *American Journal of Psychiatry, 151*(2), 169–176.

Muller, A. A., & Stoll, K. D. (1984). Carbamazepine and oxycarbazepine in the treatment of manic syndromes: Studies in Germany. In H. M. Emrich, T. Okuma, & A. A. Muller (Eds.), *Anticonvulsants in affective disorders* (pp. 139–147). Amsterdam: Elsevier.

Naylor, G. J., Martin, B., Hopwood, S. E., & Watson, Y. (1986). A two-year double-blind crossover trial of the prophylactic effect of methylene blue in manic–depressive psychosis. *Biological Psychiatry, 21,* 915–920.

Okuma, T., Inanaga, K., Otsuki, S., Sarai, K., Takahashi, R., Hazama, H., Mori, A., & Watanabe, M. (1979). Comparison of the antimanic efficacy of carbamazepine and chlorpromazine: A double-blind controlled study. *Psychopharmacology* (Berlin), *66,* 211–217.

Okuma, T., Inanaga, K., Otsuki, S., Sarai, K., Takahashi, R., Hazama, H., Mori, A., & Watanabe, M. (1981). A preliminary double-blind study on the efficacy of carbamazepine in prophylaxis of manic–depressive illness. *Psychopharmacology* (Berlin), *73,* 95–96.

Okuma, T. (1983). Therapeutic and prophylactic effects of carbamazepine in bipolar disorders. *Psychiatric Clinics of North America, 6,* 157–173.

Okuma, T., Yamashita, I., Takahashi, R., Itoh, H., Kurihara, M., Otsuki, S., Watanabe, M., Sarai, K., Hazama, H., & Inanaga, K. (1989). Clinical efficacy of carbamazepine in affective, schizoaffective, and schizophrenic disorders. *Pharmacopsychiatry, 22,* 47–53.

Patsalos, R. S., Stephenson, T. J., Krishna, S., Elyas, A. A., Laselles, P. T., & Wiles, C. M. (1985). Side effects induced by carbamazepine 10,11 epoxide [Letter]. *Lancet, ii,* 496.

Placidi, G. F., Lenzi, A., Lazzerini, F., Cassano, G. B., & Akiskal, H. S. (1986). The comparative efficacy and safety of carbamazepine versus lithium: A randomized, double-blind 3-year trial in 83 patients. *Journal of Clinical Psychiatry, 47,* 490–494.

Pope, J. G., McElroy, S. L., Keck, P. E., & Hudson, J. I. (1991). Valproate in the treatment of acute mania. *Archives of General Psychiatry, 48*(1), 62–68.

Post, R. M. (1990). Alternatives to lithium for bipolar affective illness. In A. Tasman, S. M. Goldfinger, & C. A. Kaufman (Eds.), *Review of psychiatry* (pp. 170–199). Washington, DC: American Psychiatric Press.

Post, R. M., Leverich, G. S., Altshuler, L., & Mikalauskas, K. (1992). Lithium discontinuation-induced refractoriness: Preliminary observations. *American Journal of Psychiatry, 149,* 1727–7129.

Post, R. M., Rubinow, D. R., Uhde, T. W., Roy-Byrne, P. P., Linnoila, M., Rosoff, A., & Cowdry, R. (1989). Dysphoric mania: Clinical and biological correlates. *Archives of General Psychiatry, 46,* 353–358.

Post, R. M., & Uhde, T. (1987). Clinical approaches to treatment-resistant bipolar illness. In R. Hales & A. Frances (Eds.), *APA annual review* (pp. 125–150). Washington, DC: American Psychiatric Press.

Post, R. M., Uhde, T. W., & Ballenger, J. (1984). The efficacy of carbamazepine in affective illness. In E. Usdin (Ed.), *Frontiers in biochemical and pharacological research in depression* (pp. 421–437). New York: Raven Press.

Poynton, A., Bridges, P. K., & Bartlett, J. R. (1988). Resistant bipolar affective disorder treated by stereotactic subcaudate tractotomy. *British Journal of Psychiatry, 152,* 354–358.

Prasad, A. J. (1984). The role of sodium valproate as an anti-manic agent. *Pharmacotherapeutica*, 4(1), 6–8.

Priebe, S., Wildgrube, C., & Müller-Oerlinghausen, B. (1989). Lithium prophylaxis and expressed emotion. *British Journal of Psychiatry*, 154, 396–399.

Prien, R. F., Klett, C. J., & Caffey, E. M. (1973). Lithium carbonate and imipramine in prevention of affective episodes. *Archives of General Psychiatry*, 29, 420–425.

Prien, R. F., Klett, C. J., & Caffey, E. M. (1974). Lithium prophylaxis in recurrent affective illness. *American Journal of Psychiatry*, 131(2), 198–203.

Prien, R. F., Kupfer, D., Mansky, P., Small, J., Tuason, V., Voss, C., & Johnson, W. (1984). Drug therapy in the prevention of recurrences in unipolar and bipolar affective disorders. *Archives of General Psychiatry*, 41, 1096–1104.

Prien, R. F., & Potter, W. Z. (1990). NIMH workshop report on treatment of bipolar disorder. *Psychopharmacology Bulletin*, 26(4), 409–427.

Quitkin, F. M., Kane, J., Rifkin, A., Ramos-Lorenzi, J. R., & Nayak, D. V. (1981a). Prophylactic lithium carbonate with and without imipramine for bipolar I patients. *Archives of General Psychiatry*, 38, 902–907.

Quitkin, F. M., McGrath, P., Liebowitz, M. R., Stewart, J., & Howard, A. (1981b). Monoamine oxidase inhibitors in bipolar endogenous depressives. *Journal of Clinical Psychopharmacology*, 1, 70–74.

Rosenbaum, J., Sachs, G., Kane, J., Keller, M., & Gelenberg, A. (1992). *High rates of relapse in bipolar patients abruptly changed from standard to low plasma lithium levels in a double-blind controlled trial*. Paper presented at the meeting of the New Clinical Drug Evaluation Unit, Boca Raton, FL.

Sachs, G. S. (1989). Adjuncts and alternatives to lithium therapy for bipolar affective disorder. *Journal of Clinical Psychiatry*, 50(12, Suppl.), 31–39.

Sachs, G. S. (1990). Use of clonazepam for bipolar affective disorder. *Journal of Clinical Psychiatry*, 51(5, Suppl.), 31–34.

Sachs, G. S. (1995a). [Unpublished raw data.]

Sachs, G. S. (1995b). [Unpublished raw data.]

Sachs, G. S., Lafer, B., Stoll, A. L., Banov, M., Thibault, A. B., Tohen, M., & Rosenbaum, J. F. (1994a). A double-blind trial of bupropion versus desipramine for bipolar depression. *Journal of Clinical Psychiatry*, 55(9), 391–393.

Sachs, G. S., Lafer, B., Truman, C. J., Noeth, M., & Thibault, A. B. (1994b). Lithium monotherapy: Miracle, myth and misunderstanding. *Psychiatric Annals*, 24(6), 299–306.

Schaff, M. R., Fawcett, J., & Zajecka, J. M. (1993). Divalproex sodium in the treatment of refractory affective disorders. *Journal of Clinical Psychiatry*, 54(10), 380–384.

Schnur, D. B., Mukherjee, S., Sackheim, H. A., Lee, C., & Roth, S. D. (1992). Symptomatic predictors of ECT response in medication-nonresponsive manic patients. *Journal of Clinical Psychiatry*, 53, 63–66.

Secunda, S. K., Swann, A., Katz, M. M., Koslow, S. H., Croughan, J., & Chang, S. (1987). Diagnosis and treatment of mixed mania. *American Journal of Psychiatry*, 144, 96–98.

Semadeni, G. W. (1976). Clinical study of the nomothymic effect of dipropylacetamide. *Acta Psychiatrica Belgica*, 76(3), 458–466.

Small, J. G., Klapper, M. H., Milstein, V., Kellams, J. J., Miller, M. J., Marhenke, J. D., & Small, I. F. (1991). Carbamazepine compared with lithium in the treatment of mania. *Archives of General Psychiatry*, 48, 915–921.

Small, J. G., Small, I. F., Milstein, V., Kellams, J. J., & Klapper, M. H. (1985). Manic symptoms: An indication for bilateral ECT. *Biological Psychiatry, 20,* 125–134.

Sovner, R. (1989). The use of valproate in the treatment of mentally retarded persons. *Journal of Clinical Psychiatry, 50*(Suppl.), 40–43.

Stancer, H. C., & Persad, E. (1982). Treatment of intractable rapid-cycling manic-depressive disorder with levothyroxine. *Archives of General Psychiatry, 39,* 311–312.

Stoll, A. L., Sachs, G. S., Cohen, B. M., Lafer, B., & Renshaw, P. F. (1994). *Choline and lithium interactions in rapid-cycling bipolar disorder.* Paper presented at the 33rd Annual Meeting of the American College of Neuropsychopharmacology, San Juan, PR.

Suppes, T., Baldessarini, R. J., Faedda, G. L., & Tohen, M. (1991). Risk of reoccurrence following discontinuation of lithium treatment in bipolar disorder. *Archives of General Psychiatry, 48,* 1082–1088.

Suppes, T., McElroy, S. L., Gilbert, J., Dessain, E. C., & Cole, J. O. (1992). Clozapine in the treatment of dysphoric mania. *Biological Psychiatry, 32*(3), 270–280.

Symonds, R., & Williams, P. (1981). Lithium and the changing incidence of mania. *Psychological Medicine, 11,* 193–196.

Thibault, A., Sachs, G. S., Lafer, B., Kokoletsky, J., & Rosenbaum, J. (1993). *Bipolar relapse rates during maintenance therapy.* Abstract Presented at the 146th Annual Meeting of the American Psychiatric Association, San Francisco.

Thomas, J., & Reddy, B. (1982). The treatment of mania: A retrospective evaluation of the effects of ECT, chlorpromazine and lithium. *Journal of Affective Disorders, 4,* 85–92.

Tohen, M., Castillo, J., Pope, H. G., & Herbstein, J. (1994a). Concomitant use of valproate and carbamazepine in bipolar and schizoaffective disorders. *Journal of Clinical Psychopharmacology, 14,* 67–70.

Tohen, M., Waternaux, C. M., & Tsuang, M. (1990). Outcome in mania: A 4-year prospective follow-up of 75 patients utilizing survival analysis. *Archives of General Psychiatry, 47,* 1106–1111.

Tohen, M., Zarate, C. A., Jr., Centorrino, F., Froeschl, M., Weiss, M., & Baldessarini, R. J. (1994b). *Risperidone in the treatment of mania.* Paper presented at the 33rd Annual Meeting of the American College of Neuropsychopharmacology, San Juan, PR.

Van Gent, E. M., Vida, S. L., & Zwart, F. M. (1988). Group therapy in addition to lithium therapy in patients with bipolar disorders. *Acta Psychiatrica Belgica, 88,* 405–418.

Vasile, R. G., Samson, J. A., Bemporad, J., Bloomindale, K. L., Creasey, D., Fenton, B. T., Gudeman, J. E., & Schildkraut, J. J. (1987). A biopsychosocial approach to treating patients with affective disorders. *American Journal of Psychiatry, 144*(3), 341–344.

Watkins, S. E., Callender, K., Thomas, D. R., Tidmarsh, S. F., & Shaw, D. M. (1987). The effect of carbamazepine and lithium on remission from affective illness. *British Journal of Psychiatry, 150,* 180–182.

Wehr, T. A., & Goodwin, F. K. (1979). Rapid cycling in manic–depressives induced by tricyclic antidepressants. *Archives of General Psychiatry, 36,* 555–559.

Wehr, T. A., Sack, D. A., Rosenthal, N. E., & Cowdry, R. W. (1988). Rapid cycling affective disorder: Contributing factors and treatment responses in 51 patients. *American Journal of Psychiatry, 145*(2), 179–184.

Wozniak, J., Biederman, J., Kiely, K., Ablon, S., Faraone, S. E., Mundy, E., & Mennin, D. (1995). Manic-like symptoms suggestive of childhood-onset bipolar disorder in clinically-referred children. *Journal of the American Academy of Child and Adolescent Psychiatry, 34,* 867–876.

Young, R. C., Biggs, J. T., Ziegler, V. E., & Meyer, D. A. (1978). A rating scale for mania: Reliability, validity, and sensitivity. *British Journal of Psychiatry, 133,* 429–435.

Zornberg, G. L., & Pope, H. G. (1993). Treatment of depression in bipolar disorder: New directions for research. *Journal of Clinical Psychopharmacology, 13,* 397–408.

Zubenko, G. S., Cohen, B. M., Lipinski, J. F., & Jonas, J. M. (1984). Clonidine in the treatment of mania and mixed bipolar disorder. *American Journal of Psychiatry, 141*(12), 1617–1618.

II

ANXIETY DISORDERS

4

Pharmacologic Approaches to Treatment-Resistant Panic Disorder

MARK H. POLLACK
JORDAN W. SMOLLER

Although a substantial body of clinical trial data and accumulating clinical experience demonstrate the efficacy of pharmacologic treatments for panic disorder, a substantial proportion of patients with this disorder respond either incompletely or not at all to acute treatment. Follow-up studies of treated patients and longitudinal observations of naturalistically treated patients suggest that many such patients improve but remain somewhat symptomatic, and that some remain significantly impaired over time (Pollack & Otto, 1994). In this chapter, we review diagnostic issues and contributing factors in the acute and long-term response to treatment of panic disorder, and suggest pharmacotherapeutic strategies to improve treatment outcome.

DIAGNOSTIC ISSUES

Panic disorder, as defined in the DSM-IV (American Psychiatric Association, 1994), is characterized by recurrent episodes of panic attacks involving stereotypic physical and affective symptoms, as well as anticipatory anxiety. The disorder is often complicated by phobic anxiety or avoidance of situations in which panic attacks previously occurred or from which ready escape may be difficult or help unavailable.

The lifetime prevalence of panic disorder in the general population is

3.5%, as reported by the National Comorbidity Survey (Kessler et al., 1994). Panic disorder occurs twice as often in women as in men, and tends to have its onset in the late third or early fourth decade of life; however, many patients report significant anxiety difficulties dating back to child-hood. Though many patients report a significant life event occurring in the year preceding the onset of panic disorder (Roy-Byrne, Geraci, & Uhde, 1986), the disorder usually persists even after the acute situation has resolved. Some patients note the onset of panic attacks in conjunction with a physiologic stressor, such as use of cocaine, marijuana or alcohol, or associated with medical illness; however, in these cases as well, the dis-order persists after the acute effects of these precipitants have dissipated.

Although panic attacks themselves are common in the general popu-lation, and may occur in up to a third of the population in a given year (Norton, Harrison, Hauch, & Rhodes, 1985), relatively few people go on to develop the full-blown disorder. This suggests that certain physiologic or cognitive-behavioral characteristics may make affected individuals vul-nerable to ongoing difficulties with panic. An underlying diathesis, or con-stitutional vulnerability to anxiety (probably familial and often first expressed in childhood), may be triggered by psychosocial or physical stres-sors or may emerge spontaneously; once triggered, this anxiety predisposi-tion may be variably manifested across the individual's life cycle (Rosenbaum et al., 1993). Treatment of the panic disorder patient is aimed at correct-ing or compensating for disturbed physiologic mechanisms and overcom-ing cognitive-behavioral aspects that may contribute to ongoing anxiety difficulties.

OUTCOME OF PHARMACOTHERAPEUTIC TREATMENT OF PANIC DISORDER

A number of pharmacologic agents have demonstrated acute and long-term efficacy in the treatment of panic disorder. These agents include an-tidepressants, such as tricyclic antidepressants (TCAs), selective seroto-nin reuptake inhibitors (SSRIs), and monoamine oxidase inhibitors (MAOIs); they also include the high-potency benzodiazepines (HPBs), such as alprazolam and clonazepam. Although the majority of patients improve with pharmacologic treatment, many continue to experience anxiety-related difficulties both acutely and over the long term. Controlled treatment trials with TCAs and HPBs suggest acute panic-free rates of 50–70% (Ballenger et al., 1988; Cross-National Collaborative Panic Study, 1992; Nagy, Krystal, Charney, Merikangas, & Woods, 1993; Nagy, Krystal, Woods, & Char-ney, 1989). In a large-scale placebo-controlled treatment trial with alprazo-lam, the Cross-National Collaborative Panic Study, 50% of patients were panic-free and 30% in remission after 4 weeks of treatment (Ballenger et al., 1988); similar findings were reported in another acute treatment study of the HPBs alprazolam and clonazepam (Tesar et al., 1991).

Follow-up studies of panic patients at 1–5 years after initiation of treatment with antidepressants or HPBs demonstrate that 40–90% of patients remain at least somewhat symptomatic (Nagy et al., 1989, 1993; Noyes, Garvey, & Cook, 1989; Pollack et al., 1993). Most patients remain on medication during a substantial proportion of the follow-up period. In a follow-up study of panic patients participating in a large multinational trial of alprazolam, Katschnig, Stolk, and Klerman (1989) reported that approximately 30% of patients were in remission 5 years after initiation of treatment, 50% had mild to moderate levels of symptomatology, and 20% had persistent severe symptoms over the follow-up period; over half the patients were on medication at follow-up, and 25% had been on medication continuously since the onset of treatment. Continued symptomatology despite improvement with treatment is more common than complete remission for pharmacologically treated panic disorder patients.

In summary, controlled studies of antidepressants and HPBs for panic disorder suggest that many patients, though improved, remain symptomatic at the end of an acute treatment trial, and that most remain somewhat symptomatic at follow-up. We now turn our attention to patient factors that may contribute to this relatively high rate of relative or absolute treatment refractoriness, and consider pharmacologic factors and treatment strategies that may improve outcome.

PATIENT FACTORS IN TREATMENT RESISTANCE

Table 4.1 summarizes the patient factors that can contribute to treatment resistance.

TABLE 4.1. Patient Factors Contributing to Treatment Resistance

- Comorbid psychiatric conditions
  Mood disorders
    Depression
    Bipolar disorder

  Anxiety disorders
    Social phobia
    Generalized anxiety disorder
    Obsessive–compulsive disorder
    Posttraumatic stress disorder

  Alcohol and substance abuse

  Personality disorders, psychosocial distress, and family dynamics

- Medical factors
    Conditions causing anxiety (e.g., hyperthyroidism, chronic obstructive pulmonary disease)
    Medications or other substances causing anxiety (e.g., bronchodilators, caffeine)
    Conditions mimicking or provoking anxiety (e.g., palpitations)

Comorbid Psychiatric Conditions

Comorbid mood, anxiety, and substance abuse disorders are common in panic patients. Although most controlled treatment trials exclude patients with significant comorbidity, this practice selects for a rarefied patient population that may not necessarily reflect the type of patients seen in general clinical practice. Comorbid anxiety disorders (Pollack, Otto, Sabatino, & Rosenbaum, 1994b), including social phobia, generalized anxiety disorder (GAD), and posttraumatic stress disorder (PTSD), as well as comorbid depression (Breier, Charney, & Heninger, 1984) and substance abuse (Helzer & Pryzbeck, 1988; Otto, Pollack, Sachs, O'Neil, & Rosenbaum, 1992b), worsen acute and long-term response to treatment in panic disorder patients. Effective antipanic pharmacotherapy targeted at the comorbid condition as well as at panic may enhance overall treatment outcome. For example, panic patients with comorbid social phobia may experience more comprehensive improvement during treatment with an MAOI, SSRI, or HPB than with a TCA (Liebowitz et al., 1992). Table 4.2 outlines possible treatment interventions for a variety of comorbid conditions.

Comorbid Depression

Approximately two-thirds of panic disorder patients have a lifetime history of major depression or other depressive syndromes such as dysthymia (Breier et al., 1984; Klerman et al., 1991); for many, the depressive symptoms are chronic or recurrent and represent a considerable source of ongoing distress. Attempts to establish a primary–secondary distinction regarding the depression and panic symptoms, based on temporal sequence or severity, are often difficult and of unclear clinical significance. Although a controlled trial examining the differential efficacy of the TCA imipramine and the HPB alprazolam for treatment of patients with panic disorder and depression found no difference in overall efficacy between the two agents, the antidepressant was more effective for the core symptoms of depression (Keller et al., 1993; Leon, Shear, Portera, & Klerman, 1993). Most antidepressants, with the possible exception of trazodone (Charney et al., 1986) and bupropion (Sheehan, Davidson, & Manschreck, 1983), have a spectrum of efficacy that covers both panic and depressive symptoms. However, benzodiazepines, though effective anxiolytics, are generally inferior antidepressants. Thus, in cases of a suspected or confirmed comorbid depressive syndrome, use of an antidepressant increases the likelihood that the relevant mood and anxiety symptoms will be addressed.

Treatment of panic patients experiencing significant depression or dysthymia is most prudently initiated with an antidepressant; adjunctive benzodiazepines may be used if the patient cannot tolerate the 3- to 4-week lag period for antidepressant efficacy or the increased anxiety associated with initiation of antidepressant treatment. Use of a benzodiazepine alone

TABLE 4.2. Treatment Interventions for Comorbid Conditions

Condition	Intervention
Depression	Antidepressants ± HPBs
Social phobia	SSRIs MAOIs HPBs
Generalized anxiety disorder	Antidepressants HPBs Buspirone
Posttraumatic stress disorder	Antidepressants Benzodiazepines Buspirone Anticonvulsants Antipsychotics
Obsessive–compulsive disorder	Serotonergic antidepressants Augmentation strategies (buspirone, trazodone, clonazepam, pergolide, fenfluramine) MAOIs
Alcohol and substance abuse	Alcohol/drug treatment Antidepressants Buspirone Long-acting, slow-onset benzodiazepines
Personality disorders/ psychosocial distress	Individual psychotherapy Group therapy Family/couple therapy
Comorbid medical factors/ conditions	Correction of medical factors Elimination of anxiogenic agents Management of side effects

may not to adequately treat the comorbid depression and may result in continued patient distress and dysfunction.

Patients with panic disorder may also have comorbid bipolar illness complicating their presentation. Because of the risk that antidepressants may increase cycling in bipolar patients, treatment of panic should be undertaken with alternative strategies. Both clonazepam and valproic acid have been used as mood stabilizers in bipolar patients (Sachs et al., 1994). Clonazepam (Pollack et al., 1993), and potentially valproic acid (Keck et al., 1993) are also effective for treatment of panic disorder and may be used alone or in combination for the comorbid patient.

Comorbid Social Phobia

Comorbid social phobia may occur in 20–50% of patients with panic disorder (Stein, Shea, & Uhde, 1989). For patients with comorbid generalized social phobia, treatment for both conditions may be best initiated with an MAOI (Liebowitz et al., 1992), an SSRI (Schneier, Liebowitz, & Davies, 1990), or an HPB (Reiter, Pollack, Rosenbaum, & Cohen, 1990), which have all been found to be effective for the treatment of social phobia. TCAs, though effective antipanic agents, are less effective than other agents for the treatment of social phobia; thus, they should generally not be used as first-line agents for the panic patient with comorbid social phobia.

Comorbid Generalized Anxiety Disorder

GAD, characterized by excessive worry, vigilance, and autonomic arousal, is a frequent comorbid condition in panic disorder patients (Pollack et al., 1990). Overanxiousness or generalized anxiety during childhood or adolescence frequently precedes the development of panic disorder (Otto, Pollack, Rosenbaum, Sachs, & Asher, 1994).

The medications typically used to treat panic disorder (i.e., antidepressants and HPBs) are usually also effective for treatment of GAD. In a controlled study, the TCA imipramine proved as effective as the benzodiazepine diazepam for the control of GAD symptoms (Rickels & Schweizer, 1993). In addition to these standard agents, panic patients, with comorbid GAD may benefit from the use of the azaspirone buspirone. One report details the use of adjunctive buspirone for panic disorder patients who continued to experience generalized and anticipatory anxiety, despite reduction of panic attacks with HPB treatment (Gastfriend & Rosenbaum, 1989). For some patients, use of adjunctive benzodiazepines—either HPBs (e.g., alprazolam or clonazepam, 1–5 mg/day) or low-potency agents (e.g., diazepam, 10–40 mg/day)—in combination with an antidepressant may confer additional benefit for the treatment of generalized anxiety symptoms that persist despite antidepressant pharmacotherapy.

Other Comorbid Anxiety Disorders

Patients with PTSD may, as part of this disorder, develop panic attacks and avoidance related to situations reminiscent of the trauma, or may also develop the typical panic disorder–agoraphobia syndrome. Conversely, patients with panic disorder may also develop PTSD if exposed to traumatic events such as assault, combat, or natural disasters. There is currently no "gold standard" for the treatment of PTSD. Treatment is typically targeted at prominent symptomatology—for example, antidepressant treatment for depressive symptoms; benzodiazepines, antidepressants, or buspirone for anxiety; mood stabilizers or serotonergic agents for impulsive or aggressive behavior; and antipsychotics for delusions or other psychosis. The SSRI fluoxetine was recently shown in a controlled study to be effective for treatment of PTSD (van der Kolk et al., 1994) In addition, cognitive-behavioral and psychosocial therapies, including group, individual, and family therapy, may be necessary to effect maximal improvement in panic patients with comorbid PTSD.

The pharmacologic treatment of panic disorder patients with comorbid obsessive–compulsive disorder (OCD) is generally best initiated with serotonergic antidepressants, such as SSRIs (e.g., fluoxetine, 20–80 mg/day) or clomipramine (25–250 mg/day). Patients failing to respond to initial pharmacotherapy may be candidates for augmentation strategies—such as the addition of buspirone (30–60 mg/day), trazodone (50–300 mg/day), clonazepam (2–8 mg/day), pergolide (0.5–2 mg/day), or fenfluramine (20–60 mg/day) or for treatment with an MAOI. The treatment of refractory OCD is covered in greater detail by Rauch, Baer, and Jenike in Chapter 8 of this volume. Cognitive-behavioral interventions aimed at the OCD and panic may also be necessary to optimize outcome.

Alcohol or Other Substance Abuse

Abuse of alcohol and/or other substances may complicate the presentation and treatment of panic disorder. For some patients, alcohol or other substance abuse may have developed as an attempt to "self-medicate" anxiety (Klein, 1981). In one study, over 80% of patients with comorbid panic disorder and alcohol dependence reported that their alcohol difficulties predated the onset of panic, although many of these patients had a history of childhood anxiety disorders (Otto et al., 1992b). For other patients the anxiety and substance abuse may develop independently, or the anxiety may result from substance withdrawal (e.g., alcohol, opiates, sedative/hypnotics), intoxication phenomena (e.g., cocaine, amphetamines), or toxic central nervous system (CNS) effects of repeated substance abuse (George, Nutt, Dwyer, & Linnoila, 1990). Regardless of the direction of causation, once alcohol or other substance abuse becomes entrenched, it must be specifically addressed as part of a comprehensive treatment plan. Treatment of the anxiety alone is often not sufficient to stimulate recovery from substance abuse. Other necessary interventions may include inpatient or outpatient detoxification, counseling and/or Twelve-Step programs (e.g., Alcoholics Anonymous), and regular toxicologic monitoring to assess progress. Although ideally it would be preferable to have the patient substance-free for at least a couple of months before the initiation of anxiolytic treatment, in order to clarify diagnosis (i.e., whether the anxiety is substance-related) and to simplify treatment, in practice the clinician may need to intervene before sobriety is achieved to alleviate severe anxiety or mood symptoms. The selection of appropriate pharmacotherapy is based on the target symptoms and the need to avoid agents with abuse potential or those that may interact adversely with alcohol or other substances. Fortunately, antidepressants can be effective for panic and other anxiety symptoms as well as for depression, and have little potential for abuse; the SSRIs have a relatively wide margin of safety when mixed with alcohol, and may decrease craving for alcohol (Naranjo, Kadlec, Sanhueza, Woodley-Remus, & Sellers, 1990) or other substances (e.g., cocaine; Pollack & Rosenbaum, 1991). Buspirone may reduce generalized anxiety, though not panic, as well as decrease alcohol consumption in anxious alcoholics (Kranzler et al., 1994). The use of benzodiazepines in substance abuse patients should generally be avoided whenever possible; however, they may be appropriate and effective when used cautiously to control severe anxiety in some substance abusers who (1) fail a number of adequate trials with other classes of agents, and (2) have demonstrated themselves to be reliable (e.g., participating in substance abuse treatment, coming regularly for appointments, taking medication as prescribed). Benzodiazepines with a gradual onset of effect and a longer duration of action (e.g., clonazepam) are preferable to rapid-onset and/or shorter-acting agents (e.g., diazepam, alprazolam), which may give patients a "buzz" shortly after ingestion and require multiple dosing during the day. Although dosing requirements for benzodiazepines in this population are unlikely to be lower than in the general population, and some patients may require higher doses than usual for effective anxiolysis, prescription of large quantities of medication at one time and recurrent prescription refills over the phone should be avoided. Patients should be assessed at frequent intervals, and anxiolytic treatment should be coordinated with substance abuse treatment as part of an ongoing treatment plan targeting the comorbid conditions.

Personality Disorders, Psychosocial Distress, and Family Dysfunction

Many studies have documented the high rates of personality disorders (especially dependent, avoidant, histrionic, obsessive–compulsive, and borderline) in patients with panic disorder; the presence of a personality disorder may negatively affect response to treatment (Mavissakalian, 1990; Pollack, Otto, Rosenbaum, & Sachs, 1992; Reich, 1988). For some patients, treatment of the anxiety disorder may improve self-esteem and confidence, and decrease interpersonal sensitivity and dependence, thus diminishing what may have appeared to be immutable personality characteristics. However, for others, intrapsychic distress and dysfunctional interpersonal patterns may persist despite treatment targeting anxiety and affective symptomatology, and may necessitate psychotherapeutic interventions to facilitate response to antipanic treatment and optimize overall functioning.

Family and couple dynamics may be paradoxically upset by a panic patient's symptomatic improvement, thus complicating the recovery process. For example, the spouse of a formerly dependent and anxious panic patient may become upset and resentful when the patient becomes more assertive and independent after anxiolytic treatment. Patients and their families may require education, exploration, and support to facilitate the patients' improvement and prevent interference with treatment. Individuals who have suffered from panic and agoraphobia for years may benefit from therapy to deal with issues of anger, guilt, and grief for the losses and limitations they have experienced because of their disorder, and to clarify their future options and decisions in the context of a more independent lifestyle.

Comorbid Medical Factors/Conditions

The presence of medical illness or other physiologic factors may complicate assessment and treatment of panic and other anxiety symptoms (Rosenbaum & Pollack, 1991). Some disorders (e.g., hyperthyroidism, chronic obstructive pulmonary disease) or medications used to treat medical conditions (e.g., bronchodilators) may directly cause anxiety. Other conditions, such as coronary artery disease with chest pain or palpitations, may provoke or mimic anxiety because of their potentially ominous significance and their association with the cascade of panic symptoms (e.g., palpitations as a typical component of panic attacks). Use of exogenous substances such as caffeine may contribute to anxiety, and their reduction or elimination may improve response in refractory patients. Medically ill or elderly patients may be more sensitive to side effects of medications and less responsive to anxiolytic treatment. Recognition and treatment of underlying medical conditions that contribute to anxiety, and substitution or elimination of potentially offending medications, may help to optimize of therapeutic interventions and reduce resistance to treatment.

TARGETING TREATMENT AT PREDOMINANT SYMPTOMS

The nature of the panic patient's refractory symptoms may direct appropriate interventions. The patient who continues to experience spontaneous panic attacks or situationally predisposed panic attacks may benefit from a higher dose of medication or addition of alternative antipanic agents (e.g., antidepressants, HPBs). If panic attacks are successfully suppressed, but the patient continues to experience significant anticipatory anxiety or avoidance that limits functioning, then adjunctive benzodiazepines or occasionally buspirone may be helpful. Although medication may reduce or eliminate panic attacks and comorbid symptomatology and may improve global functioning, conditioned phobic distress and disability may persist. For some patients, the scope of their avoidance behavior may only become apparent after the dramatic improvement in panic symptoms experienced during an acute medication trial. Agoraphobic symptoms may persist even after panic attacks recede, as long as the fear of anxiety symptoms (anxiety sensitivity) and propensity to avoidance are incompletely treated (Reiss, Peterson, Gursky, & McNally, 1986). This assertion is consistent with results from a follow-up study of HPB-treated panic patients, in which the baseline predictors of poorer long-term outcome included manifestations of increased avoidance as characterized by agoraphobic avoidance and comorbid social phobia (Pollack et al., 1993). Addition of interoceptive and *in vivo* cognitive-behavioral therapy, targeted at reducing sensitivity to anxiety and avoidance behavior, may lessen patient distress and extend treatment gains in pharmacologically treated patients (Pollack & Otto, 1994).

PHARMACOLOGIC FACTORS AFFECTING TREATMENT RESPONSE

Although there are no definitive guidelines as to what constitutes an adequate pharmacologic trial for panic disorder, accumulating clinical and research experience point to ways of optimizing the pharmacotherapy of panic disorder. Table 4.3 presents a pharmacopoeia for panic disorder; aspects of this pharmacopoeia are discussed here.

Dosing

Tricyclic Antidepressants

Dosing with the TCAs should be initiated at low "test" doses of 10 mg of imipramine or its equivalent, in order to minimize increased anxiety early in treatment; the dose can then be titrated up to therapeutic levels, as tolerated, over the first few weeks of treatment in increments of 25–50 mg/day. Recommendations for target dose levels of TCAs for the treatment of panic disorder have typically paralleled those for depression— that is, 150–300 mg/day of imipramine or its equivalent (Rosenbaum & Pollack, 1991). For instance, some reports suggest better responses associated with higher doses and blood levels of TCAs (Mavissakalian & Perel, 1985). In one study, responders to desipramine had therapeutic blood levels greater than 125 ng/ml, and initial nonresponders became responders once their dose was increased to achieve levels above that figure (Lydiard, 1987). However, Ballenger et al. (1984) reported that some agoraphobics responded better to imipramine levels in the range of 100–150 ng/ml than to higher levels, consistent with other reports (Mavissakalian & Perel, 1989). As part of his ongoing investigations in this area, Mavissakalian and Perel (1994) has reported that a reasonable target dose of imipramine for treatment of panic disorder and agoraphobia is about 2.25 mg/kg/day (usually between 100 and 200 mg/day for most patients), generally producing a total plasma level of 75-150 ng/ml for imipramine and its metabolite desipramine. The response rate among patients whose plasma level was in the range of 75–150 ng/ml in Mavissakalian's study of 63 patients with moderate to severe panic disorder was 80%, with lower response and more treatment dropouts at higher plasma levels. Thus, patients with plasma levels above 150 ng/ml who remain symptomatic may derive benefit from a dose *reduction* to achieve plasma levels in the range of 75–150 ng/ml.

TABLE 4.3. Pharmacopoeia for Panic Disorder

Agent	Usual initial dose (mg)	Usual dosage range (mg)	Chief limitations	Comorbid disorders[a]
TCAs				
Imipramine (Tofranil)	10–25	100–300	Jitteriness	GAD, DEP,
Desipramine (Norpramin)	10–25	100–300	TCA side effects	PTSD,
Nortriptyline (Pamelor)	10–25	50–150		
MAOIs				
Phenelzine (Nardil)	15–30	45–90	Diet	SP, OCD,
Tranylcypromine (Parnate)	10–20	30–60	MAOI side effects	DEP, PTSD GAD
SSRIs				
Fluoxetine (Prozac)	5–10	20–80	Jitteriness	SP, OCD,
Sertraline (Zoloft)	25	50–200	SSRI side effects	PTSD, DEP, GAD
Paroxetine (Paxil)	10	10–50		
Fluvoxamine (Luvox)	50	50–300		
Clomipramine (Anafranil)	25	25–250	Sedation Weight gain TCA side effects	OCD, GAD, DEP PTSD
HPBs				
Alprazolam (Xanax)	0.25 t.i.d.–q.i.d.[b]	2–10/day	Sedation	GAD, SP,
Clonazepam (Klonopin)	0.25 h.s.[b]	1–5/day	Discontinuation syndrome Abuse Psychomotor and memory impairment	OCD, PTSD, SpP

[a]GAD, generalized anxiety disorder; DEP, depression; PTSD, posttraumatic stress disorder; SP, social phobia; OCD, obsessive–compulsive disorder; SpP, specific phobia.
[b]t.i.d., three times a day; q.i.d., four times a day; h.s., bedtime.

Mavissakalian and Perel (1992a) also examined the issue of maintenance dosing for panic patients with TCAs. They reported that a group of patients with a good and stable response to a 6-month trial of full-dose imipramine (mean = 168 mg/day) remained in remission over a 1-year maintenance period after their dose was reduced by 50%. This study suggests that lower-dose TCA therapy may be adequate to maintain remission during maintenance treatment of panic patients; however, it should be emphasized that the patients in this study had responded robustly to acute therapy and met strict criteria for remission prior to the dose reduction. Whether patients who remain symptomatic during acute treatment with full doses will maintain any significant benefit with lower levels during maintenance treatment has not yet been systematically studied. Clinicians should generally use full doses of TCAs in attempts to produce remission, before considering dose reduction over the maintenance period.

Monoamine Oxidase Inhibitors

Dose–response relationships for MAOI treatment of panic disorder have not been well studied. Clinically, many patients respond to phenelzine (60–90 mg/day) or tranylcypromine (30–60 mg/day), although some may benefit from higher doses (e.g., 90–105 mg/day of phenelzine, 60–120 mg/day of tranylcypromine), as have been reported to be effective for refractory depression (Amsterdam & Berwish, 1989).

Selective Serotonin Reuptake Inhibitors

In the absence of definitive data from controlled studies, dosing recommendations for SSRIs in panic patients parallel those for depression (i.e., 20–80 mg/day of fluoxetine, 50–200 mg/day of sertraline, 20–50 mg/day of paroxetine, and 50–300 mg/day of fluvoxamine). The SSRIs, like the TCAs, may cause increased anxiety at the initiation of therapy in some patients; thus, dosing should be initiated at lower levels to prevent increased distress and premature discontinuation of treatment. For instance, treatment can be initiated with 5–10 mg/day of fluoxetine (the dose can be created by using the elixir or by dissolving a 10- or 20-mg capsule in some juice and aliquoting out an appropriate amount over a 2- to 4-day period). Patients should also be started on low doses of the other SSRIs (e.g., 25 mg of sertraline, 10 mg of paroxetine, 25 mg of fluvoxamine), and these should be increased up to typical therapeutic doses over 1–2 weeks. Although clinical experience suggests that some panic patients may respond to very low doses of SSRIs, most patients readily tolerate a dose increase after a few days or a week; until data on the dose–response relationship for the SSRIs and panic are available, it may be prudent to raise the SSRI dose to typical antidepressant levels in patients who can tolerate it, in order to maximize treatment response.

High-Potency Benzodiazepines

Treatment with HPBs should be initiated at 0.25 mg of alprazolam three times a day, or 0.25 mg of clonazepam at bedtime; doses should be titrated up by 0.25 to 0.5 mg every 3–4 days, as tolerated, until therapeutic dose levels are reached. Adequate dosing of panic patients with alprazolam and clonazepam may be critical to maximize treatment response. In the Cross-National Collaborative Panic Study (Ballenger et al., 1988), the mean prescribed dose was 4.9 ± 1.5 mg/day at week 4 and 5.7 ± 2.2 mg/day by week 8; panic attacks appeared to respond to 2–3 mg/day of alprazolam, whereas phobic avoidant behaviors required higher doses, approximately 6 mg/day. Although a fixed-dose study of alprazolam found no statistically significant differences in efficacy between patients treated with 2 and 6 mg/day, there was a trend toward greater efficacy on some measures with the higher doses (Lydiard et al., 1992). In addition, the interpretation of this latter study is complicated by the high proportion of patients in the 2 mg/day dosage who were surreptitiously using other benzodiazepines, suggesting that they may have been experiencing more anxiety than was showing up on the study assessments. Uhlenhuth, Matuzas, Glass, and Easton (1989) demonstrated greater improvement in panic patients and fewer dropouts during treatment with 6 mg/day versus 2 mg/day of alprazolam. Gradual upward dose titration is often necessary to minimize sedation and other side effects associated with the higher dose levels of the benzodiazepines.

Despite evidence from acute studies suggesting better outcome associated with higher doses of HPBs, follow-up studies and naturalistic observation of panic patients demonstrate that doses of HPBs often decrease over time. This decrease in dose during maintenance therapy may be one important explanation for the persistence of symptoms or diminution of acute treatment effects in follow-up studies of HPB-treated patients (Nagy et al., 1989; Pollack et al., 1993). It is not clear why HPB doses do not increase and often actually decline over the maintenance period, despite persistent symptomatology. In clinical practice, early dramatic response during acute treatment may result in premature termination of dose escalation and limit further dose adjustment, despite the presence of persistent residual symptomatology. In one study of treatment-refractory panic patients, inadequate dosing despite persistent symptomatology was often a result of the patients' desire to minimize the use of medication, particularly the benzodiazepines (Pollack, Otto, Kaspi, Hammerness, & Rosenbaum, 1994a). Such issues may be based on moralistic attitudes, concerns about withdrawal difficulties, and fear about dose escalation and abuse (Clinthorne, Cisin, Balter, Mellinger, & Uhlenhuth, 1986; Mellinger, Balter, & Uhlenhuth, 1984).

The consistent reports of relatively modest dose levels of benzodiazepines (e.g., alprazolam or clonazepam, 1–2 mg/day) during long-term treatment, despite the presence of continued symptomatology, suggest (1) that dose adjustments should not be prematurely terminated until a patient's symptomatology is well controlled, and (2) that residual distress may require dose escalation beyond the level needed to achieve acute therapeutic response. In clinical practice, it may take 3–6 months or more to achieve a well-tolerated dose level (e.g., 4–10 mg/day of alprazolam, 2–5 mg/day clonazepam) that blocks panic attacks and provides comprehensive relief of anticipatory and phobic anxiety and avoidance. Parallel to recommendations for the use of antidepressants in the treatment of depression (Thase, 1992), we suggest that dose levels for the HPBs during the maintenance treatment of panic disorder should be kept at the full dose levels required to achieve maximal acute response, in order to facilitate continued improvement in some patients and persistence of initial gains in others. In the Massachusetts General Hospital Naturalistic Study of the course of panic disorder (Pollack et al., 1990), patients in remission maintained with low doses of benzodiazepines relapsed sooner than patients treated with pharmacotherapeutic agents at higher levels of intensity (Pollack et al., 1994b). Patients on lower doses of benzodiazepines are still likely to develop physiologic dependence and are at risk for withdrawal symptoms during acute discontinuation, but often do not receive the maximal therapeutic benefits afforded by use of more therapeutic dose levels. Patients or clinicians with marked reservations about using adequate doses of benzodiazepines for treatment of panic should consider alternate forms of pharmacotherapy or cognitive-behavioral therapies, in order to maximize their acute and long-term response to treatment.

Pharmacokinetic Issues

Dosing Frequency

Dosing frequency may affect response to treatment. Agents with shorter half-lives (e.g., alprazolam) need to be administered four to five times per day, whereas longer-acting agents (e.g., clonazepam) generally require twice-a-day dosing. Interdose rebound anxiety may arise 4–6 hours after the last dose of a short-half-life agent, with patients experiencing withdrawal symptoms associated with declining benzodiazepine plasma levels. A decrease in dosing frequency (e.g., from four to three times daily) or precipitous decrease in total dose may also result in marked interdose rebound anxiety, particularly with shorter-acting agents. The effects of shorter-half-life agents may also wear off overnight, leading to early morning anxiety or nocturnal panic attacks. Interdose rebound anxiety may increase a patient's somatic preoccupation and lead to increased anticipatory anxiety and phobic behavior. From a cognitive-behavioral perspective, recurrent episodes of interdose rebound anxiety and the need for frequent dosing promote continued anxiety and psychologic dependency on the medication, as the patient associates increased anxiety with the absence of medication and acute relief of symptoms with taking pills (Otto, Pollack, Meltzer-Brody, & Rosenbaum, 1992a). Longer-acting agents such as clonazepam are often easier for patients to use over time, because less frequent dosing is possible and interdose rebound anxiety occurs less often.

Duration of Treatment

There is a relative paucity of systematic data addressing the issue of what constitutes an adequate duration of treatment for panic disorder. In one report (Muskin & Fyer, 1981), it took a group of patients on TCAs 3–9 months to become panic-free, and as long as 2 years to substantially reduce anticipatory anxiety. In a study of patients with panic disorder and depression who were treated with imipramine or alprazolam, the degree of phobic avoidance was a negative predictor of response at 4 weeks but not at 16 weeks, suggesting that phobic avoidance may require a period of months to respond to treatment (Pollack et al., 1994c). Whereas suppression of panic attacks may occur relatively quickly after initiation of treatment, relief from anticipatory anxiety and phobic avoidance may only occur over longer periods of time, with reversal of conditioned anxiety and avoidance associated with panic. Phobic avoidance may improve as patients test the protective antipanic and antianxiety effects of medication and expose themselves to feared situations.

In a study by Mavissakalian and Perel (1992b) examining maintenance treatment with imipramine for panic disorder, 80% of patients who demonstrated a marked, stable response to 6 months of active treatment with imipramine (150 mg/day) relapsed within 6 months of discontinuing drug therapy, while only 25% who stayed on half the dose for another year (i.e., a total of 18 months) relapsed over the 6 months subsequent to discontinuation.

Between one-half and three-quarters of patients who discontinue pharmacotherapy (whether antidepressants or HPBs) relapse at some point and require reinitiation of medication or other treatments (Pollack & Otto, 1994). Thus, as is the case for other disorders (e.g., depression, bipolar disorder, schizophrenia), long-term ongoing pharmacotherapy for panic disorder is often necessary to maintain benefit and prevent relapse. In the absence of definitive data, we recommend that treated patients remain in remission for at least a year prior to attempting discontinuation of medication. For patients with a history of recurrent relapse after treatment discontinuation, ongoing maintenance pharmacotherapy is appropriate. For some patients, the addition of cognitive-behavioral treatment during the discontinuation process may increase the likelihood of successful discontinuation and offer some protection against later relapse (Otto et al., 1993).

Side Effects and Compliance

Treatment-emergent adverse effects may limit a patient's willingness or capacity to receive an adequate pharmacotherapy trial. In a study of TCA-treated panic patients followed over a 2½-year period, treatment-emergent adverse effects (e.g., increased anxiety early in the course of treatment, weight gain over the long term) contributed to treatment discontinuation in a substantial proportion of treated patients, and limited dose escalation in 40% of patients requiring increased medication (Noyes et al., 1989). The newer antidepressants, including the SSRIs, have a more favorable side effect profile and are generally easier for patients to take at adequate doses over the long term. HPBs are also well tolerated, but patient and clinician ambivalence about their use may result in inadequate dosing and submaximal response over time. Educating patients about the need for adequate intensity and frequency of dosing, the often chronic course of panic disorder, and discussion of the reassuring evidence regarding lack of dose escalation or abuse over time with benzodiazepines may increase compliance with adequate treatment and improve overall outcome.

STRATEGIES FOR THE MEDICATION-REFRACTORY PANIC PATIENT

Combining Antidepressants and Benzodiazepines

Relatively few systematic data are available to guide clinicians on the management of patients who remain symptomatic, despite an adequate trial of an antipanic agent. Although not subjected to evaluation in a controlled study, one commonly employed strategy for a refractory patient receiving monotherapy with either an antidepressant or an HPB alone is to proffer combined treatment with these classes of agents. Thus, if the patient is being treated with a TCA, an SSRI, or an MAOI, addition of an HPB may reduce continued panic attacks, anticipatory anxiety, or phobic avoidance. Conversely, patients on HPBs alone may benefit from addition of an adequate trial of an antidepressant. Clinical experience suggests that patients benefit most from combined treatment when one or both of the agents are used at adequate dosage levels, rather than when two low-intensity interventions are employed.

Other Uses of Antidepressants

There are no systematic data demonstrating benefit from switching within or between classes of antidepressants, although this is frequently done and may be helpful. However, patients with atypical depressed features (i.e., hypersomnia, hyperphagia, rejection sensitivity) or social phobia may respond preferentially to an MAOI, and perhaps to the SSRIs, relative to the TCAs. Though data supporting this assertion are sparse, many experienced clinicians believe that no panic patients should be considered truly refractory to pharmacotherapy until they have had an adequate trial of an MAOI. In an open study of panic patients, 95% of phenelzine-treated patients were panic-free at the end of a 6-month trial (Buigues & Vallejo, 1987). However, a placebo-controlled study reported that up to 40% of phenelzine-treated patients rated themselves as only partially improved or no better after 12 weeks of treatment (Sheehan, Ballenger, & Jacobsen, 1980).

Clomipramine, a TCA that potently inhibits serotonin reuptake and is commonly used for the treatment of OCD, is also effective for patients who are refractory to standard antipanic treatments. Reports suggest that clomipramine may be more effective than imipramine (Modigh, Westberg, & Eriksson, 1992) for some panic patients. However, because it is a heterocyclic agent, its side effect profile may be daunting for some. Treatment should be initiated at 25–50 mg/day; this may be an effective dose range for some, whereas others may benefit from gradual dose escalation up to 250 mg/day.

Accumulating clinical experience and a recent report (Tiffon, Coplan, Papp, & Gorman, 1994) suggest that combined treatment with a TCA and an SSRI may be effective for patients with refractory panic. The potential for a drug interaction between the SSRIs and TCAs, which can result in increased TCA plasma levels, necessitates initiation of treatment with low doses of the TCA (e.g., 25 mg/day of desipramine) and monitoring of plasma levels to avoid toxicity. If the SSRI is being added to a TCA, the dose of the TCA should be decreased by at least half at the initiation of combined treatment.

Anticonvulsants

In addition to the considerations described above, a variety of adjunctive strategies have been reported helpful in small case studies and open reports for the treatment of the refractory panic patient. Anticonvulsants, particularly valproic acid, have been successfully used for some patients failing to respond to standard antipanic pharmacotherapies (Keck et al., 1993). Typical doses are on the order of 500–2000 mg/day, and in the absence of conclusive dose–response data, most clinicians aim for blood levels in the typical range for seizure control (i.e., 50–100 ng/ml).

For some patients, panic attacks may be manifestations of partial complex seizures, especially when they are associated with atypical features (e.g., auditory, olfactory, or visual hallucinations, micropsia or macropsia, unilateral paresthesias, *déjà vu* experiences, or absence periods). These patients are best treated with anticonvulsants such as carbamazepine or valproic acid at standard anticonvulsant levels (Weilburg et al., 1993). Clonazepam also has anticonvulsant properties and may be useful alone or as an adjunctive treatment in the seizure patient. The presence of seizures in patients with panic attacks should be suspected when the atypical features noted above are present, when anxiety symptoms start after head trauma or other CNS insult, or when patients have a strong family or personal history of seizures.

Other Adjunctive Strategies

The addition of lithium at both low (e.g., 300–900 mg/day) and typical therapeutic levels has been helpful for some refractory panic patients when added to an antidepressant or a benzodiazepine, although there are no clear predictors of response (Feder, 1988). The addition of buspirone (30–60 mg/day) may be helpful for some patients treated with benzodiazepines or antidepressants who continue to have interpanic anticipatory anxiety or marked general anxiety (Gastfriend & Rosenbaum, 1989).

In some patients, the use of lower-potency benzodiazepines alone or adjunctively can be helpful. For example, two controlled studies have indicated that diazepam can be effective for patients with panic attacks (Dunner, Ishiki, Avery, Wilson, & Hyde, 1986) or panic disorder (Noyes, Anderson, & Clancy, 1984). Patients sometimes require relatively high doses of these agents (e.g., 30–60 mg/day of diazepam) to achieve relief of panic, and sedation can be a dose-limiting side effect. Beta-adrenergic blockers (e.g., propranolol, 30–240 mg/day) are potentially useful in targeting specific anxiety symptoms (e.g., palpitations, tremor), although there are no convincing data showing that they have specific antipanic activity.

The addition of cognitive-behavioral therapy may also be very effective for the partial responder or nonresponder to pharmacotherapy (Pollack et al., 1994a). One difficulty in "prescribing" cognitive-behavioral therapy is that the availability of experienced clinicians able to provide structured treatment may be limited. However, some features of cognitive-behavioral treatment can be easily integrated into an efficient psychopharmacologic visit. The psychopharmacologist can encourage patients to initiate self-directed, gradual, step-by-step exposure to feared situations, in order to decrease phobic anxiety and avoidance. As patients experience fewer panic attacks and less anxiety with pharmacologic treatment, they should be encouraged to enter feared situations. Patients should be counseled to expect some symptoms of anxiety when first entering a phobic situation, and should be instructed to continue exposure until the anxiety levels off and recedes. Even self-directed exposure with minimal therapist contact has been demonstrated to facilitate maintenance of acute therapeutic gains at long-term follow-up of antidepressant-treated panic patients (Mavissakalian & Michelson, 1986). Self-help books and manuals are available that enable patients to guide their exposure and behavioral treatment with minimal therapist input (Clum, 1990). For some patients, self-directed exposure may be adequate to restore full functioning (Gould, Clum, & Shapiro, 1993), whereas other patients may require a more structured behavioral program to achieve full benefit. The integration of cognitive-behavioral therapy and pharmacotherapy for panic disorder is addressed in greater detail by Otto and Gould in Chapter 5 of this volume.

A POTENTIAL ALGORITHM
FOR TREATMENT OF PANIC DISORDER

At this point, no clear consensus exists on the optimal approach to the treatment of panic disorder. What follows is one potential treatment algorithm that attempts to integrate available data and clinical experience.

1. Patients should be assessed for physical illness, medication use, or substance use that may be exacerbating anxiety. These factors should be appropriately treated or eliminated.

2. The selection of an initial pharmacologic agent should be based on the presence of comorbid conditions, previous treatment history, and level of distress. For example, treatment should be initiated with an antidepressant for patients with comorbid depression, and for those at significant risk for depression as indicated by a strong personal or family history of mood disorder. Although almost all antidepressants are effective for the

treatment of panic disorder as well as depression, the favorable side effect profile of the SSRIs has led to their increasing use as first-line agents for the treatment of panic disorder, despite the relative paucity of data from controlled studies to date demonstrating their efficacy. For patients who have either failed or been unable to tolerate an SSRI trial, use of a TCA is reasonable. Clomipramine may be particularly effective among the TCAs for the treatment of panic disorder. Because of dietary restrictions and the risk of hypertensive reactions, MAOIs are most typically used after more easily managed interventions are unsuccessful. For patients with comorbid social phobia or atypical depression, treatment should be initiated with the SSRIs or MAOIs in preference to the TCAs. For patients with comorbid OCD, treatment should be initiated with a serotonergic agent such as an SSRI or clomipramine.

3. For patients without comorbid depression or substance abuse, treatment can usually be initiated with either an HPB or an antidepressant. The HPBs have the advantage of a more rapid onset of effect than the antidepressants, with generally fewer side effects. The antidepressants are less likely to cause dependence or acute withdrawal effects during discontinuation. However, given the findings suggesting that (a) many patients who receive HPBs are inadequately treated, (b) the newer antidepressants are generally well tolerated at therapeutic doses, and (c) low levels of HPBs may not be as protective against relapse as therapeutic levels of antidepressants (Pollack et al., 1994a), it may be better to initiate treatment with an antidepressant alone or in combination with an HPB if the patient or clinician is unwilling to use adequate amounts of a benzodiazepine.

Although misuse of HPBs among panic patients without a history of substance abuse is exceedingly rare in clinical practice, patients with a personal or strong family history of alcohol or other substance abuse may be at increased risk for abuse; their treatment should be initiated with an antidepressant whenever possible. However, patients who are in need of rapid anxiolysis, or who have failed to respond to or been unable to tolerate antidepressant treatment, are candidates for treatment initiation with an HPB.

4. For patients failing monotherapy with either an antidepressant or an HPB combined treatment with adequate doses of an HPB *and* an antidepressant may prove beneficial.

5. Strategies such as the use of a TCA–SSRI combination, adjunctive buspirone, or adjunctive lithium may be useful for some patients, although there are few systematic data to guide the selection of appropriate candidates. The use of anticonvulsants may be helpful in patients with symptoms suggestive of underlying complex partial seizures or those patients with a history of marked impulsiveness, aggressiveness, or mood instability; in addition, some reports suggest that valproate may be effective for nonictal panic. Cognitive-behavioral techniques should be considered in all patients who fail to respond to initial first-line pharmacologic treatment.

CONCLUSIONS

Many patients with panic disorder, though improved after initial treatment, remain symptomatic. Careful assessment and a systematic treatment approach will facilitate optimal treatment of the panic patient. Selection of appropriate initial and adjunctive interventions from the pharmacopoeia, and integration of cognitive-behavioral strategies, will improve outcome in clinical practice and are critical issues warranting further systematic study.

REFERENCES

Amsterdam, J. D., & Berwish, N. J. (1989). High dose tranylcypromine therapy for refractory depression. *Pharmacopsychiatry, 22*, 21–25.

American Psychiatric Association. (1994). *Diagnostic and statistical manual of mental disorders* (4th ed.). Washington, DC: Author,

Ballenger, J. C., Burrows, G., DuPont, R., Lesser, I. M., Noyes, R., Pecknold, J., Rifkin, A., & Swinson, R. (1988). Alprazolam in panic disorder and agoraphobia: Results from a multicenter trial. I. Efficacy in short-term treatment. *Archives of General Psychiatry, 45*, 413–422.

Ballenger, J. C., Peterson, G. A., Laraia, M. A. H., Lake, C., Jimerson, D., Cox, D., Trockman, C., Shipe, J., & Wilkinson, C. A (1984). Study of plasma catecholamines in agoraphobia and the relationship of serum tricyclic levels to treatment response. In J. C. Ballenger (Ed.), *Biology of agoraphobia.* Washington, DC: American Psychiatric Press.

Breier, A., Charney, D. S., & Heninger, G. R. (1984). Major depression in patients with agoraphobia and panic disorder. *Archives of General Psychiatry, 41*, 1129–1135.

Buigues, J., & Vallejo, J. (1987). Therapeutic response to phenelzine in patients with panic disorder and agoraphobia with panic attacks. *Journal of Clinical Psychiatry, 48*, 55–59.

Charney, D., Woods, S., Goodman, W., Rifkin, B., Kinch, M., Aiken, B., Quadrino, M. S., & Heninger, G. R. (1986). Drug treatment of panic disorder: The comparative efficacy of imipramine, alprazolam, and trazodone. *Journal of Clinical Psychiatry, 47*, 580–586.

Clinthorne, J. K., Cisin, I. H., Balter, M. B., Mellinger, G. D., & Uhlenhuth, E. H. (1986). Changes in popular attitudes and beliefs about tranquilizers. *Archives of General Psychiatry, 43*, 527–532.

Clum, G. A. (1990). *Coping with panic.* Pacific Grove, CA: Brooks/Cole.

Cross-National Collaborative Panic Study (S.P.I.). (1992). Drug treatment of panic disorder: Comparative efficacy of alprazolam, imipramine, and placebo. *British Journal of Psychiatry, 160*, 191–202.

Dunner, D. L., Ishiki, D., Avery, D. H., Wilson, L. G., & Hyde, T. S. (1986). Effect of alprazolam and diazepam on anxiety and panic attacks in panic disorder: A controlled study. *Journal of Clinical Psychiatry, 47*, 458–460.

Feder, R. (1988). Lithium augmentation of clomipramine. *Journal of Clinical Psychiatry, 49*, 458.

Gastfriend, D. R., & Rosenbaum, J. F. (1989). Adjunctive buspirone in benzodiazepine treatment of four patients with panic disorder. *American Journal of Psychiatry, 146*, 914–916.

George, D. T., Nutt, D. J., Dwyer, B. A., & Linnoila, M. (1990). Alcoholism and panic disorder: Is the comorbidity more than a coincidence? *Acta Psychiatrica Scandinavica, 81,* 97–107.

Gould, R. A., Clum, G. A., & Shapiro, D. (1993). The use of bibliotherapy in the treatment of panic: A preliminary investigation. *Behavior Therapy, 24,* 241–252.

Helzer, J. E., & Pryzbeck, T. R. (1988). The co-occurrence of alcoholism and other psychiatric disorders in the general population and its impact on treatment. *Journal of Studies on Alcohol, 49,* 219–224.

Katschnig, H., Stolk, J., & Klerman, G. L. (1989). *Long-term follow-up of panic disorder: I. Clinical outcome of a large group of patients participating in an international multicenter clinical drug trial.* Paper presented at the 27th Annual Meeting of the American College of Neuropsychopharmacology, San Juan, PR.

Keck, P. E., McElroy, S. L., Tugrul, K. C., Bennett, J. A., & Smith, J. M. R. (1993). Antiepileptic drugs for the treatment of panic disorder. *Neuropsychiatry, 27,* 150–153.

Keller, M. B., Lavori, P. W., Goldenberg, I. M., Baker, L. A., Pollack, M. H., Sachs, G. S., Rosenbaum, J. F., Deltito, J. A., Leon, A., Shear, M. K., & Klerman, G. L. (1993). Influence of depression on the treatment of panic disorder with imipramine, alprazolam and placebo. *Journal of Affective Disorders, 28,* 27–38.

Kessler, R. C., McGonagle, K. A., Zhao, S., Nelson, C. B., Hughes, M., Eshleman, S., Wittchen, H.-U., & Kendler, K. S. (1994). Lifetime and 12-month prevalence of DSM-III-R psychiatric disorders in the United States. *Archives of General Psychiatry, 51,* 8–19.

Klein, D. F. (1981). Anxiety reconceptualized. In D. F. Klein & J. Rabkin (Eds.), *Anxiety: New research and concepts.* New York: Raven Press.

Klerman, G., Shear, M., Leon, A., Keller, M., Lavori, P., Deltito, J., Rosenbaum, J., Pollack, M., & Sachs, G. (1991). *Treating the depression secondary to panic disorder.* Paper presented at the meeting of the New Clinical Drug Evaluation Unit, Key Biscayne, FL.

Kranzler, H. R., Burleson, J. A., Del Boca, F. K., Babor, T. F., Korner, P., Brown, J., & Bohn, M. J. (1994). Buspirone treatment of anxious alcoholics: A placebo-controlled trial. *Archives of General Psychiatry, 51,* 720–731.

Leon, A. C., Shear, M. K., Portera, L., & Klerman, G. L. (1993). Effect size as a measure of symptom specific drug change in clinical trials. *Psychopharmacology Bulletin, 29,* 163–167.

Liebowitz, M. R., Schneier, F., Campeas, R., Hollander, E., Hatterer, J., Fyer, A., Gorman, J. M., Papp, L., Davies, S., Gully, R., & Klein, D. F. (1992). Phenelzine vs. atenolol in social phobia: A placebo controlled comparison. *Archives of General Psychiatry, 49,* 290–300.

Lydiard, R. B. (1987). Desipramine in agoraphobia with panic attacks: An open fixed-dose study. *Journal of Clinical Psychopharmacology, 7,* 258–260.

Lydiard, R. B., Lesser, I. M., Ballenger, J. C., Rubin, R. T., Laraia, M., & Dupont, R. (1992). Fixed dose study of alprazolam 2 mg., alprazolam 6 mg., and placebo in panic disorder. *Journal of Clinical Psychopharmacology, 12,* 96–103.

Mavissakalian, M. (1990). The relationship between panic disorder/agoraphobia and personality disorders. *Psychiatric Clinics of North America, 13,* 661–684.

Mavissakalian, M., & Perel, J. M. (1994). Imipramine doses and plasma-level-response relationships in panic disorder with agoraphobia. *American Journal of Psychiatry, 152,* 673–682.

Mavissakalian, M., & Michelson, L. (1986). Two year follow up of exposure in imipramine treatment of agoraphobia. *American Journal of Psychiatry, 143,* 1106–1112.

Mavissakalian, M., & Perel, J. (1985). Imipramine in the treatment of agoraphobia: Dose–response relationships. *American Journal of Psychiatry, 142,* 1032–1036.

Mavissakalian, M., & Perel, J. M. (1989). Imipramine dose–response relationship in panic disorder with agoraphobia. *Archives of General Psychiatry, 46,* 127–131.

Mavissakalian, M., & Perel, J. M. (1992a). Clinical experiments in maintenance and discontinuation of imipramine therapy in panic disorder with agoraphobia. *Archives of General Psychiatry, 49,* 318–323.

Mavissakalian, M., & Perel, J. M. (1992b). Protective effects of imipramine maintenance treatment in panic disorder with agoraphobia. *American Journal of Psychiatry, 149,* 1053–1057.

Mellinger, G. D., Balter, M. B., & Uhlenhuth, E. H. (1984). Prevalence and correlates of the long-term regular use of anxiolytics. *Journal of the American Medical Association, 251,* 375–379.

Modigh, K., Westberg, P., & Eriksson, E. (1992). Superiority of clomipramine over imipramine in the treatment of panic disorder: A placebo-controlled trial. *Journal of Clinical Psychopharmacology, 12,* 251–261.

Muskin, P. R., & Fyer, A. J. (1981). Treatment of panic disorder. *Journal of Clinical Psychopharmacology, 1,* 81–90.

Nagy, L. M., Krystal, J. H., Charney, D. S., Merikangas, K. R., & Woods, S. W. (1993). Long-term medical and panic disorder after short-term behavioral group treatment: 2.9 year naturalistic follow-up study. *Journal of Clinical Psychopharmacology, 13,* 16–24.

Nagy, L. M., Krystal, J. H., Woods, S. W., & Charney, D. S. (1989). Clinical and medication outcome after short-term alprazolam and behavioral group treatment of panic disorder. *Archives of General Psychiatry, 46,* 993–999.

Naranjo, C. A., Kadlec, K. E., Sanhueza, P., Woodley-Remus, D., & Sellers, E. M. (1990). Fluoxetine differentially alters alcohol intake and other consummatory behaviors in problem drinkers. *Clinical Pharmacology and Therapeutics, 47,* 490–498.

Norton, G., Harrison, B., Hauch, J., & Rhodes, L. (1985). Characteristics of people with infrequent panic attacks. *Journal of Abnormal Psychology, 94,* 216–221.

Noyes, R., Anderson, D., & Clancy, J. (1984). Diazepam and propranolol in panic disorder and agoraphobia. *American Journal of Orthopsychiatry, 41,* 287–292.

Noyes, R., Garvey, M., & Cook, B. (1989). Follow up study of patients with panic attacks treated with tricyclic antidepressants. *Journal of Affective Disorders, 16,* 249–257.

Otto, M. W., Pollack, M. H., Meltzer-Brody, S., & Rosenbaum, J. F. (1992a). Cognitive-behavioral therapy for benzodiazepine discontinuation in panic disorder patients. *Psychopharmacology Bulletin, 28,* 123–130.

Otto, M. W., Pollack, M. H., Rosenbaum, J. F., Sachs, G. S., & Asher, R. H. (1994). Childhood history of anxiety in adults with panic disorder: Association with anxiety sensitivity and avoidance. *Harvard Review of Psychiatry, 1,* 288–293.

Otto, M. W., Pollack, M. H., Sachs, G. S., O'Neil, C. A., & Rosenbaum, J. F. (1992b). Alcohol dependence in panic disorder patients. *Journal of Psychiatric Research, 26,* 29–38.

Otto, M. W., Pollack, M. H., Sachs, G. S., Reiter, S. R., Meltzer-Brody, S., & Rosenbaum, J. F. (1993). Discontinuation of benzodiazepine treatment: Efficacy of cognitive-behavioral therapy for patients with panic disorder. *American Journal of Psychiatry, 150,* 1485–1490.

Pollack, M. H., & Otto, M. W. (1994). Long-term pharmacological treatment of panic disorder. *Psychiatric Annals, 24,* 291–298.

Pollack, M. H., Otto, M. W., Kaspi, S. P., Hammerness, P. G., & Rosenbaum, J. F. (1994a). Cognitive-behavioral therapy for medication refractory panic disorder. *Journal of Clinical Psychiatry, 55,* 200–205.

Pollack, M. H., Otto, M. W., Rosenbaum, J. F., & Sachs, G. S. (1992). Personality disorders in panic patients: Relationship to childhood anxiety disorders, early trauma, comorbidity and chronicity. *Comprehensive Psychiatry, 33,* 78–83.

Pollack, M. H., Otto, M. W., Rosenbaum, J. F., Sachs, G. S., O'Neil, C., Asher, R., & Meltzer-Brody, S. (1990). Longitudinal course of panic disorder: Findings from the Massachusetts General Hospital Naturalistic Study. *Journal of Clinical Psychiatry, 51,* 12–16.

Pollack, M. H., Otto, M. W., Sabatino, S. A., & Rosenbaum, J. F. (1994b). *Predictors of time to relapse in a longitudinal study of panic disorder.* Paper presented at the 33rd Annual Meeting of the American College of Neuropsychopharmacology, San Juan, PR.

Pollack, M. H., Otto, M. W., Sachs, G. S., Leon, A., Shear, M. K., Deltito, J. A., Keller, M. B., & Rosenbaum, J. R. (1994). Anxiety psychopathology predictive of outcome in patients with panic disorder treated with imipramine, alprazolam and placebo. *Journal of Affective Disorders, 30,* 273–281.

Pollack, M. H., Otto, M. W., Tesar, G. E., Cohen, L. S., Meltzer-Brody, S. M., & Rosenbaum, J. F. (1993). Long-term outcome after acute treatment with clonazepam and alprazolam for panic disorder. *Psychiatric Annals, 13,* 257–263.

Pollack, M. H., & Rosenbaum, J. F. (1991). Fluoxetine for treatment of cocaine abuse in intravenous drug users. *Journal of Clinical Psychiatry, 52,* 31–33.

Reich, J. F. (1988). DSM-III personality disorders and the outcome of treated panic disorder. *American Journal of Psychiatry, 145,* 1149–1152.

Reiss, S., Peterson, R., Gursky, M., & McNally, R. (1986). Anxiety sensitivity, anxiety frequency, and the prediction of fearfulness. *Behaviour Research and Therapy, 24,* 1–8.

Reiter, S. R., Pollack, M. H., Rosenbaum, J. F., & Cohen, L. S. (1990). Clonazepam for the treatment of social phobia. *Journal of Clinical Psychiatry, 51,* 470–472.

Rickels, K., & Schweizer, E. (1993). The treatment of generalized anxiety disorder in patients without depressive symptomatology. *Journal of Clinical Psychiatry, 54*(Suppl.), 20–23.

Rosenbaum, J. F., Biederman, J., Bolduc-Murphy, E. A., Faraone, S. V., Chaloff, J., Hirshfeld, D. R., & Kagan, J. (1993). Behavioral inhibition in childhood: A risk factor for anxiety disorders. *Harvard Review of Psychiatry, 1,* 2–16.

Rosenbaum, J. F., & Pollack, M. H. (1991). Anxiety. In N. Cassem (Ed.), *The Massachusetts General handbook of general hospital psychiatry.* St Louis, MO: C. V. Mosby.

Roy-Byrne, P. P., Geraci, M., & Uhde, T. (1986). Life events and the onset of panic disorder. *American Journal of Psychiatry, 143,* 1424–1427.

Sachs, G. S., Lafer, B., Truman, C. J., Noeth, M., & Thibault, A. B. (1994). Lithium monotherapy: Miracle, myth and misunderstanding. *Psychiatric Annals, 24,* 299–306.

Schneier, F. R., Liebowitz, M. R., & Davies, S. O. (1990). Fluoxetine in panic disorder. *Journal of Clinical Psychopharmacology, 10,* 119–121.

Sheehan, D. V., Ballenger, J., & Jacobsen, E. (1980). Treatment of endogenous anxiety with phobic, hysterical and hypochondriacal symptoms. *Archives of General Psychiatry, 37,* 51–62.

Sheehan, D. V., Davidson, J., & Manschreck, T. (1983). Lack of efficacy of a new antidepressant (bupropion) in the treatment of panic disorder with phobias. *Journal of Clinical Psychopharmacology, 3,* 28–31.

Stein, M. B., Shea, C. A., & Uhde, T. W. (1989). Social phobic symptoms in patients with panic disorder: Practical and theoretical implications. *American Journal of Psychiatry, 146,* 235–238.

Tesar, G. E., Rosenbaum, J. F., Pollack, M. H., Otto, M. W., Sachs, G. S., Herman, J. B., Cohen, L. S., & Spier, S. A. (1991). Double blind, placebo controlled comparison of clonazepam and alprazolam for panic disorder. *Journal of Clinical Psychiatry, 52,* 69–76.

Thase, M. E. (1992). Long-term treatments of recurrent depressive disorders. *Journal of Clinical Psychiatry, 53*(9, Suppl.), 32–44.

Tiffon, L., Coplan, J. D., Papp, L. A., & Gorman, J. M. (1994). Augmentation strategies with tricyclic or fluoxetine treatment in seven partially responsive panic disorder patients. *Journal of Clinical Psychiatry, 55,* 66–69.

Uhlenhuth, E. H., Matuzas, W., Glass, R. M., & Easton, C. (1989). Response of panic disorder to fixed dose of alprazolam or imipramine. *Journal of Affective Disorders, 17,* 261–270.

van der Kolk, B. A., Dreyfuss, D., Michaels, M., Shera, D., Berkowitz, R., Fisler, R., & Saxe, G. (1994). Fluoxetine in posttraumatic stress disorder. *Journal of Clinical Psychiatry, 55,* 517–522.

Weilburg, J. B., Schacter, S., Sachs, G. S., Worth, J., Pollack, M. H., Ives, J. R., & Schomer, D. L. (1993). Focal EEG changes during atypical panic attacks. *Journal of Neuropsychiatry and Clinical Neuroscience, 5,* 50–55.

5

Maximizing Treatment Outcome for Panic Disorder: Cognitive-Behavioral Strategies

MICHAEL W. OTTO
ROBERT A. GOULD

Cognitive-behavioral therapy (CBT) for anxiety disorders has become increasingly specialized in the last decade. Advances in the conceptualization of individual anxiety disorders have brought a refinement of interventions to target the particular core fears and dominant behavior patterns that characterize each disorder. Central to these treatments are exposure and cognitive restructuring interventions. Cognitive restructuring incorporates a variety of procedures to challenge the inaccurate and maladaptive cognitions that increase the anxiety and help maintain the disorder. Exposure interventions hasten the extinction of learned fears, and provide an additional means for patients to challenge anxiogenic beliefs by providing corrective experiences. Although treatments for anxiety disorders commonly utilize these interventions, procedures for their application may differ significantly among the disorders because of differences in the behavioral patterns the treatments target. For example, panic disorder is characterized by a pervasive pattern of fear of panic attacks. Accordingly, current forms of CBT for panic disorder target catastrophic misinterpretations of somatic sensations of panic and their perceived consequences, and exposure procedures focus directly on the fear of somatic sensations.

The same sort of specificity of interventions can be found for CBT

for social phobia. Diagnostic criteria for social phobia emphasize the patient's fears of negative evaluation by others. Likewise, cognitive restructuring for social phobia focuses on the modification of these fears, and
exposure treatments emphasize the completion of feared activities and interactions in front of others. For generalized anxiety disorder (GAD), treatments focus on the worry process itself, with the substitution of cognitive
restructuring and problem solving for self-perpetuating worry patterns, and
the use of imaginal exposure for select worries and fears.

For each of these interventions, the intensity of exposure is modulat-
ed so that patients do not become overwhelmed during initial trials. In
addition, symptom management strategies (e.g., breathing retraining or
muscle relaxation) or social skills training (e.g., assertiveness or problem-
solving training) are valuable adjuncts to exposure and cognitive restructuring interventions for many anxiety conditions.

The success of these strategies ranges from encouraging to striking.
For most of the anxiety disorders, CBT interventions are among the most
efficacious in the treatment literature. Recent reviews of the literature and
meta-analyses indicate that CBT is equal to or surpasses pharmacologic
interventions for the treatment of panic disorder (Clum, Clum, & Surls,
1993; Gould, Otto, & Pollack, 1995), social phobia (Gould, Otto, Yap,
& Pollack, 1994), obsessive–compulsive disorder (Christensen, Hadzi-
Pavlovic, Andrews, & Mattick, 1987), GAD (Hunt & Singh, 1991), and
posttraumatic stress disorder (PTSD; Otto, Penava, Pollock, & Smoller,
Chapter 9, this volume). In addition, CBT has long been considered the
standard intervention for specific phobias (Barlow, 1988). However, despite
the relative success of these treatments, a variety of patients continue to
respond poorly and suffer residual symptoms.

In this chapter, we review treatment elements and outcome for panic
disorder; we do the same for social phobia and GAD in Chapter 7 of this
volume. For each disorder, the nature of the disorder as conceptualized
from a cognitive-behavioral perspective is discussed, to provide a rationale for CBT interventions. Standard treatment packages are reviewed, as
are strategies for treatment-resistant patients.

THE NATURE OF PANIC DISORDER:
A COGNITIVE-BEHAVIORAL PERSPECTIVE

The 1991 National Institute of Health Consensus Development Conference on Panic Disorder concluded that the available evidence supports
the short-term efficacy of both CBT and pharmacologic treatments for
panic disorder, and identified an absence of evidence for the efficacy of
psychodynamic psychotherapy (National Institutes of Health, 1991). The
conference also encouraged the evaluation of treatment efficacy after 6–8
weeks, with consideration of alternative treatment if no response is evident. Given the success of CBT and pharmacologic treatments for panic

disorder, a focus on delineating the active elements in these treatments and on identifying variables that predict the maintenance of treatment gains offers the potential for maximizing treatment response, and/or for devising optimal combinations of treatment strategies.

CBT and pharmacologic treatments of panic disorder rest on different assumptions about the nature of panic disorder, and studies examining the biologic provocation of panic attacks provide a useful starting point for discussing differences between a primarily biologic account and an integrated cognitive-behavioral account of panic disorder. In provocation studies, any of a number of provocation procedures have been found to produce panic attacks in individuals with panic disorder, and few attacks in individuals without the disorder (Rapee, 1995; Shear, 1986). Over the years, the list of these agents and procedures has expanded to include the administration of sodium lactate, yohimbine, caffeine, norepinephrine, isoproterenol, metachlorophenyl piparazine, and cholecystokinin; carbon dioxide inhalation, hyperventilation, and exercise (for reviews, see McNally, 1994; Rapee, 1995). These findings have been marshaled in support of neurophysiologic theories of panic disorder, but given the wide diversity of effective provocation agents, it is difficult to provide a unified biochemical account of these provocation effects (Clark, 1986; Margraf, Ehlers, & Roth, 1986; McNally, 1994).

An alternative account of the provocation effects focuses not on the biochemical systems directly affected by the procedures, but on the interoceptive sensations they produce. Provocation procedures share the ability to produce somatic sensations similar to the sensations encountered in panic disorder. According to cognitive-behavioral theories of the disorder, the experience of unexpected sensations similar to those encountered in anxiety and panic has the potential to induce a panic attack. To clarify this position, it is helpful to review more generally the cognitive-behavioral account of panic disorder (see Barlow, 1988; Clark, 1986; Goldstein & Chambless, 1978; McNally, 1990).

Panic attacks are assumed to be a manifestation of the emergency fight-or-flight response that is triggered when no external danger is present. The initial panic episode often occurs during or after a period of stress, and may be influenced by individual differences in biologic reactivity. However, the occurrence of the initial panic attack does not appear to be pathognomonic in itself; up to one-third to one-half of samples of nonpatients may experience a single panic-like episode each year, and approximately 10% experience an unexpected episode that meets the four-symptom criterion required for a definable panic attack (Norton, Cox, & Malan, 1992). Instead, the occurrence of regular panic attacks, and the development of fear and avoidance of situations or events associated with panic attacks, are what define the disorder; indeed, the fear of panic and anxiety symptoms appears to be crucial in maintaining this pattern. This point receives emphasis in the fourth edition of the *Diagnostic and Statistical Manual of Mental Disorders* (DSM-IV), where the criteria for panic disorder require not only recurrent unexpected panic attacks, but persistent concerns about having a panic attack, worry about the consequences of a panic attack, or behavior changes related to the attacks (American Psychiatric Association, 1994).

If concerns and worry about the possibility of recurrent attacks are defining features of panic disorder, what then determines and maintains these concerns? Certainly part of the answer is the aversiveness of the physiologic storm that is a panic attack. Patients report that these symptoms feel bad and are frightening. However, the catastrophic misinterpretations of the meaning of these symptoms are especially noteworthy. To a patient, the symptoms appear to herald some of the most frightening events imaginable: disability, death, insanity, or humiliation. The natural response to these fears is increased anxiety, and this reaction to symptoms helps to insure a self-perpetuating cycle (see Barlow, 1988; Clark, 1986; McNally, 1990). According to cognitive-behavioral theories, fears and catastrophic interpretations of internal sensations associated with panic help maintain high levels of anticipatory anxiety and cue repeated attacks. With each attack, perceptions of danger are strengthened, helping to foster a stronger phobic response to the symptoms. A patient's apprehension about the possibility of another panic episode directs attention to the feared bodily sensations; anticipatory anxiety and anxiogenic responses to fear (increased muscle tension or hyperventilation) help insure that anxiety sensations will be present. Following repeated attacks, individuals may directly respond to even small signs of arousal (e.g., a quickened heartbeat) with conditioned fear, eliciting another panic episode. This fear-of-fear cycle is summarized in Figure 5.1.

For many patients with panic disorder, the fear of anxiety sensations may generalize to similar bodily sensations. For example, the natural sensations of arousal associated with exercise or caffeine intake may take on the ability to induce fear, avoidance, or panic in many patients with panic disorder. This phenomenon is a naturalistic manifestation of the provocation effect. Biologically induced sensations (those resulting from exercise or caffeine, in this example) have the capacity to induce anxiety, avoidance, or panic in sensitized individuals, but are considered normal sensations by the majority of the population. This is the explanation of the provocation effect: Any procedure that unexpectedly produces feared somatic sensations may provoke anxiety and panic.

If fears of anxiety sensations were fully confounded with a history of panic disorder, the explanatory value of focusing on cognitions could be questioned. However, fears of anxiety sensations, occurring independently of a history of panic disorder or panic attacks, have been documented and are effective predictors of who will respond to provocation procedures (Donnell & McNally, 1989; Telch & Harrington, 1992). That is, individuals with preexisting fears of anxiety sensations, as assessed by self-report inventories, have been found to respond to provocation procedures with anxiety and panic. In addition, fears of anxiety sensations appears to be

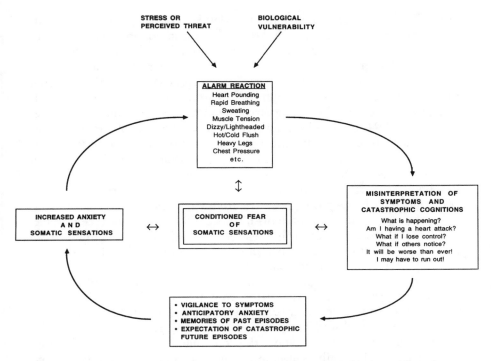

FIGURE 5.1. The fear-of-fear cycle. From Otto, Pollack, Meltzer-Brody, and Rosenbaum (1992).

important predictors of who will develop an anxiety or panic disorder over time (Maller & Reiss, 1992).

Taken together, this evidence provides an important alternative to neurophysiologic explanations of the provocation effect. Provocation procedures have in common the ability to produce unexpected, feared somatic sensations. As suggested by case reports (Cohen, Barlow, & Blanchard, 1985), it does not appear to matter whether these sensations are the result of increases or decreases in physiologic arousal; relaxation procedures are also able to induce panic episodes, presumably because they have the ability to induce odd sensations (e.g., warmth or heaviness in the limbs) that can be misinterpreted as loss of control.

COMPONENTS AND EFFECTIVENESS
OF CBT FOR PANIC DISORDER

Treatment Components

Corresponding to this analysis of the nature of panic disorder and the provocation effect, current forms of CBT for the disorder target the elimination of fears of somatic sensations of anxiety as a primary element of treatment. Treatment typically includes four basic components delivered over the course of 12 to 15 sessions. The first is an informational intervention that provides patients with a model of the disorder and a rationale for the interventions to follow. A recent study suggests that an informational intervention, provided at the outset of treatment may have significant effects. In comparing CBT to supportive treatment, Shear, Pilkonis, Cloitre, and Leon (1994) included a cognitive-behavioral model of panic disorder in the supportive treatment intervention. Surprisingly, the outcome for the supportive treatment intervention rivaled that obtained for CBT—a finding that is inconsistent with previous reports (see Beck, Sokol, Clark, Berchick, & Wright, 1992). One mitigating factor may be that therapists' compliance with the protocol was relatively low for the CBT condition, raising the possibility that patients in this condition did not receive a full dose of CBT. Nonetheless, the Shear et al. (1994) study does draw attention to the potential importance of a strong informational intervention for non-CBT treatments for panic disorder.

The second, and complementary, component of treatment is cognitive restructuring. "Cognitive restructuring" refers to a broad array of techniques designed to help patients identify and change maladaptive thinking patterns. In panic disorder, the focus of cognitive restructuring is on the patients' catastrophic beliefs about the consequences of panic attacks (e.g., see Table 5.1). Typically, self-monitoring procedures are used to help patients identify the content of their thoughts in anxiety- or panic-provoking situations. Once identified, individual thoughts can be challenged for their veracity. In particular, distortions of the degree of catastrophe and probability of feared outcomes are examined (see Barlow & Craske, 1989). The accuracy of cognitions may also be examined in "behavioral experiments," where patients have the opportunity to examine predictions about the consequences of anxiety and panic symptoms. Exposure-based procedures provide the basis for many of these behavioral tests, in which patients use their own experiences to modify their thinking. Hence, interoceptive or situational exposure procedures are true extensions of cognitive restructuring, because they allow patients to test their beliefs regarding the dangerousness of symptoms or their ability to cope in various scenarios.

A third component of treatment is training in skills for reducing anxiogenic responses to symptoms. These skills commonly include training in diaphragmatic and slow breathing techniques and in muscle relaxation. Relative to other components of CBT, this training may be of least importance. Barlow, Craske, Cerny, and Klosko (1989), in a study of components of treatment for panic disorder, found that adding relaxation to treatment emphasizing cognitive restructuring and interoceptive exposure appeared to *reduce* treatment efficacy over the long term. One explanation for the decrement in efficacy may be that patients overuse relaxation as an anxiety management technique, to the exclusion of fully learning not to fear anxiety sensations. That is, patients may incorporate anxiety

TABLE 5.1. Cognitions Associated with Panic Disorder

Fears of death or disability
  What if I have a stroke?

  Am I having a heart attack?

  If these sensations get worse, I am sure to die.

  There must be something seriously wrong with my body.

Fears of losing control/insanity
  I am going to lose control and scream.

  I must be about to have a nervous breakdown.

  I will have to leap out of my car and start running.

  What if I go insane?

  What if I can't control my car?

  What if I faint and no one comes to help me?

Fears of humiliation or embarrassment
  People will notice that I am anxious and will think something is wrong with me.

  They will know that I am not in control.

  If I tremble, everyone will notice and will think I am weird.

  I will fall down and be embarrassed.

  They will reject me and I will be alone.

  I won't be able to swallow at lunch, and they will know something is wrong.

Note. Adapted from Otto, Pollack, and Barlow (1995). Copyright 1995 by Graywind Publications. Adapted by permission.

management strategies into avoidance strategies, rather than fully learning to eliminate fears of both mild and strong anxiety sensations. However, depending on the way relaxation strategies are applied, it is clear that these procedures can offer clear benefit to patients with panic disorder, sometimes rivaling alternative CBT procedures (Öst & Westling, 1995).

The fourth component of treatment, exposure, includes both interoceptive and *in vivo* exposure procedures. Interoceptive exposure uses a variety of procedures and exercises (e.g., hyperventilation, exercise, or spinning in a chair; see Barlow & Craske, 1989; Otto, Pollack, & Barlow, 1995a) to expose patients to feared internal bodily sensations. Through repeated exposure to these sensations, the patients are helped to decrease their fear and anxiogenic responses to these stimuli. With repeated exposure, patients learn that the sensations are not harmful and need not be feared, thereby breaking a crucial aspect of the fear-of-fear cycle that is maintaining the panic disorder.

For patients with agoraphobic avoidance, therapist-paced or self-paced exposure to feared situations is important. In our clinical and research application of these procedures, interoceptive exposure is used as the primary exposure strategy and as a means of moving toward situational exposure procedures. Patients begin their exposure with interoceptive exposure procedures completed in therapy sessions (e.g., with hyperventilation). They are next assigned home practice of these procedures. As patients become comfortable and confident with the exposure procedures at home, interoceptive exposure is assigned in less "safe" surroundings (e.g., in a patient's office at work) to help insure that learned safety to symptoms is not situation-dependent. Finally, we replace the formal interoceptive exposure procedures with more naturalistic exposure, using naturally occurring events to achieve interoceptive exposure. For example, chair-spinning procedures to produce dizziness may be replaced by other activities (e.g., play with a patient's children on a merry-go-round or on swings) that induce symptoms but are also congruent with personal or role demands. Situational (*in vivo*) exposure represents a further extension of this theme. Rather than using specialized activities to induce symptoms, patients are encouraged to use feared situations to induce the once-feared sensations. If anxiety sensations are encountered, patients are to respond to these sensations in just the same manner as they respond to the sensations produced by the formal interoceptive exposure procedures; this should prevent the escalation of initial anxiety into panic. Regardless of whether or not anxiety sensations are encountered, patients achieve their goal: reentry into avoided situations without panic.

Treatment Efficacy

It is important to note that CBT for panic disorder does not simply target the goal of helping patients endure panic-related distress; it targets the elimination of panic attacks by eliminating sensitivity to and fear of symptoms and situations that help cue the next panic attack. An increased ability to tolerate the somatic sensations of a panic attack with less distress is an intermediate step in this process, but the final goal is to eliminate fears and anxiogenic responses to even mild symptoms, thereby helping end the regular evocation of limited or full-blown panic attacks. Treatment protocols including the elements discussed above (e.g., Barlow et al., 1989; Beck et al., 1992; Clark et al., 1994; Margraf, Barlow, Clark, & Telch, 1993) have been associated with marked treatment response, with panic-free rates following short-term treatment ranging from 74% to 85%. There is also evidence of maintenance of these treatment gains over follow-up periods of 1–2 years (Beck et al., 1992; Craske, Brown, & Barlow, 1991).

The significance of these outcome rates is nicely documented by reviews of the treatment literature (Chambless & Gillis, 1993; Clum et al., 1993). For example, in a recently completed meta-analysis we examined the outcomes of 43 studies (there were 78 separate comparisons) published or presented between 1974 and January 1994 (Gould et al., 1995). All studies examined treatment outcome for patients with panic disorder with or without agoraphobia that employed a control group (no treatment, waiting list, pill placebo, or psychologic placebo) and random assignment to treatments. Effect sizes were computed in such a manner that a positive effect size represented the number of standard deviation units by which an active treatment surpassed a control treatment. In this analysis, forms of CBT may have enjoyed some advantage, because a relatively greater percentage of these studies (than of pharmacologic treatment studies) employed a waiting-list control rather than a placebo control group.

Table 5.2 summarizes the findings. CBT interventions yielded the highest mean effect size (0.68), followed by combined pharmacologic and CBT interventions (0.56) and pharmacological treatments alone (0.47). There was no significant difference between antidepressant and benzodiazepine treatment. Among the CBT interventions studied, treatments that combined cognitive restructuring with interoceptive exposure yielded the strongest mean effect size (0.88). This mean effect size was significantly higher than that obtained for pharmacologic treatments. In addition, patient attrition in forms of CBT (5.6%) tended to be less than in either pharmacological (19.8%) or combined (22.0%) treatments. Finally, analysis of the cost of treatment over time indicated that the lowest-cost interventions were imipramine treatment and group CBT. In summary, our review of the outcome literature provides evidence that CBT on average results in larger treatment effects, lower attrition rates, and lower costs than pharmacologic interventions for panic disorder (Gould et al., 1995).

Examination of treatment effects over follow-up periods also supports the efficacy of CBT. Table 5.2 provides a summary of the slippage in treatment effects between acute outcome and the end of follow-up periods ranging from 6 months to 2 years. In general, medications were withdrawn during this time period; hence, slippage estimates do not represent the effects of maintenance pharmacologic treatment. Patients treated briefly with medications tended to lose treatment benefits over the follow-up periods, although the degree of loss appeared to be attenuated by the addition of behavior therapy (typically emphasizing exposure) during the treatment period. Slippage was not evident for CBT alone. Indeed, in select studies there is evidence of further improvements in outcome over follow-up periods for patients treated with CBT (Beck et al., 1992; Craske et al., 1991).

We have suggested that two factors may underlie the long-term effectiveness of CBT relative to medication treatments of panic disorder (Otto, Gould, & Pollack, 1994). First, CBT emphasizes the treatment of fears of somatic sensations of anxiety, and we believe that this treatment is central to long-term success. Second, CBT relies on skill development, which helps insure that patients retain the effects of therapy after termination of the formal treatment process. Because of the emphasis on informational interventions, skill acquisition, and independent practice, patients are provided with a model of the disorder and skills for its management, should symptoms recur at a later time. In contrast, pharmacologic interventions, despite their ability to decrease anxiety and block panic, do not necessarily decrease the tendency to fear and catastrophically interpret somatic sensations of anxiety or lead to an increase in personal coping skills. As

TABLE 5.2. **Meta-Analysis of Treatments for Panic Disorder (43 Studies; 78 Separate Comparisons)**

Treatment strategy	Effect size	Panic-free
Acute treatment effects (effect size relative to controls)		
Pharmacotherapy	0.47	
ADM	0.55	58%
BZD	0.40	61%
CBT	0.63	70%
IE + CR	0.88	
Slippage of treatment effects (posttreatment to follow-up)		
Pharmacotherapy	− 0.46	
Pharmacotherapy + exposure	− 0.07	
CBT	+ 0.06	

Note. ADM, antidepressant medications; BZD, benzodiazepine treatment; IE + CR, treatments emphasizing interoceptive exposure and cognitive restructuring. Data from Gould, Otto, and Pollack (1995).

a result, when anxiety symptoms emerge as a consequence of other life events or during or after medication tapering, patients with untreated fears of anxiety sensations may more easily reenter a cycle of catastrophic interpretations of symptoms, increasing vigilance, fear, and panic.

This conceptualization has been applied to the problems that arise upon medication discontinuation, particularly upon the discontinuation of benzodiazepine treatment for panic disorder (Otto, Pollack, Meltzer-Brody, & Rosenbaum, 1992). Benzodiazepine tapering is associated with the emergence of withdrawal symptoms that mimic many of the symptoms of anxiety and panic. When the fears of anxiety symptoms have not been treated, benzodiazepine discontinuation insures that patients are exposed to feared somatic sensations at a time when they are concerned about a worsening of their disorder. Increased anxiety and panic, and the inability to complete the taper, are frequently the results (Fyer et al., 1987; Noyes, Garvey, Cook, & Suelzer, 1991).

CBT that targets the elimination of fears and catastrophic interpretations of somatic sensations, while providing skills for decreasing the intensity of these symptoms, has been found to be effective for aiding benzodiazepine discontinuation. In a recent trial, we found that 76% of patients who received a 10-session program of CBT successfully completed benzodiazepine tapering, compared to only 25% of patients receiving slow tapering and a physician support program (Otto et al., 1993). Notably, patients successfully discontinuing their medication achieved a lower level of symptoms off medication. These findings suggest that with treatment targeting fears of anxiety symptoms, patients were able to tolerate symptoms induced by medication tapering and were able to reduce panic symptoms overall.

The success of CBT for panic disorder, both in general and in specific application to benzodiazepine discontinuation, suggests that treatment emphasizing exposure and cognitive restructuring may improve response rates or prevent relapse among patients treated with medications. Indeed, CBT for panic disorder has been found to benefit patients who respond poorly to medication (Pollack, Otto, Kaspi, Hammerness, & Rosenbaum, 1994a), and to improve response and maintenance of treatment gains among patients undergoing brief benzodiazepine treatment (Hegel, Ravaris, & Ahles, 1994; Spiegel, Bruce, Gregg, & Nuzzarello, 1994). Hence, patients failing to respond or responding incompletely to pharmacologic interventions should be considered for referral to CBT. In addition, referral should be considered at the point of medication discontinuation.

In many locations (and in many health maintenance organizations), however, access to experienced cognitive-behavioral therapists is limited. In situations where referral to an experienced therapist is not practical, a number of CBT strategies can be incorporated into pharmacologic treatment. Studies indicate that the simple addition of a self- or therapist-guided program of stepwise exposure to avoided situations can improve the outcome of medication treatment (Mavissakalian & Michelson, 1986a; Telch, Agras, Taylor, Roth, & Gallen, 1985). Studies have also documented the benefits of written, self-help programs of CBT (Gould, Clum, & Shapiro, 1993; Gould & Clum, 1993), as well as reduced-therapist-contact programs of treatment (Côte, Gauthier, Laberge, Cormier, & Plamondon, 1994). Consequently, prescribing physicians have the options of assigning self-guided exposure or recommending adjunctive self-guided treatment to help maximize the benefits of pharmacologic regimens.

THE ISSUE OF COMBINED TREATMENTS

Although there is fairly consistent evidence that CBT strategies are a useful adjunct to medication treatment (Mavissakalian, Michelson, & Dealy, 1983; Mavissakalian, 1990a; Telch et al., 1985), it is not clear whether combined treatment is more effective than CBT alone. Studies have found some initial benefits of combined treatment, but these advantages appear to wane over follow-up periods (Mavissakalian & Michelson, 1986b; Telch et al., 1985). In our meta-analysis (Gould et al., 1995), combined treatments were associated with a lower effect size than that for CBT alone. This finding is consistent with suggestions that the combination of CBT and medications, particularly benzodiazepine treatment, may interfere with the beneficial effects of exposure. Apparent deleterious effects of benzodiazepine treatment on exposure have been documented for patients who are subsequently withdrawn from medication treatment (Marks et al., 1993). However, the interfering effects of benzodiazepine treatment may be specific to more chronic treatment, as limited use of benzodiazepines does not appear to have a negative effect on exposure treatment for agoraphobia

(Wardle et al., 1994), and may even aid exposure sessions under the right conditions (Marks, Viswanathan, Lipsedge, & Gardner, 1972).

Elsewhere, we have discussed some of the potential problems for the combination of pharmacotherapy and CBT (Otto et al., 1994). These difficulties include (1) potential conflict between models of the disorder provided to patients by caregivers; (2) use of a dosing schedule that encourages pill taking rather than use of behavioral skills as a coping response to anticipatory anxiety or panic attacks; and (3) the emergence of state-dependent learning and the attribution of therapeutic gains to medications rather than to skill acquisition. To minimize these difficulties and maximize the involvement of patients in learning cognitive-behavioral skills, we suggest that patients receive an integrated model of panic disorder that acknowledges a possible biologic diathesis for the disorder but stresses the self-perpetuation cycles discussed above. Discussion of treatment options should include a review of the evidence suggesting that either medications or CBT can be used to treat these cycles successfully, but that maintenance of treatment gains appears to be higher with CBT unless medication is maintained over the long term. In addition, to help insure that patients learn cognitive-behavioral skills for managing symptoms, all medications should be prescribed on a fixed-dose basis, and patients must be provided with opportunities to apply CBT strategies when symptomatic. Interoceptive and in vivo exposure procedures provide opportunities for skill development, but to guard against the possibility of state-dependent learning, behavioral skills must be practiced independently of both the therapist and medication treatment. Hence, for optimal treatment, behavioral skills should be practiced during or after a period of medication discontinuation. When this is not possible and patients continue to take medications to "control" panic attacks, we fear that treatment with CBT will not be as successful as possible. Consistent with this concern, we recently found in a survival analysis of patients in our ongoing longitudinal study of panic disorder (Pollack et al., 1990) that patients who achieved remission with combined treatment (CBT and pharmacotherapy) and continued their pharmacologic treatment tended to relapse sooner than patients who achieve remission after CBT treatment alone (Otto, Pollack, & Sabatino, 1995c). Nonetheless, the success of adding CBT to short-term benzodiazepine treatment (and the continuation of CBT during the medication discontinuation phase; e.g., Hegel et al., 1994; Spiegel et al., 1994) suggests that pharmacologic treatments and CBT can be combined successfully under the right conditions, and that this should be considered an effective strategy for patients who require medication treatment.

PREDICTORS OF RESPONSE TO CBT

Research on predictors of response to CBT has been marked by inconsistent findings over the last 15 years, leading Keijsers, Hoogduin, and Schaap

(1994) to conclude in their review of the literature that there is no well-documented single predictor of poor CBT outcome for panic disorder. Nonetheless, a number of variables have received mixed support for predicting poorer outcome, and in combination these variables appear to have a more pronounced effect. Variables that have received moderate support as predictors of poorer outcome include the severity of agoraphobic avoidance, fears of anxiety sensations, depressed mood, and personality psychopathology (Keijsers et al., 1994). Marital discord and the severity and frequency of panic symptoms have been inconsistent predictors (Keijsers et al., 1994). It is important to note that negative predictors of outcome for CBT tend to be the same as those for pharmacologic treatment. For example, predictors of poor response to pharmacotherapy include the severity of the panic disorder and agoraphobia, comorbid depression, comorbid anxiety disorders, and high levels of personality disorder traits (Mavissakalian, 1990b; Pollack et al., 1993, 1994b).

Care needs to be taken in interpreting the role of these negative predictors in moderating outcome. The relationship between agoraphobia severity and treatment outcome provides an interesting example. Although severity of pretreatment agoraphobia predicts posttreatment outcome (Chambless & Gracely, 1989; de Beurs, 1993), patients with more severe agoraphobia have been found to make the greatest *gains* in treatment (Jansson, Öst, & Jerremalm, 1987). That is, baseline severity of agoraphobic avoidance identifies patients who are the furthest from remission, although it appears that more avoidant patients change at a rate greater than or equal to that of less avoidant patients. As such, treatment may work as well with more severely agoraphobic patients, but these patients may require a stronger dose or duration of CBT to achieve remission.

The importance of full treatment of avoidance patterns must be underscored, given the importance of avoidance in predicting ongoing anxiety difficulties, as well as the return of panic attacks in remitted patients (Ehlers, 1995). As noted by Craske et al. (1991), the success of CBT in the treatment of panic attacks should not overshadow the importance of fully treating agoraphobic avoidance to insure that patients return to a high quality of life. Furthermore, residual avoidance should be considered as a risk factor for relapse, and should be targeted for vigorous attention (e.g., *in vivo* exposure) before the acute phase of treatment is concluded.

Comorbid Depression

Depressed mood has been an inconsistent predictor of treatment outcome for CBT and pharmacotherapy for panic disorder. However, evaluation of the role of depression in treatment outcome is made difficult by the frequent exclusion from studies of patients with symptoms severe enough to meet criteria for major depression. In contrast, patients with panic disorder and comorbid major depression are common in clinical practice, with estimates that approximately two-thirds of patients with panic disorder meet criteria for past or present major depression (Clark, 1989). Patients may also develop major depression during the course of treatment. In a recent longitudinal study investigating this issue, Ball, Otto, Pollack, and Rosenbaum (1994) examined the emergence of major depression in a 2-year prospective study of 90 patients with panic disorder who were free of depression at baseline evaluation. Despite ongoing treatment for panic disorder, primarily with pharmacotherapy, 24% of these patients developed a prospective episode of major depression. Predictors of the occurrence of depression included a past history of depression, comorbid GAD, low assertiveness, and baseline depressive symptoms. Comorbid GAD and low assertiveness continued to be significant predictors after the influence of depression history and baseline depression symptoms were statistically controlled. Interestingly, pharmacologic treatment, including treatment with antidepressants, was not associated with a protective effect—a finding replicating previous research.

Comorbid depression may influence the treatment of panic disorder in a number of important ways. Depression typically affects an individual's motivation, activity level, and style of thinking. Neurovegetative symptoms may sap strength and motivation, and the high levels of dysfunctional cognitions characteristic of depression may engender negative evaluations about progress or the likelihood of improvement. These negative evaluations may also lower motivation, slowing the rate of practice of new skills and negatively biasing the evaluation of performance in homework assignments. Depression appears to have specific effects on anxiogenic cognitions as well. For example, scores on the Anxiety Sensitivity Index, a measure of fears of anxiety sensations (Peterson & Reiss, 1992), have been found to be elevated in depressed patients without anxiety disorders, and to decrease with effective treatment of the depression (Otto, Pollack, Fava, Uccello, & Rosenbaum, 1995b). Associations between anxiety-related cognitions and depression have also been found for other anxiety disorders, particularly social phobia (Ball, Otto, Pollack, Uccello, & Rosenbaum, 1995; Bruch, Mattia, Heimberg, & Holt, 1993). Together, these findings suggest that depression may help engender or maintain elevated levels of beliefs and thinking styles that perpetuate anxiety disorders. In addition, there is evidence that depression may interfere with anxiety habituation, making it more difficult for patients to achieve extinction of their fears in exposure sessions (Foa & Kozak, 1986; Salkovskis & Mills, 1994).

Table 5.3 summarizes some of these depression-associated difficulties and strategies to minimize them. In our clinical program for panic disorder, patients with comorbid depression receive information during initial sessions on the cognitive biases that accompany depression. Subsequently, they are asked to monitor the emergence of these biases, and to apply cognitive restructuring skills. We also devote extra attention to encouraging compliance with homework assignments, and help patients prepare for and then challenge mood-specific biases in self-evaluation after homework as-

TABLE 5.3. Problems and Corresponding Clinical Strategies
for Patients with Comorbid Major Depression

Problems	Strategies
Greater fears of anxiety sensations Greater fears of negative evaluation from others	Provide information on cognitive distortions in depression ("Depression is biasing your view")
Negative evaluation of self (and progress)	Practice countering negative cognitive biases for homework outcome and progress
Lowered activity level	Provide greater monitoring and reinforcement of homework.

signments. These strategies are viewed as adjunctive to the standard clinical program for panic disorder, and it is expected that treatment of the panic disorder alone will have a variety of antidepressant effects, as has been documented in research trials (e.g., Chambless & Gillis, 1993; Clark et al., 1994; Woody, 1994). In contrast to these procedures for patients with primary panic disorder and secondary depression, we first target treatment of the mood disorder when depression dominates the clinical picture (see Otto, Pava, & Sprich-Buckminster, Chapter 2, this volume), and then introduce antipanic treatment as the anxiety symptoms become the dominant residual problem.

Combined pharmacologic treatment and CBT may also be of use for comorbid depression. Like CBT, pharmacologic treatment of panic disorder is associated with reductions in depressed mood (e.g., Tesar et al., 1991). It is tempting to assume that antidepressant medications offer an advantage over benzodiazepines for the treatment of comorbid panic disorder and depression; however, a recent study did not support this proposition (Keller et al., 1993). Also, there is an absence of research addressing the question of whether combined treatment is more effective than CBT alone for patients with comorbid depression. As a result, clinicians are left on their own to choose between CBT alone and CBT with medications for patients with panic disorder who are also depressed.

Comorbid Anxiety Disorders

Comorbid anxiety conditions are also common in panic disorder and may attenuate treatment response. As noted in the introduction to this chapter, current forms of CBT for anxiety disorders tend to be specific, involving a different sets of procedures for different anxiety disorders. The implication of the specificity of these approaches is that comorbid anxiety conditions will probably require additional strategies and a longer course of treatment. However, recent evidence suggests some generalization of benefits of the treatment of panic disorder to other comorbid conditions, although the enduring presence of a comorbid anxiety disorder still appears to attenuate the long-term outcome of treatment for panic disorder (Brown, Antony, & Barlow, 1995).

Medications have good efficacy across a range of individual anxiety conditions; as such, combined CBT and pharmacologic treatment is viewed as a tempting strategy for patients with significant anxiety comorbidity. Nonetheless, anxiety comorbidity tends to be a negative predictor of outcome for pharmacologic interventions as well (Pollack et al., 1993, 1994b). As a result, the clinician is left without clear guidance from the empirical literature for choosing CBT, pharmacologic treatments, or combination treatments for patients with anxiety comorbidity. It is clear, though, that enduring comorbid anxiety conditions are likely to require a broader range of CBT interventions.

Comorbid Personality Disorders

Degree of personality psychopathology has been a fairly consistent predictor of poor treatment response or poor maintenance of treatment gains for both pharmacologic treatments and CBT (Chambless, Renneberg, Goldstein, & Gracely, 1992; Green & Curtis, 1988; Mavissakalian, 1990b; Mavissakalian & Hamann, 1988; Reich, 1988). For example, Mavissakalian and Hamann (1988) examined the association between treatment response and personality disorder traits in a sample of patients with panic disorder receiving behavioral and pharmacologic treatment. Only 25% of patients with high scores on personality disorder traits responded to treatment, compared with 75% in the group with low scores on these traits.

As evaluated by self-report questionnaires, rates of Axis II pathology are commonly in the range of 40–70% in patients with panic disorder, with avoidant, dependent, histrionic, and borderline personality disorders emerging as the most common diagnoses (Diaferia et al., 1993; Mavissakalian & Hamann, 1988; Pollack, Otto, Rosenbaum, & Sachs, 1992; Reich & Troughton, 1988a). Rates of personality pathology in panic disorder patients tend to be approximately equal to or less than those reported for other anxiety and affective disorders, including social phobia, obsessive–compulsive disorder, and major depression (Alnaes & Torgersen, 1988; Brooks, Baltazar, & Munjack, 1989; Mavissakalian, 1990b; Reich, Noyes, Hirschfeld, Coryell, & O'Gorman, 1987; Sciuto et al., 1991). As compared to nonpatient control groups, patients with panic disorder had higher rates of DSM-III and DSM-III-R Cluster B disorders (the "dramatic" cluster—antisocial, borderline, histrionic, and narcissistic personality disorders) and Cluster C disorders (the "anxious" cluster—avoidant, dependent, obsessive–compulsive, and passive–aggressive personality disorders) (Diaferia et al., 1993; Reich & Troughton, 1988a).

In many cases, apparent Axis II difficulties are not independent of the primary Axis I disorder. For example, treatment studies of patients with major depression (Reich et al., 1987), obsessive–compulsive disorder

(Ricciardi et al., 1992), and panic disorder (Mavissakalian, 1990b) have each documented the reduction in Axis II pathology with treatment of the Axis I disorder. For these reasons, we recommend the general strategy of deferring treatment of the Axis II condition, and, whenever possible, first engaging in vigorous treatment ot the Axis I disorder. However, this strategy may be impractical with more severely impaired patients, because of the regular emergence of disruptive clinical issues or distress that demand therapeutic attention.

In some cases, a patient's chronic adjustment may be characterized by frequent interpersonal or life crises that require therapeutic attention. In other cases, a patient's panic disorder may be one part of a broader deficit in emotional regulation skills, requiring a broader set of interventions than treatment of the panic disorder can provide. In both cases, it is tempting to forgo treatment of the panic disorder and devote greater attention to characterologic issues. However, the cost of this approach is the loss of the more immediate reduction in distress and improvement in functioning that may be obtained by treatment of the panic disorder. Conversely, the potential cost of ignoring weekly crises is the escalation of a patient's emotional distress, demoralization, or acting-out behaviors.

To enhance treatment of panic disorder in patients with chaotic lifestyles and unstable interpersonal relationships, we often schedule at least two sessions a week. In each week, one session is devoted to current areas of distress or broader life issues, and one session is fully devoted to the treatment of panic disorder. Although it may take several weeks for some patients to adjust to this schedule, we have had fairly good success in maintaining progress and a good therapeutic alliance with this sort of arrangement. Nonetheless, we have encountered two situations in which progress tends to stall. In the first case, patients appear to have difficulties completing homework or employing cognitive restructuring strategies because of a broader deficit in self-care skills. For example, when confronted by situations that call for increased self-care and the application of cognitive restructuring or other skills, some patients tend to respond with self-criticism and self-punishment. Consequently, to help such patients utilize the treatment for panic disorder, treatment first must target the modification of distorted belief systems and the development of appropriate self-care responses to distress. Treatment interventions developed for patients with borderline personality disorder appear to be helpful in this process (Beck, Freeman, & Associates, 1990; Farrell & Shaw, 1994; Linehan, 1993).

A second situation that poses a problem for the standard application of CBT for panic disorder occurs when patients have a trauma history and untreated PTSD (which are often associated with personality disorders; e.g., see Linehan, 1993). Diagnosis of comorbid PTSD may be made difficult by the tendency for some patients to stress panic symptomatology and minimize their trauma history and trauma-related symptoms in initial interviews. Although treatment for panic disorder may ameliorate some of the PTSD symptoms, treatment may break down if interoceptive exposure exercises cue trauma-related memories. As discussed in more detail in Chapter 9 of this volume, interoceptive sensations of anxiety can provoke trauma-related flashbacks in patients with PTSD. As a result, informational interventions and discussion of the trauma may be crucial for treatment of the panic disorder to proceed. Because interoceptive exposure can be used as a component treatment for PTSD as well as panic disorder, treatment of the primary panic disorder and the comorbid PTSD can proceed simultaneously for many patients (see Otto et al., Chapter 9, this volume). Table 5.4 summarizes these and other strategies for patients with Axis II disorders.

Finally, treatment goals may be much harder to reach in patients with avoidant and dependent Axis II traits (Mavissakalian, 1990b). For these patients, treatment of agoraphobia must take into account chronic levels of avoidance and restrictions in lifestyle. As a consequence, the identification of goals for treatment must be carefully considered in ongoing collaboration with each patient. In each stage of treatment, the patient may require additional skills to help insure success upon entry into avoided situations, and may want to reevaluate goals as initial objectives are achieved. As the treatment of these patients is likely to affect their current role functioning, a collaborative approach with the patient's partner, friends, or family members may be required. Involvement of the spouses of patients has been found to have beneficial effects on the treatment of agoraphobia (Barlow, O'Brien, & Last, 1984; Cerny, Barlow, Craske, & Himadi, 1987), and encourages the regular involvement of spouses in at least one conjoint session. For example, in our clinical treatment programs, each patient is encouraged to bring a significant other to a treatment

TABLE 5.4. Problems and Corresponding Clinical Strategies
for Patients with Comorbid Axis II Disorders

Problems	Strategies
Intrusion of life issues	Scheduling of dual sessions
Poor emotional regulation skills	Shaping of self-care skills: 　Identification of core beliefs 　Cognitive restructuring 　Affective regulation 　Problem solving
Trauma history/PTSD	Information on emotion-cued recall Additional treatment for PTSD
Chronic patterns of avoidance	Defining goals—how much avoidance to target Longer course of treatment Couple/family sessions

session, to help insure that treatment goals and methods will be supported in the patient's home life. For a patient with avoidant or dependent characteristics, this process may need to be expanded to include regular conjoint sessions to evaluate the impact of change on ongoing relationships, and to maximize support of the patient's goals and new behaviors whenever possible.

ADDITIONAL CONSIDERATIONS FOR MAXIMIZING TREATMENT OUTCOME

Controlled trials suggest that approximately 15–20% of patients may not achieve a panic-free status by the end of acute treatment, and that a larger subsample (30–46%) will not fully return to a high state of functioning (Brown & Barlow, 1995). In addition to the issues of comorbid disorders described above, we have encountered a number of specific issues that may limit response to treatment (Otto et al., 1994). Current forms of CBT for panic disorder are directed at the core fear-of-fear patterns described earlier in this chapter. However, at times the fears of anxiety sensations that typify panic disorder may be linked to broader concerns, requiring additional exposure strategies. For example, we have encountered several patients who had fears of emotional vulnerability and expression, in addition to the fears of disability or loss of control associated with panic sensations. These patients tended to believe that any unplanned emotional expression represented an embarrassing and threatening loss of emotional control. To fully target concerns about anxiety sensations, treatment in these cases was broadened to include additional cognitive restructuring and exposure to emotional mood states (e.g., through exposure to emotional memories or emotional films). These interventions are consistent with cognitive-behavioral principles for the treatment of panic disorder. To eliminate recurrent patterns of panic attacks, the core fears associated with symptoms must be eliminated. In the special cases described here, core fears included fears of emotional expression; accordingly, exposure and cognitive restructuring interventions were adjusted to target these fears.

Additional exposure and cognitive restructuring procedures may also be required for patients who have experienced a panic attack of such magnitude that it qualifies as a traumatic stressor. McNally and Lukach (1992) have documented that for some patients the traumatic experience of a select panic episode meets criteria for PTSD. Accordingly, some patients appear to have an independent fear of cues of a specific panic episode, with vigilance to these cues and intrusive thoughts occurring much as in PTSD. To fully target these patterns, exposure and cognitive restructuring procedures may need to target the memories of this traumatic panic episode, in addition to treatment of the more typical fear-of-fear patterns associated with the disorder.

Finally, exposure procedures may sometimes need to include additional training to help patients distinguish between the panic sensations themselves and the interpretation of the sensations. In some cases, patients are unable to identify cognitions that accompany panic sensations; in other cases, patients define panic sensations as simply "intolerable" and are unable to elaborate on why this is the case. For patients in both categories, we provide training in discriminating the somatic sensations of panic and other experiences from the interpretation of these experiences.

This process can be aided by the combination of cognitive strategies with interoceptive exposure. For example, it is common in our clinic for interoceptive exposure procedures to be introduced with head rolling (rolling the head in a circle to induce dizziness). After completion of two initial interoceptive exposure trials, we ask patients to recall whether they ever tried to induce dizziness as children (e.g., by spinning in a circle or rolling down a hill). If the patients have had such experiences, they are asked to recall them in detail, and are provided with imagery cues to help this recall (e.g., of a childhood episode of inducing dizziness while playing with friends on a summer day), with particular attention to the experience of enjoyment of the induced sensations. With these memories in mind, the patients are again asked to induce dizziness. After completion of this induction trial, the patients are asked to compare the aversiveness of their sensations to that in previous trials. If the trial was more tolerable than previous trials (and indeed it is often experienced as not only tolerable but pleasurable by some patients), the therapist has provided an important demonstration of the role of thoughts in determining whether a sensation is experienced as positive or aversive. Such procedures are useful for aiding patients in discriminating sensations from their interpretation of sensations as intolerable.

Additional procedures to aid this discrimination include asking patients to compare sensations from interoceptive exposure to other somatic sensations (e.g., those from a headache or stomachache). In this procedure, patients are asked to compare the intensity of the actual physical sensations with the intensity of their emotional response and desire to escape the sensation. It has been common in our experience for patients to identify sensations induced by initial interoceptive exposure as less intense than other sensations, although they respond to anxiety sensations with greater fear. By helping patients identify that their anxious responses to sensations are independent of the sensations' intensity, this sensory training provides a useful experience for the introduction of cognitive restructuring procedures. Therapist-assisted exposure to avoided situations is sometimes helpful in the same way: It provides the therapist with a context for helping patients examine the evidence for the perceived intolerability of symptoms or their potential consequences. When *in vivo* exposure is structured as an empirical test of a patient's assumptions about his or her ability to tolerate symptoms, this procedure is termed a "behavioral experiment." The therapist and patient utilize reality to challenge assumptions about the dangerousness or tolerability of anxiety sensations.

In summary, these strategies share the goal of helping patients discover their biases in interpreting anxiety sensations by examining their response to current sensations relative to other personal experiences (including their historical reality of enjoying the same sensations at a different stage of life), other intense but non-anxiety-producing sensations (e.g., muscle pain), or their actual ability to tolerate sensations *in vivo* (behavioral experiments). In all cases, these procedures are used as aids to cognitive restructuring in patients who may otherwise have difficulty identifying the role of misinterpretations of anxiety symptoms in their own fear-of-fear cycle. Table 5.5 summarizes some of these strategies. Again, improving tolerance to symptoms is only the first step of treatment; the goal is elimination of panic attacks and anticipatory anxiety by eliminating the fear-of-fear cycle.

RELAPSE PREVENTION

Earlier in this chapter, we have suggested that CBT has advantages over pharmacologic treatment because it treats the fear of anxiety symptoms and provides patients with a model of the disorder and skills for its management if symptoms should recur at a later time. In particular, we assume that periods of anxiety are characteristic of normal functioning, but that full treatment of the panic disorder helps insure that these episodes of anxiety do not escalate into patterns of apprehension, avoidance, or panic. Relapse prevention efforts are aided by full treatment of fears of anxiety symptoms during initial treatment. We have observed that many patients and some clinicians have a tendency to "leave well enough alone" when patients improve early in treatment. This strategy, characterized by waning efforts in symptom induction or *in vivo* exposure exercises, has the potential to deprive patients of full treatment of fears of anxiety sensations and/or phobic patterns, which may place them at risk for relapse if anxiety symptoms increase in the future. Instead, clinicians should be reminded that the goal of exposure and cognitive restructuring procedures is not only

TABLE 5.5. Problems and Corresponding Clinical Strategies for Patients with Atypical Core Fears

Problems	Strategies
Fears of emotional vulnerability	Exposure to emotional events
	Cognitive restructuring
Fears of a past traumatic panic episode (panic as a traumatic stressor)	Exposure to the traumatic memory
A cognitive panic and nonresponse to interoceptive exposure	Sensory discrimination training
	In vivo behavioral experiments

to provide acute cessation of panic, but to establish behavioral skills to eliminate risk for panic recurrence. Presumably, the full treatment of fears of anxiety symptoms is what helps achieve this goal. After treatment, patients should not be relying on overt or covert escape strategies as a means of preventing panic; they should have been provided with experiences assuring them that they can cope with anxiety symptoms, should these arise.

During the acute treatment phase, clinicians must be alert for subtle avoidance or "safety" behaviors used by patients to provide themselves with safety cues. For example, patients may brace themselves against the leg of a chair when completing interoceptive exposure, to provide themselves with a sense of safety if sensations of dizziness become strong. This provision of a "safety cue" may have the unfortunate consequence of depriving the patients of the opportunity to learn fully that symptom induction is safe; instead, they may be left in the anxiogenic position of believing that symptoms are safe only if a safety behavior or escape option is readily available. Under these conditions, elimination of fears of symptoms would be expected to be incomplete, leaving patients at a higher risk for relapse. Consequently, to help insure full treatment, clinicians should be alert for such safety behaviors, and should seek to eliminate them during the course of exposure treatment (see Wells et al., 1995, for an empirical demonstration of the effects of safety cues on exposure).

In addition to safety cues, we have observed that some patients experience a temporary resurgence of panic symptoms when they are exposed to rare or seasonal phobic events that were not present during treatment. For example, patients achieving remission during a course of treatment in the winter may have an increase in symptoms in the summer when exposed to situations (e.g., a swimming pool) or other contextual cues (heat and humidity) that have been long-standing phobic or panic cues. The goal of acute treatment is to prepare patients for such future episodes, so that panic control skills can be effectively reapplied if they are needed.

In the initial stage of treatment, patients are treated as collaborators in the treatment process, so that they will become skilled in analyzing and selecting interventions for their own particular anxiety patterns. We try to maximize this training by giving patients greater responsibility for reviewing symptoms and planning cognitive restructuring and exposure assignments in the final weeks of treatment (Otto et al., 1994a). This training is formalized when the frequency of clinic sessions is decreased; patients are asked to hold their own self-directed sessions when clinic treatment is not scheduled. In subsequent clinic sessions, these self-directed sessions are reviewed, with a therapist assuming the role of training supervisor of a patient's own self-help efforts. Efforts are also made to help patients return to an active lifestyle that insures continued mild exposure to various somatic sensations (e.g., those induced by such normal activities as exercising, drinking caffeinated beverages, playing with children, climbing stairs, etc.).

Written treatment manuals (e.g., Barlow & Craske, 1989; Otto et al.,

1995a) provide another way of insuring that patients have the treatment rationale and methods available for future reference. In addition, Öst (1989) has documented the efficacy of written follow-up procedures to further improvement and reduce relapse, as well as the need for additional treatment during follow-up periods. Booster sessions may also be of help during periods of worsening, to help patients reestablish treatment skills.

In all cases, these interventions are guided by the cognitive-behavioral model of panic disorder, which stresses the importance of treating the fears of anxiety sensations and the anxiogenic cognitive and behavioral responses to symptoms that characterize this cycle. Cognitive restructuring, exposure, and symptom management skills provide patients with the means to disrupt this cycle. Relapse prevention training is aimed at insuring that these cognitive and behavioral responses are well learned and emerge as part of a patient's behavioral repertoire, should symptoms or phobic cues be encountered in the future.

REFERENCES

Alnaes, R., & Torgersen, S. (1988). The relationship between DSM-III symptom disorders (Axis I) and personality disorders (Axis II) in an outpatient population. *Acta Psychiatrica Scandinavica, 78,* 485–492.

American Psychiatric Association. (1994). *Diagnostic and statistical manual of mental disorders* (4th ed.). Washington, DC: Author.

Ball, S. G., Otto, M. W., Pollack, M. H., & Rosenbaum, J. F. (1994). Predicting prospective episodes of depression in patients with panic disorder: A longitudinal study. *Journal of Consulting and Clinical Psychology, 62,* 359–365.

Ball, S. G., Otto, M. W., Pollack, M. H., Uccello, R., & Rosenbaum, J. F. (1995). Differentiating social phobia and panic disorder: A test of core beliefs. *Cognitive Therapy and Research, 18,* 473–482.

Barlow, D. H. (1988). *Anxiety and its disorders: The nature and treatment of anxiety and panic.* New York: Guilford Press.

Barlow, D. H., & Craske, M. G. (1989). *Mastery of your anxiety and panic.* Albany, NY: Graywind.

Barlow, D. H., Craske, M. G., Cerny, J. A., & Klosko, J. S. (1989). Behavioral treatment of panic disorder. *Behavior Therapy, 20,* 261–282.

Barlow, D. H., O'Brien, G. T., & Last, C. G. (1984). Couples treatment of agoraphobia. *Behavior Therapy, 15,* 41–58.

Beck, A. T., Freeman, A., & Associates. (1990). *Cognitive therapy of personality disorders.* New York: Guilford Press.

Beck, A. T., Sokol, L., Clark, D. A., Berchick, R., & Wright, F. (1992). A crossover study of focused cognitive therapy for panic disorder. *American Journal of Psychiatry, 149,* 778–783.

Brooks, R. B., Baltazar, P. L., & Munjack, D. J. (1989). Co-occurrence of personality disorders with panic disorder, social phobia, and generalized anxiety disorder: A review of the literature. *Journal of Anxiety Disorders, 3,* 259–285.

Brown, T. A., Antony, M. M., & Barlow, D. H. (1995). Diagnostic comorbidity in panic disorder: Effect on treatment outcome and course of comorbid diagnoses following treatment. *Journal of Consulting and Clinical Psychology, 63,* 408–418.

Brown, T. A., & Barlow, D. H. (1995). Long-term outcome in cognitive-behavioral treatment of panic disorder: Clinical predictors and alternative strategies for assessment. *Journal of Consulting and Clinical Psychology, 63,* 754–765.

Bruch, M. A., Mattia, J. I., Heimberg, R. G., & Holt, C. S. (1993). Cognitive specificity in social anxiety and depression: Supporting evidence and qualifications due to affective confounding. *Cognitive Therapy and Research, 17,* 1–21.

Cerny, J. A., Barlow, D. H., Craske, M. G., & Himadi, W. G. (1987). Couples treatment of agoraphobia: A two-year follow-up. *Behavior Therapy, 18,* 401–416.

Chambless, D. L., & Gillis, M. M. (1993). Cognitive therapy of anxiety disorders. *Journal of Consulting and Clinical Psychology, 61,* 248–260.

Chambless, D. L., & Gracely, E. J. (1989). Fear of fear and the anxiety disorders. *Cognitive Therapy and Research, 13,* 9–20.

Chambless, D. L., Renneberg, B., Goldstein, A., & Gracely, E. J. (1992). MCMI-diagnosed personality disorders among agoraphobic outpatients: Prevalence and relationship to severity and treatment outcome. *Journal of Anxiety Disorders, 6,* 193–211.

Christensen, H., Hadzi-Pavlovic, D., Andrews, G., & Mattick, R. (1987). Behavior therapy and tricyclic medication in the treatment of obsessive–compulsive disorder: A quantitative review. *Journal of Consulting and Clinical Psychology, 55*(5), 701–711.

Clark, D. M. (1986). A cognitive approach to panic. *Behaviour Research and Therapy, 24,* 461–470.

Clark, D. M., Salkovskis, P. M., Hackmann, A., Middleton, H., Pavlos, A., & Gelder, M. (1994). A comparison of cognitive therapy, applied relaxation and imipramine in the treatment of panic disorder. *British Journal of Psychiatry, 164,* 759–769.

Clark, L. A. (1989). The anxiety and depressive disorders: Descriptive psychopathology and differential diagnosis. In P. Kendall & D. Watson (Eds.), *Anxiety and depression: Distinctive and overlapping features.* New York: Academic Press.

Clum, G. A., Clum, G. A., & Surls, R. (1993). A meta-analysis of treatments for panic disorder. *Journal of Consulting and Clinical Psychology, 61,* 317–326.

Cohen, A. S., Barlow, D. H., & Blanchard, E. B. (1985). The psychophysiology of relaxation-associated panic attacks. *Journal of Abnormal Psychology, 94,* 96–101.

Côte, G., Gauthier, J. G., Laberge, B., Cormier, H. H., & Plamondon, J. (1994). Reduced therapist contact in the cognitive behavioral treatment of panic disorder. *Behavior Therapy, 25,* 123–145.

Craske, M. G., Brown, T. A., & Barlow, D. H. (1991). Behavioral treatment of panic: A two year follow-up. *Behavior Therapy, 22,* 289–304.

de Beurs, E. (1993). *The assessment and treatment of panic disorder and agoraphobia.* Amsterdam: Thesis.

Diaferia, G., Sciuto, G., Pernal, G., Bernardeschi, L., Battaglia, M., Rusmini, S., & Bellowdi, L. (1993). DSM-III-R personality disorders in panic disorder. *Journal of Anxiety Disorders, 7,* 153–161.

Donnell, C. D., & McNally, R. J. (1989). Anxiety sensitivity and history of panic as predictors of response to hyperventilation. *Behaviour Research and Therapy, 27*, 325–332.

Ehlers, A. (1995). A 1-year prospective study of panic attacks: Clinical course and factors associated with maintenance. *Journal of Abnormal Psychology, 104*, 164–172.

Farrell, J. M., & Shaw, I. A. (1994). Emotional awareness training: A prerequisite to effective cognitive-behavioral treatment of borderline personality disorder. *Cognitive and Behavioral Practice, 1*, 71–91.

Foa, E. B., & Kozak, M. J. (1986). Emotional processing of fear: Exposure to corrective information. *Psychological Bulletin, 99*, 20–35.

Fyer, A. J., Liebowitz, M. R., Gorman, J. M., Campeas, R., Levin, A., Davies, S. O., Goetz, D., & Klein, D. F. (1987). Discontinuation of alprazolam treatment in panic patients. *American Journal of Psychiatry, 144*, 303–308.

Goldstein, A. J., & Chambless, D. L. (1978). A reanalysis of agoraphobia. *Behavior Therapy, 9*, 47–59.

Gould, R. A., & Clum, G. A. (1993). A meta-analysis of self-help treatment approaches. *Clinical Psychology Review, 13*, 169–186.

Gould, R. A., Clum, G. A., & Shapiro, D. (1993). The use of bibliotherapy in the treatment of panic disorder. *Behavior Therapy, 24*, 241–252.

Gould, R. A., Otto, M. W., & Pollack, M. H. (1995). A meta-analysis of treatment outcome for panic disorder. *Clinical Psychology Review, 15*, 819–844.

Gould, R. A., Otto, M. W., Yap, L., & Pollack, M. H. (1994). *Cognitive-behavioral and pharmacological treatment of social phobia: A meta-analysis.* Paper presented at the 28th Annual Meeting of the Association for the Advancement of Behavior Therapy, San Diego, CA.

Green, M. A., & Curtis, G. (1988). Personality disorders in panic patients: Response to termination of antipanic medication. *Journal of Personality Disorders, 2*, 303–314.

Hegel, M. T., Ravaris, C. L., & Ahles, T. A. (1994). Combined cognitive-behavioral and time-limited alprazolam treatment of panic disorder. *Behavior Therapy, 25*, 183–195.

Hunt, C., & Singh, M. (1991). Generalized anxiety disorder. *International Review of Psychiatry, 3*, 215–229.

Jansson, L., Öst, L.-G., & Jerremalm, A. (1987). Prognostic factors in the behavioral treatment of agoraphobia. *Behavioral Psychotherapy, 15*, 31–44.

Keijsers, G. P. J., Hoogduin, C. A. L., & Schaap, C. P. D. R. (1994). Prognostic factors in the behavioral treatment of panic disorder with and without agoraphobia. *Behavior Therapy, 25*, 689–708.

Keller, M. B., Lavori, P. W., Goldenberg, I. M., Baker, L. A., Pollack, M. H., Sachs, G. S., Rosenbaum, J. F., Deltitio, J. A., Leon, A., Shear, K., & Klerman, G. L. (1993). Influence of depression on the treatment of panic disorder with imipramine, alprazolam and placebo. *Journal of Affective Disorders, 28*, 27–38.

Linehan, M. M. (1993). *Cognitive-behavioral treatment of borderline personality disorder.* New York: Guilford Press.

Maller, R. G., & Reiss, S. (1992). Anxiety sensitivity in 1984 and panic attacks in 1987. *Journal of Anxiety Disorders, 6*, 241–247.

Margraf, J., Barlow, D. H., Clark, D. M., & Telch, M. J. (1993). Psychological treatment of panic: Work in progress on outcome, active ingredients, and follow-up. *Behaviour Research and Therapy, 31*, 1–8.

Margraf, J., Ehlers, A., & Roth, W. T. (1986). Biological models of panic disorder and agoraphobia: A review. *Behaviour Research and Therapy, 24*, 553–567.

Marks, I. M., Swinson, R. P., Basoglu, M., Kuch, K., Noshirvani, H., O'Sullivan, G., Lelliott, P. T., Kirby, M., McNamee, G., Sengun, S., & Wickwire, K. (1993). Alprazolam and exposure alone and combined in panic disorder with agoraphobia: A controlled study in London and Toronto. *British Journal of Psychiatry, 162*, 776–787.

Marks, I. M., Viswanathan, R., Lipsedge, M. D., & Gardner, R. (1972). Enhanced relief of phobias by flooding during waning diazepam effect. *British Journal of Psychiatry, 121*, 493–505.

Mavissakalian, M. (1990a). Sequential combination of imipramine and self-directed exposure in the treatment of panic disorder with agoraphobia. *Journal of Clinical Psychiatry, 51*, 184–188.

Mavissakalian, M. (1990b). The relationship between panic disorder/agoraphobia and personality disorders. *Psychiatric Clinics of North America, 13*(4), 661–684.

Mavissakalian, M., & Hamann, M. S. (1988). Correlates of DSM-III personality disorder in panic disorder and agoraphobia. *Comprehensive Psychiatry, 29*, 535–544.

Mavissakalian, M., & Michelson, L. (1986a). Agoraphobia: Relative and combined effectiveness of therapist-assisted *in vivo* exposure and imipramine. *Journal of Clinical Psychiatry, 47*(3), 117–122.

Mavissakalian, M., & Michelson, L. (1986b). Two year follow up of exposure in imipramine treatment of agoraphobia. *American Journal of Psychiatry, 143*(9), 1106–1112.

Mavissakalian, M., Michelson, L., & Dealy, R. S. (1983). Pharmacological treatment of agoraphobia: Imipramine versus imipramine with programmed practice. *British Journal of Psychiatry, 143*, 348–355.

McNally, R. J. (1990). Psychological approaches to panic disorder: A review. *Psychological Bulletin, 108*, 403–419.

McNally, R. J. (1994). *Panic disorder: A critical analysis.* New York: Guilford Press.

McNally, R. J., & Lukach, B. M. (1992). Are panic attacks traumatic stressors? *American Journal of Psychiatry, 149*, 824–826.

National Institutes of Health. (1991, September). Treatment of panic disorder. *NIH Consensus Development Conference Consensus Statement* (Technical report), 9(2).

Norton, G. R., Cox, B. J., & Malan, J. (1992). Nonclinical panickers: A critical review. *Clinical Psychology Review, 12*, 121–139.

Noyes, R., Garvey, M. J., Cook, B., & Suelzer, M. (1991). Controlled discontinuation of benzodiazepine treatment for patients with panic disorder. *American Journal of Psychiatry, 148*, 517–523.

Öst, L. G. (1989). A maintenance program for behavioural treatment of anxiety disorders. *Behaviour Research and Therapy, 27*, 123–130.

Öst, L. G., & Westling, B. E. (1995). Applied relaxation vs. cognitive behaviour therapy in the treatment of panic disorder. *Behaviour Research and Therapy, 33*, 145–158.

Otto, M. W., Gould, R. A., & Pollack, M. H. (1994). Cognitive-behavioral treatment of panic disorder: Considerations for the treatment of patients over the long term. *Psychiatric Annals, 24*, 307–315.

Otto, M. W., Pollack, M. H., & Barlow, D. H. (1995a). *Stopping anxiety medication: A workbook for patients wanting to discontinue benzodiazepine treatment for panic disorder.* Albany, NY: Graywind Publications.

Otto, M. W., Pollack, M. H., Fava, M., Uccello, R., & Rosenbaum, J. F. (1995b). Elevated Anxiety Sensitivity Index scores in patients with major depression: Correlates and changes with antidepressant treatment. *Journal of Anxiety Disorders, 9,* 117–123.

Otto, M. W., Pollack, M. H., Meltzer-Brody, S., & Rosenbaum, J. F. (1992). Cognitive-behavioral therapy for benzodiazepine discontinuation in panic disorder patients. *Psychopharmacology Bulletin, 28,* 123–130.

Otto, M. W., Pollack, M. H., & Sabatino, S. A. (1995c, November). *Maintenance of remission in panic disorder: Cognitive-behavior therapy alone or in combination with medications.* Paper presented at the 29th meeting of the Association for Advancement of Behavior Therapy, Washington, DC.

Otto, M. W., Pollack, M. H., Sachs, G. S., Reiter, S. R., Meltzer-Brody, S., & Rosenbaum, J. F. (1993). Discontinuation of benzodiazepine treatment: Efficacy of cognitive-behavior therapy for patients with panic disorder. *American Journal of Psychiatry, 150,* 1485–1490.

Pecknold, J. C., Swinson, R. P., Kuch, K., & Lewis, C. P. (1988). Alprazolam in panic disorder and agoraphobia: Results from a multicenter trial: III. Discontinuation effects. *Archives of General Psychiatry, 45,* 429–436.

Peterson, R. A., & Reiss, S. (1992). *Anxiety Sensitivity Index revised test manual.* Worthington, OH.

Pollack, M. H., Otto, M. W., Kaspi, S. P., Hammerness, P. G., & Rosenbaum, J. F. (1994a). Cognitive-behavior therapy for treatment-refractory panic disorder. *Journal of Clinical Psychiatry, 55,* 200–205.

Pollack, M. H., Otto, M. W., Rosenbaum, J. F., & Sachs, G. S. (1992). Personality disorders in patients with panic disorder: Association with childhood anxiety disorders, early trauma, comorbidity and chronicity. *Comprehensive Psychiatry, 33,* 78–83.

Pollack, M. H., Otto, M. W., Rosenbaum, J. F., Sachs, G. S., O'Neil, C., Asher, R., & Meltzer-Brody, S. (1990). Longitudinal course of panic disorder: Findings from the Massachusetts General Hospital Naturalistic Study. *Journal of Clinical Psychiatry, 51,* 12–16.

Pollack, M. H., Otto, M. W., Sachs, G. S., Leon, A., Sher, M. K., Deltito, J. A., Keller, M. B., & Rosenbaum, J. R. (1994b). Anxiety psychopathology predictive of outcome in patients with panic disorder and depression treated with imipramine, alprazolam and placebo. *Journal of Affective Disorders, 30,* 273–281.

Pollack, M. H., Otto, M. W., Tesar, G. E., Cohen, L. S., Meltzer-Brody, S., & Rosenbaum, J. F. (1993). Long-term outcome after acute treatment with clonazepam and alprazolam for panic disorder. *Journal of Clinical Psychopharmacology, 13,* 257–263.

Rapee, R. M. (1995). Psychological factors influencing the affective response to biological challenge procedures in panic disorder. *Journal of Anxiety Disorders, 9,* 59–74.

Reich, J. (1988). DSM-III personality disorders and the outcome of treated panic disorder. *American Journal of Psychiatry, 245,* 1149–1152.

Reich, J., Noyes, R., Hirschfeld, R., Coryell, W., & O'Gorman, T. (1987). State and personality in depressed and panic patients. *American Journal of Psychiatry, 144*(2), 181–187.

Reich, J., & Troughton, E. (1988a). Personality disorders in patients with panic disorder: Comparison with psychiatric and normal control subjects. *Psychiatry Research, 26*, 89–100.

Ricciardi, J. N., Baer, L., Jenike, M. A., Fischer, S. C., Sholtz, D., Buttolph, M. L. (1992). Changes in DSM-III-R Axis II diagnoses following treatment of obsessive–compulsive disorder. *American Journal of Psychiatry, 149*(6), 829–831.

Salkovskis, P., & Mills, I. (1994). Induced mood, phobic responding and the return of fear. *Behaviour Research and Therapy, 32*, 430–445.

Sciuto, G., Diaferia, G., Battaglia, M., Perna, G. P., Gabriele, A., & Bellodi, L. (1991). DSM-III-R personality disorders in panic and obsessive–compulsive disorder: A comparison study. *Comprehensive Psychiatry, 32*(5), 450–457.

Shear, M. K. (1986). Pathophysiology of panic: A review of pharmacologic provocation tests and naturalistic monitoring data. *Journal of Clinical Psychiatry, 47*(Suppl.), 18–26.

Shear, K. S., Pilkonis, P. A., Cloitre, M., & Leon, A. C. (1994). Cognitive behavioral treatment compared with nonprescriptive treatment of panic disorder. *Archives of General Psychiatry, 51*, 395–401.

Spiegel, D. A., Bruce, T. J., Gregg, S. F., & Nuzzarello, A. (1994). Does cognitive behavior therapy assist slow-taper alprazolam discontinuation in panic disorder? *American Journal of Psychiatry, 151*, 876–881.

Telch, M. J., Agras, W. S., Taylor, C. B., Roth, W. T., & Gallen, C. (1985). Combined pharmacological and behavioral treatment for agoraphobia. *Behaviour Research and Therapy, 23*, 325–335.

Telch, M. J., & Harrington, P. J. (1992). *Anxiety sensitivity and expectedness of arousal in mediating affective response to 35% carbon dioxide inhalation.* Paper presented at the 26th Annual Meeeting of the Association for Advancement of Behavior Therapy, Boston.

Tesar, G. E., Rosenbaum, J. F., Pollack, M. H., Otto, M. W., Sachs, G. S., Herman, J. B., Cohen, L. S., & Spier, S. A. (1991). Double-blind placebo-controlled comparison of clonazepam and alprazolam for panic disorder. *Journal of Clinical Psychiatry, 52*, 69–76.

Wardle, J., Hayward, P., Higgitt, A., Stabl, M., Blizard, R., & Gray, J. (1994). Effects of concurrent diazepam treatment on the outcome of exposure therapy in agoraphobia. *Behaviour Research and Therapy, 32*, 203–215.

Wells, A., Clark, D. M., Salkovskis, P., Ludgate, J., Hackmann, A., & Gelder, M. (1995). Social phobia: The role of in-situation safety behaviors in maintaining anxiety and negative beliefs. *Behavior Therapy, 26*, 153–161.

Woody, S. (1994, August) *Comorbidity of panic and depression: Implications for cognitive therapy.* Paper presented at the 102nd Annual Meeting of the American Psychological Association, Los Angeles.

6

Pharmacologic Approaches to Treatment-Resistant Social Phobia and Generalized Anxiety Disorder

JORDAN W. SMOLLER
MARK H. POLLACK

Although the idea of pathologic anxiety as a cause of significant morbidity is as old as psychiatry itself, the current diagnostic conceptualization of anxiety disorders—which includes panic disorder, generalized anxiety disorder (GAD), social phobia, posttraumatic stress disorder (PTSD), and others—has only existed since the publication of the *Diagnostic and Statistical Manual of Mental Disorders*, third edition (DSM-III; American Psychiatric Association, 1980). Since then, a great deal of research has helped to identify effective first-line treatments for these disorders, although studies of long-term management have been rare. Even rarer have been studies addressing the management of patients who do not respond to an initial trial of pharmacotherapy or psychotherapy. In this chapter, we review the use of first-line pharmacotherapies for social phobia and GAD and provide guidelines for the management of the treatment-resistant patient. The management of refractory panic disorder and PTSD is addressed elsewhere in the volume (Chapter 4 and 9, respectively). Although the clinical presentation and course of these disorders vary considerably, we suggest a generally applicable approach to the refractory anxiety patient.

PRINCIPLES OF MANAGING PATIENTS WITH TREATMENT-RESISTANT ANXIETY

A systematic approach to the patient with treatment-resistant anxiety can be achieved with attention to the factors that most commonly interfere with therapeutic response and consideration of treatment strategies that can be used to address them (see Table 6.1). Reconsideration of the differential diagnosis of a patient's symptoms is an important first step. The anxiety symptoms may be attributable to another anxiety disorder, a mood disorder, substance use or withdrawal, medication side effects, or an occult medical illness. When an error in diagnosis can be identified and corrected, more appropriate therapy can be given. For example, hyperthyroidism masquerading as refractory GAD may respond far better to methimazole than to benzodiazepines.

In some patients, poor treatment response may be attributable to concurrent psychiatric disorders, so that the identification and treatment of comorbidity may be essential. For social phobia and GAD, the most common comorbid Axis I disorders are other anxiety disorders, depression, and substance use disorders. Each of these may require independent treatment. Concurrent Axis II pathology can also complicate treatment by, for example, interfering with the treatment alliance and affecting medication compliance. In discussing the individual disorders we focus on comorbid Axis I disorders, but the contribution of personality disorders can be substantial and may need to be addressed with concurrent psychosocial interventions.

The possibility of medication noncompliance and/or intolerance should be considered in patients who show poor response to pharmacotherapy. Tricyclic and selective serotonergic antidepressants used for the treatment of anxiety can initially exacerbate anxiety, so that the maxim "Start low, go slow" is appropriate for many patients. The short-term addition of benzodiazepines in the initial stages of therapy with these agents may also be helpful. Medications with anticholinergic side effects may produce intolerable dry mouth, constipation, or urinary hesitancy—all of which can be ameliorated with adjunctive agents or dose adjustments (Coplan, Tiffon, & Gorman, 1993; Pollack & Rosenbaum, 1987).

A frequent cause of treatment resistance to a medication trial is inadequate dosing, frequency, or duration of treatment. Optimizing therapy may mean increasing the dose of a tricyclic up to 300 mg/day, increasing the dosing schedule of a short-half-life benzodiazepine from three to five times per day, or continuing a trial of a serotonergic antidepressant for at least 8–12 weeks before concluding that it is ineffective.

When first-line agents produce only a partial response, it is appropriate to augment or combine them with other agents or with psychotherapies. In some cases, agents can be added to target specific symptoms that have not responded to an initial medication. For example, beta-adrenergic blockers may provide substantial relief to patients with social phobia whose

TABLE 6.1. Principles of Managing Patients with Treatment-Resistant Anxiety

I. Review the differential diagnosis, with attention to:
   A. Anxiety and depressive disorders

   B. Substance abuse and withdrawal

   C. Medication-induced anxiety

   D. Medical or neurologic illnesses

   E. Personality disorders and psychosocial factors

II. Identify and treat comorbidity
   A. Anxiety and depressive disorders, substance abuse

   B. Personality disorders

III. Identify and address medication noncompliance or medication intolerance
   A. Use adjunctive medications to treat side effects

   B. "Start low, go slow" with activating medication

IV. Optimize therapeutic trials
   A. Dose

   B. Frequency

   C. Duration

V. Use combination therapy
   A. Combine medication with cognitive-behavioral therapy or other psychotherapy

   B. Combine classes of medications (e.g., antidepressant and benzodiazepine)

   C. Augment first-line agent with one that targets specific symptoms (e.g., add beta-adrenergic blocker for sympathetic hyperarousal)

VI. Switch to another class of medication

VII. When symptoms return after an initially favorable response:
   A. Consider loss of initial placebo response

   B. Consider role of acute psychosocial stressors and make appropriate intervention

   C. Consider altered drug action (receptor up- or down-regulation, metabolic enzyme induction, adverse interaction with concurrent medications); may respond to dose adjustment

somatic anxiety symptoms have not resolved with an antidepressant. When a first-line agent has produced virtually no response, switching from one class of medication to another can be tried. Unfortunately, for the disorders we discuss here, the outcome of combining or switching among therapies has not been well studied.

In patients who demonstrate an initial response to therapy but whose symptoms relapse or worsen, several other factors should be considered. Some patients may experience a "honeymoon period" in which rapid and dramatic reduction in some symptoms (e.g., panic attacks) may mask the presence of other, more subtle dysfunction (e.g., phobic avoidance). The loss of an initial placebo response may appear as "breakthrough" symptoms in the face of what appeared to be effective treatment (Coplan et al., 1993). The presence of acute psychosocial stressors can exacerbate anxiety symptoms and may be best managed by psychotherapy or crisis intervention. Finally, when a medication loses its clinical effectiveness, pharmacodynamic factors (e.g., tolerance) or pharmacokinetic factors (e.g., the induction of metabolic enzymes) may be at work (Coplan et al., 1993), and raising dosage may be effective.

In this chapter, we address the management of patients with social phobia or GAD who demonstrate an inadequate response to a trial of one of the first-line therapies. Several of the principles in Table 6.1 apply to all psychiatric disorders and are not specifically discussed (i.e., the role of noncompliance, medication intolerance, Axis II pathology, acute psychosocial stressors, placebo responses, and pharmacodynamic/pharmacokinetic considerations). We focus instead on the diagnostic issues (differential diagnosis and comorbidity) and therapeutic issues (optimization of therapy, combination therapy, and switching agents) that are specific to social phobia and GAD.

SOCIAL PHOBIA

General Considerations

The central feature of social phobia is a fear of humiliation in situations in which an individual may be exposed to evaluation and scrutiny by others. This fear persists despite the individual's awareness that it is unreasonable or excessive, and leads to avoidant behavior that may severely impair social or occupational functioning. A variety of social activities may provoke an intense anxiety reaction, including attending parties, public speaking, signing one's name in front of others, and eating in public. A distinction has been made between the "generalized" and "discrete" subtypes of social phobia (Liebowitz, Gorman, Fyer, & Klein, 1985). Individuals with generalized social phobia have fear or avoidance of most social situations, whereas those with discrete social phobias experience anxiety when exposed to only a particular performance situation (most commonly public speaking). The value of this distinction is supported by evidence that the two subtypes may respond differentially to pharmacotherapy (Liebowitz et al., 1992). For example, beta-adrenergic blockers may be useful in discrete social phobia but do not have significant efficacy for generalized social phobia (Liebowitz et al., 1992). In addition, generalized social phobia is associated with more severe comorbidity and functional impairment (Heimberg, Hope, Dodge, & Becker, 1990b; Mannuzza et al., 1995).

Social phobia appears to have a relatively early age of onset, with a mean of 15.5 years in a recent large-scale epidemiologic study (Schneier, Johnson, Hornig, Liebowitz, & Weissman, 1992b). Recent investigations suggest that biologically based temperamental factors (i.e., "behavioral inhibition to the unfamiliar") may predispose children to the later development of social phobia and panic disorder (Rosenbaum et al., 1993). Social phobia appears to be a prevalent disorder, with estimates of lifetime prevalence ranging from 2.4% across four sites in the Epidemiologic Catchment Area (ECA) study (Schneier et al., 1992b) to as high as 13.3% in the National Comorbidity Survey (Kessler et al., 1994). The diagnosis is complicated by significant morbidity, including financial dependency, impaired relationships, and suicide attempts (Schneier et al., 1992b, 1994). Controlled studies tend to show low placebo response rates in patients with social phobia, suggesting that the disorder is unlikely to remit without treatment (Davidson et al., 1993). Nevertheless, only about 5% of individuals with uncomplicated social phobia may seek specific treatment (Schneier et al., 1992b).

An important consideration in the treatment of social phobia is the high rate of comorbid Axis I disorders (Rosenbaum & Pollock, 1994). Data from a sample of 13,000 adults from the ECA study (Schneier et al., 1992b) indicate a high lifetime rate of comorbid anxiety disorders in individuals with social phobia: Comorbidity with simple phobia occurred in 59% of social phobics, agoraphobia in 44.9%, obsessive–compulsive disorder (OCD) in 11.1%, and panic disorder in 4.7%. Other studies have suggested much higher rates of comorbid panic disorder (Stein, Shea, & Uhde, 1989; Van Ameringen, Mancini, Styan, & Donison, 1991). In addition, depression and alcoholism may coexist with or be sequelae of social phobia (Liebowitz et al., 1985; Otto, Pollack, Sachs, O'Neil, & Rosenbaum, 1992; Reiter, Otto, Pollack, & Rosenbaum, 1991; Schneier et al., 1992b; Van Ameringen et al., 1991). For example, in the ECA study (Schneier et al., 1992b) the lifetime rate of depression among social phobia patients was 16.6%, and the lifetime rate of alcohol abuse was 18.8%. In general, social phobia appears to precede the onset of many comorbid disorders and may in fact be a risk factor for other psychopathology (Schneier et al., 1992b; Van Ameringen et al., 1991). As discussed below, the identification of comorbid conditions in patients with social phobia can help guide the selection of pharmacologic interventions.

Pharmacotherapy: First-Line Treatments

With the growing appreciation of the prevalence and morbid sequelae of social phobia, there has been increasing attention to the treatment, including pharmacotherapy, of this disorder. Four classes of medication have been most extensively studied—monoamine oxidase inhibitors (MAOIs), serotonin reuptake inhibitors (SSRIs), benzodiazepines, and beta-adrenergic blockers—and all have demonstrated some efficacy.

Monoamine Oxidase Inhibitors

Phenelzine has been the medication most extensively studied for the treatment of social phobia, and its efficacy has been demonstrated in several reports, including three double-blind placebo-controlled studies (Gelernter et al., 1991; Liebowitz et al., 1992; Versiani et al., 1992). Liebowitz et al. (1988, 1992) compared phenelzine to atenolol and placebo in 74 social phobia patients. At 8 weeks, significant improvement was seen in 64% of phenelzine-treated patients, compared with 30% of those treated with atenolol—a response rate not significantly different from that for placebo (23%). In a comparison among phenelzine, alprazolam, cognitive-behavioral therapy (CBT), and placebo (Gelernter et al., 1991), all of the active treatments were comparably effective, although the phenelzine-treated group had a nonsignificantly higher response rate (63%). Finally, Versiani et al. (1992) compared phenelzine and moclobemide, a reversible inhibitor of monoamine oxidase type A (RIMA), in a placebo-controlled trial with 78 subjects. Although phenelzine was superior to moclobemide at week 4, 82% of the moclobemide group and 91% of the phenelzine group had almost complete resolution of their symptoms by week 16. In an open trial, the MAOI tranylcypromine (40–60 mg/day) was also found to be effective for social phobia (Versiani, Mundim, & Nardi, 1988).

The development of RIMAs holds promise for exploiting the benefits of MAOIs without the need for dietary restriction, since MAOIs have a reduced risk of causing a tyramine-induced hypertensive crisis. In the study mentioned above, moclobemide was better tolerated than phenelzine. Trials of another RIMA, brofaromine, suggest that it also may be effective for social phobia (Marshall, Schneier, Fallon, Feerick, & Liebowitz, 1994; Van Vliet, Den Boer, & Westenberg, 1992). Although moclobemide is available abroad, results from clinical trials in the United States have precluded further development in this country.

Overall, MAOIs are well-substantiated treatments for social phobia, but their utility is limited by the need for dietary proscriptions and their side effect profiles. Dosing for phenelzine is in the range of 60–90 mg/day and for tranylcypromine is 30–60 mg/day, although some patients may require higher doses to achieve maximal benefit.

Selective Serotonin Reuptake Inhibitors

The favorable side effect profile of the SSRIs has made them attractive therapeutic options for the treatment of social phobia and other mood and anxiety disorders. Case reports and open trials suggest that fluoxetine may be effective in social phobia. Schneier, Chin, Hollander, and Liebowitz (1992a) reported moderate to marked improvement in 7 of 12 patients, who responded at a mean dose of 25.7 mg/day of fluoxetine. Black, Uhde, and Tancer (1992) found moderate to marked improvement in 10 out of 14 patients (71%) treated with 10–80 mg/day of fluoxetine. In another open trial (Van Ameringen, Mancini, & Streiner, 1993), 10 of 13 patients (81%) who completed 12 weeks of treatment with fluoxetine (mean dose 53.6 mg/day) showed at least moderate improvement in global ratings of social phobia symptoms. Uncontrolled reports have suggested that sertraline and paroxetine may also be effective (Ringold, 1994; Van Ameringen, Mancini, & Streiner, 1994; Munjack, Flowers, & Eagan, 1994/1995; Czepowicz et al., 1995). For example, in an open 12-week trial of sertraline (Van Ameringen et al., 1994), 16 of 20 patients (80%) who completed 8 weeks of treatment were considered responders based on clinical global impression ratings. The mean dose of sertraline at end point was 147.5 mg/day. In a small, placebo-controlled crossover study, 6 of 12 patients (50%) were rated as moderately or markedly improved on sertraline (mean dose 133.5) compared with one patient (9%) on placebo (Katzelnick et al., 1995). Finally, a double-blind placebo-controlled study of fluvoxamine (Van Vliet, Den Boer, & Westenberg, 1994) found marked improvement in social anxiety (but not avoidance) in 46% of fluvoxamine-treated patients (150 mg/day), compared with 7% of patients on placebo. In this study, a significant decrease in social anxiety was not seen until week 12. It is unclear whether higher doses would have produced a more rapid or robust response.

Because they are well tolerated and generally effective for both social phobia and its common comorbid conditions, SSRIs are a reasonable first-line treatment choice, particularly for generalized social phobia. Compared with panic disorder patients, individuals with social phobia may be less susceptible to excessive jitteriness when starting SSRIs (Schneier et al., 1992a; Van Vliet et al., 1994); however, they too may benefit from treatment initiation at low doses (e.g., 10 mg/day of fluoxetine, 25 mg/day of sertraline, 10 mg/day of paroxetine), with escalation to typical therapeutic doses after 1 week as tolerated.

Benzodiazepines

The high-potency benzodiazepines alprazolam and clonazepam have also demonstrated efficacy in social phobia. Several case reports and open studies suggest that alprazolam reduces social phobics' anxiety and avoidance behavior (Gelernter et al., 1991; Lydiard, Laraia, Howell, & Ballenger, 1988; Reich, Noyes, & Yates, 1989; Reich & Yates, 1988). In a controlled trial comparing alprazolam (mean dose 4.2 mg/day), phenelzine (mean dose 55 mg/day), CBT, and placebo plus exposure instruction, alprazolam was as effective as the other active treatments although phenelzine was more likely to produce "unequivocal" improvement based on self-report measures of anxiety and avoidance (Gelernter et al., 1991). Therapeutic effects do not appear to be maintained when alprazolam is discontinued, however (Gelernter et al., 1991; Reich et al., 1989).

Clonazepam also appears to provide significant symptomatic relief in social phobia (Munjack, Baltazar, Bohn, Cabe, & Appleton, 1990; Reiter,

Pollack, Rosenbaum, & Cohen, 1990). In a double-blind placebo-controlled trial of 75 patients with social phobia, Davidson et al. (1993) found a response rate of 78% for clonazepam (mean dose 2.4 mg/day) compared with 20% for placebo, with therapeutic benefit demonstrable within a week. Both performance and generalized anxiety symptoms (including fear, avoidance, and disability) were improved, and response was sustained for the full 10 weeks of the trial.

Benzodiazepines have the advantage of relatively rapid onset of symptomatic relief (generally within 1–2 weeks), but their use is complicated by the risks of physiologic dependence and discontinuation-related difficulties. The frequent presence of substance abuse (particularly alcohol abuse) in social phobics may complicate the use of benzodiazepines in affected patients (Marshall, 1994).

Beta-Adrenergic Blockers

Beta-adrenergic blockers may minimize patients' self-perceptions of anxiety by decreasing peripheral symptoms of anxiety (tremor, quavering voice, palpitations), which can themselves be anxiety-provoking and impair performance (Gorman, Liebowitz, Fyer, Campeas, & Klein, 1985). In a series of studies, these agents have been found to be effective for performance anxiety (e.g., anxiety related to musical performances and public speaking) (Liebowitz et al., 1985), but they are less effective than MAOIs and may be no better than a placebo for patients with generalized social phobia (Liebowitz et al., 1992; Turner, Beidel, & Jacob, 1994). Individuals with public speaking phobia in particular appear to have an exaggerated tachycardic response to phobic stimuli, and this may in part account for the effectiveness of beta-adrenergic blockers in this group (Heimberg et al., 1990).

Propranolol and atenolol are probably equally effective for patients with discrete performance-related social phobia, and may be used either routinely or on an as-needed basis. Atenolol may cause less sedation and other adverse central nervous system effects, and can be used in once-a-day dosing during maintenance treatment. Depending on individual requirements, 10–80 mg of propranolol or 25–100 mg of atenolol may be taken 60–90 minutes prior to an anxiety-provoking event. Patients should test themselves initially with low doses (e.g., 10–20 mg of propranolol) during nonperformance situations to determine tolerability before using the agent for the first time in a performance situation.

Other Agents

In two open trials of buspirone, at least moderate improvement was found at doses of 45 mg/day or more (Munjack et al., 1991; Schneier et al., 1993). For example, Schneier et al. (1993) reported on 17 patients who completed at least two weeks of treatment in a 12-week trial of buspirone. At week

12, 47% were rated as much to very much improved on the Clinical Global Impressions Scale. The mean dose for responders was 56.9 mg/day. Tricyclic antidepressants have shown only modest effectiveness for social phobia, although they have not been well studied (Liebowitz et al., 1985); the SSRI's and MAOIs are generally the preferred agents for social phobia when antidepressant treatment is indicated.

Nonpharmacologic Treatment

The best-studied nonpharmacologic treatment modalities for social phobia have been behavior therapy and CBT. These approaches include a variety of techniques, including cognitive restructuring, relaxation, exposure, and social skills training. Behavioral and cognitive approaches appear to be about equally effective (Chambless & Gillis, 1993) and compare favorably with drug treatment. In the controlled study of Gelertner et al. (1991), CBT provided substantial relief of symptoms, comparable to that found with phenelzine and alprazolam in the same study. Of particular interest is the finding that the CBT group, unlike the comparison groups, showed evidence of continued improvement at a 2-month follow-up. The form of CBT used in this study was the cognitive-behavioral group treatment for social phobia developed by Heimberg and colleagues (see Heimberg & Juster, 1994, for a review). This method involves 12 weeks of group therapy focusing on cognitive restructuring and situational exposure. In studies comparing it with a placebo therapy control, the group treatment was associated with a 75% response rate, compared to 40% for the placebo condition; at a 5-year follow-up, these gains appeared to be maintained (Heimberg, Dodge, Hope, Kennedy, & Zollo, 1990a; Heimberg, Salzman, Holt, & Blendell, 1993). Cognitive-behavioral approaches to social phobia are discussed in greater detail by Gould and Otto in Chapter 7 of this volume.

Treatment Resistance

Little more than 10 years ago, Liebowitz et al. (1985) noted that social phobia was a relatively "neglected anxiety disorder." Since then, a great deal has been learned about the phenomenology and treatment of the disorder. However, the management of patients who remain symptomatic after a trial of first-line therapy remains largely unstudied. In general, though, the systematic approach to treatment resistance outlined earlier in the chapter can be applied to social phobia.

Differential Diagnosis

The differential diagnosis of social phobia includes both psychiatic disorders (especially panic disorder with agoraphobia and avoidant personality disorder) and medical conditions capable of producing anxiety symptoms.

In common with social phobia patients, agoraphobic individuals may suffer from panic attacks, intense anticipatory anxiety related to social situations, and avoidance behavior. Distinguishing the two conditions may be important, since they may differ in treatment responsiveness (particularly to tricyclic antidepressants, which are less effective for social phobia). The two conditions can be distinguished by the nature of the situations that are anxiety-provoking. Social phobia is associated with intense anxiety in situations where an individual may encounter unfamiliar people or be subjected to the scrutiny of others. The anxiety and even panic attacks that may occur in social phobia are situationally bound and are often reactions to concerns about public embarrassment or humiliation. Patients with panic disorder are generally more focused on the fear of the attack itself and may experience attacks spontaneously or in situations other than those involving public scrutiny. When confronted with an unfamiliar situation, patients with social phobia may be more anxious in the presence of other people, whereas those with panic and agoraphobia may be comforted by the presence of others and fear being left alone. Recently, Page (1994) empirically derived a diagnostic algorithm to distinguish social phobia from panic disorder with agoraphobia. He found that five clinical variables were particularly discriminating: (1) Feeling dizzy or lightheaded in a panic attack and (2) avoiding traveling alone on public transportation favored a diagnosis of panic disorder with agoraphobia over social phobia, whereas (3) avoiding speaking to strangers, (4) fear of blushing, shaking, or feeling foolish, and (5) fear of eating with others favored a diagnosis of social phobia over panic disorder with agoraphobia.

There is a great deal of overlap in the clinical presentation of patients with social phobia and those with avoidant personality disorder who are often viewed as having more pervasive degrees of social constriction. However, the precise nature of the distinction between these conditions remains uncertain, and its clinical relevance (if any) is unclear. Moreover, studies which have assessed comorbid avoidant personality disorder have found that it improves and may remit with successful treatment of social phobia (Liebowitz et al., 1992; Versiani et al., 1992). Like those with social phobia, individuals with schizoid personality disorder may avoid social interaction, but the latter are motivated by a lack of interest in, rather than fear of, social contact.

The presence of severe, persistent anxiety despite treatment may suggest an unrecognized medical condition, although a history of anxiety that is only related to social situations makes this possibility less likely. Nevertheless, medical illness may exacerbate anxiety, and a physical exam and laboratory screening (including thyroid function tests) would be appropriate in a refractory patient. Similarly, the possibility that ingested substances (e.g., caffeine, stimulants, theophylline) may be contributing to the anxiety should be considered, and corrective measures should be instituted if this is found to be the case.

Comorbidity

Nearly 70% of social phobia patients may have comorbid psychiatric conditions over their lifetimes (Schneier et al., 1992b). Comorbidity may be associated with treatment resistance in a number of ways: Comorbidity may reflect a greater loading for psychopathology (Rosenbaum et al., 1992); the presence of comorbidity may exacerbate the severity of the individual disorders; and residual symptoms of untreated comorbid disorders (e.g., panic disorder) may mimic symptoms of social phobia. An example of the adverse interaction of comorbid disorders is the greater rate of depression in patients with comorbid panic disorder and social phobia, compared with patients with panic disorder alone (Reiter et al., 1991). Comorbidity may also interfere with the effectiveness of certain pharmacologic approaches. For example, Carrasco, Hollander, Schneier, and Liebowitz (1992) reported on a series of patients with comorbid OCD and social phobia whose symptoms were poorly responsive to SSRIs but who responded well to phenelzine. The identification and successful treatment of comorbid disorders may therefore be useful when a patient appears to be refractory to treatment for social phobia.

The most common comorbid conditions in patients with social phobia are other anxiety disorders (particularly specific phobia, panic disorder, and agoraphobia, and OCD), depressive disorders (dysthymia and major depression), and alcohol or other substance abuse (which sometimes results from attempts to "self-medicate" anxiety).

Rosenbaum and Pollock (1994) have recently reviewed strategies for treating social phobia and comorbid disorders. In some cases, a single agent may be used for both social phobia and a comorbid disorder (e.g., SSRIs for social phobia with comorbid depression, panic disorder, or OCD); in others, adjunct medications targeted at the comorbid disorder may be necessary (e.g., mood stabilizers for comorbid bipolar disorder). The nature of the comorbid disorder may also restrict the use of some treatments of social phobia. For example, coexisting alcohol dependence would be a relative contraindication to the use of an MAOI because of the risk of an adverse interaction, and to the use of benzodiazepines because of concerns about abuse.

It is often appropriate for clinicians to use combinations of agents when treating comorbid conditions. For example, patients whose depression responds better to a tricyclic antidepressant than to an SSRI or an MAOI may require a benzodiazepine for treatment of their social phobia. In general, CBT can be useful for both social phobia and the common comorbid Axis I disorders (depression, other anxiety disorders, substance abuse).

Optimization of Therapy

There is a relative paucity of available data to guide the discussion of optimization of dose or duration of pharmacotherapeutic interventions for social phobia. The absence of fixed-dose comparison studies makes it difficult to assess dose–response relationships for any available pharmacotherapies. Nevertheless, information from several studies may suggest tentative guidelines. Liebowitz et al. (1992) found that a significant response to phenelzine was observed by week 8 but not yet at week 4, suggesting that a minimum of 2 months may be necessary to demonstrate response to an MAOI. In clinical practice, patients may demonstrate improvement after 12–16 weeks of treatment. The mean dose among responders in the Liebowitz et al. (1992) study was 73 mg/day, although this was not different from the mean dose for nonresponders.

Studies of SSRIs suggest that the onset of benefit does not occur for some patients until 8–12 weeks of therapy. Patients should not be considered refractory to SSRIs until they have completed at least a 12-week trial (Van Ameringen et al., 1993; Van Vliet et al., 1994). Moreover, some patients who ultimately respond to fluoxetine may require doses as high as 80 mg/day or more (Black et al., 1992; Schneier et al., 1992a; Van Ameringen et al., 1993); presumably, patients on other SSRIs may require relatively higher doses as well.

Studies of benzodiazepine therapy provide limited data on optimal dosing and treatment duration. In studies of alprazolam for social phobia, the effective dose has ranged from about 3 to 5 mg/day, but some patients may require doses of 6–10 mg/day to achieve optimal response (Gelernter et al., 1991; Lydiard et al., 1988; Reich et al., 1989; Reich & Yates, 1988). An additional consideration with refractory patients taking short-half-life benzodiazepines such as alprazolam is the possibility that dosing frequency is inadequate. Breakthrough or rebound anxiety may occur if the drug effect wears off before the next scheduled dose (especially before the first morning dose). Patients on alprazolam or other short-acting benzodiazepines who complain of persistent anxiety with three-times-a-day or less frequent dosing may experience more persistent improvement with less interdose rebound anxiety when switched to four-times-a-day dosing or to a longer-acting agent such as clonazepam. For clonazepam, reported mean effective doses have generally been under 3 mg/day, but doses of 4–6 mg/day have been associated with improvement in some patients (Davidson, Ford, Smith, & Potts, 1991; Munjack et al., 1990; Ontiveros & Fontaine, 1990).

The question of when to decide that a benzodiazepine trial has been unsuccessful has not been answered. In one controlled study of clonazepam (Davidson et al., 1993), improvement was seen as early as 1–2 weeks, but the number of responders continued to increase throughout the 10-week study period. Practically speaking, patients may continue to improve over the first 8–12 weeks of treatment, and a therapeutic trial should generally be maintained at least that long before it is deemed ineffective.

The optimal duration of pharmacologic treatment also remains unclear. Most patients maintain benefit over years of treatment; clinically, relapse rates appear high when pharmacologic treatment is discontinued (comparable to what is seen with panic disorder), but this is an area warranting further controlled study.

Augmentation and Switching

After a reasonable trial (e.g., 8 weeks) of adequate doses of a medication, it may be useful to augment medications in patients who remain symptomatic, prior to switching treatments; however, there are few systematic data on which to base the choice of augmentation strategies. Addition of a high-potency benzodiazepine to an antidepressant (MAOI or SSRI), or vice versa, may benefit some patients. The benzodiazepines may be particularly useful for patients with prominent anticipatory anxiety and avoidant traits (Reich et al., 1989), and patients in whom these symptoms persist after treatment with an antidepressant may benefit from the addition of alprazolam or clonazepam. The addition of a beta-adrenergic blocker may be useful for targeting autonomic symptoms such as tachycardia or tremor, or used on an as-needed basis for patients with persistent performance anxiety. MAOIs and SSRIs should not be combined because of a potentially fatal interaction, and a washout period is required before a switch between these classes (5 weeks when switching from fluoxetine, 2–3 weeks when switching from sertraline, paroxetine, or fluvoxamine). The combination of pharmacotherapy with CBT often provides synergistic benefit, and patients who fail to respond to either one of these interventions should be offered a trial of the other or of combination therapy.

Case reports and open trials suggest that patients who fail to respond to any one of the classes of medications described above may respond to any other (Black et al., 1992; Reiter et al., 1990; Schneier et al., 1992a; Versiani et al., 1988). Reports of SSRIs in particular have often noted that patients responded to these agents after a history of poor response to other treatments, including benzodiazepines, MAOIs, tricyclics, buspirone, beta-adrenergic blockers, and CBT (Black et al., 1992; Schneier et al., 1992a; Van Ameringen et al., 1993, 1994; Van Vliet et al., 1994). Moreover, patients who do not respond to one SSRI may respond to another (Ringold, 1994; Van Ameringen et al., 1994). It should be noted, however, that there have not been any systematic investigations of the utility of SSRIs or any other agents for refractory social phobia.

In patients who do not respond to the more established agents for social phobia, less well-studied alternatives may be considered. Buspirone at doses of 45 mg/day or more may be helpful in some patients (Munjack et al., 1991; Schneier et al., 1993). A single case report supports the use of bupropion (Emmanuel et al., 1991) and another case report found that clonidine 0.1 mg bid relieved social phobia symptoms in a patient who had failed trials of alprazolam, phenelzine, and propranolol (Goldstein, 1987).

Summary

First-line treatments for social phobia include MAOIs, benzodiazepines, SSRIs, and CBT, all of which may be effective in 60–80% of patients. The choice of initial treatment depends on comorbidity, prior treatment history, patient preference, cost, and side effect profiles. One approach to the pharmacotherapy of social phobia is given in Figure 6.1. The sequence of steps outlined in the figure is based on clinical experience and the results of available studies, but it should be reemphasized that an optimal strategy for managing social phobia has not been established. Although MAOIs have been the most extensively studied agents for the treatment of social phobia, their risks and side effects often limit their use as first-line agents. Most patients with generalized social phobia for whom pharmacotherapy is appropriate can be started on either a high-potency benzodiazepine or (particularly for patients with comorbid substance abuse or depression) an SSRI. Nonresponders to a 4- to 6-week trial of a benzodiazepine or an 8- to 12-week trial of an SSRI may then be treated with combined benzodiazepine–antidepressant therapy, may be switched to an MAOI with or without benzodiazepine augmentation, or may receive a trial of CBT (alone or in combination with medication). For patients with significant autonomic symptoms and those with discrete performance anxiety, beta-adrenergic blockers may be useful alone or as augmenting agents for other therapies.

GENERALIZED ANXIETY DISORDER

General Considerations

According to DSM-IV (American Psychiatric Association, 1994), a diagnosis of GAD is made when an individual experiences anxiety and worry that (1) occur more often than not for at least 6 months and concern a number of activities or events; (2) are difficult to control; (3) are linked with somatic symptoms; and (4) cause significant functional impairment. Three of six associated symptoms (restlessness/feeling keyed up; easy fatiguability; impairment of concentration; irritability; muscle tension; sleep disturbance) must be present. In addition, the anxiety and worry cannot be attributable to another Axis I disorder (e.g., worry about gaining weight in anorexia nervosa), substance use, or a general medical condition. Many of the studies on this disorder used the earlier DSM-III and DSM-III-R criteria, which did not emphasize that the anxiety and worry have to be excessive and hard to control, or that significant functional impairment must be present. This fact, combined with the inclusion of patients with comorbid anxiety and mood disorders in many studies, makes it difficult to interpret much of the early literature on the pharmacotherapy of GAD (Swinson, Cox, & Fergus, 1993).

Patients with GAD may report a range of nonspecific symptoms as-

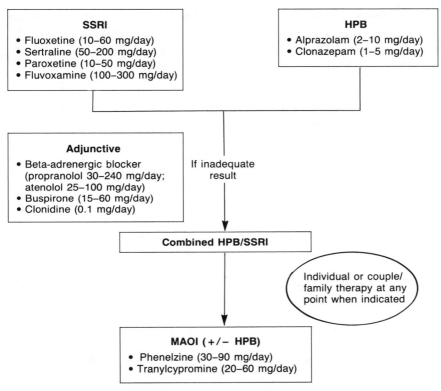

If comorbid depression, OCD, or substance abuse, initiate with:

SSRI
- Fluoxetine (10–60 mg/day)
- Sertraline (50–200 mg/day)
- Paroxetine (10–50 mg/day)
- Fluvoxamine (100–300 mg/day)

HPB
- Alprazolam (2–10 mg/day)
- Clonazepam (1–5 mg/day)

Adjunctive
- Beta-adrenergic blocker (propranolol 30–240 mg/day; atenolol 25–100 mg/day)
- Buspirone (15–60 mg/day)
- Clonidine (0.1 mg/day)

If inadequate result

Combined HPB/SSRI

Individual or couple/ family therapy at any point when indicated

MAOI (+/− HPB)
- Phenelzine (30–90 mg/day)
- Tranylcypromine (20–60 mg/day)

Note: Cognitive-behavioral therapy may be useful at any point in treatment.

FIGURE 6.1. An approach to the pharmacotherapy of social phobia. HPB, high-potency benzodiazepine (see text for other abbreviations).

sociated with anxiety (e.g., muscle tension, GI distress, diaphoresis, or dizziness) and often present initially to primary care physicians seeking diagnosis and relief of their multiple somatic complaints. The course of the disorder is generally chronic, although its onset and exacerbations may be related to stressful life events. Recent data from the National Comorbidity Survey indicate that the lifetime prevalence of GAD is 5.1%, with a female-to-male predominance of 1.8:1 (Kessler et al., 1994). Comorbidity appears to be common in GAD, and it has been estimated that the prevalence of individuals with "pure" GAD (i.e., individuals with GAD who have no other psychiatric diagnosis during their lifetimes) is less than 10% (Wittchen, Zhao, Kessler, & Eaton, 1994).

Pharmacotherapy: First-Line Treatments

Both pharmacologic and nonpharmacologic approaches have been shown to be effective in the treatment of GAD, so the decision to initiate pharmacotherapy may depend on patient preference, treatment history, comorbidity, and degree of distress experienced by the individual patient. Benzodiazepines have been the mainstay of the pharmacologic treatment of GAD, but other agents have also demonstrated effectiveness, including antidepressants and buspirone. The interpretation of trials without placebo comparison in GAD requires caution because of the high placebo response rate in this condition (on the order of 50% in some controlled trials) (Bjerrum, Allerup, Thunedborg, Jakobsen, & Bech, 1992; Rickels, Downing, Schweizer, & Hassman, 1993).

Benzodiazepines

The utility of benzodiazepines for anxiolysis has been demonstrated in numerous studies (Shader & Greenblatt, 1993). These agents may be particularly indicated for patients who are in significant distress and require rapid anxiolysis, who have not responded to antidepressant therapy, or for whom nonpharmacologic approaches (e.g., CBT stress management programs, counseling) have failed or are not available. They are relatively contraindicated in patients with a history of substance abuse or medical conditions in which sedation should be avoided (e.g., sleep apnea or severe pulmonary disease). The choice of which benzodiazepine to use is often based on half-life and potency, since there is no conclusive evidence to suggest that the members of this drug class differ in anxiolytic efficacy (Shader & Greenblatt, 1993). Both low potency (e.g., diazepam) and high potency (e.g., alprazolam) benzodiazepines have been effective in controlled studies of patients with GAD (Chouinard, Annable, Fontaine, & Solyom, 1982; Rickels et al., 1982). The short-half-life agents (e.g., alprazolam, oxazepam, lorazepam) have no active metabolites and are less likely to accumulate over time, causing excessive sedation or ataxia. However, compared with longer-acting agents (e.g., clonazepam, diazepam, and clorazepate), they require more frequent dosing to achieve a sustained effect and may be associated with interdose rebound anxiety and more severe discontinuation syndromes if treatment is abruptly discontinued (Shader & Greenblatt, 1993). Specific dosing information for the benodiazepines is presented in Table 6.2.

Since GAD is a chronic disorder, long-term use of benzodiazepines is often indicated, although the optimal duration of therapy in responders has not been established (Rickels & Schweizer, 1990). There are few data on maintenance treatment lasting more than 6 months, although follow-up studies suggest that patients who respond to benzodiazepines relapse when they are discontinued. In a follow-up of patients in a 6-month diazepam trial, Rickels, Case, Downing, and Fridman (1986) found that 63%

TABLE 6.2. Characteristics of Commonly Used Benzodiazepines

Drug	Half-life (hr)	Dose equivalent (mg)	Onset	Significant metabolites	Typical route of administration[a]
Midazolam (Versed)	1–12	2.0	Fast	No	i.v., i.m.
Oxazepam (Serax)	5–15	15	Slow	No	p.o.
Lorazepam (Ativan)	10–20	1.0	Intermed.	No	i.v., i.m., p.o.
Alprazolam (Xanax)[b]	12–15	0.5	Intermed.–fast	No	p.o.
Chlordiazepoxide (Librium)	5–30	10	Intermed.	Yes	p.o., i.v.
Clonazepam (Klonopin)[b]	15–50	0.25	Intermed.	No	p.o.
Diazepam (Valium)	20–100	5.0	Fast	Yes	p.o., i.v.
Flurazepam (Dalmane)	40	5.0	Fast	Yes	p.o.
Clorazepate (Tranxene)	30–200	7.5	Fast	Yes	p.o.

[a]i.v., intravenous; i.m., intramuscular; p.o., oral.
[b]Commonly used to treat panic disorder.

of patients experienced a relapse of their anxiety within a year following discontinuation of diazepam. Similarly, 57% of patients treated for 6 months with clorazepate had relapsed at a 40-month follow-up (Rickels & Schweizer, 1990). These data suggest that many patients may require long-term or even continuous therapy to remain free of significant anxiety. On the other hand, the same data have been used to support the approach of using benzodiazepines for brief periods of time and reinstituting therapy as needed, since 40–50% of patients will achieve sustained remission after 6 months or less of treatment. In general, it is advisable to use doses sufficient to effect marked relief of symptoms and to attempt gradual discontinuation after a sustained improvement has been achieved. However, patients who relapse shortly after discontinuation or who cannot tolerate the discontinuation process may be maintained on a benzodiazepine for longer periods of time and often indefinitely before another taper is attempted. CBT, treatment targeted at comorbid conditions (e.g., antidepressants for depression), and psychotherapy directed toward psychosocial difficulties may facilitate attempts to discontinue benzodiazepine therapy. However, repeated attempts to discontinue treatment that is effective and well tolerated may be counterproductive and distressing to patients. Many anxious patients clearly benefit from long-term treatment, as do patients with other chronic medical and psychiatric disorders.

Tricyclic Antidepressants

A number of open and controlled trials have demonstrated the efficacy of tricyclic antidepressants in the treatment of generalized anxiety. In a double-blind, placebo-controlled study of 242 anxious patients, Kahn, McNair, and Lipman (1986) found that imipramine (at doses of approximately 100–150 mg/day) was more effective than chlordiazepoxide for nonphobic anxiety, independent of baseline levels of depression. Hoehn-Saric, McLeod, and Zimmerli (1988) compared alprazolam (mean dose 2.2 mg) and imipramine (mean dose 90 mg) in 60 patients with GAD. Alprazolam was effective earlier, but after the second week the two drugs produced similar levels of improvement. Interestingly, the medications appeared to target different symptoms, with alprazolam having a greater effect on somatic symptoms and imipramine affecting predominantly "psychic" symptoms (e.g., interpersonal sensitivity, negative anticipation, dysphoria, and rumination). Similar results were reported in a recent placebo-controlled 8-week study of imipramine (mean dose 143 mg), trazodone (mean dose 255 mg), and diazepam (mean dose 26 mg) in 230 patients with DSM-III GAD (Rickels, Downing, Schweizer, & Hassman, 1993). Of the active drugs, diazepam was effective earliest, but imipramine produced the most consistent and sustained improvement, particularly in psychic symptoms of anxiety (e.g., worry and tension).

In an 8-week open trial of clomipramine (50–250 mg/day), 5 of 10 patients with GAD showed moderate to marked improvement in symptoms; however, the other 5 patients discontinued the medication because of severe side effects, predominantly overstimulation and increased anxiety (Wingerson, Nguyen, & Roy-Byrne, 1992). Because patients with GAD, like patients with panic disorder, may be sensitive to somatic side effects, tricyclics may be best initiated at low doses (the equivalent 10–25 mg of imipramine) and titrated up slowly to therapeutic doses (which are frequently in the range used to treat depression).

Buspirone

Another agent that has been shown to be effective in GAD is buspirone, an azapirone serotonin (5-HT_{1A}) receptor partial agonist. In controlled comparisons, buspirone has shown efficacy equivalent to that of various benzodiazepines: diazepam (Feighner, Merideth, & Hendrickson, 1982; Rickels et al., 1982), clorazepate (Rickels, Schweizer, Csanalosi, Case, & Chung, 1988), alprazolam (Enkelmann, 1991), lorazepam (Petracca et al., 1990), and oxazepam (Strand et al., 1990). Mean doses of buspirone in these studies have been in the range of 15–45 mg/day, although in clinical practice higher doses (60–90 mg/day) may be necessary for some patients. Overall response rates tend to be in the range of 50–60%. Compared with the benzodiazepines, buspirone has a slower onset of action (2–4 weeks); this may lead some patients with GAD, particularly those with a history of benzodiazepine treatment, to drop out of treatment prematurely (Enkelmann, 1991; Rickels et al., 1988). Buspirone does not cause physical dependence or discontinuation syndromes (Petracca et al., 1990; Rickels et al., 1988; Strand et al., 1990), and thus may be useful for some anxious patients with a history of alcohol or other substance abuse. Perhaps because benzodiazepine discontinuation effects can include rebound and withdrawal anxiety, relapse rates seem to be higher after discontinuation of benzodiazepines than of buspirone (Rickels & Schweizer, 1990; Rickels et al., 1988).

The side effect profile of buspirone is generally benign and includes headache, nausea, dizziness, and restlessness. There is evidence that other azapirones (e.g., ipsapirone) are effective for GAD, but these agents are not clinically available at present (Cutler, Sramek, Wardle, Keppel Hesselink, & Roeschen, 1993).

Other Agents

In addition to the report that the serotonergic heterocyclic antidepressant clomipramine may be effective in GAD, increasing clinical experience suggests that other serotonin reuptake inhibitors may be helpful. Although they have not been widely studied for this indication, the favorable side effect profile of SSRIs makes them useful agents for the anxious patient.

In a placebo-controlled trial of 230 patients, the antidepressant trazodone (mean dose 255 mg) produced moderate to marked global improvement in GAD symptoms (69% response rate), comparable to that achieved with imipramine (73%) and diazepam (66%) (Rickels et al., 1993). Because of its sedating properties, trazodone may be a useful alternative to benzodiazepines in patients with prominent sleep disturbance. Finally, beta-adrenergic blockers can be useful adjunctively in minimizing certain troubling somatic symptoms of anxiety (e.g., palpitations, tremor), but they are generally not used as first-line agents because they usually do not reduce the subjective experience of anxiety as well as other available agents do.

Nonpharmacologic Treatment

A variety of nonpharmacologic approaches may be effective for patients with generalized anxiety, including exercise, meditation, and stress management programs. Patients with greater degrees of distress, however, are candidates for psychodynamic, supportive, or interpersonal psychotherapies CBT. The best-studied of these are behavioral approaches and CBT, which are covered in greater detail in Chapter 7 of this volume. As in drug studies of GAD, placebo responses in the CBT studies tend to be high, but controlled studies have repeatedly demonstrated CBT to be more effective than waiting-list or pill placebo controls (Chambless & Gillis, 1993). A recent controlled study found that both CBT and a behavioral relaxation training program were superior to nonspecific, nondirective therapy (Borkovec & Costello, 1993). Importantly, for patients who respond to these treatments, improvements appear to be maintained at 6- to 12-month follow-up (Borkovec & Costello, 1993; Chambless & Gillis, 1993; Zinbarg, Barlow, Brown, & Hertz, 1992).

Treatment Resistance

The overall response rate with the first-line approaches discussed above is on the order of 40–70%, so that a substantial proportion of GAD patients remain symptomatic and may be considered "treatment-resistant." As with social phobia, there is a paucity of systematic data on which to base an approach to treatment-resistant GAD. However, attention to issues of differential diagnosis and comorbidity is of critical importance, since the symptoms of GAD may overlap or coexist with those of several medical and psychiatric disorders.

Differential Diagnosis

The most important considerations in the psychiatric differential diagnosis of GAD are other anxiety disorders, depression or dysthymia, and substance use or withdrawal states. Though both GAD and panic disorder are characterized by somatic symptoms and worry, the somatic symptoms in patients with panic occur during discrete attacks, and the worry is primarily focused on anticipation of another attack. The ruminative obsessions of some patients with OCD may mimic the excessive worry of GAD, but they are usually felt to be intrusive and senseless and are often accompanied by compulsive behavior. The presence of obsessions argues for the initiation of treatment with the SSRIs or clomipramine.

The symptoms of major depression and dysthymia also overlap with features of GAD, particularly the symptoms of ruminative worry, poor concentration, insomnia, and fatigue. Indeed, it has been suggested that depression and GAD represent phenotypic variants of a common genetic substrate (Kendler, Neale, Kessler, Heath, & Eaves, 1992). To complicate matters further, it has been proposed that the syndrome of "mixed anxiety–depression" may be a distinct diagnostic entity, and comorbidity of GAD and mood disorders occurs in a significant subset of patients (Brown, Barlow, & Liebowitz, 1994). Patients without the GAD symptoms of hypervigilance, autonomic hyperactivity, and muscle tension may be primarily suffering from a mood disorder, and may thus do poorly on benzodiazepines and better on antidepressants. In cases of diagnostic uncertainty, it is best to initiate treatment with antidepressants, in order to ensure appropriate treatment of affective symptomatology.

Symptoms related to substance use and withdrawal can be identical to those of GAD. In particular, generalized anxiety is a common symptom associated with longstanding alcohol use and withdrawal; the presence of alcohol and other substance use disorders should always be assessed in anxious patients. Patients should also be routinely questioned about their use of common anxiogenic agents, including caffeine, decongestants, and other sympathomimetics. Patients being treated for concomitant medical conditions may be on medications capable of producing anxiety—for example, theophylline, beta-adrenergic agonists, and glucocorticoids in pulmonary patients, or thyroid hormones in hypothyroid patients. The DSM-IV diagnosis of "substance-induced anxiety disorder with generalized anxiety" includes anxiety caused by either prescribed medications (e.g., theophylline, bronchodilators) or "recreational" drugs (e.g., alcohol, cocaine, amphetamines). In such cases, the treatment of choice would be removal of the offending drug—either detoxification from abusable substances, or the use of alternatives to medically prescribed drugs.

Patients with somatoform disorders may present with chronic, uncontrollable worry about having an illness (hypochondriasis) or about multiple somatic complaints (somatization disorder). This differential diagnosis may be difficult, but the restriction of worry to medical concerns may favor a somatoform disorder over GAD.

Patients whose GAD does not respond to initial treatment should be reevaluated for the presence of occult medical illness. The list of neurologic and medical conditions that can produce anxiety is extensive (Rosenbaum & Pollack, 1991). Although it is neither possible nor necessary to rule out each and every one before initiating treatment for patients thought to have GAD, a focused evaluation to assess likely culprits may be efficient and may yield important information. A screening physical exam and routine laboratory studies (electrolytes, blood urea nitrogen and creatinine, glucose, calcium, thyroid functions, liver functions, electrocariogram) should be undertaken in treatment-resistant patients. Further studies may be indicated if patients present with atypical or suspicious signs or symptoms. For example, anxiety associated with alterations in consciousness, olfactory hallucinations, or macropsia/micropsia would warrant an electroencephalogram to rule out complex partial seizures. Patients complaining of unremitting headaches or those exhibiting focal neurologic signs may require neuroimaging (computed tomography or magnetic resonance imaging) to rule out space-occupying lesions or multiple sclerosis (Coplan et al., 1993).

Comorbidity

Data from the National Comorbidity Survey suggest that the prevalence of concurrent comorbid disorders in patients with GAD is approximately 65% (Wittchen et al., 1994). The most common comorbid disorders in patients with GAD are other anxiety disorders (especially social phobia, specific phobias, and panic disorder), mood disorders (most commonly depression and dysthymia), and substance use disorders (Brawman-Mintzer et al., 1993; Brown et al., 1994). As discussed previously, social phobia and panic disorder, like GAD, may be responsive to benzodiazepines, but nonresponders may benefit from treatments targeted at each disorder (e.g., an SSRI for social phobia or panic). The presence of comorbid depressive symptoms would argue for treatment with antidepressants, which, unlike benzodiazepines, have both substantial anxiolytic and antidepressant effects (Kahn, McNair, & Frankenthaler, 1987; Rickels & Schweizer, 1993). Buspirone may also be helpful for some patients with GAD and milder degrees of depression. However, in patients who fail a trial of these medications, combined treatment with a benzodiazepine (for GAD) and an antidepressant may be warranted.

Anxious patients with substance abuse problems present particular difficulties, both because treatment options are more limited (by the need to avoid benzodiazepines whenever possible) and because the substance use/withdrawal may exacerbate or mimic anxiety symptoms. Aggressive efforts to treat the substance use disorder are important and may be undertaken simultaneously with treatment of the anxiety. The efficacy and lack of abuse potential of antidepressants (i.e., tricyclics and SSRIs) and of buspirone make them useful agents for patients with alcohol abuse and GAD (Tollefson, Montague-Clouse, & Tollefson, 1992); nonresponders should be given additional treatment trials with antidepressants and considered for CBT and/or psychotherapy when appropriate. Benzodiazepine use in these patients is best reserved for patients who have failed multiple adequate trials of antidepressants, and who have demonstrated good compliance with treatment and a commitment to reduction of substance use over time.

Optimization of Therapy

The optimal dosing and duration of pharmacotherapies for GAD have not been established. Patients treated with benzodiazepines usually show a response within 1–2 weeks, but a 4- to 6-week trial, with progressively increasing doses as tolerated, may be necessary in patients who do not respond initially. On average, studies have suggested that daily doses equivalent to 20 mg of diazepam are effective for responders, but doses equaling up to 40 mg of diazepam may be used if tolerated.

The slower onset of action of antidepressants and buspirone suggest that patients should be treated at therapeutic doses of these agents for at least 8 weeks before being considered refractory. Since patients may expect rapid relief of symptoms, it is important to provide education and reassurance about the expected delay in treatment effects with antidepressants and buspirone, so that patients do not prematurely terminate treatment. Available data suggest that doses of tricyclics should be titrated up to the equivalent of 100–200 mg/day of imipramine (Hoehn-Saric et al., 1988; Kahn et al., 1986). Because patients with GAD may be sensitive to antidepressant side effects, treatment should be initiated with test doses of antidepressants (e.g. 10 mg/day of imipramine, 10 mg/day of fluoxetine), which should be gradually titrated up to therapeutic levels as tolerated.

The addition of benzodiazepines or beta-adrenergic blockers may be helpful in patients who have difficulty with early jitteriness. Patients who do not respond to doses of buspirone of 5–10 mg three times daily may benefit from titration up to 20 mg thrice daily; occasionally, higher doses (e.g., 30 mg three times daily) may be helpful.

Augmentation and Switching

There have been no systematic studies designed to determine the most effective "next step" for patients who fail to respond to an adequate trial of one of the first-line agents for GAD (i.e., benzodiazepines, buspirone, or antidepressants). In theory, patients who do not respond to any one of these agents can be given sequential trials of the others. In practice, however, it is common that patients who fail to respond or partially respond to buspirone or a tricyclic will have a benzodiazepine added to their regimen. In patients who show a response, it may then be possible to discontinue the original agent. For patients refractory to an initial trial of benzodiazepines, the situation may be more difficult. There is evidence that patients with a history of prior benzodiazepine treatment may be less responsive to buspirone (Olajide & Lader, 1987; Schweizer, Rickels, & Lucki, 1986), perhaps because they have come to associate anxiolysis with the rapid onset and sedative properties of benzodiazepines. To minimize confusion between recurrent anxiety and benzodiazepine discontinuation effects, buspirone can be added for a period of 2–4 weeks before the benzodiazepine is gradually tapered. This strategy may limit rebound anxiety (Delle Chiaie et al., 1995). The addition of beta-adrenergic blockers may be helpful for patients who partially respond to other treatments but have persistent symptoms of autonomic hyperarousal. Clomipramine may be useful in patients who fail to respond to these combinations of medications; two of the five responders in the small open trial by Wingerson et al. (1992) had previously failed to respond to benzodiazepines. Although no published trials exist to support their use, SSRIs and the newer antidepressants venlafaxine and nefazodone have been used successfully in patients with GAD. For patients who fail a medication trial, the clinician should consider a trial of nonpharmacologic therapies (e.g., CBT, interpersonal psychotherapy, or psychodynamic therapies), all of which can be combined with drug therapy.

Summary

More than half of patients with GAD treated with first-line therapies (benzodiazepines, buspirone, antidepressants, and CBT) may experience substantial improvement. Although benzodiazepines have long been the mainstay of pharmacotherapy for generalized anxiety, an increasing variety of medications appear to be effective in GAD. In particular, antidepressants and the serotonergic anxiolytic buspirone have demonstrated ef-

ficacy comparable to benzodiazepines. The choice of an initial drug treatment will depend mainly on the patients' level of distress and need for
rapid anxiolysis (favoring benzodiazepines) and the presence of comorbid
depression or substance abuse (favoring buspirone or antidepressants). For
most patients, a trial of a benzodiazepine (10–40 mg/day diazepam equivalent), a tricyclic (e.g., imipramine, 75–300 mg/day), or buspirone (15–
60 mg/day) is an appropriate first choice. Nonresponders should be

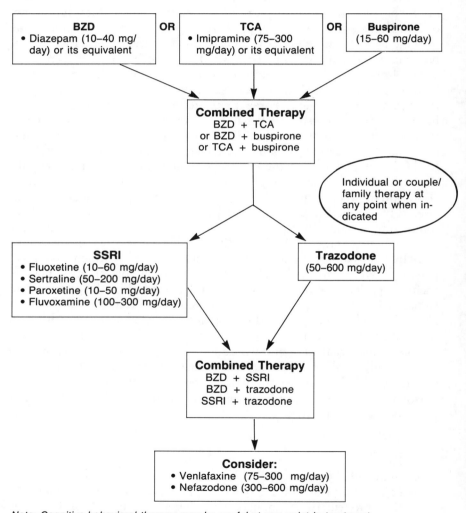

Note: Cognitive-behavioral therapy may be useful at any point in treatment.

FIGURE 6.2. An approach to the pharmacotherapy of generalized anxiety disorder. BZD,
benzodiazepine (see text for other abbreviations).

reevaluated for comorbid disorders and substance-induced or medically related anxiety. Patients with unremitting GAD may benefit from CBT, augmentation, or combination therapy (e.g., combining an antidepressant with buspirone or a benzodiazepine), or switching to an alternative antidepressant (e.g., SSRI, trazodone, venlafaxine, or nefazodone). Figure 6.2 depicts an approach to the treatment of GAD.

REFERENCES

American Psychiatric Association. (1980). *Diagnostic and statistical manual of mental disorders* (3rd ed.). Washington, DC: Author.

American Psychiatric Association. (1994). *Diagnostic and statistical manual of mental disorders* (4th ed.). Washington, DC: Author.

Black, B., Uhde, T. W., & Tancer, M. E. (1992). Fluoxetine for the treatment of social phobia [Letter]. *Journal of Clinical Psychopharmacology, 12,* 293–295.

Bjerrum, H., Allerup, P., Thunedborg, K., Jakobsen, K., & Bech, P. (1992). Treatment of generalized anxiety disorder: Comparison of a new beta-blocking drug (CGP361A), low-dose neuroleptic (flupenthixol), and placebo. *Pharmacopsychiatry, 25,* 229–233.

Borkovec, T. D., & Costello, E. (1993). Efficacy of applied relaxation and cognitive-behavioral therapy in the treatment of generalized anxiety disorder. *Journal of Consulting and Clinical Psychology, 61,* 611–619.

Brawman-Mintzer, O., Lydiard, R. B., Emmanuel, N., Payeur, R., Johnson, M., Roberts, J., Jarrell, M. P., & Ballenger, J. C. (1993). Psychiatric comorbidity in patients with generalized anxiety disorder. *American Journal of Psychiatry, 150,* 1216–1218.

Brown, T. A., Barlow, D. H., & Liebowitz, M. R. (1994). The empirical basis of generalized anxiety disorder. *American Journal of Psychiatry, 151,* 1272–1280.

Carrasco, J. L., Hollander, E., Schneier, F. R., & Liebowitz, M. R. (1992). Treatment outcome of obsessive compulsive disorder with comorbid social phobia. *Journal of Clinical Psychiatry, 53,* 387–391.

Chambless, D. L., & Gillis, M. M. (1993). Cognitive therapy of anxiety disorders. *Journal of Consulting and Clinical Psychology, 61,* 248–260.

Chouinard, G., Annable, L., Fontaine, R., & Solyom, L. (1982). Alprazolam in the treatment of generalized anxiety and panic disorders: A double-blind placebo-controlled study. *Psychopharmacology, 77,* 229–233.

Coplan, J. D., Tiffon, L., & Gorman, J. M. (1993). Therapeutic strategies for the patient with treatment-resistant anxiety. *Journal of Clinical Psychiatry, 54*(5, Suppl.), 69–74.

Cutler, N. R., Stramek, J. J., Wardle, T. S., Keppel Hesselink, J. M., & Roeschen, J. K. (1993). The safety and efficacy of ipsapirone vs. lorazepam in outpatients with generalized anxiety disorder (GAD): Single site findings from a multicenter trial. *Psychopharmacological Bulletin, 29,* 303–308.

Czepowicz, V. D., Johnson, M. R., Lydiard, R. B., Emmanuel, N. P., Ware, M. R., Mintzer, O. B., Walsh, M. D., & Ballenger, J. C. (1995). Sertraline in social phobia. *Journal of Clinical Psychopharmacology, 15,* 372–373.

Davidson, J. R. T., Ford, S. M., Smith, R. D., & Potts, N. L. S. (1991). Long-term treatment of social phobia with clonazepam. *Journal of Clinical Psychiatry, 52*(11, Suppl.), 16–20.

Davidson, J. R. T., Potts, N., Richichi, E., Krishnan, R., Ford, S. M., Smith, R., & Wilson, W. H. (1993). Treatment of social phobia with clonazepam and placebo. *Journal of Clinical Psychopharmacology, 13,* 423–428.

Delle Chiaie, R., Pancheri, P., Casacchia, M., Stratta, P., Kotzalidis, G. D., & Zibellini, M. (1995). Assessment of the efficacy of buspirone in patients affected by generalized anxiety disorder, shifting to buspirone from prior treatment with lorazepam: A placebo-controlled, double-blind study. *Journal of Psychopharmacology, 15,* 12–19.

Emmanuel, N. P., Lydiard, R. B., & Ballenger, J. C. (1991). Treatment of social phobia with bupropion [Letter]. *Journal of Clinical Psychopharmacology, 11,* 276–277.

Enkelmann, R. (1991). Alprazolam versus buspirone in the treatment of outpatients with generalized anxiety disorder. *Psychopharmacology, 105,* 428–432.

Feighner, J. P., Merideth, C. H., & Hendrickson, G. A. (1982). A double-blind comparison of buspirone and diazepam in outpatients with generalized anxiety disorder. *Journal of Clinical Psychiatry, 43*(12, Sec. 2), 103–107.

Gelernter, C. S., Uhde, T. W., Cimbolic, P., Arnkoff, D. B., Vittone, B. J., Tancer, M. E., & Bartko, J. J. (1991). Cognitive-behavioral and pharmacological treatments of social phobia: A controlled study. *Archives of General Psychiatry, 48,* 938–945.

Goldstein, S. (1987). Treatment of social phobia with clonidine. *Biological Psychiatry, 22,* 369–372.

Gorman, J. M., Liebowitz, M. R., Fyer, A. J., Campeas, R., & Klein, D. F. (1985). Treatment of social phobia with atenolol. *Journal of Clinical Psychopharmacology, 5,* 298–301.

Heimberg, R. G., Dodge, C. S., Hope, D. A., Kennedy, C., & Zollo, L. (1990a). Cognitive behavioral treatment of social phobia: Comparison to a credible placebo control. *Cognitive Therapy and Research, 14,* 1–23.

Heimberg, R. G., Hope, D. A., Dodge, C. S., & Becker, R. (1990b). DSM-III-R subtypes of social phobia: Comparison of generalized social phobics and public speaking social phobics. *Journal of Nervous and Mental Disease, 178,* 172–179.

Heimberg, R. G., & Juster, H. R. (1994). Treatment of social phobia in cognitive-behavioral groups. *Journal of Clinical Psychiatry, 55*(6, Suppl.), 38–46.

Heimberg, R. G., Salzman, D. G., Holt, C. S., & Blendell, K. (1993). Cognitive behavioral group treatment for social phobia: Effectiveness at five-year follow-up. *Cognitive Therapy and Research, 17,* 325–339.

Hoehn-Saric, R., McLeod, D. R., & Zimmerli, W. D. (1988). Differential effects of alprazolam and imipramine in generalized anxiety disorder: Somatic versus psychic symptoms. *Journal of Clinical Psychiatry, 49,* 293–301.

Kahn, R. J., McNair, D. M., & Frankenthaler, L. M. (1987). Tricyclic treatment of generalized anxiety disorder. *Journal of Affective Disorders, 13,* 145–151.

Kahn, R. J., McNair, D. M., & Lipman, R. S. (1986). Imipramine and chlordiazepoxide in depressive and anxiety disorders: II. Efficacy in anxious outpatients. *Archives of General Psychiatry, 43,* 79–85.

Katzelnick, D. J., Kobak, K. A., Greist, J. H., Jefferson, J. W., Mantle, J. M., & Serlin, R. C. (1995). Sertraline for social phobia: A double-blind, placebo-controlled crossover study. *American Journal of Psychiatry, 152,* 1368–1371.

Kendler, K. S., Neale, M. C., Kessler, R. C., Heath, A. C., & Eaves, L. J. (1992).

Major depression and generalized anxiety disorder: Same genes, (partly) different environments? *Archives of General Psychiatry, 49,* 716–722.

Kessler, R. C., McGonagle, K. A., Zhao, S., Nelson, C. B., Hughes, M., Eshleman, S., Wittchen, H.-U., & Kendler, K. S. (1994). Lifetime and 12-month prevalence of DSM-III-R psychiatric disorders in the United States. *Archives of General Psychiatry, 51,* 8–19.

Liebowitz, M. R., Gorman, J. M., Fyer, A. J., Campeas, R., Levin, A. P., Sandberg, D., Hollander, E., Papp, L., & Goetz, D. (1988). Pharmacotherapy of social phobia: An interim report of a placebo-controlled comparison of phenelzine and atenolol. *Journal of Clinical Psychiatry, 49,* 252–257.

Liebowitz, M. R., Gorman, J. M., Fyer, A. J., & Klein, D. F. (1985). Social phobia: Review of a neglected anxiety disorder. *Archives of General Psychiatry, 42,* 729–736.

Liebowitz, M. R., Schneier, F., Campeas, R., Hollander, E., Hatterer, J., Fyer, A., Gorman, J., Papp, L., Davies, S., Gully, R., & Klein, D. F. (1992). Phenelzine vs. atenolol in social phobia: A placebo-controlled comparison. *Archives of General Psychiatry, 49,* 290–300.

Lydiard, R. B., Laraia, M. T., Howell, E. F., & Ballenger, J. C. (1988). Alprazolam in the treatment of social phobia. *Journal of Clinical Psychiatry, 49,* 17–19.

Mannuzza, S., Schneier, F. R., Chapman, T. F., Liebowitz, M. R., Klein, D. F., & Fyer, A. J. (1995). Generalized social phobia: Reliability and validity. *Archives of General Psychiatry, 52,* 230–237.

Marshall, J. R. (1994). The diagnosis and treatment of social phobia and alcohol abuse. *Bulletin of the Menninger Clinic, 58*(2, Suppl. A), A58–A66.

Marshall, R. D., Schneier, F. R., Fallon, B. A., Feerick, J., & Liebowitz, M. R. (1994). Medication therapy for social phobia. *Journal of Clinical Psychiatry, 55*(6, Suppl), 33–37.

Munjack, D. J., Baltazar, P. L., Bohn, P. B., Cabe, D. D., & Appleton, A. A. (1990). Clonazepam in the treatment of social phobia: A pilot study. *Journal of Clinical Psychiatry, 5*(5, Suppl.), 35–40.

Munjack, D. J., Bruns, J., Baltazar, P. L., Brown, R., Leonard, M., Nagy, R., Koek, R., Crocker, B., & Schafer, S. (1991). A pilot study of buspirone in the treatment of social phobia. *Journal of Anxiety Disorders, 5,* 87–98.

Munjack, D. J., Flowers, C., & Eagan, T. V. (1994/1995). Sertraline in social phobia. *Anxiety, 1,* 196–198.

Olajide, D., & Lader, M. (1987). A comparison of buspirone, diazepam, and placebo in patients with chronic anxiety states. *Journal of Clinical Psychopharmacology, 7,* 148–152.

Ontiveros, A., & Fontaine, R. (1990). Social phobia and clonazepam. *Canadian Journal of Psychiatry, 35,* 439–441.

Otto, M. W., Pollack, M. H., Sachs, G. S., O'Neil, C. A., & Rosenbaum, J. F. (1992). Alcohol dependence in panic disorder patients. *Journal of Psychiatric Research, 26,* 29–38.

Page, A. C. (1994). Distinguishing panic disorder and agoraphobia from social phobia. *Journal of Nervous and Mental Disease, 182,* 611–617.

Petracca, A., Nisita, C., McNair, D., Melis, G., Guerani, G., & Cassano, G. B. (1990). Treatment of generalized anxiety disorder: Preliminary clinical evidence with buspirone. *Journal of Clinical Psychiatry, 51*(9, Suppl.), 31–39.

Pollack, M. H., & Rosenbaum, J. F. (1987). Management of antidepressant-induced side effects: A practical guide for the clinician. *Jounal of Clinical Psychiatry, 48,* 3–8.

Reich, J., Noyes, R., Jr., & Yates, W. (1989). Alprazolam treatment of avoidant personality traits in social phobic patients. *Journal of Clinical Psychiatry, 50,* 91–95.

Reich, J., & Yates, W. (1988). A pilot study of treatment of social phobia with alprazolam. *American Journal of Psychiatry, 145,* 590–594.

Reiter, S. R., Otto, M. W., Pollack, M. H., & Rosenbaum, J. F. (1991). Major depression in panic disorder patients with comorbid social phobia. *Journal of Affective Disorders, 22,* 171–177.

Reiter, S. R., Pollack, M. H., Rosenbaum, J. F., & Cohen, L. S. (1990). Clonazepam for the treatment of social phobia. *Journal of Clinical Psychiatry, 51,* 470–472.

Rickels, K., Case, W. G., Downing, R. W., & Fridman, R. (1986). One-year follow-up of anxious patients treated with diazepam. *Journal of Clinical Psychopharmacology, 6,* 32–36.

Rickels, K., Downing, R., Schweizer, E., & Hassman, H. (1993). Antidepressants for the treatment of generalized anxiety disorder. *Archives of General Psychiatry, 50,* 884–895.

Rickels, K., & Schweizer, E. (1990). The clinical course and long-term management of generalized anxiety disorder. *Journal of Clinical Psychopharmacology, 10,* 101S–110S.

Rickels, K., & Schweizer, E. (1993). The treatment of generalized anxiety disorder in patients with depressive symptomatology. *Journal of Clinical Psychiatry, 54*(1, Suppl.), 20–23.

Rickels, K., Schweizer, E., Csanalosi, I., Case, G., & Chung, H. (1988). Long-term treatment of anxiety and risk of withdrawal. *Archives of General Psychiatry, 45,* 444–450.

Rickels, K., Weisman, K., Norstad, N., Singer, M., Stoltz, D., Brown, A., & Danton, J. (1982). Buspirone and diazepam in anxiety: A controlled study. *Journal of Clinical Psychiatry, 43*(12, Sec.2), 81–86.

Ringold, A. L. (1994). Paroxetine efficacy in social phobia [Letter]. *Journal of Clinical Psychiatry, 55,* 363–364.

Rosenbaum, J. F., Biederman, J., Bolduc, E. A., Hirshfeld, D. R., Faraone, S. V., & Kagan, J. (1992). Comorbidity of parental anxiety disorders as risk for childhood-onset anxiety in inhibited children. *American Journal of Psychiatry, 149,* 475–481.

Rosenbaum, J. F., Biederman, J., Bolduc-Murphy, E. A., Faraone, S. V., Chaloff, J., Hirshfeld, D., & Kagan, J. (1993). Behavioral inhibition in childhood: A risk factor for anxiety disorders. *Harvard Review of Psychiatry, 1,* 2–16.

Rosenbaum, J. F., & Pollack, M. H. (1991). Anxiety. In N. H. Cassem (Ed.), *Massachusetts General Hospital handbook of general hospital psychiatry* (pp. 158–190). St. Louis, MO: C. V. Mosby.

Rosenbaum, J. F., & Pollock, R. A. (1994). The psychopharmacology of social phobia and comorbid disorders. *Bulletin of the Menninger Clinic, 58*(2, Suppl A), A67–A83.

Schneier, F. R., Chin, S. J., Hollander, E., & Liebowitz, M. R. (1992a). Fluoxetine in social phobia [Letter]. *Journal of Clinical Psychopharmacology, 12,* 62–63.

Schneier, F. R., Heckelman, L. R., Garfinkel, R., Campeas, R., Fallon, B. A.,

Gitow, A., Street, L., Del Bene, D., & Liebowitz, M. R. (1994). Functional impairment in social phobia. *Journal of Clinical Psychiatry, 55,* 322–331.

Schneier, F. R., Jihad, B. S., Campeas, R., Fallon, B. A., Hollander, E., Coplan, J., & Liebowitz, M. R. (1993). Buspirone in social phobia. *Journal of Clinical Psychopharmacology, 13,* 251–256.

Schneier, F. R., Johnson, J., Hornig, C. D., Liebowitz, M. R., & Weissman, M. M. (1992b). Social phobia: Comorbidity and morbidity in an epidemiologic sample. *Archives of General Psychiatry, 49,* 282–288.

Schweizer, E., Rickels, K., & Lucki, I. (1986). Resistance to the antianxiety effect of buspirone in patients with a history of benzodiazepine use [Letter]. *New England Journal of Medicine, 314,* 719–720.

Shader, R. I., & Greenblatt, D. J. (1993). Use of benzodiazepines in anxiety disorders. *New England Journal of Medicine, 328,* 1398–1405.

Stein, M. B., Shea, C. A., & Uhde, T. W. (1989). Social phobic symptoms in patients with panic disorder: Practical and theoretical implications. *American Journal of Psychiatry, 146,* 235–238.

Strand, M., Hetta, J., Rosen, A., Sorensen, S., Malmstrom, R., Fabian, C., Marits, K., Vetterskog, K., Liljestrand, A.-G., & Hegen, C. (1990). A double-blind, controlled trial in primary care patients with generalized anxiety: A comparison between buspirone and oxazepam. *Journal of Clinical Psychiatry, 51*(9, Suppl.), 40–45.

Swinson, R. P., Cox, B. J., & Fergus, K. D. (1993). Diagnostic criteria in generalized anxiety disorder treatment studies [Letter]. *Journal of Clinical Psychopharmacology, 13,* 455.

Tollefson, G. D., Montague-Clouse, J., & Tollefson, S. L. (1992). Treatment of comorbid generalized anxiety in a recently detoxified alcoholic population with a selective serotonergic drug (buspirone). *Journal of Clinical Psychopharmacology, 12,* 19–26.

Turner, S. M., Beidel, D. C., & Jacob, R. G. (1994). Social phobia: A comparison of behavior therapy and atenolol. *Journal of Consulting and Clinical Psychology, 62,* 350–358.

Van Ameringen, M., Mancini, C., & Streiner, D. L. (1993). Fluoxetine efficacy in social phobia. *Journal of Clinical Psychiatry, 54,* 27–32.

Van Ameringen, M., Mancini, C., & Streiner, D. L. (1994). Sertraline in social phobia. *Journal of Affective Disorders, 31,* 141–145.

Van Ameringen, M., Mancini, C., Styan, G., & Donison, D. (1991). Relationship of social phobia with other psychiatric illness. *Journal of Affective Disorders, 21,* 93–99.

Van Vliet, I. M., Den Boer, J. A., & Westenberg, H. G. M. (1992). Psychopharmacological treatment of social phobia: Clinical and biochemical effects of brofaromine, a selective MAO-A inhibitor. *European Neuropsychopharmacology, 2,* 21–29.

Van Vliet, I. M., Den Boer, J. A., & Westenberg, H. G. M. (1994). Psychopharmacological treatment of social phobia: A double blind placebo controlled study with fluvoxamine. *Psychopharmacology, 115,* 128–134.

Versiani, M., Mundim, F. D., & Nardi, A. E. (1988). Tranylcypromine in social phobia. *Journal of Clinical Psychopharmacology, 8,* 279–283.

Versiani, M., Nardi, A. E., Mundim, F. D., Alves, A. B., Liebowitz, M. R., & Amrein, R. (1992). Pharmacotherapy of social phobia: A controlled study with moclobemide and phenelzine. *British Journal of Psychiatry, 161,* 353–360.

Wingerson, D., Nguyen, C., & Roy-Byrne, P. P. (1992). Clomipramine treat-
    ment for generalized anxiety disorder. *Journal of Clinical Psychopharmacology,*
    12, 214–215.
Wittchen, H.-U., Zhao, S., Kessler, R., & Eaton, W. W. (1994). DSM-III-R gener-
    alized anxiety disorder in the National Comorbidity Survey. *Archives of General*
    Psychiatry, 51, 355–364.
Zinbarg, R. E., Barlow, D. H., Brown, T. A., & Hertz, R. M. (1992). Cognitive-
    behavioral approaches to the nature and treatment of anxiety disorders. *An-*
    nual Review of Psychology, 43, 235–267.

7

Cognitive-Behavioral Treatment of Social Phobia and Generalized Anxiety Disorder

ROBERT A. GOULD
MICHAEL W. OTTO

Relative to panic disorder, social phobia and generalized anxiety disorder (GAD) have received considerably less empirical attention over the last decade. Social phobia was identified in the mid-1980s as a "neglected anxiety disorder" that was expected to move into the limelight during the 1990s (Liebowitz, Gorman, Fyer, & Klein, 1985); and, despite characterizations of GAD as the "basic" anxiety disorder, it has continued to receive less attention than other disorders. Nonetheless, specialized forms of cognitive-behavioral treatment (CBT) for these disorders have been developed and validated, and these offer promising outcome to patients with these problems. This chapter reviews the nature and efficacy of CBT for social phobia and GAD, and discusses strategies for optimizing treatment outcome.

SOCIAL PHOBIA

General Considerations

In many ways, social phobia represents an extreme form of the shyness, performance anxiety, or stage fright that most individuals have experienced at some point in their lives. It is characterized by fears of humiliation or embarrassment in social or performance situations—fears that result in the regular provocation of anxiety and interference in such situations. Social phobia may include physical symptoms resembling those of panic disorder: increased heart rate, hot flashes, sweating, shaking, trembling, shortness of breath, and abdominal distress. Although anxiety in social situations may quickly crescendo into a "panic attack," social phobia and panic disorder are distinguished by the focus of the fears in each disorder (Ball, Otto, Pollack, Uccello, & Rosenbaum, 1995; Mannuzza, Fyer, Liebowitz, & Klein, 1990). The panic attack and its perceived consequences are the focus of the fear in panic disorder, whereas concerns about humiliation and embarrassment in front of others are dominant in social phobia, and there is typically no fear when activities are performed alone.

Often these physical symptoms are preceded and triggered by maladaptive cognitions in which patients may (1) underestimate their ability to cope in social situations (e.g., "I am certain that my mind will go blank when I try to give this speech"); (2) exaggerate the perceived consequences of performing inadequately in social situations (e.g., "If my face turns red when I ask Bonnie out for a date, she will never want to go out with me"); and/or (3) rehearse self-defeating and global attributions about themselves and their future social behavior (e.g., "I am a social failure and am destined to be a misfit"). Behavioral correlates typically consist of avoidance behaviors (e.g., skipping class, avoiding calling someone for a date, or avoiding a party or a conversation).

Data from three epidemiologic studies indicate that the prevalence of social phobia in the general population is 2–3% (Myers et al., 1984; Pollard & Henderson, 1988; Schneier, Johnson, Hornig, Liebowitz, & Weissman, 1992). As such, it is the most common anxiety disorder and one of the most common psychiatric disorders. An even larger percentage of individuals (20%) report problems with social anxiety, but do not meet the diagnostic criteria for social phobia (Pollard & Henderson, 1988). It is not uncommon for individuals with social phobia to suffer from comorbid problems. Liebowitz et al. (1985) reported that roughly 20% of the social phobics in their study sample met the criteria for alcohol dependence or abuse, and that approximately one-third presented with major depression. Ross (1994a) paints an equally disturbing picture of the lives of social phobia patients and describes individuals who avoid jobs that require social contact, fail to develop sustained friendships and relationships, forgo career promotions that may potentially require increased social contact, and isolate themselves from others outside of their immediate families. Turner, Beidel, Dancu, and Keys (1986) found that 92% of a sample of social phobia patients felt that their anxiety has interfered with occupational performance, and that 69% were unable to attend common social events. Some social phobics describe years of extensive and unnecessary medical examinations to find the cause of symptoms associated with the disorder, such as excessive sweating or difficulties in urinating (Craske, Barlow, & O'Leary, 1993).

The age of onset for social phobia is generally between 15 and 20 years (Liebowitz et al., 1985; Turner, Beidel, & Townsley, 1992). The increasing social pressures and social scrutiny during adolescence may contribute to onset during this life phase. Although onset of social phobia is early relative to other anxiety disorders, treatment-seeking behavior is not. In a review of 17 studies, Heimberg (1989) found that the mean age of subjects seeking treatment ranged from 27 to 41 years, and that the mean duration of phobia ranged from 8.2 to 22.1 years. Individuals presenting for treatment are as likely to be men as women (Öst, 1987; Heimberg, 1989).

Subtypes and Diagnostic Issues

Clinical researchers have noted that some individuals with social phobia tend to have fears about social interaction that extend across a variety of situations (e.g., public speaking, introducing themselves to others, eating in front of others) and individuals (e.g., authority figures, dates, strangers) (McNeill & Lewin, 1986; Spitzer & Williams, 1985). Both the revised third and fourth editions of the *Diagnostic and Statistical Manual of Mental Disorders* (DSM-III-R and DSM-IV; American Psychiatric Association, 1987, 1994) have incorporated this "subtype" into their diagnostic nomenclature and designated it "social phobia, generalized." Patients who do not have generalized social phobia tend to present on a continuum of severity, ranging from those who have problems in one circumscribed area (e.g., public speaking) to those with increasing numbers of problem areas. Research has suggested that generalized social phobics report greater fear of negative evaluation, greater social avoidance, and more depression than social phobics with more discrete problems (Heimberg, Hope, Dodge, & Becker, 1990b). Turner et al. (1992) also found that generalized social phobics tended to be more severely impaired and to perform more poorly on behavioral avoidance tests. Collectively, these findings suggest that generalized social phobics may have greater difficulty responding to treatment, and may require more specialized or intensive treatment interventions.

A second diagnostic issue relates to the relationship between social phobia and avoidant personality disorder. Avoidant personality disorder is defined as a pervasive pattern of social discomfort and fear of negative evaluation in which individuals avoid social and interpersonal contact and are easily hurt by criticism and disapproval of others. Studies have suggested that there is a large degree of overlap between the two disorders. The percentage of social phobics who also meet the criteria for avoidant personality disorder has ranged from 20% to 90% (Heimberg, 1989), with the highest rates evident for generalized social phobics. This marked overlap blurs the diagnostic distinctiveness of these two disorders and raises questions of whether avoidant personality disorder simply represents a more extreme version of generalized social phobia.

Cognitive-Behavioral Models of the Disorder

Early behavioral treatments for social phobia were grounded in the belief that the disorder reflected a behavioral deficit that could be rectified with social skills training. Lacking social skills, patients were presumed to find interpersonal interactions more aversive; this was believed to prompt avoidance, which would further undermine the acquisition of more effective social repertoires. Training typically involved use of instruction, participant modeling, corrective feedback, role plays, and therapist-assisted *in vivo* practice.

Research on the effectiveness of social skills training alone has suggested only modest outcome. Some studies have found no differences between social skills training and attention placebo controls (Marzillier, Lambert, & Kellett, 1976), and have found that social skills training does not generalize well to *in vivo* performance tasks (Falloon, Lloyd, & Harpin, 1981). Others have had more promising results, in which patients receiving social skills training exhibit modest decreases in social anxiety, avoidance, and distress at posttreatment (Lucock & Salkovskis, 1988; Stravynski, Marks, & Yule, 1982). In general, conceptualizations of social phobia as a skills deficit problem may fail to incorporate cognitive and affective aspects of the disorder that may be important for treatment.

Within the past 5–10 years, cognitive-behavioral models of social phobia have become increasingly multidimensional, and the treatments associated with them have accordingly become more comprehensive. Heimberg and Barlow (1991; Barlow, 1988) have proposed a model of social dysfunction in social phobia that focuses on the interaction of negative affect, expectancies, and cognitions in the maintenance of the disorder. This model purports that an individual with social phobia enters social situations with a real or perceived history of negative social interactions, which can contribute to negative affect and to expectancies of failure or embarrassment. Negative expectancies may occur in the form of perceived lack of control (e.g., "I am going to be unable to stop myself from sweating and shaking") or in more general forms (e.g., "I am going to embarrass myself," "She will notice that I am sweating and think that there is something wrong with me"). These predictions of negative outcome are likely to result in heightened autonomic arousal in social situations. As the individual enters the social situation, his or her attentional focus then shifts away from appropriate social cues and toward the adverse consequences of poor social performance or other distracting issues. Rather than focusing on the social cues in the situation and the ongoing social interactions, the person focuses on anxiety symptoms (e.g., the level of heart rate, the level of sweating, the trembling of the hands) or on cognitive cues of perceived failure (e.g., "I can feel my face turning red," "I will never get another date in my life"). This shift in turn leads to greater increases in autonomic arousal, thereby raising anxiety and motivating avoidance or escape. Because the individual is not focusing on appropriate social cues, this may in turn lead to dysfunctional or suboptimal social performance. Lastly, the social phobic adopts avoidance as the primary method of coping with future social situations, and maintains his or her negative expectancies with regard to these situations.

For the socially functional person, this pattern is quite different. Social performance is considerably less connected to dysfunctional expectancies and negative affect in such individuals. Instead, they approach these situations with generally positive expectancies, based on their past social histories. Within the social situation, they focus on appropriate social cues and are able to compensate for increased autonomic arousal with increased attentional focus on such cues. This aids them in social performance and provides them with generally positive feedback. The result is an adequate and nonaversive social performance, which encourages these individuals to approach future social interactions (Heimberg & Barlow, 1991).

The marked contrast between these two patterns of social behavior emphasizes the level of impairment in many social phobics. Their patterns of severe self-evaluation and overwhelming anxiety create a self-fulfilling prophecy of poor performance, anxiety, and avoidance. Given these sorts of negative cognitive biases, it is easy to see why dysthymia and depression may well co-occur with social phobia. Comorbid alcohol problems are also not uncommon. Not surprisingly, social phobics may at times turn to alcohol as an apparent attempt to self-medicate their anxiety by decreasing their own social awareness and self-evaluation (Kushner, Sher, & Beitman, 1990; Otto et al., 1992). Unfortunately, the effects of alcohol are short-lived and, because of state-dependent learning, do not generalize well beyond a nonintoxicated state.

Cognitive-Behavioral Treatment

The general goal of CBT for social phobia is to help patients break out of their self-defeating patterns and behave more adaptively in social situations. Consistent with the model described above, treatment focuses on helping patients eliminate their anxiogenic cognitions and redirect their attention to more relevant cues. Avoidance is also targeted, because of its role in denying patients the opportunity to challenge maladaptive anxiogenic thoughts and receive corrective feedback. Group treatment may be particularly effective because of the built-in exposure that it provides and the opportunities for observational learning and contact with individuals having similar concerns and goals. Programmed simulations of the events that provoke social phobia are more accessible within a group format. When these general strategies are used, the fear and avoidance cycle can be broken, and the patient can develop more functional cognitive and behavioral responses to social situations.

One of the more comprehensive and empirically based forms of CBT for social phobia was developed by Heimberg and his colleagues (Heimberg, 1989; Heimberg & Barlow, 1988; Heimberg et al., 1990a). This 12-week cognitive-behavioral group treatment (CBGT) has four basic components. First, patients are educated about social phobia and presented with a model (described above) of how their problem is maintained. The interaction among cognitive, physiologic, and behavioral components is described, as well as how these components escalate during a problematic social situation. Particular emphasis is placed on the notion that social phobia is a learned response, and as such can be unlearned through behavioral exposure and cognitive restructuring. Group members are asked to share examples of how social phobia has influenced their lives, and to develop a hierarchy of aversive social situations that will be used for later exposure simulations. For many patients, adjustment to the group setting is the first aspect of exposure treatment, and open discussion of their anxiety about participating in the group is encouraged by the group leader.

In weeks 2 and 3, patients are taught the fundamentals of cognitive restructuring that will be used in the remaining treatment sessions. Patients are instructed on how to recognize distortions in their thinking during social situations and social performance (e.g., fortune-telling errors, mind reading, all-or-nothing thinking), and to develop cognitive responses to their thoughts that credibly challenge these errors. Hypothesis-testing procedures are used to encourage patients to come up with more accurate and honest appraisals of their performance and public perception. These techniques are designed to help patients identify and change their expectations of negative social outcomes and their relatively severe evaluations of themselves in social situations. Patients rehearse identifying these errors and creating countering thoughts in session; they are also asked to monitor their thoughts during social interactions in the course of the subsequent week.

The remaining nine sessions of CBGT consist of completing exposure simulations of personally relevant situations and assignments of in vivo exposure homework. Exposure simulations require that patients role-play increasingly difficult feared situations in the group setting, using other group members to try to make these situations as true to life as possible. These exposures are designed to provide patients with opportunities to experience arousal in social situations, to learn to respond differently to this arousal, and to learn that their anxiety will decrease with practice. Patients also have the opportunity to challenge cognitive distortions in these situations and to practice adaptive coping statements. The group setting provides an audience and role players for these interventions, which may include simulations of conversations, giving a speech, or eating a messy food. With successful treatment, patients learn of the severity of their cognitive distortions about feared situations, develop skills for identifying and correcting these distortions, and gain experience at performing in such situations (with particular practice in correcting and identifying distortions before, during, and after these programmed exposure simulations). As the group continues, exposure practice is expanded, helping patients develop confidence and competence in a wider variety of social situations and helping them change the cognitive biases that led to anxiety in the first place. Homework assignments require that patients practice their newly acquired skills between sessions and report back to the group on their successes and difficulties. Group size is typically five to seven patients, and sessions last for 2½ hours to insure that each patient will experience several exposure simulations by the end of treatment (Heimberg & Barlow, 1991).

Treatment Outcome Findings

Outcome for CBGT and Other Forms of CBT

Studies assessing the effectiveness of CBGT have reported favorable results. In a comparison of CBGT to an educational–supportive psychotherapy program, improvements were found for both groups, but the patients receiving CBGT were significantly more improved than the treatment control at both posttreatment and follow-up (Heimberg et al., 1990b). Seventy-five percent of patients undergoing CBGT met criteria for clinical improvement based on a phobia severity rating scale; by the educational–supportive program resulted in a 40% improvement rate. Clinical benefit was maintained and, in fact, increased over the 6-month follow-up period: 81% of CBGT-treated patients met the clinical criteria for improvement at the follow-up assessment. Consistent with a cognitive-behavioral formulation of the disorder, decreases in phobic severity for social situations were associated with the decreases in negative self-evaluations.

A number of other studies have examined the effectiveness of other cognitive and behavioral techniques, used either alone or in combination. Studies employing social skills training have found that these procedures are associated with improvement in patients who are defined as both socially phobic and socially inadequate, but they may be more efficacious for unskilled than for overanxious patients (Heimberg & Barlow, 1991; Öst, Jerremalm, & Johansson, 1981). Interventions employing relaxation training techniques have obtained mixed results. Alstrom, Nordlund, Persson, Harding, and Ljungqvist (1984) compared relaxation training to exposure, supportive therapy, and a control condition. The authors reported that relaxation training was ineffective, doing more poorly than the exposure and supportive therapy conditions, and no better than the control condition. Studies using applied relaxation have fared better. Öst et al. (1981) compared applied relaxation to standard progressive muscle relaxation and found that subjects receiving applied relaxation were significantly more improved on most measures than the group receiving progressive muscle relaxation.

Studies comparing the effectiveness of behaviorally based exposure treatments to CBT have failed to demonstrate consistent superiority of the latter. Butler, Cullington, Munby, Amies, and Gelder (1984) compared exposure therapy to exposure therapy plus anxiety management training and to a waiting-list control group. At posttreatment, both treatment groups were significantly different from the waiting-list control on measures of phobic severity, anticipatory anxiety, social avoidance and distress, and depression. Emmelkamp, Mersch, Vissia, and van der Helm (1985) assigned subjects randomly to *in vivo* exposure, rational–emotive therapy, and self-instruction training in which subjects practiced generating adaptive cognitive responses. Results indicated that all three treatments were equally effective at reducing social fear and distress. Mattick, Peters, and Clarke (1989) found that patients receiving exposure alone performed better on measures of behavioral approach than did patients receiving cognitive restructuring alone, but worse on measures of attitudinal change. Other studies have also indicated that exposure treatments yield reductions in social phobics' anxiety and avoidance (Biran, Augusto, & Wilson, 1981; Mattick & Peters, 1988).

CBT versus Pharmacologic Interventions

Few comparisons between CBT and pharmacologic interventions are available. Gelernter et al. (1991) compared a group form of CBT (not Heimberg et al.'s CBGT) to pharmacotherapy (with alprazolam, phenelzine, or a pill placebo) plus instructions for exposure to phobic stimuli. All of the treatments were associated with significant improvement (measured by changes in self-report instruments and physician rating scales), and no one treatment was consistently superior to the others. Interpretations of these findings are limited, however, because patients in all of the drug treatment conditions were instructed to complete self-directed exposure to fearful social situations. This instruction helped to insure that exposure interventions were common to all treatment conditions, thus raising the possibility that exposure was the active treatment element for this study. In another study, exposure alone, in the form of 20 sessions of imaginal and *in vivo* flooding, was compared to the drug atenolol and to a drug placebo condition (Turner, Beidel, & Jacob, 1994). These researchers found that flooding was consistently superior to placebo, whereas atenolol was not. In addition, flooding was superior to atenolol on behavioral and composite outcome measures. More recently, Heimberg et al. (1994) compared CBGT to phenelzine and to a pill placebo. At posttreatment (12 weeks), both CBGT and phenelzine were superior to placebo, but not different from each other. Phenelzine had a faster onset of therapeutic effect than CBGT by week 6, but this difference was eliminated by the end of treatment.

Meta-Analytic Findings

Meta-analysis is a statistical technique that allows comparison of treatment results in terms of quantifiable units (called "effect sizes") based on the normal curve. The advantage of meta-analytic procedures is that they yield standardized scores (effect sizes) that can be used as a common metric across several treatment outcome studies using different treatment outcome measures. To provide a summary of the literature to date, we recently conducted a meta-analysis of 24 studies that used psychosocial or pharmacologic interventions for social phobia (Gould, Buckminster, Pollack, Otto, & Yap, 1994). All studies employed treatment control conditions, and between-group effect sizes were calculated relative to these control conditions. In addition, in order to reduce measurement bias, effect sizes were only derived from self-report questionnaires. Three effect sizes were calculated for each social phobia study to capture three symptom dimensions of social phobia: social anxiety or avoidance, cognitive change, and depression. Results of this meta-analysis are presented in Table 7.1.

Ten studies provided data on the efficacy of pharmacotherapy relative to pill placebo ($n = 8$ studies), pill placebo plus exposure instructions ($n = 1$ study), or a no-treatment control group ($n = 1$ study). The mean effect size for social anxiety was 0.62 and for depression was 0.83. Measures of cognitive change were assessed in only one study. Comparisons of the social anxiety and depression effect sizes to the null hypothesis (effect size = 0.0) were statistically significant. In addition, eliminating the two studies that did not use pure pill placebo control groups did little to change the overall effect sizes (0.52 for social anxiety; 0.88 for depression). The mean dropout rate for these studies was 14.9%.

Monoamine oxidase inhibitors (MAOIs) in this meta-analysis included phenelzine ($n = 4$ studies) and moclobemide ($n = 1$ study), and their mean social anxiety effect size was 0.64 with a dropout rate of 14%. Two controlled studies assessed the efficacy of high potency benzodiazepines (BZDs; alprazolam and clonazepam); their mean effect size was 0.72, and their dropout rate was 12%. Promising results were obtained from SSRIs

TABLE 7.1. Meta-Analysis of Acute Treatment Outcome for Social Phobia

Treatment intervention	Mean social anxiety effect size
Pharmacotherapy vs. pill placebo	
MAOIs (5 studies)	0.64
Benzodiazepines (2 studies)	0.72
SSRIs (2 studies)	1.89
Beta-adrenergic blockers (3 studies)	− 0.09
Buspirone (1 study)	− 0.50
CBT vs. controls	
Cognitive restructuring alone (3 studies)	0.60
Exposure techniques alone (6 studies)	0.89
Exposure plus cognitive restructuring (8 studies)	0.80

Note. The number of studies providing outcome comparisons is noted for each treatment listed. From Gould, Otto, Yap, and Pollack (1994).

including fluvoxamine (n = 1 study) (effect size = 2.73; dropout rate = 3%) and sertraline (n = 1 study) (effect size = 1.05; dropout rate = 0%). The beta-adrenergic blocker atenolol (n = 3 studies) (effect size = 0.09) and buspirone (n = 1 study) (effect size = −0.50) did not appear to be effective for social phobia because they did worse than a pill placebo condition.

Studies of cognitive-behavioral therapy utilized cognitive restructuring, situational exposure, social skills training, systematic desensitization, flooding, and anxiety management techniques. A total of 16 studies used cognitive-behavioral interventions without pharmacotherapy, and their mean social anxiety effect size was 0.71, the mean cogntive change effect size was 0.74, and the mean depression effect size was 0.67. The mean dropout rate for CBT interventions in these studies was 11.5%. In general, there were no significant differences between types of CBT interventions, and all were superior to the null hypothesis (effect size = 0.0). Studies using cognitive restructuring alone (effect size = 0.60) did not differ significantly in efficacy from studies using exposure techniques alone (effect size = 0.89) or the combination of exposure plus cognitive restructuring (effect size = 0.80), nor did they differ in terms of dropout rates.

Comparisons of studies utilizing cognitive-behavioral treatments (effect size = 0.71) to those using pharmacotherapy (effect size = 0.62) were not statistically significant. In addition, mean attrition rates were not significantly different among subjects receiving a cognitive-behavioral intervention (11.5%) and those receiving a medication intervention (14.9%). CBT interventions may also enjoy a small advantage in terms of these comparisons due to their use of wait-list controls, which tend to be weaker control conditions relative to pill placebo conditions.

Results from our meta-analysis are similar to findings by Chambless and Gillis (1993). These authors derived effect sizes based on within-group change from pre- to posttreatment in 10 studies of CBT for social phobia. They found large effect sizes for CBT at the end of treatment. In addition, their review of controlled research studies indicated that CBT-treated patients did significantly better on most measures than did their control cohorts. For measures of social phobia, the pre-to-post effect size was 0.68; for measures of fear of negative evaluation, the effect size was 0.70.

Long-Term Results

Only four studies using cognitive and behavioral techniques have included data with follow-up periods of 1 year or longer. Fava, Grandi, and Canestrari (1989), in an uncontrolled trial of the effects of exposure treatment alone for 10 social phobia patients, reported that 7 of the 10 had maintained their posttreatment gains at a 1-year follow-up. Mersch, Emmelkamp, and Lips (1991) used a 14-month follow-up on a study that originally compared social skills training with rational–emotive therapy. At posttreatment, both groups showed improvement on a number of outcome measures.

Although subjects generally maintained their treatment gains at follow-up, 44% of them sought and obtained additional treatment for their social phobia during this time period.

Wlazlo, Schroeder-Hartwig, Hand, Kaiser, and Munchau (1990) compared a social skills training program to individual and group-administered *in vivo* exposure treatments. Results suggested no significant differences between the two conditions and general improvement for the majority of patients. Long-term assessments were conducted between 1 and 5.5 years (mean = 2.5 years), and the authors reported additional improvements on several measures for both groups at follow-up. It should be noted, however, that methodologic problems existed in this study: Patients were not randomly assigned to groups, and patients in the social skills training condition were also taught exposure techniques.

Heimberg et al. (1990a) compared a credible placebo (an education–support group) to CBGT and found that 75% of CBGT patients met the criteria for clinical improvement at posttreatment, compared to 40% of the placebo group. Data from this study represent the longest mean follow-up period (mean = 5.5 years; range = 4.5 to 6.25 years) and were derived from 19 of the 40 original subjects (Heimberg, Salzman, Holt, & Blendell, 1993). The authors indicated that their follow-up subsample may have been less impaired before treatment than nonparticipating subjects, but also noted that CBGT and the placebo treatment were equivalent in terms of participant–nonparticipant differences. At follow-up, 89% of CBGT patients were judged to be clinically improved by independent assessors, compared to 44% of the education–support group members. More recently, Heimberg et al. (1994) reported that although CBGT and phenelzine were equivalent and superior to a placebo at posttreatment, at 6-month follow-up the CBGT subjects had maintained their improvement, whereas one-half of phenelzine patients had relapsed. In summary, results from these studies suggest that the benefit from CBT generally endures over time.

Treatment Resistance/Maximizing Treatment Outcome

From the perspective of clinical research, relatively little is known about what kinds of patients tend to be resistant to standard forms of CBT for social phobia. There is some evidence that patients with discrete social phobia tend to benefit more from CBGT than do those with generalized social phobia (Heimberg, 1989). It is also evident that patients who have relatively more skills deficits will benefit more from an approach that emphasizes skills than from an approach that emphasizes anxiety reduction (for a review, see Heimberg, 1989). Hence, package treatment approaches that are able to stress either anxiety reduction, skills acquisition, or a combination of these interventions may offer the best benefit to a heterogeneous sample of patients.

The overlap between social phobia and avoidant personality disorder suggests that patients with the generalized subtype of social phobia may have prominent and fixed patterns of avoidance in social situations, and hence that treatment may necessarily require a longer course of intervention. In addition, nearly one-third to one-half of some samples of patients with social phobia have been found to have comorbid panic disorder (Barlow, 1988; Rosenbaum & Pollack, 1994). Often this comorbidity manifests itself in the form of situationally bound panic attacks, in which a panic attack becomes increasingly common under specific social conditions and then generalizes to other social situations. As such, patients experience anticipatory anxiety not only with regard to fears of humiliation, but also with regard to the experience of uncontrollable panic symptoms. Because standard CBGT focuses the most attention on cognitive restructuring, patients with comorbidity may benefit from the addition of techniques found to be useful for panic disorder, particularly interoceptive exposure techniques. Interoceptive exposure—that is, exposing patients to the somatic sensations of anxiety (see Otto & Gould, Chapter 5, this volume)—offers the therapist the ability to include in exposure assignments not just the extensive cues of a social situation, but also relevant internal sensations of arousal. Treatment can thus focus on decreasing anxiogenic responses to both internal and external cues. The addition of other symptom management skills and cognitive restructuring for panic attacks may also be of use for these patients.

Comorbid depression has been identified as a negative predictor of treatment outcome (Barlow, 1994). Brown and Barlow (1992) reported that 35% of patients with social phobia had experienced at least one episode of major depression. Stein, Tancer, Gelertner, Vittone, and Uhde (1990) reported that 20% of patients with social phobia presented with an additional mood disorder (either major depression or dysthymia). Comorbid dysthymic disorder has been found in 15% of social phobics (Van Ameringen, Mancini, Styan, & Donison, 1991). In more than 80% of cases of social phobia with comorbid depression, the depressive symptoms develop after the onset of social fear and avoidance (Brooks, Baltazar, & Munjack, 1989; Turner, Beidel, Borden, Stanley, & Jacob, 1991). Because comorbid depression tends to increase the severity of fears of negative evaluation (Ball et al., 1995; Bruch, Mattia, Heimberg, & Holt, 1993), the addition of supplemental cognitive restructuring and activity assignments may be necessary for these patients. In particular, we have noticed in our clinical practice that patients with comorbid depression easily become preoccupied with global depressive thoughts about themselves and their performance. For patients with such comorbidity, we routinely apply additional cognitive restructuring skills, as well as informational interventions to caution them about cognitive biases that emerge from depression and to help them develop ways of restructuring these biases. However, whenever depression dominates the clinical picture, we refer patients for CBT for depression prior to referral for social phobia treatment.

In summary, social phobia treatment is just now receiving the research attention that it deserves. Treatment studies conducted to date affirm that

CBT is a powerful intervention, producing results that rival the outcomes obtained with antidepressant interventions. CBT interventions have borrowed the same principles as those identified for treating other anxiety disorders; these include identifying behavioral excesses and deficits, and providing corrective skills training and exposure experiences to eliminate patterns that maintain the anxiety disorder. It appears that cognitive restructuring and exposure interventions provide a powerful combination of interventions for the treatment of social phobia. For a subsample of patients who are poorly skilled in social situations, additional training in social skills may provide further benefits. As with other anxiety disorders, comorbidity is likely to require additional and broader treatment interventions that include components of treatments found to be effective for other Axis I disorders (e.g., panic disorder or depression).

GENERALIZED ANXIETY DISORDER

General Considerations

Although GAD has been described as the "basic" anxiety disorder, it has received only minimal research attention. This phenomenon may have stemmed originally from the lack of well-defined diagnostic criteria for GAD and from its origins as a residual diagnostic category. With the advent of DSM-III (American Psychiatric Association, 1980), panic disorder was separated from the anxiety neuroses, and GAD was defined as a discrete diagnostic category. Identification of GAD as a separate disorder has encouraged systematic collection of data with regard to the phenomenology and treatment of this condition.

GAD is conceptualized as a disorder of excessive worry that manifests itself in cognitive, physiologic, and behavioral components. The cognitive and physiologic components provide the core diagnostic criteria for the disorder. As defined in DSM-IV, the cognitive component includes unrealistic or excessive worry about several life circumstances occurring more often than not for at least 6 months (American Psychiatric Association, 1994). For example, a patient may worry about money when his or her finances are sound; a mother may agonize over the health of a robust child; or a husband may worry about low-probability catastrophic events (e.g., "My wife's plane will crash"). Individuals with GAD often feel unable to control this anxious apprehension and it causes significant distress or impairment in social or occupational functioning.

In accordance with these apprehensive thoughts, patients with GAD suffer from physiologic symptoms of anxiety. These symptoms include muscle tension, increased irritability, difficulty concentrating, and increased vigilance (e.g., difficulty sleeping, feeling restless or keyed up). Although some of these symptoms overlap with those of panic disorder, they have a different profile: They tend to be associated with worry thoughts and are much less likely to occur spontaneously. In addition, GAD patients without panic disorder are less likely to be fearful of the physical symptoms themselves, despite finding them uncomfortable. Patients with GAD tend to report anxiety during protracted periods each day, and are also more likely to experience anxiety on more days of the week than panic sufferers. Barlow (1988) found that patients with GAD suffered from anxiety 56% of the time, which was considerably more than for patients with panic disorder (16%). In addition, the majority of individuals with GAD are symptomatic from the time that they acquire the disorder, with only 25% reporting episodes of remittance of 3 months or longer (Noyes, Clarkson, Crowe, Yates, & McChesney, 1987).

Although such behaviors are not part of the formal diagnostic criteria, individuals with GAD tend to engage in behaviors that reinforce and perpetuate their anxious worry (Craske et al., 1993). Behavioral manifestations of worry often include checking, avoidance, and vigilance. Specific examples include repeatedly calling the family physician about a child's runny nose; staying at home when it is raining lightly for fear of a car accident; and instructing children who are outside playing to come in the house every 15 minutes in order for the anxious parent to check on their safety. Functionally, such behaviors provide immediate relief of anxiety. In the long term, however, they do not allow the normal habituation of anxiety to occur. In this way, worry behaviors and worry thoughts reinforce each other and can evolve into a chronic pattern.

GAD is one of the more common anxiety disorders, with prevalence rates varying from 1.6% to 4.0% (Wittchen, Zhao, Kessler, & Eaton, 1994; Weissman & Merikangas, 1986). Estimates of prevalence for individuals who experience excessive worry that does not meet formal Axis I criteria may be as high as 10% (Shepherd, Cooper, & Brown, 1966). Findings regarding gender differences have been inconsistent, although the most recent National Comorbidity Survey found that the disorder was twice as common in women than in men (Wittchen et al., 1994). Age of onset is typically in the late teens or early 20s (Anderson, Noyes, & Crowe, 1984; Rickels & Schweizer, 1990; Rapee, 1991); however, patients tend to seek initial treatment later than patients with panic disorder (Nisita et al., 1990). This delay may be attributable to a paucity of adequate diagnostic and referral procedures at the level of primary care; poor diagnostic and referral procedures at this level; or a belief on the part of the patients that their anxiety problem is a fixed trait that is not treatable.

Relatively few patients with GAD are seen in anxiety disorder clinics (Dubovsky, 1990). The majority are seen by general practitioners, to whom they often initially report complaints of physical anxiety symptoms. Dubovsky (1990) estimated that only 25% of patients with GAD receive specific treatments tailored to the disorder. This percentage may be even smaller in more rural settings with fewer mental health professionals. Patients with GAD are more likely to have experienced some recent stressful life event (e.g., marriage, job promotion, loss of parent) at the time that they present for treatment (Blazer, Hughes, & George, 1987). The percentage of patients diagnosed with GAD who report having received previous psychologic or psychiatric treatment varies widely; it ranges from 29% (Power, Jerrom, Simpson, & Swanson, 1989) to 94% (Durham & Turvey, 1987).

Etiology and Nature of the Disorder

As in the other anxiety disorders, a combination of genetic, personality trait, and life event factors seems to be implicated in the genesis of GAD. However, identification of the true etiologic mechanisms of this disorder is hampered by the absence of prospective studies examining its onset. Barlow and his colleagues have described a number of characteristics in their GAD patients that they believe predispose patients to developing the disorder as well as other anxiety disorders (Barlow, 1988). First, these patients are characterized by higher levels of diffuse arousal and sensitivity than are nonanxious normals. Second, they possess a cognitive bias to view the world as a dangerous place, and this view is often precipitated by past life experiences. Other researchers have confirmed that a history of negative life experiences may predict later development of GAD (Nisita et al., 1990). Torgerson (1986) found that GAD patients were more likely than panic disorder subjects to have experienced the death of a parent prior to the age of 16. Third, they are more likely to have heightened beliefs about responsibility, control, and perfectionism. However, it is not clear whether these personality characteristics are causes or consequences of GAD, because of the retrospective bias of this finding.

Other researchers have also looked at genetic mediators of GAD. They report evidence that the frequency of GAD is higher in relatives of GAD probands than it is in relatives of control or panic disorder probands, and the frequency of panic disorder is higher in relatives of panic disorder probands than it is in relatives of control or GAD probands (Crowe, Noyes, Pauls, & Slymen, 1983; Noyes et al., 1987). However, relatives of panic disorder, agoraphobia, and control probands were found to be equally at risk for GAD (Noyes et al., 1986). It may be that individuals with GAD and panic disorder inherit a diathesis to develop anxiety disorders in general.

How GAD is maintained after its onset has been the subject of some theoretical debate. A number of authors have looked to cognitive factors as the core mechanism of action for this disorder. Borkovec and his colleagues have hypothesized that worry is primarily characterized by verbal thoughts rather than images and is mediated by avoidance of potentially distressing emotional imagery (Borkovec & Inz, 1990). They cite evidence that during relaxation nonanxious controls showed a predominance of imagery, whereas GAD subjects showed equal amounts of thought and imagery. After successful therapy, GAD subjects showed thought and image frequencies that resembled those of normals. Accordingly, worry is hypothesized to allow the GAD sufferer to escape distressing imagery; because of this lack of exposure, the anxiety associated with such imagery is never allowed to habituate. Other authors have questioned this conceptualization and point out that other kinds of thinking are at least as effective as worry thinking in suppressing emotional imagery (East & Watts, 1994).

A number of cognitive biases may trigger the worry process. These may include patients' tendency to overestimate the likelihood of the occurrence of negative events and the negative consequences of these events, and to underestimate their ability to cope with these events (Barlow, 1988). In addition, information-processing research suggests biases in the way that GAD patients attend to information in their environments. Butler and Mathews (1987) found that individuals with GAD were more likely to make threatening interpretations of ambiguous materials than were normal controls, and more likely to rate the probability that dangerous events would occur as high. Mathews and McLeod (1985, 1986) used modified Stroop and dichotic listening tasks to study these information-processing biases, and confirmed that patients with GAD allocate proportionally greater resources for detecting threatening material than normal controls and can detect this material more rapidly.

Individuals with GAD may also have a tendency to misinterpret common negative events that are part of the human condition (e.g., occasional accidents, the death of an elderly relative) as evidence that the world is a dangerous place and that their worrying is justified. This world view is hypothesized to contribute to heightened vigilance and to the belief that their worrying is adaptive and prophylactic. In more severe cases, GAD sufferers may develop a superstitious cognitive schema that they actually can prevent future negative events by worrying (Borkovec, 1985). The worry process may be further exacerbated by the sufferers' tendency to shift from one worry thought or belief to another very rapidly, without giving themselves the chance to test the veracity of these thoughts. As such, they become so preoccupied with worry that they cannot focus their attention on finding solutions to their problems, or are unable to try out potential solutions to their problems (Craske et al., 1993). In other cases, patients with GAD recognize that they are worrying excessively, and this leads them to resist worrying or to distract themselves from worrying. Paradoxically, this strategy may have the opposite effect, in the way that trying to resist thinking about something often makes it stronger.

In summary, although the exact mechanism or mechanisms mediating GAD are still open to debate, the components of GAD that appear to contribute to the cycle of worry include (1) emotional arousal and information-processing biases to threatening stimuli; (2) belief that worry prevents future negative events; (3) ineffective problem solving; and (4) attempts to resist and distract negative imagery without reaching alternative solutions.

Cognitive-Behavioral Treatment

There are three basic strategies for CBT of GAD: cognitive restructuring of anxiogenic thoughts, relaxation training, and worry exposure assignments. Each of these strategies attempts to target elements of the worry cycle that trigger and maintain the disorder. Cognitive restructuring of anxiogenic thoughts is at the foundation of treatment for GAD. The components of cognitive restructuring are as follows: education about the role of cognitions in increasing anxiety; the logical examination of thoughts; probability estimations; and the use of behavioral assignments and monitoring to challenge the veracity of anxiety-related beliefs. Approximately one-third of the patients presenting with GAD to our clinic do not understand the relationship between cognitive and emotional processes. They do not understand that their anxious mood states are often triggered by cognitions, and that this relationship is reciprocal (i.e., how they feel can also affect what they think). Education about these processes is a first step for such patients.

The core elements of cognitive restructuring focus on teaching patients a systematic method for examining the veracity of their thinking and estimating the probability of negative events. Patients are first instructed to use thought records to write down their anxiogenic thoughts, in order to examine these thoughts more objectively. Patients are next instructed in uncovering cognitive distortions in their thinking (e.g., catastrophizing, mind reading, all-or-nothing thinking) and examining the evidence supporting and refuting anxiogenic thoughts. Because individuals with GAD are likely to underestimate their ability to cope in situations, and to overestimate both the potential for negative events to occur and the negative consequences related to these events, probability estimation techniques are taught to allow patients to measure the actual likelihood of these events more accurately. Patients are also taught to generate alternative explanations and rational responses that challenge distorted anxiogenic thoughts (e.g., "My son did not call me because he lost track of time" instead of "My son did not call me because he must have had an accident"). Finally, patients are taught problem-solving techniques so that they can be proactive about generating and implementing solutions to their problems.

A second basic CBT strategy is relaxation training. Reduction in autonomic arousal has been targeted with a variety of relaxation strategies, ranging from progressive muscle relaxation to biofeedback-assisted procedures (Barlow et al., 1984; Cragan & Deffenbacher, 1984; Townsend, House, & Addario, 1975). Progressive muscle relaxation is probably the most commonly employed strategy; it consists of having patients learn to systematically relax progressively larger groups of muscles until they can ultimately relax all the muscles at once by using a single cued word like "relax" or "calm." This type of relaxation is often initially taught in treatment sessions and then assigned as a homework activity with a cassette tape. Merely giving patients a tape without demonstrating these techniques has been associated with less than optimal treatment outcome (Borkovec & Sides, 1979). Patients are encouraged to apply their relaxation skills when they are engaged in worry and experiencing physical symptoms of anxiety. Research has suggested that progressive muscle relaxation is helpful to patients with GAD, but it should be implemented early in treatment, because it often takes 4–8 weeks for its benefits to be realized by patients (Craske et al., 1993).

Many individuals with GAD attempt to mentally block negative or catastrophic images and to distract themselves from such images. As a result, the anxiety associated with these images is never allowed to habituate. Worry exposure is a CBT procedure developed specifically to counteract this problem; it involves having patients focus on frightening or catastrophic images (e.g., "I will lose my job and be living on the street") for discrete periods of time, usually between 25 and 50 minutes. Patients are instructed to try to make the images as vivid and anxiety-provoking as possible. Because of their habitual tendency toward distraction and avoidance, patients may at first have difficulty staying focused on the images; it is therefore often helpful initially to complete exposures in a treatment session, and then later to assign them as homework. It may be helpful for patients to make "subjective units of distress" ratings of their anxiety at 5-minute intervals during the exposures, in order to have a more tangible measure of whether their anxiety is decreasing. These ratings are made on a scale of 0 to 100, with 100 reflecting extreme anxiety and 0 reflecting no anxiety at all.

Some patients may find that self-directed treatments, such as bibliotherapy, are helpful adjuncts to individual therapy. Some materials are also designed to be used by motivated patients independently of professionals. The advantages to self-directed treatments include decreased cost, increased dissemination, and decreased stigmatization. Self-directed treatments vary from general inspirational works (e.g., Ross, 1994b) to specific forms of CBT with explicit homework exercises (e.g., Craske et al., 1993).

Treatment Outcome Findings

Outcome for Forms of CBT

How effective are standard CBT techniques in terms of empirical treatment outcome? In general, results have been promising. Treatment outcome studies have varied in their design, comparing CBT to no-treatment or waiting-list controls, to relaxation alone, to pill placebo conditions, and to standard pharmacotherapy treatments. A number of studies have found that CBT treatments are superior to no-treatment and waiting-list control conditions in the short term (less than 6 months) (Woodward & Jones, 1980; Barlow et al., 1984; Blowers, Cobb, & Mathews, 1987; Butler, Cullington, Hibbert, Klimes, & Gelder, 1987; Butler, Fennell, Robson, & Gelder, 1991; Lindsay, Gamsu, McLaughlin, Hood, & Espie, 1987; Barlow, Rapee, & Brown, 1992). Some studies have employed a technique called "anxiety management training" (Suinn & Richardson, 1971), in which anxiety symptoms are elicited in the therapy office and the patient employs applied relaxation techniques to cope with them. Two studies have found these techniques to be superior to a no-treatment control (Jannoun, Oppenheimer, & Gelder, 1982; Tarrier & Main, 1986).

Research comparing CBT techniques to medication interventions have found generally that CBT is equivalent or superior to medications. Lindsay et al. (1987) found greater initial gains in patients receiving the benzodiazepine lorazepam, but no differences between these subjects and subjects receiving CBT at 4 weeks. In addition, because of the lack of sustained improvement among lorazepam-treated subjects, over half of them refused to wait without treatment until the follow-up assessment. A study comparing the effectiveness of diazepam to CBT interventions found that CBT was superior at posttreatment, and that subjects receiving this treatment were less likely to have used subsequent psychotropic medications or pursued other psychologic treatments at a 12-month follow-up (Power et al., 1989). Power and his colleagues later replicated this finding and also found that diazepam was no more effective than placebo (Power, Simpson, Swanson, & Wallace, 1990).

Studies demonstrating the superiority of CBT techniques to nondirective treatment have been mixed. Blowers et al. (1987) found that an intervention combining cognitive therapy with relaxation training was not significantly better than nondirective counseling. Similarly, Borkovec and Mathews (1988) found no differences between three treatment groups that employed progressive muscle relaxation training plus either nondirective therapy, coping desensitization, or cognitive therapy. This finding challenged the results of an earlier study by these authors (Borkovec et al., 1987), in which they found that cognitive therapy with relaxation was superior to nondirective therapy with relaxation. In general, these findings suggest that at least part of the effectiveness of CBT treatment can be attributed to nonspecific treatment effects, such as the instillation of hope, the expectation of improvement, and participation in a treatment study.

There is somewhat more evidence for the benefit of CBT when a return to normal functioning is the outcome criterion. In a review of the treatment literature using this criterion, Durham and Allan (1993) found that roughly half (57%) of patients in CBT achieved a return to normal functioning, compared to only 22% in relaxation treatment alone. These authors also reported that psychologic treatments of GAD in general yielded a 50% reduction in the severity of somatic symptoms and a 25% decrease in measures of trait anxiety. In addition, these positive changes were likely to be maintained at 6-month follow-up.

There is a paucity of long-term treatment outcome results for GAD. Four studies using CBT approaches have demonstrated maintenance of treatment gains over a 3- to 6-month follow-up (Lindsay et al., 1987; Power et al., 1990; White & Keenan, 1990; Butler et al., 1991). Interventions that include cognitive restructuring appear to provide more stable long-term outcome and better retention in treatment than relaxation treatments alone (Barlow et al., 1992; Butler et al., 1991; Durham & Turvey, 1987). In a review of psychosocial treatments, Durham and Allan (1993) found an average reduction of 54% in Hamilton Rating Scale for Anxiety (HAM-A; Hamilton, 1959) scores at the end of treatment and 50% at longer-term follow-up assessments. The tendency to worry was itself reduced by 25%.

Pharmacologic and Combined Techniques

The class of drugs long associated with anxiety relief has been the benzodiazepines, and results on their efficacy for treating GAD have been generally favorable. A number of studies have found that benzodiazepines are superior to pill placebo controls (Ansseau, Doumont, Thiry, von Frenckell, & Collard, 1985; Cohn, Rickels, & Steege, 1989; Rickels et al., 1982). Roughly 35% of patients with GAD treated with benzodiazepines show marked improvement, and 40% demonstrate moderate improvement but are still symptomatic (Uhlenhuth, Dewitt, Balter, Johanson, & Mellinger, 1988). Table 7.2 presents data comparing psychosocial and benzodiazepine treatment for GAD. In a review of nine studies of benzodiazepine treatment of GAD, Barlow (1988) found an average reduction in HAM-A scores of 48%. By way of comparison, placebo treatment was associated with an average 30% reduction in these scores. Hence, like the results from CBT studies, these results suggest the difficulties of obtaining an outcome through active treatment that significantly exceeds nonspecific or placebo treatment effects.

Although benzodiazepines have demonstrated their effectiveness in providing symptomatic relief for GAD patients, a number of drawbacks have been cited; these include side effects (e.g., impaired cognitive performance, lethargy), drug tolerance, drug dependence, and relapse upon withdrawal (Shader & Greenblatt, 1993). Dubovsky (1990) has reported

TABLE 7.2. Mean Percentage Reduction in Hamilton Rating Scale for Anxiety (HAM-A) Scores in Studies of Patients with GAD

Treatment	Percentage reduction in scores	
	Mean	Range
Psychosocial treatment[a]	50%	20–76%
Benzodiazepine treatment[b]	48%	22–62%
Placebo treatment[b]	30%	18–48%

[a]Data from Durham and Allan (1993).
[b]Data from Barlow (1988).

a relapse to baseline symptoms in 63–81% of individuals who discontinue their benzodiazepine medications. Buspirone, an azapirone anxiolytic agent, has the advantages of fewer sedative side effects and less potential for rebound anxiety upon withdrawal. The limited research on treatment effectiveness with buspirone suggests that it may be as useful as benzodiazepines (Cohn et al., 1989; Feighner & Cohn, 1989; Sussman, 1987).

Only one study in the GAD treatment literature combined psychologic and pharmacologic treatment strategies. Power et al. (1990) found that CBT plus diazepam was no better than CBT alone, but that both of these treatments were superior to diazepam alone. Future outcome research should further investigate the efficacy of combined treatments.

Meta-Analytic Findings

Some researchers have used meta-analytic techniques to assess differences in treatment outcome more objectively. Chambless and Gillis (1993) reported a large within-group pre-to-post effect size (1.69) for CBT in seven GAD studies; these treatment gains were maintained at 6- and 12-month follow-ups. By comparison, the effect size for control groups that were used in some of these studies was considerably smaller (0.60). Hunt and Singh (1991) also used meta-analytic techniques to evaluate treatment outcome in 42 studies. Results based on short-term outcome indicated that on measures of anxiety, short- and long-acting benzodiazepines and buspirone were all roughly equivalent. All three drugs were superior to drug placebo conditions. CBT that included cognitive restructuring and relaxation training were equivalent to drug interventions and superior to waiting-list controls. In addition, CBT interventions had better long-term results than did drug therapies. Finally, relaxation techniques alone were not as effective as drug or CBT interventions and were not different from waiting-list controls. Hunt and Singh have endorsed CBT as the treatment of choice because of its short- and long-term benefits.

In a more recent meta-analysis Gould et al. (1995) compared CBT to pharmacotherapy in 27 studies that employed a control comparison condition. Subjects in these studies were required to meet DSM (III, III-R, or IV) criteria for GAD, or would have met these criteria had they been applied. Effect sizes for anxiety were calculated only from validated self-report questionnaires and clinician-rated measures. Pharmacotherapy studies (n = 15) yielded an acute (less than 6 months) mean effect size of 0.57 relative to placebo and subjects dropped out at the rate of 15.4%. Benzodiazepines were the drug most commonly employed for GAD treatment (n = 11 studies) and their mean effect size was 0.67; however, several authors reported difficulties with tapering these agents and relapse upon taper. Buspirone was employed in 6 studies and its mean effect size was 0.44. Three controlled studies assessed the efficacy of antidepressants and their mean effect size was 0.57.

Cognitive-behavioral interventions included studies that utilized cognitive restructuring, relaxation training, exposure, anxiety management training, or combinations of these. A total of 14 studies used CBT without pharmacotherapy, and their mean anxiety effect size was 0.71. The mean dropout rate for CBT interventions in these studies was 11.6%. In general, there were no significant differences between subtypes of CBT interventions, and all were superior to the null hypothesis (effect size = 0.0). Interventions that used both cognitive and behavioral techniques yielded strong effect sizes (0.90) as did Anxiety Management Training (0.74). Pure cogntive therapy (0.59) and relaxation training (0.63) appeared to be effective interventions. Studies employing behavioral techniques alone appeared to be least effective (0.48).

Comparisons of studies utilizing cognitive-behavioral treatments (0.71) to those using pharmacotherapy (0.57) were not statistically significant. In addition, mean attrition rates were not significantly different between the two forms of treatment. Only one study (Power et al., 1990) attempted to combine CBT and medication, and results from this study were promising.

In summary, the available data suggest that CBT and benzodiazepine treatment for GAD are both effective in the short term; however, problems with drug side effects and tolerance make benzodiazepines a less attractive first-line intervention. Treatment gains appear to be better maintained over long follow-up periods (1 to 2 years) with CBT. CBT is also associated with decreased concomitant medication use over follow-up periods (Barlow et al., 1992; Hunt & Singh, 1991; White, Keenan, & Brooks, 1991).

Treatment Resistance/Maximizing Treatment Effectiveness

A number of patients with GAD may respond only modestly to standard CBT strategies (Barlow et al., 1992). Unfortunately, research on GAD is less advanced than that on other anxiety disorders, and data indicating clinical predictors of treatment response are not abundant. Some authors have reported that comorbid depression in GAD patients is a predictor of suboptimal treatment outcome and is positively correlated with the chronicity and severity of anxiety symptoms (Breslau & Davis, 1985; Butler et al., 1987). This finding is particularly troubling, given the fact that one-third to one-half of GAD patients presenting for treatment suffer from comorbid depression or dysthymia (de Ruiter, Rijken, Garssen, van Schaik, & Kraaimaat, 1989; Butler et al., 1987). For GAD patients receiving CBT, comorbid depression can be particularly problematic because of the number and variety of homework tasks (e.g., practicing relaxation techniques, completing thought records) that are essential to this intervention. Several strategies that we have suggested in Chapter 5 of this volume for treating comorbid panic disorder and depression may also be useful for helping GAD patients with comorbid depression. These include (1) educating patients about the cognitive biases that accompany depression; (2) having patients monitor these biases and apply cognitive restructuring skills that target them; and (3) devoting extra time in sessions to encouraging compliance with homework assignments. CBT for GAD alone may help to reduce depressive symptomatology (Chambless & Gillis, 1993). In patients with more severe depression, a standard trial of CBT for depression or use of antidepressant medication may be necessary prior to GAD treatment.

Patients with GAD may also present with comorbid panic disorder, social phobia, and alcohol abuse (Barlow, 1988; Tyrer, 1984). Butler et al. (1987) reported that 29% of their GAD study sample suffered from panic disorder. Similarly, Jannoun et al. (1982) reported that one-third of their sample suffered from comorbid agoraphobia. For patients with comorbid panic disorder whose main focus of worry is having a panic attack, a standard course of CBT for panic prior to GAD treatment may be most helpful. For patients having panic disorder with mild agoraphobia, we find that an early introduction to breathing retraining skills, along with interoceptive exposure exercises, can enhance GAD treatment. In many instances, self-help books about panic disorder and agoraphobia (e.g, Clum, 1990; Barlow & Craske, 1993) may be employed concurrently with GAD treatment. For patients with comorbid social phobia, extra sessions may need to be devoted to cognitive restructuring training that teaches them how to challenge and change thoughts associated with fear of negative evaluation. In addition, *in vivo* homework assignments requiring systematic exposure to feared social situations may be beneficial.

When standard CBT techniques for GAD are not successful, patients may benefit from treatment strategies appropriate for more severely obsessional conditions. Some patients report that they try to push these obsessive worries away by using distraction techniques, but find that this strategy is only helpful in the short term. For patients with obsessive–compulsive disorder characterized by primary obsessional symptoms, benefits have been reported for exposure strategies utilizing a loop tape, which allows patients to listen to their obsessive thoughts repeatedly in an exposure format (Salkovskis, 1983; Thyer, 1985). With repeated exposure, the tendency to respond to these thoughts with anxiety or rituals is broken.

An additional aspect of treatment that may influence longer-term outcome is relapse prevention training. CBT interventions for anxiety generally include instruction in the nature of the disorder and encouragement of patients to learn new responses to anxiety with cognitive restructuring and exposure exercises. Patients are instructed to apply this new learning to situations in their own lives, and this learning is designed to continue to occur after the completion of formal treatment. In all of our anxiety treatment programs, we encourage patients to continue to practice somatic symptom management skills (e.g., relaxation) and cognitive restructuring and exposure techniques after the short-term CBT intervention. Patients are also instructed in a model of relapse prevention that stresses the reapplication of treatment procedures when high-risk situations are encountered and/or if symptoms return. Such procedures have been shown to be helpful at improving long-term outcome (Öst, 1987).

REFERENCES

Alstrom, J. E., Nordlund, C. L., Persson, G., Harding, M., & Ljungqvist, C. (1984). Effects of four treatment methods on social phobic patients not suitable for insight-oriented psychotherapy. *Acta Psychiatrica Scandinavica, 70,* 97–110.

American Psychiatric Association. (1980). *Diagnostic and statistical manual of mental disorders* (3rd ed.). Washington, DC: Author.

American Psychiatric Association. (1987). *Diagnostic and statistical manual of mental disorders* (3rd ed., rev.). Washington, DC: Author.

American Psychiatric Association. (1994). *Diagnostic and statistical manual of mental disorders* (4th ed.). Washington, DC: Author.

Anderson, D. J., Noyes, R., & Crowe, R. R. (1984). A comparison of panic disorder and generalized anxiety disorder. *American Journal of Psychiatry, 141,* 572–575.

Ansseau, M., Doumont, A., Thiry, D., von Frenckell, R., & Collard, J. (1985). Initial study of methylclonazepam in generalized anxiety disorder. *Psychopharmacology, 87,* 130–135.

Ball, S. G., Otto, M. W., Pollack, M. H., Uccello, R., & Rosenbaum, J. F. (1995). Differentiating social phobia and panic disorder: A test of core beliefs. *Cognitive Therapy and Research, 19,* 473–482.

Barlow, D. H. (1988). *Anxiety and its disorders: The nature and treatment of anxiety and panic.* New York: Guilford Press.

Barlow, D. H. (1994). Comorbidity in social phobia: Implications for cognitive-behavioral treatment. *Bulletin of the Menninger Clinic, 58,* A43–A52.

Barlow, D. H., Cohen, A. S., Wadell, M. T., Vermilyea, B. B., Kosko, J. S., Blanchard, E. B., & DiNardo, P. A. (1984). Panic and generalized anxiety disorder: Nature and treatment. *Behavior Therapy, 15,* 431–449.

Barlow, D. H., & Craske, M. G. (1993). *Mastery of your anxiety and panic II.* Albany, NY: Graywind.

Barlow, D. H., Rapee, R. M., & Brown, T. A. (1992). Behavioral treatment of generalized anxiety disorder. *Behavior Therapy, 23,* 551–570.

Biran, M., Augusto, F., & Wilson, G. T. (1981). *In vivo* exposure versus cognitive restructuring in the scriptophobia. *Behaviour Research and Therapy, 19,* 525–532.

Blazer, D., Hughes, D., & George, L. K. (1987). Stressful life events and the onset of generalized anxiety syndrome. *American Journal of Psychiatry, 144,* 1178–1183.

Blowers, C., Cobb, J., & Mathews, A. (1987). Generalised anxiety: A controlled treatment study. *Behaviour Research and Therapy, 25,* 493–502.

Borkovec, T. D. (1985). Worry: A potentially valuable concept. *Behaviour Research and Therapy, 23,* 481–482.

Borkovec, T. D., & Inz, J. (1990). The nature of worry in generalised anxiety disorder: A predominance of thought activity. *Behaviour Research and Therapy, 28,* 153–158.

Borkovec, T. D., & Mathews, A. (1988). Treatment of non-phobic anxiety disorders: A comparison of non-directive, cognitive, and coping desensitization therapy. *Journal of Consulting and Clinical Psychology, 56,* 877–884.

Borkovec, T. D., Mathews, A. M., Chambers, A., Ebrahimi, S., Lytle, R., & Nelson, R. (1987). The effects of relaxation training with cognitive therapy or nondirective therapy and the role of relaxation-induced anxiety in the treatment of generalized anxiety. *Journal of Consulting and Clinical Psychology, 55,* 883–888.

Borkovec, T. D., & Sides, J. R. (1979). Critical procedural variables related to the physiological effects of progressive relaxation: A review. *Behaviour Research and Therapy, 17,* 119–125.

Breslau, N., & Davis, G. C. (1985). DSM-III generalized anxiety disorder: An empirical investigation of more stringent criteria. *Psychiatry Research, 5,* 231–238.

Brooks, R. B., Baltazar, P. L., & Munjack, D. J. (1989). Co-occurrence of personality disorders with panic disorder, social phobia, and generalized anxiety disorder: A review of the literature. *Journal of Anxiety Disorders, 3,* 259–285.

Brown, T. A., & Barlow, D. N. (1992). Comorbidity among anxiety disorders: Implications for treatment and DSM-IV. *Journal of Consulting and Clinical Psychology, 60,* 835–844.

Bruch, M. A., Mattia, J. I., Heimberg, R. G., & Holt, C. S. (1993). Cognitive specificity in social anxiety and depression: Supporting evidence and qualifications due to affective confounding. *Cognitive Therapy and Research, 17,* 1–21.

Butler, G., Cullington, A., Hibbert, G., Klimes, I., & Gelder, M. (1987). Anxiety management for persistent generalised anxiety. *British Journal of Psychiatry, 151,* 535–542.

Butler, G., Cullington, A., Munby, M., Amies, P., & Gelder, M. (1984). Exposure and anxiety management in the treatment of social phobia. *Journal of Consulting and Clinical Psychology, 52*(4), 642–650.

Butler, G., Fennell, M., Robson, P., & Gelder, M. (1991). Comparison of behavior therapy and cognitive behavior therapy in the treatment of generalized anxiety disorder. *Journal of Consulting and Clinical Psychology, 59,* 167–175.

Butler, G., & Mathews, A. (1987). Anticipatory anxiety and risk perception. *Cognitive Therapy and Research, 11,* 551–565.

Chambless, D. L., & Gillis, M. M. (1993). Cognitive therapy of anxiety disorders. *Journal of Consulting and Clinical Psychology, 61*(2), 248–260.

Clum, G. A. (1990). *Coping with panic.* Pacific Grove, CA: Brooks/Cole.

Cohn, J. B., Rickels, K., & Steege, J. F. (1989). A pooled, double-blind comparison of the effects of buspirone, diazepam and placebo in women with chronic anxiety. *Current Medical Research Opinion, 11,* 304–320.

Cragan, M. K., & Deffenbacher, J. L. (1984). Anxiety management training and relaxation as self-control in the treatment of generalized anxiety in medical outpatients. *Journal of Consulting and Clinical Psychology, 31,* 123–131.

Craske, M. G., Barlow, D. H., & O'Leary, T. A. (1993). *Mastery of your anxiety and worry.* Albany, NY: Graywind.

Crowe, R. R., Noyes, R., Pauls, D. L., & Slymen, D. (1983). A family study of panic disorder. *Archives of General Psychiatry, 40,* 1065–1069.

Davidson, J. R. T., & Versiani, M. (1994). International advances in the treatment of social phobia. *Journal of Clinical Psychiatry, 55*(3), 123–369.

de Ruiter, C., Rijken, H., Garssen, B., van Schaik, A., & Kraaimaat, F. (1989). Cormorbidity among anxiety disorders. *Journal of Anxiety Disorders, 3,* 57–68.

Dubovsky, S. L. (1990). Generalized anxiety disorder: New concepts and psychopharmacologic therapies. *Journal of Clinical Psychiatry, 51*, 3–10.

Durham, R. C., & Allan, T. (1993). Psychological treatment of generalised anxiety disorder: A review of the clinical significance of results in outcome studies since 1980. *British Journal of Psychiatry, 163*, 19–26.

Durham, R. C., & Turvey, A. A. (1987). Cognitive therapy versus behaviour therapy in the treatment of chronic generalised anxiety. *Behaviour Research and Therapy, 25*, 229–234.

East, M. P., & Watts, F. N. (1994). Worry and the suppression of imagery. *Behaviour Research and Therapy, 32*, 851–856.

Emmelkamp, P. M. G., Mersch, P. P., Vissia, E., & van der Helm, M. (1985). Social phobia: A comparative evaluation of cognitive and behavioural interventions. *Behaviour Research and Therapy, 23*, 365–369.

Falloon, I. R. H., Lloyd, G. G., & Harpin, R. E. (1981). The treatment of social phobia: Real life rehearsal with nonprofessional therapists. *Journal of Nervous and Mental Disease, 169*, 180–184.

Fava, G. A., Grandi, S., & Canestrari, R. (1989). Treatment of social phobia by homework exposure. *Psychotherapy and Psychosomatics, 52*, 209–213.

Feighner, J. P., & Cohn, J. B. (1989). Analysis of individual symptoms in generalized anxiety: A pooled multi-study, double-blind evaluation of buspirone. *Neuropsychobiology, 21*, 124–130.

Gelernter, C. S., Uhde, T. W., Cimbolic, P., Arnkoff, D. B., Vittone, B. J., Tancer, M. E., & Bartko, J. J. (1991). Cognitive-behavioral and pharmacological treatments of social phobia: A controlled study. *Archives of General Psychiatry, 48*, 938–945.

Gould, R. A., Otto, M. W., Yap, L., & Pollack, M. H. (1994, November). *Cognitive-behavioral and pharmacological treatment of social phobia: A meta-analysis.* Paper presented at the 28th Annual Meeting of the Association for Advancement of Behavior Therapy, San Diego, CA.

Gould, R. A., Otto, M. W., Yap, L., & Pollack, M. H. (1995, November). *A meta-analysis of treatment outcome for generalized anxiety disorder.* Paper presented at the 29th Annual Meeting of the Association for Advancement of Behavior Therapy, Washington, DC.

Hamilton, M. (1959). The measurement of anxiety states by rating. *British Journal of Medical Psychology, 32*, 50–55.

Heimberg, R. G. (1989). Cognitive and behavioral treatments for social phobia: A critical analysis. *Clinical Psychology Review, 9*, 107–128.

Heimberg, R. G., & Barlow, D. H. (1988). Psychosocial treatments for social phobia. *Psychosomatics, 29*(1), 27–37.

Heimberg, R. G., & Barlow, D. H. (1991). New developments in cognitive-behavioral therapy for social phobia. *Journal of Clinical Psychiatry, 52*(11, Suppl.), 21–30.

Heimberg, R. G., Dodge, C. S., Hope, D. A., Kennedy, C. R., Zollo, L. J., & Becker, R. E. (1990a). Cognitive behavioral group treatment for social phobia: Comparison with a credible placebo control. *Cognitive Therapy and Research, 14*(1), 1–23.

Heimberg, R. G., Hope, D. A., Dodge, C. S., & Becker, R. E. (1990b). DSM-III-R subtypes of social phobia: Comparison of generalized social phobics and public speaking phobics. *Journal of Nervous and Mental Disease, 178*, 172–179.

Heimberg, R. G., Juster, H. R., Brown, E. J., Holle, C., Makris, G. S., Leung,

A. W., Schneier, F. R., Gitow, A., & Liebowitz, M. R. (1994, November). *Cognitive-behavioral versus pharmacological treatment of social phobia: Posttreatment and follow-up effects.* Poster presented at the 28th Annual Meeting of the Association for Advancement of Behavior Therapy, San Diego, CA.

Heimberg, R. G., Salzman, D. G., Holt, C. S., & Blendell, K. A. (1993). Cognitive-behavioral group treatment for social phobia: Effectiveness at five-year follow-up. *Cognitive Therapy and Research, 17*(4), 325–339.

Hunt, C., & Singh, M. (1991). Generalized anxiety disorder. *International Review of Psychiatry, 3,* 215–229.

Jannoun, L., Oppenheimer, C., & Gelder, M. (1982). A self-help treatment program for anxiety state patients. *Behavior Therapy, 13,* 103–111.

Kushner, M. G., Sher, K. J., & Beitman, B. D. (1990). The relation between alcohol problems and the anxiety disorders. *American Journal of Psychiatry, 147,* 685–695.

Liebowitz, M. R., Gorman, J. M., Fyer, A. J., & Klein, D. F. (1985). Social phobia: Review of a neglected anxiety disorder. *Archives of General Psychiatry, 42,* 729–736.

Lindsay, W. R., Gamsu, C. V., McLaughlin, E., Hood, E. M., & Espie, C. A. (1987). A controlled trial for treatments of generalised anxiety. *British Journal of Clinical Psychology, 26,* 3–15.

Lucock, M., & Salkovskis, P. M. (1988). Cognitive factors in social anxiety and its treatment. *Behaviour Research and Therapy, 26,* 297–302.

Mannuzza, S., Fyer, A. J., Liebowitz, M. R., & Klein, D. F. (1990). Delineating the boundaries of social phobia: Its relationship to panic disorder and agoraphobia. *Journal of Anxiety Disorders, 4,* 41–59.

Marzillier, J. S., Lambert, C., & Kellett, J. (1976). A controlled evaluation of systematic desensitization and social skills training for socially inadequate psychiatric patients. *Behaviour Research and Therapy, 14,* 225–238.

Mathews, A., & MacLeod, C. (1985). Selective processing of threat cues in anxiety states. *Behaviour Research and Therapy, 23,* 563–569.

Mathews, A., & MacLeod, C. (1986). Discrimination of threat cues without awareness in anxiety states. *Journal of Abnormal Psychology, 95,* 131–138.

Mattick, R. P., & Peters, L. (1988). Treatment of severe social phobia: Effects of guided exposure with and without cognitive restructuring. *Journal of Consulting and Clinical Psychology, 56,* 251–260.

Mattick, R. P., Peters, L., & Clarke, J. C. (1989). Exposure and cognitive restructuring for social phobia: A controlled study. *Behavior Therapy, 20,* 3–23.

McNeill, D. W., & Lewin, M. R. (1986). *Public speaking anxiety: A meaningful subtype of social phobia?* Paper presented at the 20th Annual Meeting of the Association for Advancement of Behavior Therapy, Chicago.

Mersch, P. P. A., Emmelkamp, P. M. G., & Lips, C. (1991). Social phobia: Individual response patterns and the long-term effects of behavioural and cognitive interventions: A follow-up study. *Behaviour Research and Therapy, 29,* 357–362.

Myers, J. K., Weissman, M. M., Tischler, G. L., Holzer, C. E., Leaf, P. J., Orvachel, H., Anthony, J. C., Boyd, J. H., Burke, J. D., Jr., & Kramer, M. (1984). Six-month prevalence of psychiatric disorders in three communities: 1980–1982. *Archives of General Psychiatry, 41,* 959–967.

Nisita, C., Petracca, A., Akiskal, H. S., Galli, L., Gepponi, I., & Cassano, G. B. (1990). Delimitation of generalized anxiety disorder: Clinical comparisons with panic and major depressive disorders. *Comprehensive Psychiatry, 31,* 409–415.

Noyes, R., Clarkson, C., Crowe, R. R., Yates, W. R., & McChesney, C. M. (1987). A family study of generalized anxiety disorder. *American Journal of Psychiatry, 144,* 1019–1024.

Noyes, R., Crowe, R. R., Harris, E. L., Hambra, B. J., McChesney, C. M., & Chuadry, D. R. (1986). Relationship between panic disorder and agoraphobia: A family study. *Archives of General Psychiatry, 43,* 227–232.

Öst, L.-G. (1987). Age of onset in different phobias. *Journal of Abnormal Psychology, 96,* 223–229.

Öst, L.-G., Jerremalm, A., & Johansson, J. (1981). Individual response patterns and the effects of different behavioural methods in the treatment of social phobia. *Behaviour Research and Therapy, 19,* 1–16.

Otto, M. W., Pollack, M. H., Sachs, G. S., O'Neil, C. A., & Rosenbaum, J. F. (1992). Alcohol dependence in panic disorder patients. *Journal of Psychiatric Research, 26,* 29–38.

Pollard, C. A., & Henderson, J. G. (1988). Four types of social phobia in a community sample. *Journal of Nervous and Mental Disease, 176,* 440–445.

Power, K. G., Jerrom, D. W. A., Simpson, R. J., & Mitchell, M. (1989). A controlled comparison of cognitive-behaviour therapy, diazepam, and placebo in the management of generalised anxiety. *Behavioural Psychotherapy, 17,* 1–14.

Power, K. G., Simpson, R. J., Swanson, V., & Wallace, L. A. (1990). A controlled study of cognitive behavior therapy, diazepam, and placebo, alone and in combination for the treatment of generalized anxiety. *Journal of Anxiety Disorders, 4,* 267–292.

Rapee, R. M. (1991). Generalized anxiety disorder: A review of clinical features and theoretical concepts. *Clinical Psychology Review. 11,* 419–440.

Rickels, K., & Schweizer, E. (1990). The clinical course and long-term management of generalized anxiety disorder. *Journal of Clinical Psychopharmacology, 10*(Suppl.), 101S–110S.

Rickels, K., Weisman, K., Norstad, N., Singer, M., Stoltz, D., Brown, A., & Danton, J. (1982). Buspirone and diazepam in anxiety: A controlled study. *Journal of Clinical Psychiatry, 43,* 81–86.

Rosenbaum, J. F., & Pollock, R. A. (1994). The psychopharmacology of social phobia and comorbid disorders. *Bulletin of the Menninger Clinic, 58,* 67–73.

Ross, J. (1994a). Social phobia: The consumer's perspective. *Journal of Clinical Psychiatry, 54*(12, Suppl.), 5–9.

Ross, J. (1994b). *Triumph over fear.* New York: Bantam Books.

Salkovskis, P. M. (1983). Treatment of an obsessional patient using habituation to an audiotaped rumination. *British Journal of Psychiatry, 22*(4), 311–313.

Schneier, F. R., Johnson, J., Hornig, C. D., Liebowitz, M. R., & Weissman, M. M. (1992). Social phobia: Comorbidity and morbidity in an epidemiological sample. *Archives of General Psychiatry, 49,* 282–288.

Shader, R. I., & Greenblatt, D. J. (1993). Use of benzodiazepines in anxiety disorders. *New England Journal of Medicine, 328,* 1398–1405.

Shepherd, M., Cooper, B., & Brown, A. C. (1966). *Psychiatric illness in general practice.* London: Oxford University Press.

Spitzer, R., & Williams, J. B. W. (1985). Proposed revisions in the DSM-III classification of anxiety disorders based on research and clinical experience. In

A. H. Tuma & J. D. Maser (Eds.), *Anxiety and the anxiety disorders* (pp. 759–773). Hillsdale, NJ: Erlbaum.

Stein, M. B., Tancer, M. E., Gelertner, C. S., Vittone, B. J., & Uhde, T. W. (1990). Major depression in patients with social phobia. *American Journal of Psychiatry, 147,* 637–639.

Stravynski, A., Marks, I., & Yule, W. (1982). Social skills problems in neurotic outpatients. *Archives of General Psychiatry, 39,* 1378–1384.

Suinn, R. M., & Richardson, F. (1971). Anxiety management training: A non-specific behavior therapy program for anxiety control. *Behavior Therapy, 2,* 498–510.

Sussman, N. (1987). Treatment of anxiety with buspirone. *Psychiatric Annals, 17,* 114–120.

Tarrier, N., & Main, C. J. (1986). Applied relaxation for generalised anxiety and panic attacks: The efficacy of a learnt coping strategy on subjective reports. *British Journal of Psychiatry, 149,* 330–336.

Thyer, B. A. (1985). Audio-taped exposure therapy in a case of obsessional neurosis. *Journal of Behavior Therapy and Experimental Psychiatry, 16,* 271–273.

Torgerson, S. (1986). Childhood and family characteristics in panic and generalized anxiety disorders. *American Journal of Psychiatry, 143,* 630–632.

Townsend, R. E., House, J. F., & Addario, D. (1975). A comparison of biofeedback mediated relaxation and group therapy in the treatment of chronic anxiety. *American Journal of Psychiatry, 132,* 598–601.

Turner, S. M., Beidel, D. C., Borden, J. W., Stanley, M. A., & Jacob, R. G. (1991). Social phobia: Axis I and II correlates. *Journal of Abnormal Psychology, 100,* 102–106.

Turner, S. M., Beidel, D. C., Dancu, C. V., & Keys, D. J. (1986). Psychopathology of social phobia and comparison to avoidant personality disorder. *Journal of Abnormal Psychology, 95,* 389–394.

Turner, S. M., Beidel, D. C., & Jacob, R. G. (1994). Social phobia: A comparison of behavior therapy and atenolol. *Journal of Consulting and Clinical Psychology, 62*(4), 350–358.

Turner, S. M., Beidel, D. C., & Townsley, R. M. (1992). Social phobia: A comparison of specific and generalized subtypes and avoidant personality disorder. *Journal of Abnormal Psychology, 101,* 326–331.

Tyrer, P. (1984). Classification of anxiety. *British Journal of Psychiatry, 144,* 78–93.

Uhlenhuth, E. H., Dewitt, H., Balter, M. B., Johanson, C. E., & Mellinger, G. D. (1988). Risks and benefits of long-term benzodiazepine use. *Journal of Clinical Psychopharmacology, 8,* 161–167.

Van Ameringen, M., Mancini, C., Styan, G., & Donison, D. (1991). Relationship of social phobia with other psychiatric illnesses. *Journal of Affective Disorders, 21,* 93–99.

Van Vliet, I. M., Den Boer, J. A., & Westenberg, H. G. M. (1992). Psychopharmacological treatment of social phobia: A double blind placebo controlled study with fluvoxamine. *Psychopharmacology, 115,* 128–134.

Weissman, M. M., & Meikangas, K. R. (1986). The epidemiology of anxiety and panic disorder. *Journal of Clinical Psychiatry, 46*(Suppl.), 11–17.

White, J., & Keenan, M. (1990). Stress control: A pilot study of large group therapy for generalized anxiety disorder. *Behavioural Psychotherapy, 18,* 143–146.

White, J., Keenan, M., & Brooks, N. (1991). *Stress control: A controlled investigation of large group therapy for generalized anxiety disorder.* Manuscript in preparation.

Wittchen, H.-U., Zhao, S., Kessler, R. C., & Eaton, W. W. (1994). DSM-III-R generalized anxiety disorder in the National Comorbidity Survey. *Archives of General Psychiatry, 51,* 355–364.

Wlazlo, Z., Schroeder-Hartwig, K., Hand, I., Kaiser, G., & Munchau, N. (1990). Exposure *in vivo* versus social skills training for social phobia: long-term outcome and differential effects. *Behaviour Research and Therapy, 28,* 181–193.

Woodward, R., & Jones, R. B. (1980). Cognitive restructuring treatment: A controlled trial with anxious patients. *Behaviour Research and Therapy, 18,* 401–407.

8

Treatment-Resistant Obsessive–Compulsive Disorder: Practical Strategies for Management

SCOTT L. RAUCH
LEE BAER
MICHAEL A. JENIKE

Obsessive–compulsive disorder (OCD) is a common illness, with lifetime prevalence estimates of ∼ 1–3% worldwide (Rasmussen & Eisen, 1992). Fortunately, a number of available therapies provide substantial symptomatic relief for the majority of OCD sufferers. Currently accepted first-line treatments for OCD include behavioral therapy (consisting of exposure and response prevention) and pharmacologic therapy with clomipramine, a tricyclic antidepressant that inhibits serotonin reuptake, or with one of the selective serotonin reuptake inhibitors (SSRIs). Nonetheless, up to 40% of patients with OCD fail to derive satisfactory response from initial therapies (Goodman, McDougle, & Price, 1992). Such patients are designated as "treatment-resistant." This chapter addresses the practical considerations involved in managing treatment-resistant OCD.

ASSESSMENT OF TREATMENT RESISTANCE

Many of the points pertaining to the assessment of apparent treatment resistance for OCD are generalizable to other disorders as well. There are three critical steps in assessing treatment-resistant OCD:

1. *Consider whether the diagnosis of OCD might be incorrect.* Often patients who appear to be treatment-resistant may have been mistakenly diagnosed with OCD when in fact they suffer from a different disorder that resembles OCD (see Table 8.1). Thus, the antiobsessional treatments invoked may lack efficacy simply because the patients' symptoms are not manifestations of OCD. If a different diagnosis is more appropriate, then first-line treatments for that diagnosis should be considered.

2. *Consider whether comorbid psychiatric diagnoses are present.* OCD symptoms are often unresponsive to treatment when a concurrent psychiatric condition remains untreated. Affective disorders, other anxiety disorders, organic mental disorders, substance abuse disorders, and personality disorders are prime offenders in this regard. Comorbid conditions, when present, must be treated *as well as* the OCD; the first-line therapies for OCD should not be abandoned.

3. *Review the adequacy of the first-line antiobsessional trials already conducted.* It is important to assess trials of both medication and behavior therapy for "dose," duration, and response.

a. *Pharmacotherapy.* We recommend that first-line pharmacotherapy include up to three separate trials with different agents, and that at least one of them be clomipramine (Pigott et al., 1990; Pigott, L'Heureux, & Murphy, 1993), barring a major contraindication. Meta-analyses provide some suggestion that efficacy among the first-line medications is actually inversely related to their serotonergic selectivity (i.e., efficacy of clomipramine > fluoxetine > fluvoxamine > sertraline > paroxetine) (Jenike et al., 1990). These results may be an artifact of the times at which these

TABLE 8.1. Differential Diagnosis of OCD

Major depression (with ruminations)

Bipolar disorder

Other anxiety disorders
  Posttraumatic stress disorder
  Generalized anxiety disorder
  Panic disorder
  Specific phobia
  Social phobia

Psychotic disorders (with intrusive thoughts, delusions)

Organic mental disorders (with intrusive thoughts, stereotypies)

Habit disorders

Impulse control disorders

Eating disorders

Borderline personality disorder (with ritualized self-injury)

Obsessive–compulsive *personality* disorder

Note. Disorders that may be related to OCD and should also be considered include Tourette's disorder, trichotillomania, and body dysmorphic disorder.

different agents have become available. The higher-selectivity agents were developed later; consequently, studies of their efficacy may have involved ever higher proportions of relatively treatment-resistant subjects. For each agent, an adequate trial entails titration to optimal or maximal tolerated doses, and a total trial duration of greater than 10 weeks.

   b. *Behavior therapy.* Behavior therapy probably has the best risk–benefit profile of any treatment available for OCD. Therefore, it must always be considered as a first-line option. An adequate trial of exposure and response prevention requires that the patient participate in earnest, be supervised by a therapist who is competent in behavioral techniques, and complete a minimum of 20 hours of actual exposure and response prevention treatment.

   c. *Assessment of treatment response.* One must distinguish trials aborted because of adverse effects from truly adequate but ineffective trials. In this regard, it can be difficult to monitor patient improvement effectively by using qualitative descriptions of global improvements. Therefore, we recommend quantification of OCD symptom severity with the Yale–Brown Obsessive Compulsive Scale (Y-BOCS; Goodman et al., 1989a, 1989b). The Y-BOCS contains 10 items, 5 pertaining to severity of obsessions and 5 to severity of compulsions, each ranked on a scale from 0 to 4. This instrument yields a score from 0 (absent symptoms) to 40 (most severe); for instance, scores of >15 are typically used as entry criteria for most clinical research studies of OCD. For our purposes, treatment resistance is operationalized as failure to achieve a 25% reduction from baseline in Y-BOCS score and a residual Y-BOCS score of >12. This reflects the reality that even "treatment responders" are usually left with some residual symptoms. Patients should be advised at the outset that complete cure of OCD is rare.

   Once a patient's diagnosis and treatment history have been reviewed in the face of treatment resistance, alternative treatment strategies can be considered.

ALTERNATIVE TREATMENT OPTIONS

For patients with OCD who are treatment-resistant, there remain three general modes of intervention: pharmacologic, behavioral, and neurosurgical.

Pharmacologic Interventions

For patients who have failed to respond to adequate trials of the first-line medications, alternative pharmacologic options include augmentation strategies, alternative monotherapies, and alternative routes of administration (see Table 8.2).

TABLE 8.2. Recommended Pharmacologic Strategies

Agent	Dose	Duration	Relative indications [contraindications] for non-first-line strategies
First-line pharmacotherapies: Serotonin reuptake inhibitors			
Clomipramine	Up to 250 mg/day	>10 weeks	—
SSRIs			
Fluoxetine	Up to 80 mg/day	>10 weeks	—
Fluvoxamine	Up to 250 mg/day	>10 weeks	—
Sertraline	Up to 200 mg/day	>10 weeks	—
Paroxetine	Up to 80 mg/day	>10 weeks	—
Augmentation strategies			
Clonazepam	Up to 5 mg/day	>4 weeks	Anxiety, insomnia, tics, akathisia, bipolar disorder
Neuroleptics	Up to 3 mg/day (pimozide)	>4 weeks	Body dysmorphic disorder, tics, trichotillomania, [cardiac dysrhythmia, akathisia]
Buspirone	Up to 30 mg/day	>8 weeks	Medical illness
Alternative monotherapies			
Clonazepam	Up to 5 mg/day	>4 weeks	Anxiety, tics, insomnia, bipolar disorder, clomipramine/SSRI intolerance
MAOIs	Up to 90 mg/day (phenelzine)	>10 weeks	Panic disorder, depression, clomipramine/SSRI intolerance
Buspirone	Up to 60 mg/day	>6 weeks	Medical illness, clomipramine/SSRI intolerance

Augmentation Strategies

Augmentation or combination therapy relies on the notion that the addition of an augmenting agent to an ongoing pharmacotherapy will enhance treatment response; that is, it will have efficacy superior to that of either agent administered alone. Research into the efficacy of augmentation for OCD has focused on the use of clomipramine or one of the SSRIs as the foundation agent, with a variety of other medications used as adjuncts. Unfortunately, the data available on augmentation are largely the products of case studies or open trials. Moreover, in several instances promising results from uncontrolled trials have not been supported by subsequent, more definitive controlled studies. Consequently, recommendations about optimal augmentation strategies must be tentative.

Given that the treatment-resistant population is probably quite heterogeneous, even the best interventions may not be deemed "effective" if efficacy is assessed on the basis of mean change across an entire cohort. Therefore, the ratio of responders to nonresponders may be the most appropriate measure of efficacy for a given strategy, rather than differences in mean Y-BOCS change scores across an entire study population.

With these caveats in mind, we recommend the following augmentation strategies, taking into account relevant relative indications or contraindications for each. In treatment-resistant OCD, second-line pharmacotherapy entails augmentation of clomipramine or an SSRI with clonazepam, a neuroleptic, or buspirone.

Clonazepam is a benzodiazepine widely used for its anxiolytic or anticonvulsant properties. Recent evidence suggests that clonazepam has preferential effects on the serotonergic system (Hewlett, 1993; Hwang & Van Woert, 1979; Jenner, Chadwick, Reynolds, & Marsden, 1975; Pratt, Jenner, Reynolds, & Marsden, 1979; Wagner, Reches, Yablonskaya, & Fahn, 1986), which may explain its apparent efficacy as an antiobsessional agent (Hewlett, 1993; Bacher, 1990; Bodkin & White, 1989; Hewlett, Vinogradov, & Agras, 1990, 1992; Pigott, L'Heureux, Rubinstein, Hill, & Murphy, 1992c), beyond its fundamental anxiolytic action. Clonazepam can be added to any of the first-line agents, beginning at doses of 0.25–0.5 mg once or twice per day. The dosage can be increased every few days until an optimal effect is achieved. We recommend that dosages not exceed 5 mg/day, except in rare circumstances (e.g., for patients who have a high tolerance for benzodiazepines). Clonazepam may be a particularly good choice for patients who have a high degree of anxiety (including comorbid anxiety disorders), motor agitation, comorbid bipolar illness, or insomnia. Because clonazepam is sedating, it may be poorly tolerated by patients who are already anergic, hypersomnic, or depressed. Furthermore, clonazepam's sedating side effects may be particularly poorly tolerated when it is combined with clomipramine. Conversely, addition of clonazepam may help patients to tolerate higher doses of fluoxetine if previous trials were limited because of akathisia, anxiety, or insomnia. An adequate trial of clonazepam augmentation should be maintained for a minimum of 4 weeks before its efficacy can be fairly assessed.

Neuroleptics have been used with some success as monotherapies for several disorders that are possibly related to OCD (i.e., Tourette's disorder and body dysmorphic disorder) (Troung, Bressman, Shali, & Fahn, 1988; Shapiro et al., 1989; Phillips, 1991; Opler & Feinberg, 1991). They may be effective as agents added to clomipramine or an SSRI in the treatment of OCD (McDougle et al., 1990). Pimozide, for instance, can be added to a first-line agent at an initial dose of 1 mg/day (or haloperidol 0.5 mg/day); this can be increased every couple of weeks to a maximum recommended dose not to exceed 3 mg/day. The usual risks associated with neuroleptics should be considered and reviewed as part of formal informed consent. The risk of tardive dyskinesia should be explicitly discussed. Anticholinergic effects may be especially prominent if a neuroleptic is added to clomipramine, whereas the likelihood of akathisia may be increased when a neuroleptic is added to fluoxetine. Also, quinidine-like cardiac effects mandate that an electrocardiogram be performed in patients over 40 years old, or at any age when a cardiac history is present or when pimozide is combined with a tricyclic antidepressant, such as clomipramine. Neuroleptics may be particularly useful in cases where OCD is accompanied by tics or frank Tourette's disorder (McDougle et al., 1990), body dysmorphic disorder, or trichotillomania (Stein & Hollander, 1992). Although it may be intuitively appealing to believe that addition of a neuroleptic to clomipramine of an SSRI is indicated for patients with a comorbid Cluster A personality disorder (i.e., schizotypal, schizoid, or paranoid personality disorder), there is little empirical evidence to support this maneuver. Certainly in cases of comorbid psychosis, or OCD that progresses to delusional intensity, a trial of an adjunctive neuroleptic is prudent. An adequate trial of neuroleptic augmentation should proceed for at least 4 weeks.

Buspirone is a serotonin (5-HT$_{1A}$) partial agonist with relatively weak anxiolytic effects. Although there is some conflicting evidence with regard to its efficacy as an antiobsessional augmenting agent, we believe that it is used optimally in combination with fluoxetine (Markovitz, Stagno, & Calabrese, 1990; Alessi & Bos, 1991; Jenike, Baer, & Buttolph, 1991b). Buspirone augmentation of other SSRIs has not been systematically studied, whereas buspirone augmentation of clomipramine has been associated with adverse effects, including exacerbation of depressive symptoms in up to 25% of patients in one study (Pigott et al., 1992a). Buspirone can be added to fluoxetine at a starting dose of 5 mg three times per day, which can be increased as tolerated to a therapeutic dose of 30–60 mg/day. It should be noted that therapeutic benefits may not become apparent before 8 weeks (Jenike et al., 1991b; Grady et al., 1993).

A number of other candidate antiobsessional augmenting strategies are worthy of mention. Because the data supporting their efficacy are sparse or inconsistent, these interventions are best reserved for the most refractory cases.

Fenfluramine is a psychostimulant, marketed as an anorectic agent, that acts via both serotonergic release and reuptake blockade. Fenfluramine may be added to clomipramine or an SSRI, starting at a dose of 5 mg/day, which can be increased to a therapeutic dose of 20–60 mg/day (Hollander & Leibowitz, 1988; Judd, Chua, Lynch, & Norman, 1991; Hollander et al., 1990). There is no clear profile of patients who selectively respond to this strategy. Fenfluramine should be avoided in cases where use of a psychostimulant is relatively contraindicated (e.g., history of seizures or bipolar disorder). Side effects may include tinnitus, impotence, and sexual impulsivity. An adequate trial of fenfluramine augmentation should proceed for at least 8 weeks.

The addition of other tricyclic antidepressants (Hollander et al., 1991) or other SSRIs (Simeon, Thatte, & Wiggins, 1990) to an ongoing trial of clomipramine or an SSRI has yielded beneficial effects in some case series. This may be an especially effective approach in cases where comorbid depression is present. Moreover, it can be an efficient way to make the transition between trials of different first-line agents. In this context, care should be exercised with regard to dosing, since the addition of SSRIs can drastically increase the blood levels of a concurrently administered tricyclic antidepressant (Aranow et al., 1989). The addition of the atypical antidepressant trazodone (Jenike, 1990; Pigott et al., 1992b) to SSRIs seems to be poorly tolerated because of excessive sedation. Nonetheless, this strategy may be helpful for patients complaining of insomnia on an SSRI alone.

Lithium is perhaps the most thoroughly studied antiobsessional augmenting agent (Stern & Jenike, 1983; Rasmussen, 1984; Eisenberg & Asnis, 1985; Feder, 1988; Golden, Morris, & Sack, 1988; Howland, 1991; McDougle, Price, Goodman, Charney, & Heninger, 1991; Pigott et al., 1991). Although the best available data speak against its reliable efficacy (McDougle et al., 1991; Pigott et al., 1991), its use in doses of 300–600 mg/day may be effective for occasional patients.

Despite an anecdotal report of antiobsessional effects from addition of L-tryptophan to clomipramine (Rasmussen, 1984), this combination has not been adequately studied. Finally, there are mixed anecdotal case reports, both for (Knesevich, 1982; Lipsedge & Prothero, 1987) and against (Hollander, Fay, & Liebowitz, 1988), the use of clonidine as a clomipramine or SSRI adjunct in doses of 0.1–0.6 mg/day.

Alternative Monotherapies

Although clomipramine and the SSRIs are the most tried and true antiobsessional agents, other medications have shown promise as monotherapies for OCD as well. Monoamine oxidase inhibitors (MAOIs) (Vallejo, Olivares, Marcos, Bulbena, & Menchon, 1992), clonazepam (Hewlett, 1993; Hewlett et al., 1992), and buspirone (Pato et al., 1991) have all been the subject of double-blind studies suggesting legitimate antiobsessional efficacy as monotherapies; dextroamphetamine has been shown to reduce obsessional symptoms acutely (Joffe, Swinson, & Levitt, 1991; Insel, Hamilton, Guttmacher, & Murphy, 1983), but its efficacy when chronically administered has never been tested.

We recommend that clonazepam or buspirone be considered as monotherapy for patients who derive partial response to either agent as an augmentor with clomipramine or an SSRI, or in cases where the first-line agents are poorly tolerated. Buspirone and clonazepam both tend to be well tolerated, and provide beneficial anxiolytic effects as well as more specific antiobsessional action.

Clonazepam can be started at doses of 0.5 mg at bedtime and increased every few days, titrated against sedation to a maximum of 5 mg/day. It is usually taken twice a day, with the majority of the dose administered at bedtime. If the patient is already on clomipramine or an SSRI plus clonazepam, the first-line agent can be tapered or discontinued, and the clonazepam increased. Although the time course of clonazepam's antiobsessional effect has not been formally studied, there is the suggestion that it may be on the order of days rather than weeks, as with clomipramine and the SSRIs. In patients without a prior history of alcohol or substance abuse, we have not observed the development of abuse with clonazepam. Nonetheless, patients maintained on this agent for more than a couple of weeks will develop physiologic dependence; despite its relatively long half-life, clonazepam should not be discontinued abruptly, because rebound anxiety or more severe withdrawal effects may ensue.

Buspirone did not yield significant antiobsessional benefits as a monotherapy in one open trial (Jenike & Baer, 1988). Nonetheless, a 6-week double-blind study comparing buspirone with clomipramine suggested that the two drugs were comparably effective at reducing OCD symptoms (Pato et al., 1991). The short duration of treatment in that study probably led to suboptimal clomipramine response. Although claims of efficacy comparable to that of clomipramine are unjustified, based on the parameters of that study, the potential efficacy of buspirone monotherapy deserves further study. Buspirone may be particularly worthwhile in patients who suffer from severe comorbid medical illness, since its side effect profile is relatively benign. Buspirone can be started at 5 mg three times per day and advanced by 5 mg every few days to a maximum total dose of 60 mg/day (20 mg three times per day). For the partial responder to combined first-line and buspirone therapy, the first-line agent can be tapered and the buspirone titrated up for a trial of maximal buspirone monotherapy.

MAOIs have been reported to relieve OCD symptoms in a few cases characterized by comorbid panic disorder (Jenike, Surman, Cassem, Zusky, & Anderson, 1983). An early double-blind study demonstrated the inefficacy of clorgyline and its inferiority to clomipramine (Insel et al., 1983). A more recent controlled trial, however, revealed that phenelzine provided significant antiobsessional effects, comparable to those of clomipramine, over a 12-week study period (Vallejo et al., 1992). There is the suggestion that MAOIs may be most effective in cases of OCD characterized by comorbid anxiety or depressive disorders. In addition to dietary restrictions, the risk of drug interactions is of paramount concern when the use of MAOIs in OCD is being considered. Hypertensive crisis or serotonergic syndrome can be induced by combining clomipramine, SSRIs, or buspirone with an MAOI, or by insufficient washout between successive trials (Sternbach, 1991; Insel, Roy, Cohen, & Murphy, 1982). Trials of a first-line agent or buspirone should not be initiated for at least 2 weeks following discontinuation of an MAOI, and adverse reactions have been reported up to 4 weeks following discontinuation of an MAOI (i.e., clorgyline), with irreversible effects on monoamine oxidase (Insel et al., 1983). Conversely, MAOIs should not be initiated for at least 2 weeks following the discontinuation of buspirone or the shorter-half-life first-line agents (e.g., sertraline, clomipramine), and not for at least 5 weeks in the case of fluoxetine. Consequently, we recommend that MAOIs not be tried until fair trials of clomipramine and SSRIs, as well as several adjuncts, have failed. It is most efficient to try an MAOI after a trial of clonazepam monotherapy, to minimize any need for extended washout. Administration of MAOIs for OCD can follow the same dosage guidelines as for major depression. Phenelzine, for instance, can be started at 15 mg once or twice per day, and increased by 15 mg every 3–4 days to a therapeutic dose of 60–90 mg/day. In general, phenelzine tends to be more sedating; tranylcypromine has greater potential for energizing effects with attendant insomnia. Both can cause orthostatic hypotension and weight gain.

Alternative Route of Administration

Intravenous clomipramine has been used to good effect in several cases of treatment-resistant OCD (Warneke, 1989; Fallon et al., 1992). One regimen involving 14 clomipramine infusions of up to 350 mg each has shown promising preliminary results (Fallon et al., 1992). Currently, this strategy must be considered experimental and is only available at a few institutions in the context of research paradigms. When all other pharmacologic and behavioral strategies have failed, intravenous clomipramine may be attempted prior to consideration of neurosurgical intervention.

Behavioral Interventions

We strongly recommend behavior therapy as a first-line treatment for OCD, and consider a combination of clomipramine or an SSRI with behavior therapy the treatment of choice for the vast majority of patients. Unfortunately, the power of behavior therapy as a treatment modality for OCD often goes unappreciated. Misconceptions about exposure and response prevention may be shared and perpetuated by clinicians, as well as patients and their families. As an example, patients often view this as "force therapy" over which they will have no control, rather than as a graduated series of practice exercises that the patients will, for the most part, complete outside of therapy sessions with the assistance of family members. Moreover, the scarcity of therapists trained in behavioral techniques can compound the situation by complicating access.

Education of clinicians, patients, and patients' families is an important first step toward a trial of behavior therapy. Self-help books (Marks, 1987; Baer, 1991) and patient-run support organizations can be valuable sources of information. When behavior therapy is considered and a patient is reluctant, the clinician should attempt to correct any misconceptions or catastrophic thoughts that may underlie the patient's fears of attempting the therapy (Salkovskis, 1993). Since by far the most common reason for failure of behavior therapy in OCD is noncompliance (Marks, 1981), treatment should only be initiated with patients who are motivated to carry out the therapist's treatment recommendations. In addition, patients should recognize that behavior therapy will not magically eliminate all their OCD symptoms overnight; rather, improvement is a gradual process requiring hard work on sequential goals, although progress should be apparent in the first few hours of practice. Treatment should be delayed for patients who are not ready or fully committed to the activities that will be required of them, since success is unlikely, and a failure experience will reduce the chances of a later attempt.

An adequate trial of behavior therapy for OCD is particularly critical when first-line pharmacotherapies alone have failed. But how is the non-behavioral clinician to determine what constitutes an "adequate trial"? Too often patients have presented or been referred to our clinic as "treatment-resistant" to behavior therapy for OCD, when in fact what they had received was relaxation training, systematic desensitization, or cognitive therapy. These treatments alone are ineffective for OCD. Research indicates that at least 20 hours of actual exposure and response prevention constitute the "active ingredient" in virtually all successful behavioral treatment of OCD (Baer & Minichiello, 1990).

Definitions and Examples of Exposure and Response Prevention

"Exposure" involves a patient's confronting a situation that triggers obsessive thoughts and/or compulsive rituals. For example, a patient who fears contamination from germs is exposed to touching water faucets or door-knobs if he or she typically avoids these objects. However, exposure alone is not effective unless it is used in conjunction with "response prevention" (also known as "ritual prevention"; Foa, Steketee, & Milby, 1980). In the preceding example, response prevention requires this patient to resist urges to wash his or her hands for at least 1 hour after exposure, and also to resist performing any other rituals that might reduce the discomfort resulting from exposure. (We tell patients, "The goal is to teach your body that nothing terrible will happen even if you don't do a ritual, and it will learn to relax on its own.") Similarly, a patient who has problems with hoarding is asked to throw objects into a trash can (exposure) without performing rituals such as staring at, checking, or shredding these objects while they are being thrown away or afterward (response prevention). Patients are told that when they repeatedly expose themselves to situations they have avoided, without performing rituals to feel better, they will gradually become used to them through the process of habituation (similar to the way children get used to the dark).

Maximizing Likelihood of Success

Once a trial of exposure and response prevention has been initiated, the clinician can take several steps to maximize the potential for success (Marks, 1993). Whenever possible, family members should be recruited to participate in the therapy to increase the likelihood of adequate compliance. Optimally, role playing under the therapist's supervision can help family members and the patient to understand which interventions are helpful and which may be counterproductive with regard to homework; that is, family members must be alerted to avoid performing vicarious rituals for the patient. The patient should also be encouraged to keep a diary of self-exposure. Such a diary will serve as a reminder, a subtle reinforcer, and a tangible means of monitoring the patient's efforts and signs of progress, while helping to identify trouble spots.

Once the therapy is underway, the clinician must watch for evidence of undoing, discounting, neutralizing, or dissociating behaviors, which can be subtle and can undermine the success of the therapy. As noted above, the most common reason for failure of behavior therapy is noncompliance. Such noncompliance is obvious when a patient simply refuses to expose himself or herself to situations that trigger obsessions or rituals. More difficult for the clinician to detect are instances of noncompliance with response prevention. For example, a patient of ours who was fearful of situations with superstitious significance was asked to go to a baseball game on Friday the 13th. Although he complied with this, we did not know that he spent most of the game mentally repeating prayers and counting. Thus, although he complied with exposure, he was noncompliant with response prevention and did not habituate until this noncompliance was detected and eliminated.

An illustration of these principles is the development of a treatment for obsessions. Recent evidence suggests that, contrary to our past negative experience, many patients with predominantly obsessive symptoms can be helped with behavior therapy as well (Salkovskis & Westbrook, 1989). Past treatment for violent, sexual, or blasphemous obsessions included asking the patient to imagine himself or herself actually engaging in the feared activities, in hopes that this would lead to habituation. Unfortunately, this approach was rarely successful, probably because of patients' avoiding these aversive thoughts (i.e., being noncompliant with exposure). As a next step, behavior therapists began presenting the obsessions recorded in the patients' own voices on a portable cassette tape recorder, which resulted in a small improvement in efficacy. However, it became clear that patients would sometimes include verbal rituals on these tapes, thereby not complying with response prevention and preventing habituation. Most recently, we have found that presentation of obsessions recorded in the patients' own voices, with any verbal rituals edited out by the therapist, results in acceptable rates of improvement.

Finally, in some cases, proper exposure and response prevention can only be carried out in special settings. Patients who only experience their symptoms in certain situations may require *in situ* therapy, such as home visits or field trips. Other patients may have sufficient difficulty with either exposure or response prevention that inpatient treatment is necessary to provide an adequate trial.

Despite clinicians' and patients' best efforts, a minority of patients will comply with exposure and response prevention for at least 20 hours, but still show no signs of habituation or of a reduction in obsessions and compulsions. In most cases, this failure of habituation appears to result from either overvalued ideation or severe depression (Foa, 1979). It appears that with overvalued ideation, in which a patient holds beliefs of a delusional intensity that something terrible will happen if he or she does not engage in rituals, habituation does not occur because the process is blocked by danger signals from higher centers in the brain. With severe depression, it appears that the actual process of habituation does not occur normally. In these cases, if pharmacotherapy has not previously been tried, it should be attempted with an effect on these target symptoms prior to another trial of behavior therapy.

Neurosurgical Intervention

Patients who have failed an exhaustive array of behavioral and pharmacologic treatments are said to be treatment-refractory. If their OCD is severe, debilitating, and chronic, neurosurgical intervention should be considered. (See Table 8.3 for the recommended course of therapy leading up to this consideration.)

Several different neurosurgical procedures have been used in efforts to treat OCD (Chiocca & Martuza, 1990). In the absence of sham-controlled double-blind studies, the efficacy of these various operations remains unproven. Many limbic system operations have been performed to date and reported in case series. The available data strongly suggest

TABLE 8.3. Recommended Course of Therapy for OCD

First:
   Three trials of first-line pharmacotherapies (including clomipramine)
   Behavior therapy (minimum of 20 hours of exposure and response prevention)

Second:
   Augmentation of clomipramine or an SSRI with clonazepam
   Two additional serial augmentation trials (i.e., buspirone and a neuroleptic)
   Consider modifications to behavior therapy (e.g., increase family involvement, check adequacy of exposure and response prevention, attempt alternative treatment targets, consider inpatient treatment)

Third:
   Consider monotherapy trial of clonazepam or buspirone

Fourth:
   Consider monotherapy trial of an MAOI

Fifth:
   Consider intravenous clomipramine (if available)

Sixth:
   If symptoms are chronic, severe, debilitating, and treatment-refractory, consider neurosurgery

that these procedures are efficacious for some patients and are also relatively safe. The neurosurgical procedures currently in use for treatment-refractory OCD include anterior cingulotomy, anterior capsulotomy, subcaudate tractotomy, and limbic leucotomy (tractotomy plus anterior cingulotomy). Response rates of 25–90% have been reported for these various procedures. Although well-designed studies directly comparing the relative efficacy of the different procedures are lacking, the suggestion is that anterior capsulotomy may be the most effective procedure and anterior cingulotomy may be the safest. Conservative estimates of anterior cingulotomy response indicate that approximately 25–30% of intractable cases are significantly improved (Jenike et al., 1991a). The procedure can be performed under a local anesthetic, with postoperative hospital stays of less than 1 week. The most common significant adverse results are postoperative seizures, which are typically well controlled with anticonvulsant medication. Cognitive sequelae have not been demonstrated in independent studies (Corkin, Twitchell, & Sullivan, 1979). Unlike the psychosurgery of an earlier era, contemporary stereotactic procedures are designed to minimize lesion size with specific circumscribed targets.

In the United States, anterior cingulotomies are performed at the Massachusetts General Hospital in Boston; anterior capsulotomies are performed at Rhode Island Hospital in Providence. Overseas, neurosurgical treatment of OCD is provided at the Karolinska Institute in Stockholm and at the Priory Hospital in London. Multidisciplinary review committees are assembled at these institutions to insure thorough scrutiny of cases before candidates are accepted for neurosurgical treatment.

With the advent of new techniques (e.g., the gamma knife and proton beam) that do not require craniotomy, sham procedures are now ethically possible, making a definitive study of efficacy plausible. Such a large-scale double-blind sham-controlled study of capsulotomy has already been proposed in a pending grant.

CONCLUSIONS

OCD is a common and sometimes debilitating disorder. Fortunately, the first-line treatments—namely, clomipramine, the SSRIs, and behavior therapy—are effective for most patients. For those patients who fail to respond to first-line therapies, other pharmacologic strategies include augmentation of clomipramine/SSRIs, alternative monotherapies, and intravenous clomipramine. Likewise, specific strategies can be invoked to enhance the efficacy of an initially unsuccessful behavioral therapy as well. Finally, neurosurgical treatment may be indicated for cases of severe, chronic OCD that is unresponsive to pharmacologic and behavioral interventions. At each step along the path of apparent treatment resistance, it is crucial to reassess primary diagnosis, comorbid diagnoses, and treatment history.

Future research may uncover new and different treatment options for OCD, further reducing the number of patients who suffer persistently. While we search for new cures, it will be important to thoroughly evaluate the tools that are currently at our disposal. Placebo-controlled double-blind trials of various augmentation strategies and alternative monotherapies are much needed. Likewise, identifying predictors of treatment response will provide practical guidance for clinicians. With such data, the order of interventions tried can proceed logically and efficiently. Finally, expanding education about OCD and its treatment will be of service to all involved.

REFERENCES

Alessi, N., & Bos, T. (1991). Buspirone augmentation of fluoxetine in a depressed child with obsessive–compulsive disorder. *American Journal of Psychiatry, 148,* 1605–1606.

Aranow, R. B., Hudson, J. I., Pope, H. G., Grady, T. A., Laage, T. A., Bell, I. R., & Cole, J. O. (1989). Elevated antidepressant plasma levels after addition of fluoxetine. *American Journal of Psychiatry, 146,* 911–913.

Bacher, N. M. (1990). Clonazepam treatment of obsessive compulsive disorder [Letter]. *Journal of Clinical Psychiatry, 51,* 168–169.

Baer, L. (1991). *Getting control.* Boston: Little, Brown.

Baer, L., & Minichiello, W. E. (1990). Behavior therapy for obsessive compulsive disorder. In G. D. Burrows, R. Noyes, & M. Roth (Eds.), *Handbook of anxiety* (Vol. 4, pp. 363–387). Amsterdam: Elsevier.

Bodkin, A., & White, K. (1989). Clonazepam in the treatment of obsessive compulsive disorder. *Journal of Clinical Psychiatry, 50,* 265–266.

Chiocca, E. A., & Martuza, R. L. (1990). Neurosurgical therapy of obsessive–compulsive disorder. In M. A. Jenike, L. Baer, & W. E. Minichiello (Eds.), *Obsessive–compulsive disorders: Theory and management* (pp. 283–294). Chicago: Year Book Medical.

Corkin, S., Twitchell, T. E., & Sullivan, E. V. (1979). Safety and efficacy of cingulotomy for pain and psychiatric disorders. In E. R. Hitchcock, H. T. Ballantine, & B. A. Myerson (Eds.), *Modern concepts in psychiatric surgery* (pp. 253–272). Amsterdam: Elsevier.

Eisenberg, J., & Asnis, G. (1985). Lithium as an adjunct treatment in obsessive–compulsive disorder. *American Journal of Psychiatry, 142,* 663.

Fallon, B. A., Campeas, R., Schneier, F. R., Hollander, E., Ferrick, J., Hatterer, J., Goetz, D., Dario, S., & Liebowitz, M. R. (1992). Open trial of intravenous clomipramine in five treatment refractory patients with obsessive compulsive disorder. *Journal of Neuropsychiatry, 4,* 70–75.

Feder, R. (1988). Lithium augmentation of clomipramine. *Journal of Clinical Psychiatry, 49,* 458.

Foa, E. B. (1979). Failure in treating obsessive compulsives. *Behaviour Research and Therapy, 17,* 169–176.

Foa, E. B., Steketee, G., & Milby, J. B. (1980). Differential effects of exposure and response prevention in obsessive–compulsive washers. *Journal of Consulting and Clinical Psychology, 48,* 71–79.

Golden, R. N., Morris, J. E., & Sack, D. A. (1988). Combined lithium–tricyclic treatment of obsessive–compulsive disorder. *Biological Psychiatry, 23*, 181–185.

Goodman, W. K., McDougle, C. J., & Price, L. H. (1992). Pharmacotherapy of obsessive compulsive disorder. *Journal of Clinical Psychiatry, 53*(Suppl.), 29–37.

Goodman, W. K., Price, L. H., Rasmussen, S. A., Mazure, C., Delgado, P., Heninger, G. R., & Charney, D. S. (1989a). The Yale–Brown Obsessive Compulsive Scale (Y-BOCS): Part II. Validity. *Archives of General Psychiatry, 46*, 1012–1016.

Goodman, W. K., Price, L. H., Rasmussen, S. A., Mazure, C., Fleischman, R. L., Hill, C. L., Heninger, G. R., & Charney, D. S. (1989b). The Yale–Brown Obsessive Compulsive Scale (Y-BOCS): Part I. Development, use, and reliability. *Archives of General Psychiatry, 46*, 1006–1011.

Grady, T. A., Pigott, T. A., L'Heureux, F., Hill, J. L., Bernstein, S. E., & Murphy, D. L. (1993). A double-blind study of adjuvant buspirone hydrochloride in fluoxetine treated patients with obsessive compulsive disorder. *American Journal of Psychiatry, 150*, 819–821.

Hewlett, W. A. (1993). The use of benzodiazepines in obsessive compulsive disorder and Tourette's syndrome. *Psychiatric Annals, 23*, 309–316.

Hewlett, W. A., Vinogradov, S., & Agras, W. S. (1990). Clonazepam treatment of obsessions and compulsions. *Journal of Clinical Psychiatry, 51*, 158–161.

Hewlett, W. A., Vinogradov, S., & Agras, W. (1992). Clomipramine, clonazepam, and clonidine treatment of obsessive compulsive disorder. *Journal of Clinical Psychopharmacology, 12*, 420–430.

Hollander, E., DeCaria, C. M., Schneiner, F. R., Schneiner, H. A., Liebowitz, M. R., & Klein, D. F. (1990). Fenfluramine augmentation of serotonin reuptake blockade antiobsessional treatment. *Journal of Clinical Psychiatry, 51*, 119–123.

Hollander, E., Fay, M., & Liebowitz, M. R. (1988). Clonidine and clomipramine in obsessive–compulsive disorder. *American Journal of Psychiatry, 145*, 388–389.

Hollander, E., & Liebowitz, M. R. (1988). Augmentation of antiobsessional treatment with fenfluramine. *American Journal of Psychiatry, 145*, 1314–1315.

Hollander, E., Mullen, L., DeCaria, C. M., Skodol, A., Schneier, F. R., Liebowitz, M. R., & Klein, D. F. (1991). Obsessive compulsive disorder, depression, and fluoxetine. *Journal of Clinical Psychiatry, 52*, 418–422.

Howland, R. H. (1991). Lithium augmentation of fluoxetine in the treatment of OCD and major depression: A case report. *Canadian Journal of Psychiatry, 36*, 154–155.

Hwang, E. C., & Van Woert, M. H. (1979). Antimyoclonic action of clonazepam: The role of serotonin. *European Journal of Pharmacology, 60*, 31–40.

Insel, T. R., Hamilton, J. A., Guttmacher, L. M., & Murphy, D. L. (1983). D-amphetamine in obsessive compulsive disorder. *Psychopharmacology, 80*, 231–235.

Insel, T. R., Murphy, D. L., Cohen, R. M., Alterman, I., Kilts, C., & Linnoila, M. (1983). Obsessive compulsive disorder: A double blind trial of clomipramine and clorgyline. *Archives of General Psychiatry, 40*, 605–612.

Insel, T. R., Roy, B. F., Cohen, R. M., & Murphy, D. L. (1982). Possible development of the serotonin syndrome in man. *American Journal of Psychiatry, 139*, 954–955.

Jenike, M. A. (1990). Approaches to the patient with treatment-refractory obsessive–compulsive disorder. *Journal of Clinical Psychiatry, 51*(2, Suppl.), 15–21.

Jenike, M. A., & Baer, L. (1988). Buspirone in obsessive-compulsive disorder: An open trial. *American Journal of Psychiatry, 145,* 1285–1286.

Jenike, M. A., Baer, L., Ballantine, H. T., Martuza, R. L., Tynes, S., Giriunas, I., Buttolph, L., & Cassem, N. H. (1991a). Cingulotomy for refractory obsessive–compulsive disorder: A long-term follow-up of 33 patients. *Archives of General Psychiatry, 48,* 548–555.

Jenike, M. A., Baer, L., & Buttolph, L. (1991b). Buspirone augmentation of fluoxetine in patients with obsessive–compulsive disorder. *Journal of Clinical Psychiatry, 52,* 13–14.

Jenike, M. A., Hyman, S. E., Baer, L., Holland, A., Minnichiello, W. E., Buttolph, L., Summergrad, P., Seymour, R., & Ricciardi, J. (1990). Fluvoxamine for obsessive–compulsive disorder: A double-blind, placebo-controlled trial in 40 patients. *American Journal of Psychiatry, 147,* 1209–1215.

Jenike, M. A., Surman, O. S., Cassem, N. H., Zusky, P., & Anderson, W. H. (1983). Monoamine oxidase inhibitors in obsessive–compulsive disorder. *Journal of Clinical Psychiatry, 44,* 131–132.

Jenner, P., Chadwick, D., Reynolds, E. H., & Marsden, C. D. (1975). Altered 5-HT metabolism with clonazepam, diazepam and diphenylhydantoin. *Journal of Pharmacology, 27,* 707–710.

Joffe, R. T., Swinson, R. P., & Levitt, A. J. (1991). Acute psychostimulant challenge in primary obsessive compulsive disorder. *Journal of Clinical Psychopharmacology, 11,* 237–241.

Judd, F. K., Chua, P., Lynch, C., & Norman, T. (1991). Fenfluramine augmentation of clomipramine treatment of obsessive compulsive disorder. *Australian and New Zealand Journal of Psychiatry, 25,* 412–414.

Knesevich, J. W. (1982). Successful treatment of obsessive–compulsive disorder with clonidine. *Journal of Clinical Psychopharmacology, 7,* 278–279.

Lipsedge, M. S., & Prothero, W. (1987). Clonidine and clomipramine in obsessive–compulsive disorder [Letter]. *American Journal of Psychiatry, 144,* 965–966.

Markovitz, P. J., Stagno, S. J., & Calabrese, J. R. (1990). Buspirone augmentation of fluoxetine in obsessive–compulsive disorder. *American Journal of Psychiatry, 147,* 798–800.

Marks, I. M. (1981). Review of behavioral psychotherapy: I. Obsessive–compulsive disorders. *American Journal of Psychiatry, 138,* 584–592.

Marks, I. M (1987). *Fears, phobias and rituals.* New York: Oxford University Press.

Marks, I. M. (1993, March). *Resistance to exposure therapy.* Paper presented at the First International Obsessive–Compulsive Disorder Conference, Capri, Italy.

McDougle, C. J., Goodman, W. K., Price, L. H., Delgado, P. O., Krystal, J. H., Charney, D. S., & Heninger, G. R. (1990). Neuroleptic addition in fluvoxamine refractory obsessive compulsive disorder. *American Journal of Psychiatry, 147,* 652–654.

McDougle, C. J., Price, L. H., Goodman, W. K., Charney, D. S., & Heninger, G. R. (1991). A controlled trial of lithium augmentation in fluvoxamine-refractory obsessive compulsive disorder: Lack of efficacy. *Journal of Clinical Psychopharmacology, 11,* 175–184.

Opler, L. A., & Feinberg, S. S. (1991). The role of pimozide in clinical psychiatry: A review. *Journal of Clinical Psychiatry, 52,* 221–233.

Pato, M. T., Pigott, T. A., Hill, J. L., Grover, G. N., Bernstein, S., & Murphy, D. L. (1991). Controlled comparison of buspirone and clomipramine in obsessive–compulsive disorder. *American Journal of Psychiatry, 148,* 127–129.

Phillips, K. A. (1991). Body dysmorphic disorder: The distress of imagined ugliness. *American Journal of Psychiatry, 148,* 1138–1149.

Pigott, T. A., L'Heureux, F., Hill, J. L., Bihari, K., Bernstein, S. E., & Murphy, D. L. (1992a). A double-blind study of adjuvant buspirone hydrochloride in clomipramine-treated patients. *Journal of Clinical Psychopharmacology, 12,* 11–18.

Pigott, T. A., L'Heureux, F. L., & Murphy, D. L. (1993, March). *Pharmacologic approaches to treatment-resistant OCD patients.* Paper presented at the First International Obsessive–Compulsive Disorder Conference, Capri, Italy.

Pigott, T. A., L'Heureux, F., Rubinstein, C. S., Bernstein, S. E., Hill, J. L., & Murphy, D. L. (1992b). Double-blind, placebo-controlled study of trazodone in patients with obsessive compulsive disorder. *Journal of Clinical Psychopharmacology, 12,* 156–162.

Pigott, T. A., L'Heureux, F., Rubenstein, C. S., Hill, J. L., & Murphy, D. L. (1992c, May). *A controlled trial of clonazepam augmentation in OCD patients treated with clomipramine or fluoxetine.* American Psychiatric Association, Annual Meeting, Washington, DC.

Pigott, T. A., Pato, M. T., Bernstein, S. E., Grover, G. N., Hill, J. L., Tolliver, T. J., & Murphy, D. L. (1990). Controlled comparison of clomipramine and fluoxetine in the treatment of obsessive–compulsive disorder: Behavioral and biological results. *Archives of General Psychiatry, 47,* 926–932.

Pigott, T. A., Pato, M. T., L'Heureux, F., L'Heureux, F., Hill, J. L., Grover, G. N., Bernstein, S. E., & Murphy, D. L. (1991). A controlled comparison of adjuvant lithium carbonate or thyroid hormone in clomipramine-treated patients with obsessive compulsive disorder. *Journal of Clinical Psychopharmacology, 11,* 242–248.

Pratt, J., Jenner, P., Reynolds, E. H., & Marsden, C. D. (1979). Clonazepam induces decreased serotoninergic activity in the mouse brain. *Neuropharmacology, 18,* 791–799.

Rasmussen, S. A. (1984). Lithium and tryptophan augmentation in clomipramine-resistant obsessive–compulsive disorder. *American Journal of Psychiatry, 141,* 1283–1285.

Rasmussen, S. A., & Eisen, J. L. (1992). The epidemiology and differential diagnosis of obsessive compulsive disorder. *Journal of Clinical Psychiatry, 53*(4, Suppl.), 4–10.

Salkovskis, P. M. (1993, March). *Cognitive techniques to limit non-compliance.* Paper presented at the First International Obsessive–Compulsive Disorder Conference, Capri, Italy.

Salkovskis, P. M., & Westbrook, D. (1989). Behavior therapy and obsessional ruminations: Can failure be turned into success? *Behaviour Research and Therapy, 27,* 149–160.

Shapiro, E., Shapiro, A. K., Fulop, G., Hubbard, M.. Mandeli, J., Norolie, J., & Phillips, R. A. (1989). Controlled study of haloperidol, pimozide and placebo for the treatment of Gilles de la Tourette's syndrome. *Archives of General Psychiatry, 46,* 722–730.

Simeon, J. G., Thatte, S., & Wiggins, D. (1990). Treatment of adolescent obsessive–compulsive disorder with a clomipramine–fluoxetine combination. *Psychopharmacology Bulletin, 26,* 285–290.

Stein, D., & Hollander, E. (1992). Low-dose pimozide augmentation of serotonin reuptake blockers in the treatment of trichotillomania. *Journal of Clinical Psychiatry, 53,* 123–126.

Stern, T. A., & Jenike, M. A. (1983). Treatment of obsessive–compulsive disorder with lithium carbonate. *Psychosomatics, 24,* 671–673.

Sternbach, H. (1991). The serotonin syndrome. *American Journal of Psychiatry, 148,* 705–713.

Troung, D. D., Bressman, S., Shali, H., & Fahn, S. (1988). Clonazepam, haloperidol, and clonidine in tic disorders. *Southern Medical Journal, 81,* 1103–1105.

Vallejo, J., Olivares, J., Marcos, T., Bulbena, A., & Menchon, J. (1992). Clomipramine versus phenelzine in obsessive–compulsive disorder: A controlled trial. *British Journal of Psychiatry, 161,* 665–670.

Wagner, H. R., Reches, A., Yablonskaya, E., & Fahn, S. (1986). Clonazepam-induced up-regulation of serotonin$_1$ and serotonin$_2$ binding sites in rat frontal cortex. *Advances in Neurology, 43,* 645–651.

Warneke, L. B. (1989). The use of intravenous chlorimipramine therapy in obsessive compulsive disorder. *Canadian Journal of Psychiatry, 34,* 853–859.

9

Cognitive-Behavioral and Pharmacologic Perspectives on the Treatment of Posttraumatic Stress Disorder

MICHAEL W. OTTO
SUSAN J. PENAVA
RACHEL A. POLLACK
JORDAN W. SMOLLER

In the absence of information about danger, most people assume that a situation is safe. For the PTSD individual, the lack of safety signals may be taken to mean that a situation is dangerous. Because it is virtually impossible to provide enough safety signals in any single situation to ensure no danger, the post-traumatic person is always on the alert.
　　　　　—FOA, STEKETEE, & ROTHBAUM (1989, p. 171)

The range and intensity of symptoms associated with posttraumatic stress disorder (PTSD) are striking. These symptoms may include intrusive memories, nightmares, dissociative episodes, marked anxiety, panic episodes, depression, substance abuse, and a host of cognitive and behavioral avoidance reactions. Despite the severity of initial anxiety symptoms, trauma victims may delay seeking treatment because of attempts to minimize evocation of trauma-related memories or emotions. When psychiatric care is sought, any of a number of symptoms may be prominent and therefore selected for intervention. At times, attention to a prominent symptom dimension (e.g., comorbid depression) may exclude full therapeutic attention to the core symptoms of PTSD. Inadequate treatment and more entrenched patterns of symptoms may be the result.

DEFINITIONS

PTSD is defined in the revised third edition of the *Diagnostic and Statistical Manual of Mental Disorders* (DSM-III-R) by three domains of symptoms: reexperiencing phenomena, avoidance reactions, and persistent high levels of autonomic arousal (American Psychiatric Association, 1987). Reexperiencing phenomena include intrusive and recurrent recollections of the trauma during waking hours or in dreams; perceptions that the trauma is recurring; and the experience of significant distress upon exposure to events representing or resembling aspects of the trauma. Avoidance symptoms include the avoidance of thoughts, feelings, and activities that may cue recollections of the trauma; difficulties in recalling important aspects of the trauma; a feeling of a foreshortened future; emotional blunting (including decreased interest in usual activities); feelings of being estranged or detached from other people; and a decreased ability to feel emotions of any kind, especially those associated with tenderness, intimacy, and sexuality. Finally, symptoms of increased arousal may include sleep difficulties, trouble concentrating, hypervigilance, an exaggerated startle response, irritability or angry outbursts, and physiologic reactivity to events representing or resembling some aspect of the trauma. The duration of these symptoms must have been at least 1 month. A delayed onset is specified if the onset of the symptoms is at least 6 months after the traumatic event.

DSM-IV (American Psychiatric Association, 1994) has brought with it several modifications to these criteria. First, the diagnosis no longer requires a stressor outside the range of usual human experience; this characterization has been found to be unreliable and inaccurate. Rather, according to DSM-IV, exposure to a traumatic event is defined by two criteria: (1) exposure to one or more events involving actual or possible death or serious injury, or a threat to one's own or others' physical integrity; and (2) an emotional response characterized by intense helplessness, fear, or horror. The three symptom domains (reexperiencing, avoidance, and increased arousal) remain relatively unchanged from DSM-III-R. Physiologic reactivity in response to cues of the trauma is redefined in DSM-IV as a reexperiencing symptom rather than as a symptom of increased arousal. In addition, a new criterion requires clinically important distress or impairment in social, job-related, or other major areas of functioning. Acute (if symptom duration is less than 3 months) and chronic (if symptom duration is 3 months or more) subtypes are also now defined, and the delayed-onset subtype has been retained from DSM-III-R.

Acute stress disorder, a new diagnostic category describing reactions to extreme stress lasting up to 1 month, is presented for the first time in DSM-IV. This disorder is characterized by reexperiencing, avoidance, and increased arousal symptoms that last for at least 2 days and no more than 4 weeks, and that occur within 4 weeks of the trauma. At least one symptom from each of the three symptom domains described for PTSD must be present, as must three or more dissociative symptoms during or after the trauma. As with PTSD, the symptoms must cause clinically important distress or impairment in social, job-related, or other major areas of functioning, or must interfere with the person's ability to perform a necessary task related to the trauma (e.g., informing family members of the trauma). Hence, a victim of violent crime or other trauma may develop acute stress disorder immediately or shortly after the trauma; however, if the symptoms persist beyond 1 month, or if there is a delayed onset of symptoms, a diagnosis of PTSD should be considered.

PREVALENCE

The Epidemiologic Catchment Area survey found the prevalence of PTSD to be 1% in the general population (Helzer, Robins, & McEvoy, 1987). Estimates of the lifetime prevalence in the general population range from 1% to 9% (Breslau, Davis, Andreski, & Peterson, 1991; Davidson, Hughes, Blazer, & George, 1991a), and appear to be in the range of 15% among psychiatric inpatients (Saxe et al., 1993). Estimates of the current prevalence of PTSD among Vietnam veterans tend to converge in the range of 13–17% (Kulka et al., 1991), with lifetime rates approximately twice as high (Keane, Litz, & Blake, 1990). In veterans, the degree of exposure to combat-related trauma greatly increases the likelihood of PTSD (Foy, Carroll, & Donahoe, 1987), with rates of 36% for men and 18% for women exposed to high stress in a war zone. Relative to civilian populations, combat veterans are more likely to have a delayed onset and greater duration of the disorder (Helzer et al., 1987). However, symptom profiles are remarkably similar among PTSD sufferers, regardless of the source of their trauma (e.g., combat, rape, physical assault, etc.; Keane & Wolfe, 1990).

Foa et al. (1989) have hypothesized that PTSD is most likely to develop when the traumatic event is perceived as both uncontrollable and life-threatening. In a community survey, a history of PTSD was diagnosed in approximately 28% of crime victims and 57% of rape victims. When assessed an average of 17 years later, 17% still met criteria for PTSD; this finding highlights the enduring nature of the disorder (Kilpatrick, Saunders, Veronen, Best, & Von, 1987). Similar rates of PTSD were found in a prospective study, with almost half of rape victims and 22% of victims of nonsexual assault developing PTSD within 3 months of the assault (Rothbaum, Foa, Riggs, Murdock, & Walsh, 1992). Among victims of crime, cognitive appraisal of life threat, physical injury, and rape were found to have independent and additive effects on the likelihood of the development of the disorder (Kilpatrick et al., 1989). In addition, more severe reactions to rape have been documented when rape occurred in situations thought to be safe, as compared to situations where danger was suspected (Schepple & Bart, 1983). Attitudinal surveys have also found that a general assumption of low controllability over aversive events is associated with greater PTSD symptom severity (Kushner, Riggs, Foa, & Miller, 1992).

Consistent relationships have not been found between trauma victims' gender, age, or ethnic background and the emergence of PTSD (Jones & Barlow, 1990). There is evidence that for rape-related traumas, symptoms are unstable for the first several months following the assault; however, there appears to be little evidence for spontaneous recovery 2–3 months following the trauma (Kilpatrick & Calhoun, 1988). Factors that may forestall the emergence of PTSD include greater social support, higher economic status, and less avoidance of trauma-related cues (Burnam et al., 1988; Jones & Barlow, 1990; Steketee & Foa, 1987). With respect to the negative effect of avoidance, Wirtz and Harrell (1987) found that victims of physical assault were less distressed 6 months after the assault if they had been naturalistically exposed (under safe conditions) to situations and/or stimuli reminiscent of the attack. Consistent with the notion that greater tendencies toward emotional arousal, negative affect, or avoidance may influence the emergence of PTSD, there are indications that individuals with higher levels of neuroticism, preexisting anxiety or depression, or a family history of anxiety, may be more susceptible to PTSD following exposure to traumatic stress (Breslau et al., 1991).

The following sections consider biologic and cognitive-behavioral perspectives on PTSD and strategies for its treatment. Pharmacologic strategies examined to date have included treatment with beta-adrenergic blockers and alpha-adrenergic agonists, benzodiazepines, antikindling agents, mood stabilizers, and various antidepressants. Exposure-based treatments have been included in a number of approaches to the disorder, but have received the most direct attention in cognitive-behavioral conceptualizations. Each of these interventions has the potential to change one aspect or a constellation of PTSD symptoms, and must be evaluated relative to the number of symptom domains that each affects.

BIOLOGIC PERSPECTIVES

Exposure to uncontrollable stress is associated with the dysregulation of a wide range of neurotransmitter and neuropeptide systems. Biologic models of PTSD receive the core of their empirical support from animal models of inescapable stress, particularly the phenomenon of learned helplessness. Exposure to an inescapable traumatic stressor (e.g., inescapable electric shock) results in depletion of noradrenergic and cholinergic neurotransmitters; in contrast, escapable stress may even lead to an increase in these neurotransmitters (Anisman, Ritch, & Sklar, 1981; see also van der Kolk, Greenberg, Boyd, & Krystal, 1985). Previous experience with inescapable stress also appears to influence norepinephrine activity in response to subsequent stressors. For example, in mice exposed to inescapable electric shock, norepinephrine depletion and deficits of escape behaviors emerged in response to subsequent exposure to electric shock, whereas the stress-naive animals demonstrated no such effects (Anisman & Sklar, 1979). One interpretation of these findings focuses on the conditionability of norepinephrine depletion. This hypothesis is consistent with kindling theories of PTSD (Lipper et al., 1986), which emphasize the conditioning of greater neuronal reactivity to traumatic cues.

Periods of norepinephrine depletion are hypothesized to give rise to subsequent periods of receptor hypersensitivity. Indeed, some accounts of the biologic basis of PTSD have suggested that periods of norepinephrine depletion and subsequent hypersensitivity coincide with the appearance of different symptom dimensions of PTSD. For example, van der Kolk et al. (1985) proposed that norepinephrine depletion may be linked to the negative symptoms of PTSD (i.e., decreased motivation and occupational functioning, and constriction of affect), and that noradrenergic hypersensitivity may be associated with startle responses, aggressive outbursts, nightmares, and intrusive recollections of the trauma. However, it is not clear whether such broad generalizations about adrenergic activity can account for the mixed constellation of symptoms that characterize the chronic adjustment of patients with PTSD, or for the emergence of specific symptoms (e.g., intrusive thoughts or dissociative experiences) following encounters with cues of the trauma; even exogenous manipulation of neurotransmitter activity with medications appears to exert its influence on emotions and behavior through intraneuronal mechanisms that take weeks to induce (Hyman & Nestler, 1993).

What is clear is that trauma has powerful effects on an organism, including the capacity to induce strong learned reactions to subsequent stressors or to cues related to the original trauma. Exposure to traumatic stressors produces a myriad of alterations in cholinergic and serotonergic activity, as well as neuroendocrine changes affecting levels of corticosteroids and endogenous opiates. Interestingly, some of these changes may alter the intensity with which memories of trauma are encoded for later retrieval (van der Kolk, 1994). In particular, recent evidence suggests that activation of the beta-adrenergic stress hormone system may play a role in enhancing memories associated with emotional arousal (Cahil, Prins, Weber, & McGaugh, 1994). Furthermore, to the extent that exposure to trauma cues is able to activate emotional responses appropriate to the original trauma, neurotransmitter and neurohormonal responses to threat will be chronically activated. Structural changes in neuronal connections are among the potential consequences (Kolb, 1987; van der Kolk, 1994).

Regardless of the particular biologic mechanisms involved, the various symptoms that may be present in PTSD provide a broad and formidable array of targets for treatment interventions. In addition, the prevalence of a number of comorbid disorders, such as major depression, substance abuse, panic disorder, generalized anxiety disorder, and personality disorders (Davidson & Foa, 1991; Keane & Wolfe, 1990; Steketee & Foa, 1987), complicates treatment approaches.

PHARMACOLOGIC TREATMENTS

In recent years, clinical trials and case reports have documented the use of a wide range of pharmacologic agents in the treatment of PTSD. As discussed in the following subsections, most of these agents have demonstrated variable efficacy for different symptom clusters of PTSD (intrusive, avoidance, and arousal). In addition, care must be taken to differentiate the effects of medication on comorbid anxiety or affective symptoms, as opposed to the treatment of the core symptoms of PTSD themselves.

Beta-Adrenergic Blockers and Alpha-Adrenergic Agonists

Beta-adrenergic blockers have varying actions on beta-1 and beta-2 receptors, and differ in their degree of lipid solubility, which determines how easily they cross the blood–brain barrier. For example, propranolol is an agent with relatively high lipid solubility, and hence may act centrally. This agent, and peripherally acting beta-adrenergic blockers such as atenolol and nadolol, have received attention for the treatment of performance anxiety. These agents are capable of blocking a number of anxiety symptoms that are commonly encountered in stage fright (e.g., trembling and heart palpitations). In addition to their direct effects in attenuating some of the outward signs of autonomic arousal, these medications may also act to interrupt cycles of increasing anxiety that result from self-focused attention on anxiety symptoms (Liebowitz, Gorman, Fyer, & Klein, 1985). Hence, these agents offer the potential for blocking some of the arousal symptoms of PTSD. In addition, recent findings suggest that beta-adrenergic blockers may help reduce the frequency of anger outbursts among patients with organic or psychotic mental conditions (Greendyke, Kanter, Schuster, Verstreate, & Wooton, 1986; Ratey et al., 1992). Consequently, these medications may help control the aggressive episodes and autonomic arousal associated with PTSD.

    Although there have been no controlled studies of beta-adrenergic blockers for PTSD, uncontrolled studies have suggested that propranolol has some efficacy in reducing peripheral autonomic activation, intrusive recollections, dream and sleep disturbances, startle responses, and explosive behavior (Birkhimer, DeVane, & Muniz, 1985; Boehnlein, Kinzie, Ben, & Flech, 1985; Kolb, Burris, & Griffiths, 1984).

    With a biologic action similar to that of beta-adrenergic blockers, alpha-adrenergic agonists, such as clonidine, act to modulate autonomic arousal by modulating noradrenergic function. These agents reduce the rate of neuronal firing in the locus coeruleus and inhibit activity of the noradrenergic system. In an open study of Cambodian refugee patients with PTSD, Kinzie and Leung (1989) found that clonidine in conjunction with the tricyclic antidepressant (TCA) imipramine was associated with improvements in depression, arousal symptoms, intrusive thoughts, nightmares, and startle reactions; however, avoidant behavior was apparently unaffected. The value of clonidine alone for PTSD (without a TCA) remains unclear.

In summary, there is preliminary evidence that alpha-adrenergic agonists and beta-adrenergic blockers may have some beneficial effects on PTSD, particularly with regard to arousal and reexperiencing symptoms. A specific role for beta-adrenergic blockers in controlling anger outbursts is supported by studies of other populations, but it is not clear whether these agents can compete with the anger management effects of serotonin selective reuptake inhibitors (SSRIs) discussed below.

Benzodiazepines

High-potency benzodiazepines have shown clear efficacy in the treatment of panic disorder, exerting effects on anticipatory anxiety, frequency of panic attacks, and in many cases phobic avoidance (Ballenger et al., 1988; Tesar et al., 1991). Successful treatment of panic disorder with high-potency benzodiazepines has also been associated with significant reductions in depressed mood (Tesar et al., 1991). These findings suggest that high-potency benzodiazepines may have similar actions on some of the symptoms of arousal and avoidance that are characteristic of PTSD. Evidence to date, however, suggests that efficacy of benzodiazepines for PTSD may be limited to its direct effects on autonomic arousal and anxiety. The only double-blind, placebo-controlled study of a benzodiazepine for PTSD compared alprazolam to placebo in 16 PTSD patients (Braun, Greenberg, Dosberg, & Lerer, 1990). There was a modest reduction of anxiety symptoms in 10 patients, but PTSD-specific avoidant and intrusive symptoms were not significantly affected by alprazolam treatment.

Given the high rate of concurrent substance abuse among some PTSD patients, benzodiazepine treatment may be problematic because of its potential for abuse (Friedman, 1988; Risse et al., 1990). In addition, discontinuation of benzodiazepines is often difficult (Schweizer, Rickels, Case, & Greenblatt, 1990). These concerns, along with evidence for limited efficacy, do not suggest a central role for benzodiazepines in the treatment of PTSD.

Antikindling Agents and Mood Stabilizers

"Kindling" is defined as progressively increasing effects on neural activity that result from repetitive subthreshold electrical or chemical brain stimulation. Drawing upon the phenomenon of kindling, Post and colleagues

(Post, Rubinow, & Ballenger, 1984; Post & Weiss, 1989) have suggested that repeated pharmacologic or stress-induced subthreshold stimulation of limbic circuits may result in sensitization, and that oversensitization of limbic circuits may influence the course of some psychiatric disorders (e.g., bipolar disorder) by increasing the frequency and severity of symptom episodes. Lipper et al. (1986) have applied this model to PTSD. They suggest that traumatic events may sensitize limbic neurons and kindle reexperiencing phenomena when an individual is exposed to cues of the traumatic event. In accordance with this conceptualization, a number of antikindling agents have been examined in open trials for the treatment of PTSD.

Lipper et al. (1986) examined the effects of carbamazepine in a 5-week trial in 10 patients with PTSD. They found that 7 out of 10 patients were judged to be moderately to very much improved by a single evaluator. Symptoms demonstrating the greatest change were nightmares, flashbacks, and intrusive recollections. In a separate preliminary trial of carbamazepine in 10 Vietnam combat veterans with PTSD, Wolf, Alavi, and Mosnaim (1988) found that symptoms of impulsivity, violent behavior, and anger outbursts improved with treatment. Other specific symptoms, such as flashbacks and intrusive recollections, were not assessed in this study.

Encouraging findings have also been reported for another antikindling agent, valproate. An open trial of valproate (Fesler, 1991) found significant effects on symptoms of hyperarousal and hyperreactivity (but not intrusive symptoms such as reexperiencing phenomena) in 10 of 16 Vietnam veterans with PTSD. Nine patients reported significant improvement in avoidance and emotional withdrawal symptoms.

The mood-stabilizing effects of lithium may also be useful in PTSD. In an open trial of lithium in 22 combat veterans, van der Kolk (1983) noticed improvement in flashbacks, anger, startle responses, sleep disturbance, alcohol abuse, and psychological distress. Fourteen subjects reported a subjective sense of control over their lives. Side effects were relatively few, and dropout rates were low; however, it is interesting to note that of the lithium responders, only those who remained in individual or group therapy continued to take the prescribed medication. This finding suggests the importance of continued adjunctive psychotherapy. Although reports of mood stabilizers in PTSD are relatively few and limited to uncontrolled trials and case reports, the results indicate a potential role for these agents in the pharmacologic treatment of PTSD. Controlled investigations are needed.

Tricyclic Antidepressants and Monoamine Oxidase Inhibitors

In addition to their traditional use in treating depression, TCAs and monoamine oxidase inhibitors (MAOIs) have been found to be effective in the treatment of panic disorder and agoraphobia (see Pollack & Smoller, Chapter 4, this volume), and TCAs in the treatment of generalized anxiety disorder (Rickels, Downing, Schweizer, & Hassman, 1993). The potential for treatment of both depressive and anxious symptoms encourages application of these agents to PTSD.

The efficacy of TCAs in PTSD has been the subject of multiple open studies (Bleich, Siegel, Garb, & Lerer, 1986; Boehnlein et al., 1985; Burstein, 1984; Falcon, Ryan, Chamberlain, & Curtis, 1985; Turchan, Holmes, & Wasserman, 1992). In general, uncontrolled studies of TCAs in PTSD have demonstrated improvements in intrusive and depressive symptoms. For example, imipramine was found to improve sleep and decrease nightmares and flashbacks in 10 nonmilitary patients with PTSD (Burstein, 1984), and in a case series examining the relatively serotonin—selective TCA clomipramine, improvements in intrusive symptoms were seen in six of seven veterans with PTSD (Chen, 1991).

Open clinical trials also support the efficacy of the MAOI phenelzine. For example, Davidson, Walker, and Kilts (1987) administered phenelzine to 11 combat veterans for 6 weeks. At the end of this treatment, 85% of patients had demonstrated improvement in intrusive recollections, constricted affect, estrangement from others, and cognitive disturbances. Other investigations of phenelzine have found a decrease in panic, anxiety, nightmares, flashbacks, and startle responses, and an improvement in concentration (Bleich et al., 1986; Hogben & Cornfield, 1981). Unfortunately, the side effect profile and dietary restrictions associated with MAOIs may limit patient acceptance and make these agents difficult to use in patients with comorbid substance abuse.

In contrast to the fairly encouraging results of open trials, results from controlled trials of TCAs (amitriptyline, desipramine, imipramine) and an MAOI (phenelzine) have been mixed. Shestatzky, Greenberg, and Lerer (1988) conducted a randomized, double-blind, crossover trial comparing phenelzine and placebo. The findings demonstrated that phenelzine did not differ from placebo in clinical response. The sample size was small ($n = 13$), however, and therapeutic dose was established by means of clinical tolerance. In contrast, Kosten, Frank, Dan, McDougle, and Giller (1991) examined the relative efficacy of phenelzine, imipramine, and placebo in 60 Vietnam veterans with PTSD. They found that both active agents improved PTSD symptoms, but that phenelzine produced greater improvement in intrusive symptoms. Neither drug significantly improved avoidance symptoms. It should be noted that the patients in this study had relatively mild PTSD symptoms and did not have comorbid major depression. Depressive symptoms that were present did not improve with either antidepressant.

Reist, Kauffman, and Haier (1989) conducted a 4-week double-blind, crossover study comparing desipramine with placebo in 18 veterans with PTSD, and observed a significant reduction in some symptoms of depression and intrusion only in patients who had initially met criteria for major depression; no changes were found in PTSD or anxiety symptoms. Finally, an 8-week randomized, double-blind, placebo-controlled trial comparing amitriptyline with placebo in veterans (Davidson et al., 1993) found significant benefit of amitriptyline over placebo for anxiety and depressive symptoms. However, efficacy for PTSD-specific symptoms was only marginally significant on avoidance measures, and nonsignificant for intrusive symptoms. At the end of the study, 64% of the amitriptyline and 72% of the placebo-treated patients still met diagnostic criteria for PTSD.

Selective Serotonin Reuptake Inhibitors

The SSRIs have been widely accepted as first-line treatments for depression and other disorders because of their efficacy and tolerability (Rosenbaum & Pollack, 1994). They also offer a promising profile of actions for the treatment of PTSD. In addition to their antidepressant effects, SSRIs have received attention as antipanic agents (Black, Wesner, Bowers, & Gabel, 1993) and antiobsessional agents (Fontaine & Chouinard, 1985; Jenike et al., 1990), and have also shown promising effects in the treatment of the anger attacks that sometimes accompany depression (Fava et al., 1993). The application of SSRIs to PTSD is supported by the putative role of serotonin in mediating responses to traumatic stress (Sutherland & Davidson, 1994; van der Kolk, 1987).

The value of SSRIs in PTSD has been investigated in several case reports and open trials, and one placebo-controlled trial (Davidson, Roth, & Newman, 1991b; March, 1992; McDougle, Southwick, Charney, & St. James, 1991; Shay, 1992; van der Kolk et al., 1994). For example, in an open trial of fluoxetine in 20 veterans with PTSD, 65% of patients who completed at least 4 weeks of treatment showed significant improvement in PTSD symptoms (including intrusive, avoidance, and hyperarousal symptoms; McDougle et al., 1991). The presence of comorbid depression was unrelated to treatment response. In another open trial (Kline, Dow, Brown, & Matloff, 1994), sertraline produced improvement in PTSD and depressive symptoms in 12 of 19 veterans with PTSD and comorbid depression.

In a 5-week randomized, double-blind trial of fluoxetine and placebo (the only controlled trial of an SSRI in PTSD), van der Kolk et al. (1994) found significant reduction of overall PTSD symptomatology in patients receiving fluoxetine. Improvement was most marked in arousal and numbing symptoms. Fluoxetine was also effective in treating concurrent depression. It is interesting to note, however, that upon site analysis, combat veterans at a Department of Veterans Affairs (VA) hospital showed no significant reduction (other than depression) in PTSD symptoms in response to fluoxetine; by contrast, outpatients at a trauma clinic showed a greater response to fluoxetine, with substantial improvement of depression and numbing symptoms. The veterans as a group had been receiving some form of therapy for their PTSD symptoms for over a decade, which suggests that they may have been treatment-resistant. Many of the trauma clinic patients were taking initial steps toward treating their disorder.

In summary, the heterogeneity of patient populations, study design, and severity of PTSD symptomatology among pharmacologic studies makes it difficult to draw firm conclusions about the utility of these agents in the treatment of PTSD. In general, the treatment of core PTSD symptoms with pharmacotherapy has been associated with modest improvements, and few agents have shown efficacy for all three symptom clusters. Because of their apparent effect on intrusive, avoidance, and hyperarousal symptoms, and their favorable side effect profiles, SSRIs may emerge as the drugs of first choice in PTSD. This issue is further discussed in an effect size analysis later in the chapter.

COGNITIVE-BEHAVIORAL PERSPECTIVES

Most psychosocial interventions for PTSD share an emphasis on exposure to memories of the trauma to aid in the emotional reprocessing of the experience. For example, in his focused, psychodynamically oriented approach to treating trauma-related disorders, Horowitz (1986) describes the importance of dosed reexperiencing of the trauma. This exposure is hierarchically arranged, so as to provide the patient with tolerable experiences of emotional abreaction to aid in the adaptive reprocessing of the experience. Accordingly, Foa and Kozak (1986) note the emphasis on the role of avoidance of disturbing experiences in psychodynamic accounts of psychopathology. For example, Perls (1969, p. 11) wrote, "If some of our thoughts, feelings are unacceptable to us, we want to disown them but only at the cost of disowning valuable parts of ourselves. . . . Your ability to cope with the world becomes less and less."

Exposure therapy can be conducted in a wide range of formats, including discussions of the trauma, guided imagery, structured review of memories (in oral or written form), hypnosis, or exposure to trauma cues *in vivo* (e.g., walking on the street where an assault occurred). Although these exposure-based interventions may be incorporated into a variety of therapeutic approaches, the behavioral therapies are the ones in which exposure is most directly and formally addressed, and for which a wealth of experimental paradigms and empirical data has been organized. At present, there are a number of cognitive-behavioral treatment approaches that combine exposure with cognitive restructuring procedures and anxiety management skills in the treatment of PTSD. These treatments have been designed for both individual (E. Frank et al., 1988; Veronen & Kilpatrick, 1983) and group (Calhoun & Resick, 1993) formats.

An important starting point for considering cognitive-behavioral accounts of PTSD is Mowrer's (1960) two-factor theory of fear and avoidance. Anxiety reactions and phobic responses to innocuous cues are thought to be the result of classical conditioning; at the time of a trauma, innocuous cues become associated with the trauma and accompanying emotional reactions (factor 1). This pairing imbues trauma cues with the ability to evoke emotional responses appropriate to the trauma itself. For example, in the case of a severe physical or sexual assault, the hour of the attack, the location, and the sights, sounds, and smells associated with the assault may develop the capability to signal danger. Stimulus generalization and higher-order conditioning are used to explain the proliferation of anxiety-provoking stimuli, so that stimuli only vaguely resembling or associated with the original trauma cues may come to elicit anxiety and avoidance (Jones & Barlow, 1990; Keane, Fairbank, Caddell, Zimering, & Bender, 1985). "Stimulus generalization" refers to the tendency for stimuli similar to trauma-related cues to become capable of eliciting symptoms over time (e.g., a trauma victim may begin to avoid all small rooms following an assault in a restricted space). "Higher-order conditioning" refers to the capability of unrelated stimuli to become cues for trauma-related symptoms through their pairing with other trauma cues. For example, police uniforms may begin to cue anxiety because of their pairing with discussions of the traumatic experience with investigating officers. The breadth of sensitivity to trauma-related cues is illustrated by the recent finding of activation of combat-related PTSD symptoms among Vietnam veterans following television coverage of the Gulf War (Long, Chamberlain, & Vincent, 1994).

Avoidance of the evocation of conditioned emotional responses to trauma cues is thought to maintain the fear reaction by preventing the opportunity for extinction of these learned associations. The avoidance itself is maintained by the temporary anxiety reduction it achieves (factor 2), but over time, the proliferation of cues that are capable of eliciting memories makes this strategy especially problematic.

From this basic account of the acquisition and maintenance of conditioned emotional reactions to trauma, individual approaches to PTSD differ in terms of the paradigms used for organizing observations and explaining the treatment process. One approach to understanding the nature of exposure treatment is provided by information-processing theories of emotion, which focus on the nature of fear memories. Exposure to a traumatic event is hypothesized to form a network of associations that includes the memory of the trauma and associated cues. According to Lang's (1977) bioinformational theory of emotion, fear networks consist of (1) stimulus elements, which represent visual, auditory, olfactory, and other sensory cues associated with the feared event; (2) response elements, which include cognitive, affective, physiologic, and behavioral responses to these cues; and (3) interpretive elements, which include information about the meaning of the event and the nature of the association between the stimulus and response elements. Once the network is formed, cues associated with the network (e.g., either stimulus or response cues) can activate the fear network, and consequently can activate anxiety and urges to avoid or escape.

Because of the catastrophic nature of traumatic events, trauma networks are thought to be large and easily activated. Trauma networks are also distinguished from other fear networks by the breadth of emotions that may be elements of the network (Pitman, Orr, Forgue, de Jong, & Claiborn, 1987; Resick & Schnicke, 1992). For example, Pitman et al. (1987) found that exposure of combat veterans with PTSD to combat cues elicited a range of emotions in addition to fear, including sadness, anger, surprise, and disgust. There is also evidence that the emotional meaning of a traumatic memory is not fixed at the time of the trauma. D. G. Kilpatrick (personal communication, cited in Foa et al., 1989) provides a case example of a rape victim who did not develop significant PTSD symptoms until months later, when she learned that her attacker had killed his next victim. Foa et al. (1989) interpret this phenomenon as the alteration of the trauma network to include a much more pronounced representation of threat, which made the memory into a stronger fear structure. In characterizing the difference between PTSD and other anxiety disorders, they emphasize the "monumental significance" of the trauma:

> We propose that what distinguishes PTSD from other anxiety disorders is that the traumatic event was of monumental significance and violated formerly held basic concepts of safety. That is to say, stimuli and responses that previously signalled safety have now become associated with danger. In this way, one's world becomes less predictable and controllable. (p. 166)

Viewed from this perspective, the purpose of exposure is not simply to loosen the association between trauma cues and the conditioned response of fear, but also to change trauma-related beliefs about the safety of one's current world.

EXPOSURE-BASED TREATMENTS

The efficacy of exposure-based treatments is supported by numerous case reports and open trials (Fairbank, Gross, & Keane, 1983; E. Frank et al., 1988; Keane & Kaloupek, 1982; Saigh, 1987), and by the limited number of controlled studies completed to date. Controlled trials examining exposure-based interventions, with or without cognitive restructuring components, have been found to be superior to waiting-list or other control conditions (Boudewyns & Hyer, 1990; Boudewyns, Hyer, Woods, Harrison, & McCranie, 1990; Brom, Kleber, & Defares, 1989; Cooper & Clum, 1989; Foa, Rothbaum, Riggs, & Murdock, 1991; Foa et al., 1994; Keane, Fairbank, Caddell, & Zimering, 1989; Peniston, 1986; Resick & Schnicke, 1992). Results from controlled trials are considered in greater detail in the effect size analysis presented later in the chapter.

In addition to studies of component treatments, two comprehensive cognitive-behavioral therapy protocols for PTSD have been described in the clinical research literature: stress inoculation training (SIT; Veronen

& Kilpatrick, 1983) and cognitive processing therapy (CPT; Calhoun & Resick, 1993; Resick & Schnicke, 1993). Both were developed specifically for use with victims of sexual assault. SIT offers a combination of educational, skills acquisition, and situational exposure interventions. Skill acquisition includes training in the modulation of autonomic arousal through diaphragmatic breathing and relaxation techniques. A cognitive restructuring treatment component includes training in guided self-dialogue about rape-related reactions. Thought-stopping techniques are also taught for managing intrusive or dysfunctional thoughts. However, it should be noted that thought-stopping procedures are falling out of favor in the treatment of other anxiety conditions (e.g., obsessive–compulsive disorder) because of their similarity to thought suppression; thought suppression itself may play a role in increasing the frequency of intrusive thoughts (Salkovskis & Campbell, 1994). For management of avoidance reactions, behavioral modeling and role playing are provided to encourage skill development. Although SIT does not utilize direct exposure to traumatic memories, exposure to trauma-related, anxiety-provoking situations is used, with emphasis on application of cognitive, symptom management, and behavioral skills in this context.

Examination of the efficacy of SIT in controlled trials supports its efficacy over waiting-list conditions (Foa et al., 1991, 1994; Resick, Jordan, Girelli, Hutter, & Marhoefer-Dvorak, 1988). Individual elements of SIT were examined in two studies by Foa and associates. In the first (Foa et al., 1991), SIT without exposure elements tended to produce better results than exposure treatment alone on most measures at the end of treatment. However, these trends reversed themselves at a 3-month follow-up. One explanation is that the nonexposure elements of SIT are effective for reducing most elements of anxiety immediately following treatment, but that exposure is necessary for longer-term change.

In a more recent study, Foa et al. (1994) examined the efficacy of SIT without exposure, exposure alone, and the combination of these treatments, relative to a waiting-list control condition. All treatments were superior to the waiting-list condition, but exposure alone tended to perform the best among the active treatments. The authors suggest that the complexity of the combined treatment, delivered in a brief therapy format, may have detracted from the efficacy of these combined elements of treatment. Hence, in clinical application, a full course of exposure and a full course of the cognitive restructuring and symptom management elements of SIT may offer the most promising outcome.

CPT is another treatment package developed specifically for victims of rape (Calhoun & Resick, 1993). CPT interventions are based on an information-processing formulation of PTSD, and imaginal exposure to the trauma memory and cognitive restructuring are crucial aspects of the program. This approach uses exposure to elicit memories of the traumatic event, and then uses cognitive techniques to challenge maladaptive beliefs. CPT is also designed for application in group treatment settings. To allow exposure in a group setting, patients are assigned the homework of writing about the trauma, including stimulus, response, and interpretive elements. When writing and subsequently reading over the account of the trauma, patients are encouraged to experience their emotions fully. Therapists help patients identify and challenge maladaptive beliefs about the trauma and the safety of their current world. Instruction in more adaptive self-statements, and interpretation of the trauma in the context of their current life and future expectations, are then stressed. These cognitive processing procedures specifically target changes in feelings of safety, trust, power, esteem, and intimacy that may have resulted from the trauma (sexual assault). As is commonplace in cognitive-behavioral therapy approaches, homework assignments are routinely given; this prompts much of the therapeutic work to be done between sessions. The application of some of these techniques to the treatment of adults who were raped in childhood is illustrated by Smucker and Niederee (1995).

Resick and Schnicke (1992) examined the efficacy of CPT delivered in a short-term group format. The treatment was found to result in significant improvement in both PTSD and depressive symptomatology. In addition, many patients reported a substantial improvement in their quality of life. These improvements in symptoms and social functioning were maintained over a follow-up period of 6-months. The control group for this study was a waiting-list group consisting of patients later assigned to the active treatment conditions. Hence, because of the use of this quasi-experimental design, this study is not described in the effect size analysis presented below.

Elements of Exposure-Based Treatment

Foa and Kozak (1986) have argued that two conditions are necessary for fear reduction via exposure: activation of the fear network, and incorporation of new information into that network. Activation of the fear network is deemed necessary to allow modification of the memory. Foa and Kozak emphasize that the memory can be modified in either a positive or a negative direction, depending on whether the new information is compatible or incompatible with the fear structure; it is the incompatible (safety) information that is crucial for effective exposure treatment.

For the goal of maximizing the accessibility and modification of a fear network, Foa and Kozak (1986) emphasize the importance of four issues: (1) the match between the trauma memory and exposure cues, (2) the medium in which the exposure is delivered, (3) the duration of exposure, and (4) adequate attention to trauma cues. Fear evocation appears to be maximized by a good match between between the trauma memory and exposure cues. This match may be aided by exposure presentation of response elements (e.g., directing the patient in imaginal exposure that includes what the patient was feeling at the time of the trauma), in addition to relevant sensory cues of the trauma (Lang, 1977). In accordance with data indicating that trauma memories are associated with a range of negative emotions, Resick and Schnicke (1992) argue that exposure treatment may alter the fear or perceptions of danger, without necessarily benefiting other emotional characteristics. Correspondingly, their treatment protocol for victims of rape includes specific cognitive restructuring and exposure interventions for a range of trauma-related emotions. Finally, because individuals may differ in their ability to generate trauma-related imagery, imagery training may be necessary to improve the quality of the exposure cues (Foa & Kozak, 1986).

The medium in which the exposure is delivered can also influence the match between the trauma memory and exposure cues. Foa and Kozak (1986) emphasize that visual displays, verbal descriptions, and lifelike enactments may act as effective exposure procedures. As a result, therapists have at their disposal a wide range of exposure choices, which vary in flexibility from easily administered imaginal exposure to more-difficult-to-arrange *in vivo* exposure. The variety of mediums and methods by which exposure can be conducted gives the therapist freedom to titrate the intensity of exposure to match the patient's coping skills at any given stage of treatment.

The duration of the exposure session has received consistent attention in the treatment of phobic conditions. A decrease in anxiety during the exposure session is thought to allow integration of new information into the fear network, in part because exposure to the cues is not accompanied by current threat or incessant anxiety. Longer exposure sessions provide greater opportunities for habituation; correspondingly, prolonged exposure (e.g., 50 minutes or more) has been found to be superior to short exposure for more severe phobic conditions (Foa & Kozak, 1986). For example, Foa et al. (1991) conduct 90-minute treatment sessions, devoting 60 minutes of each session to imaginal exposure. Patients are also assigned imaginal and *in vivo* exposure homework between sessions.

Finally, the objective presentation of trauma cues does not insure that these cues will be processed (Foa & Kozak, 1986). Patients may try to reduce their emotional response to exposure by minimizing their attention to the exposure stimuli with either passive or active avoidance strategies, such as focusing on nonfearful images, distorting the trauma images, or focusing on less relevant aspects of the trauma memory. A clinical manifestation of this cognitive avoidance is seen in the patient who reports "just the facts" of his/her trauma, without attention to the emotional significance of the events.

Another and more pervasive manifestation of cognitive avoidance may be the emotional numbing associated with the disorder. As noted above, emotional responses and feelings of autonomic arousal are thought to be relevant cues for activation of the trauma network. Correspondingly, in an effort to prevent the activation of such memories, patients may attempt to reduce emotional arousal altogether; these attempts promote symptoms of emotional numbing. In fact, the negative symptoms of PTSD (e.g., emotional numbness, distractibility, depersonalization, and memory loss) have been hypothesized to be the products of habitual cognitive avoidance of cues that have the potential to activate trauma memories. One potential consequence of these avoidance strategies is restriction of the opportunity to develop or use skills of problem solving, assertiveness, or emotional regulation. Figure 9.1 illustrates some of the common patterns in PTSD.

Habitual avoidance of emotionality is not specific to PTSD; it has

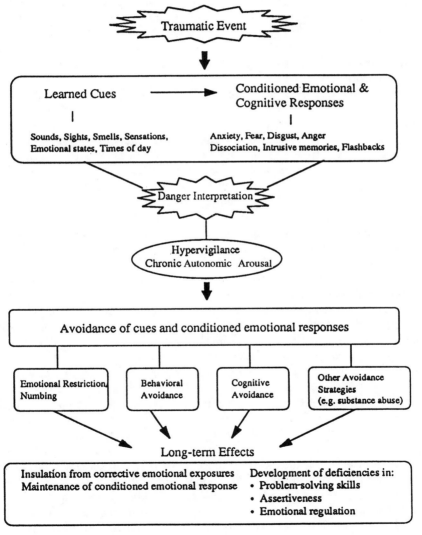

FIGURE 9.1. Symptom development in PTSD.

been described in other anxiety disorders. For example, patients with panic disorder may avoid exercise, caffeine use, or emotionally evocative situations (e.g., arguments with a spouse or emotionally laden films), in an attempt to avoid the potential elicitation of feared sensations of anxiety (see Otto & Gould, Chapter 5, this volume). The costs of such avoidance strategies to therapeutic exposure are significant. Although decreased attention to the phobic cues during exposure has no significant effects on in-session habituation, it appears to decrease fear reduction across sessions (Foa & Kozak, 1986), thereby attenuating the beneficial effects of exposure. Foa et al. (1989) argue that fears of emotional symptoms often decrease across exposure sessions as patients learn that these reactions are not interminable or dangerous, but patients may nonetheless have significant difficulties approaching initial exposure sessions. As will be reviewed below, treatment refusal is a significant issue in patients with PTSD; correspondingly, patients' ability to tolerate exposure sessions without avoidance is an important clinical issue on its own.

Regarding this issue, we are especially alert to the way in which symptoms may "fold back upon themselves" in the context of exposure sessions. Exposure to traumatic material induces autonomic arousal (e.g., rapid heart rate, muscle tension, flushing) in patients, and may also induce feelings of dissociation. These feelings may be interpreted as threatening in their own right (e.g., "I am about to lose control," "I'll go crazy if I keep this up"); more significantly, they may be experienced as additional cues of the original trauma (at which time the patients may have experienced autonomic arousal, dissociation, and/or fears of loss of control or death). This rush of additional, interoceptive cues of the trauma may lead the patients to feel that the trauma is going to happen again, or that they cannot tolerate the memories. This experience may increase the patients' sense that trauma-related memories are uncontrollable, unpredictable, and dangerous; thus, it may lead to increased cognitive avoidance.

There is evidence that such interoceptive anxiety cues may be powerful elicitors of flashbacks. Rainey et al. (1987) examined the response to sodium lactate infusion in a small sample of combat veterans with PTSD. Sodium lactate infusion produces a range of somatic sensations reminiscent of anxiety, and is capable of inducing panic attacks in individuals with fears of these sensations (e.g., patients with panic disorder; for a review, see Clark, 1986). Like patients with panic disorder, patients with PTSD are characterized by marked fears of anxiety sensations and their imagined consequences (Peterson & Reiss, 1992; Taylor, Koch, & McNally, 1992). Rainey et al. (1987) found that in patients with PTSD, lactate infusion resulted in flashbacks (and subsequent panic attacks). The hospital setting for the provocation trial also appeared to influence the type of flashbacks experienced (i.e., medical situations)—a finding suggesting the potential importance of environmental context in determining flashback content. Provocation of flashbacks has also been reported for provocation with yohimbine injections (Southwick et al., 1993). These findings support the hypothesis that interoceptive sensations of anxiety serve as cues that activate trauma memories (Jones & Barlow, 1990).

Interoceptive Exposure

Identification of the role of interoceptive cues of anxiety in both activating trauma memories and motivating avoidance offers the potential of expanding approaches to exposure treatment. The development of therapeutic strategies for panic disorder may provide an analogy. For years, behavioral treatment of panic disorder and agoraphobia emphasized exposure to avoided situations, despite the long-held belief that agoraphobia was a result of the *fear of having a panic attack* in the avoided situation. Although exposure to agoraphobic situations has useful effects on panic frequency, current treatments of panic disorder have focused more directly on modifying the fears of anxiety sensations and panic attacks. This is achieved with a program of exposure to panic-like sensations (termed "interoceptive exposure" because the patient is exposed to internal sensations rather than environmental cues; see Otto & Gould, Chapter 5, this volume). In the treatment of agoraphobic avoidance, interoceptive exposure may be applied as a prelude to *in vivo* exposure; the goal is first to decrease fears of anxiety sensations, and then to eliminate fears of situations where these sensations have been elicited in the past.

Interoceptive exposure may offer a similar benefit to the treatment of PTSD by eliminating fears of anxiety symptoms and the salience of anxiety symptoms as cues for flashbacks or cognitive avoidance. The procedure can be used to aid initial exposure to trauma cues by reducing the perceived aversiveness of the anxiety sensations produced by exposure. That is, interoceptive exposure and cognitive restructuring (e.g., "This feeling of anxiety does not mean I am about to lose control or be attacked") can be used early in treatment to decrease fears of anxiety sensations and the likelihood that these sensations will serve as independent cues of the trauma. Feelings of derealization and dissociation can be induced successfully with interoceptive exposure methods (Miller, Brown, DiNardo, & Barlow, 1994), providing an opportunity for direct exposure to these symptoms in the treatment of PTSD. Although other clinical researchers (e.g., Resnick & Newton, 1992) have encouraged the use of interoceptive exposure in the treatment of PTSD, the additive value of the application of this technique awaits empirical validation. Nonetheless, this approach for treating the fear of anxiety symptoms, independent of the fear of environmental stimuli, has been applied successfully in the treatment of specific phobias (Zarate, Rapee, Craske, & Barlow, 1988).

BIOLOGIC MODELS REVISITED

LeDoux, Romanski, and Xagoraris (1989) have provided evidence that subcortical connections—specifically, thalamo-amygdala connections—may

mediate the acquisition of conditioned fear responses. LeDoux et al. conclude that once formed, these neuronal manifestations of fear reactions
are indelible. Nonetheless, it appears that the emotional and behavioral
responses to fear may be altered by the formation of an alternate thalamo-
cortico-amygdala pathway, which mediates the extinction of conditioned
fears.

Shalev, Rogel-Fuchs, and Pitman (1992) have applied these and other
observations to the conceptualization of PTSD and its treatment. They
suggest that the modification of conditioned emotional responses to trauma does not involve their structural undoing. Instead, control of conditioned responses is hypothesized to be the result of cortical inhibition of
their expression. Shalev et al.'s rendering of this observation conveys a
pessimistic message about the potential for effective treatment of PTSD.
They emphasize, as do LeDoux et al. (1989), that emotional memories
may last forever because of their "indelible" subcortical traces. This proposal
(but perhaps not the accompanying pessimism) is consistent with exposure-
based, information-processing accounts of PTSD treatment.

Exposure-based treatments do not operate by eliminating emotional
memories of the trauma, but by modifying the trauma network so that
current cues no longer have the capacity to activate aversive emotional
responses and avoidance behavior. Consistent with the notion of build-
ing an alternate thalamo-cortico-amygdala pathway, exposure seeks to reac-
tivate the trauma network and form new associations. These new
safety-related associations presumably allow a patient to discriminate
trauma-related cues from an actually dangerous situation. That is, exposure
trains patients to discriminate current environmental and interoceptive
cues from the original and dangerous trauma. The result of effective treatment is that innocuous cues associated with the trauma no longer auto-
matically induce anxiety and defensive behavior. In treatment, the exposure
and cognitive restructuring elements are repeated with enough emphasis
to help insure that current, safety-related associations are the more strongly
held ones. This emphasis on exposure and cognitive restructuring is in
direct opposition to the natural tendency toward avoidance behaviors.
Avoidance insulates patients from corrective experiences, helping ensure
that the only active associative pathway is the trauma-related thalamo-
amygdala connection.

One implication of this theoretical account is that treatment that does
not incorporate some form of exposure is likely to be inadequate; without
exposure to help develop an alternate thalamo-cortico-amygdala pathway,
the original thalamo-amygdala pathway may remain dominant. Although
the emotional and behavioral effects of limbic activation may be attenuated by pharmacologic or other interventions (e.g., symptom management
skills), an additional emphasis on naturalistic or therapist-assisted exposure
to trauma cues is theoretically important for full treatment of PTSD. This
proposition is consistent with evidence from the study of other anxiety
disorders (e.g., panic disorder with agoraphobia) indicating that anti-

exposure instructions attenuate the beneficial effects of pharmacotherapy (Telch, Agras, Taylor, Roth, & Gallen, 1985). Correspondingly, we suggest that pharmacologic interventions may help reestablish a sense of safety in patients with PTSD, but that the development of alternative associative pathways is what helps solidify this change. Treatment elements that are designed to maximize learning of alternative responses to trauma-related cues may provide the best means of achieving this goal.

COMBINED PHARMACOLOGIC AND COGNITIVE-BEHAVIORAL TREATMENT

In discussing pharmacologic treatment of PTSD, van der Kolk (1994) emphasizes that the goal is to help people live in the present by differentiating past traumatic experiences from current reality. He notes that symptoms of hyperarousal, intrusive reliving, dissociation, and numbing interfere with this process, and he suggests that medications "are often essential for patients to begin to achieve a sense of safety and perspective from which to approach their tasks" (p. 261). From a cognitive-behavioral perspective, both medications and affect regulation skills provide a means to control the number and aversiveness of symptoms, thereby facilitating the constructive application of exposure and cognitive restructuring procedures.

Control of depressed mood may be especially important. Depression has been found to attenuate the effectiveness of exposure treatment for anxiety disorders (Foa & Kozak, 1986). In particular, depression has been identified as interfering with the effects of habituation, leading to a relatively greater return of fear in subsequent exposure sessions (Salkovskis & Mills, 1994). Control of depressive symptoms with medication also appears to influence the modulation of negative cognitions. For example, studies of the pharmacologic treatment of depression indicate that antidepressants are effective in altering dysfunctional and catastrophic thinking styles and beliefs (Fava, Bless, Otto, Pava, & Rosenbaum, 1994; Otto, Pollack, Fava, Uccello, & Rosenbaum, 1995). Antidepressant agents with relatively higher serotonergic potential have been identified as having efficacy for obsessional states as well (Jenike et al., 1990). Hence, antidepressant treatment used as an adjunct to exposure-based therapies offers the potential of direct effects on negative thinking patterns in PTSD, as well as potential benefit from the treatment of any comorbid depressive conditions.

In our own experience, adjunctive pharmacologic treatments are very helpful for controlling affective disturbances while an exposure-based treatment is implemented. One crucial issue, however, for the combination of medications with exposure-based treatments is the potential for pharmacologic agents to interfere with the benefits of exposure. This question has been discussed in more detail in regard to panic disorder by Otto and Gould in Chapter 5 of this volume. However, at present there is only limited evidence for disruptive effects of combination treatments for panic disorder. There has been particular concern in this regard about the use of benzodiazepines, although it appears that any disruptive effects may be minimized or eliminated by short-term use and continued behavior therapy throughout a medication discontinuation period. Until similar questions for the treatment of PTSD are empirically tested, a conservative approach is to use medications during the initial treatment process to control the severity of anxiety and affective symptoms. Once acute exposure work has been completed, additional cognitive-behavioral interventions can be substituted for medications for longer-term management (e.g., as discussed for depression by Otto, Pava, & Sprich-Buckminster in Chapter 2, this volume).

OUTCOMES OF RANDOMIZED, CONTROLLED TRIALS

The paucity of well-controlled treatment trials for PTSD is exemplified by a recent review of treatment studies published or presented between 1987 and 1991 (Solomon, Gerrity, & Muff, 1992). Of the 255 studies identified, only 11 met criteria for a clear DSM-III or DSM-III-R diagnosis and random assignment to treatment conditions. The vast majority of studies were case reports, with relatively few open trials. Of the 11 controlled studies, 5 examined pharmacologic treatments and 6 examined exposure-based interventions. Four of the 11 examined group differences with fewer than 10 subjects per cell. Our own review of studies published or presented between 1991 and December 1994 identified five additional reports of randomized, controlled trials of PTSD with adequate posttreatment measures, although three of the five were extensions of earlier preliminary reports. Table 9.1 presents a summary of the outcomes achieved in these 16 reports. Because of the small sample sizes frequently used in these studies (resulting in low power to detect treatment differences), outcomes are presented as effect sizes, which reflect the improvement shown by the active treatment group(s) relative to the control group. For many of the individual interventions reviewed below, effect sizes are based on the findings from a very limited number of studies (e.g., a single study for many of the medications discussed below). As a result, the following analysis should not be approached as a meta-analysis of treatment outcome, but as an accounting of the small number of controlled trials currently available.

Effect sizes were calculated by subtracting the mean of the posttreatment experimental group(s) from the mean of the posttreatment control group, and then dividing by the standard deviation of the control group at posttreatment. Alternative procedures (Glass, McGaw, & Smith, 1981) were used if the means and standard deviations of a comparison group were not reported (e.g., if the t statistic was reported, the effect size was calculated as follows: $\text{ES} = t \sqrt{(1/N_t + 1/N_c)}$.

TABLE 9.1. Effect Size Analysis of Treatments for PTSD

Study	Treatment group [Control group]	Trauma type	% Male	Number refused/ excluded	Initial n	Dropout rate	Depression effect size	Anxiety effect size	PTSD effect size	Intrusion effect size	Avoidance effect size	Arousal effect size	Overall effect size
	Pharmacologic intervention studies												
Frank et al. (1988)	Imipramine (50–300 mg) (8 wk) Phenelzine (15–75 mg) [Placebo]	Vietnam veterans	100%	10	36	53%	0.48 0.43	0.52 0.5	0.42 1.12	0.45 1.24	0.24 0.60	NR NR	0.42 0.78
Shestatzky et al. (1988)	Phenelzine (45–75 mg) (5 wk) [Placebo]	Varied traumas	NR	NR	13	53.8%	-0.31	-0.04	-0.17	-0.22	-0.17	NR	-0.18
Reist et al. (1989)	Desipramine (100–200 mg) (4wk) [Placebo]	Vietnam veterans (1 WWII veteran)	100%	NR	27	33.3%	0.21	0.10	NR	0.05	0.15	NR	0.14
Braun et al. (1990)	Alprazolam (2.5–6 mg) (5 wk) [Placebo]	Varied traumas	100%	NR	16	37.5%	0.11	0.51	0.25	0.36	0.05	NR	0.24
Davidson et al. (1990)	Amitriptyline (50–300 mg)(8 wk) [Placebo]	Veterans (WWII, Korea, Vietnam)	100%	56	46	28.3%	1.09	0.92	1.0	1.0	1.23	NR	1.04
Kosten et al. (1991)	Imipramine (50–300 mg) (8wk) Phenelzine (15–75 mg) (8 wk) [Placebo]	Vietnam veterans	100%	42	60	50%	0.30 0.49	0.37 0.53	0.26 0.95	0.23 0.99	0.25 0.75		0.28 0.70
Davidson et al. (1993)	Amitriptyline (50–300 mg) (8wk) [Placebo]	Combat veterans	100%	NR	62	25.8%	0.83	0.66	0.37	NR	NR	NR	0.56
van der Kolk et al. (1994)	Fluoxetine (20–60 mg) (5 wk) [Placebo]	Varied traumas	65%	NR	64	26.6%	1.08	NR	0.77	0.46	0.32	0.61	0.65

(continued)

TABLE 9.1. (cont.)

Study	Treatment group [Control group]	Trauma type	% Male	Number refused/ excluded	Initial n	Dropout rate	Depression effect size	Anxiety effect size	PTSD effect size	Intrusion effect size	Avoidance effect size	Arousal effect size	Overall effect size
	Psychosocial intervention studies												
Peniston (1986)	Desensitization (48 30-min sessions) [No tx. control]	Vietnam veterans	100%	NR	16	0	NR	NR	NR	1.57	NR	NR	NR
Brom et al. (1989)	Desensitization (15 sessions) Hypnotherapy (14.4 sessions) Psychodynamic tx. (18.8 sessions) [Waiting list]	Varied traumas	21%	NR	112	11%	NR NR NR	0.24 0.25 0.62	1.22 0.84 0.91	1.19 0.81 0.61	1.13 0.87 0.98	NR NR NR	0.95 0.69 0.78
Cooper & Clum (1989)	Flooding & standard tx. (6–14 90-min sessions) [Standard tx.]	Vietnam veterans	100%	4	22	27.3%	0.41	0.46	0.83	NR	NR	NR	0.57
Keane et al. (1989)	Flooding (exposure) (14–16 90-min sessions) [Waiting list]	Vietnam veterans	100%	NR	24	0	0.81	0.86	0.85	NR	NR	NR	0.84
Boudewyns & Hyer (1990)	Flooding (exposure) (10–12 50-min sessions) [Indiv. psych. tx.]	Vietnam veterans	100%	NR	51	25.5%	NR	0.19	NR	NR	NR	0.03	—
Boudewyns et al. (1990)	Flooding (exposure) (up to 12 50-min sessions) [Indiv. psych. tx.]	Vietnam veterans	100%	NR	58	0	NR	NR	NR	NR	NR	NR	0.79
Foa et al. (1991)	Stress inoc. tx. (SIT) (9 biweekly 90-min sessions) Prolonged exp. (PE) Supp. counseling [Waiting list]	Rape victims	0%	11	55	18.2%	0.57 0.21 0.004	0.92 0.61 0.45	1.17 0.57 0.20	1.56 0.34 0.06	1.36 0.73 0.31	0.55 0.34 0.06	1.02 0.47 0.18
Foa et al. (1994)	Stress inoc. tx. (SIT) (9 biweekly 90-min sessions) Prolonged exp. (PE) SIT & PE [Waiting list]	Assault victims	0%	NR	76	NR	NR NR	NR NR	NR NR	NR NR	NR NR	NR NR	1.77 0.83 1.15

Whenever possible, effect sizes were computed for each of seven different symptom dimensions associated with PTSD: a total PTSD score, PTSD intrusion symptoms, PTSD avoidance symptoms, PTSD arousal symptoms, depression, anxiety, and an overall study effect size that encompassed all of these variables. Two psychosocial studies (Resick et al., 1988; Resick & Schnicke, 1992) used quasi-experimental designs, and hence were excluded from the effect size analysis. In all cases, overall PTSD effect sizes were determined from the best overall measure of PTSD symptomatology. Overall study effect sizes were determined by taking the average of the anxiety, depression, total PTSD, and PTSD symptom dimension effect sizes.

Pharmacologic Treatment Results

Eight reports of placebo-controlled drug trials were found in our search of the pharmacotherapy literature. In total, these studies examined the efficacy of six different agents: imipramine, desipramine, amitriptyline, phenelzine, fluoxetine, and alprazolam. Of these reports, two were preliminary accounts of later-published full data sets. Preliminary results of the full trial of Kosten et al. (1991) were presented by J. B. Frank, Kosten, Giller, and Dan (1988), and preliminary results of the full trial by Davidson et al. (1993) were presented by Davidson et al. (1990). All studies are presented in Table 9.1, but the summary effect sizes presented in the text below exclude the preliminary studies' results.

Each of the medication studies, with the exception of van der Kolk et al. (1994), utilized the Impact of Events Scale as an outcome measure for PTSD symptomatology; van der Kolk et al. used the Clinician Administered PTSD Scale. The total PTSD effect size, calculated from the total score for these measures, was 0.41 across all medication trials. The strongest PTSD symptom effect size was for fluoxetine at 0.77, followed in order by phenelzine at 0.39, TCAs at 0.32, and alprazolam at 0.25.

Across all medication trials, the effect size for intrusion symptoms was 0.41, and for avoidance symptoms it was 0.37. Effect sizes for intrusion symptoms varied little among the medications under study, ranging from 0.36 to 0.46 for each class of medication. There was greater variation for avoidance symptoms, with effect sizes ranging from 0.05 to 0.54, depending on the medication class being considered. TCAs had the highest effect size (0.54) for avoidance symptoms, followed by fluoxetine at 0.32, phenelzine at 0.29, and alprazolam at 0.05. Only van der Kolk et al. (1994) reported on arousal symptoms independent of general anxiety effects, finding an effect size of 0.61 for the influence of fluoxetine on these symptoms.

The overall depression effect size across all medications was 0.39. The largest effect size found was for fluoxetine at 1.08. The TCAs were the next most efficacious medications in relieving depression, with a depression effect size of 0.45. However, we found a large difference in effect sizes among the TCAs themselves, with depression effect sizes of 0.83, 0.30, and 0.21 for amitriptyline, imipramine, and desipramine, respectively. Phenelzine effect sizes varied widely, with one study reporting an effect size of 0.49 and one reporting an increase in depression (ES = − 0.31). Alprazolam was found to have the modest effect size of 0.11 for depression.

The overall anxiety effect size across all classes of medications was 0.36. The largest effect size was for alprazolam at 0.51, followed by the TCAs at 0.38 and phenelzine at 0.25. A specific measure of anxiety was not reported in the van der Kolk et al. (1994) study of fluoxetine. Again, when TCAs were considered independently, amitriptyline demonstrated the strongest effect at 0.66, followed by imipramine at 0.37 and by desipramine at 0.10.

Overall Study Effect Sizes: Pharmacotherapy

To provide an overall study effect size, individual effect sizes for depression, anxiety, overall PTSD symptom severity, and PTSD symptom dimension measures were averaged. Ancillary measures (e.g., psychosocial functioning or hostility) were not included in these calculations. Clinical global impression scores were also not included because of the variability of inclusion of this measure in the studies. The mean study effect size for pharmacologic treatments was 0.34. When considered more specifically by medication class, the SSRI fluoxetine demonstrated the largest overall study effect size at 0.65, followed by TCAs at 0.33, phenelzine at 0.26, and alprazolam at 0.24. On all measures, amitriptyline did better than the other TCAs. The overall effect size for amitriptyline was 0.56, whereas the overall effect sizes for imipramine and desipramine were 0.28 and 0.14, respectively.

In summary, the most consistently strong pharmacologic effect sizes in our analysis were those for fluoxetine and amitriptyline. Although there are no clear guidelines regarding adequate dosing for PTSD, the mean doses used in these studies fell within generally accepted levels of adequacy for the treatment of depression. Thus, differential adequacy of treatment trials (in terms of drug doses) is an unlikely explanation for differences in the effectiveness of the agents studied. In general, the efficacy of the antidepressant agents were in order of increasing serotonergic relative to noradrenergic potential; that is, more serotonin-specific agents were more effective. This finding, plus the promising data from open trials of SSRI agents, encourages further application of the more strongly serotonergic agents for PTSD. This conclusion should be considered tentative, however, because effect sizes for pharmacologic treatments were based for the most part on single controlled studies. Also, data for the treatment of obsessive–compulsive disorder indicate that the most extremely serotonergic agents are less efficacious than agents with a more mixed profile of serotonergic and noradrenergic action (Jenike et al., 1990). Hence, more balanced serotonergic–noradrenergic agents such as fluoxetine or clomipramine may offer the most promising pharmacologic alternative for conditions marked by anxiety, intrusive thoughts, and depressed mood.

Psychosocial Treatment Results

Eight reports of randomized, controlled trials for psychosocial interventions were found in our search of the psychologic literature. These studies examined the efficacy of the following types of therapeutic interventions: SIT, prolonged exposure, imaginal exposure (flooding), systematic desensitization, hypnotherapy, structured dynamic therapy, and supportive counseling. All studies compared a primary exposure-based treatment to a control (either no treatment or a supportive treatment). Two other treatments, Horowitz's (1986) brief dynamic treatment and hypnotherapy, were also based on exposure, but are reported separately. Supportive counseling was examined as an experimental condition in one study, and SIT was examined in two trials. Two studies (Boudewyns & Hyer, 1990; Boudewyns et al., 1990) presented results on patient samples drawn from a single, larger patient population; each study reported on different aspects of treatment outcome.

Comparisons among psychosocial treatments were made difficult by the wide variability in the types of outcome measures used. As can be seen in Table 9.1, psychosocial interventions frequently did not report on the individual symptom domains of PTSD, or results were not presented in a way that allowed effect size calculations. The controlled trials of psychosocial treatments were also characterized by less consistency in the outcome measures used, as compared to pharmacologic treatment studies. To maximize comparisons between psychosocial and pharmacologic treatments, measures for the effect size analysis were chosen to match or approximate the measure most often used in the pharmacologic studies (i.e., the Impact of Events Scale for intrusive and avoidant symptoms). Because of their idiosyncratic use and application, behavioral avoidance tests, personality measures, and social adjustment measures were excluded from analysis. Likewise, only state measures of anxiety were used. Results from all eight reports are presented in Table 9.1; however, the studies by Peniston (1986) and Boudewyns and Hyer (1990) were excluded from the effect size analysis because effect sizes could be calculated only for limited symptom domains.

The overall PTSD effect size across all psychologic treatment interventions was 0.82 relative to control conditions. The strongest overall PTSD effect size was found for SIT at 1.17, followed by specific exposure treatments and by structured dynamic interventions/hypnotherapy, both at a mean of 0.87; lastly, supportive counseling had an overall effect size of 0.20. For psychosocial interventions taken as a whole, the largest effect sizes were for avoidance (0.90) and intrusive (0.76) symptoms, followed by arousal symptoms (0.32).

The depression effect size across all psychosocial treatment studies was 0.40—a level almost identical to the average depression effect size for the pharmacologic treatments (0.39). SIT demonstrated the largest depression effect size at 0.57, followed by exposure-based treatments at 0.48 and by supportive counseling at 0.004. No effect size for brief dynamic treatment could be calculated from the results presented. A similar pattern of results was obtained for the anxiety effect size. The anxiety effect size was 0.55, with the strongest contributor being SIT at 0.92, followed by exposure-based treatments (0.54), and finally by structured dynamic therapy/hypnotherapy 0.44. Considered separately, a structured dynamic program of treatment and hypnotherapy had effect sizes of 0.62 and 0.25, respectively.

Overall Study Effect Sizes: Psychosocial Treatments

Unlike the individual effect size computations, our analysis of the overall study effect size included the most recent Foa et al. (1994) study, which provided a global outcome score for SIT without exposure, prolonged exposure alone, and the combination of these conditions compared to a waiting-list control condition. Considered independently, this study suggested greatest efficacy for the exposure condition, which had an effect size of 1.77. The combined treatment condition was not as effective as the exposure condition alone (ES = 1.15), perhaps as a function of an overloaded treatment itinerary for a short-term program. SIT was the least effective of the three active treatments (ES = 0.83). When the Foa et al. (1994) study was included, the overall study effect size for all psychosocial interventions was 0.84. Exposure treatments and SIT (without a specific exposure component) were approximately equal contributors, with overall effect sizes of 0.90 and 0.93, respectively. Somewhat smaller overall effect sizes were obtained for the short-term psychodynamic and hypnotherapy conditions (0.78 and 0.69, respectively). Supportive treatment alone was associated with a very modest effect size (0.18).

Comparison of Pharmacologic and Psychosocial Interventions

The grand average for all pharmacotherapy interventions was 0.41 for the PTSD effect size and 0.34 for the overall study effect size. In contrast, the overall PTSD effect size was 0.82 and the overall study effect size was 0.84 for all psychosocial interventions. Indeed, of psychosocial interventions, four of five exceeded the best overall effect size for pharmacotherapy (0.65 for fluoxetine). Hence, the available evidence is most strongly supportive of the efficacy of exposure-based and cognitive-behavioral treatments, followed by promising findings for fluoxetine.

Across the six double-blind, placebo-controlled pharmacologic studies, the overall dropout rate was 38% at study completion. The dropout rates across medication classes were quite similar, ranging from 36% to 43%. Alprazolam had the highest dropout rate for any one class of medication (43%). Studies of TCAs, phenelzine, and fluoxetine reported dropout rates of approximately 37%. Within the TCA class there was extreme variability, with desipramine and amitriptyline at fairly low rates (22% and 27%, respectively), and imipramine at a high of 61%. As is common for anxiety disorder treatment studies in general, attrition in psychosocial treatment studies of PTSD was less than that for pharmacotherapy studies. The overall dropout rate for psychosocial treatments ranged from 14% to 22%, with an average rate of 19%.

Refusal of treatment by patients with PTSD also appears to be a significant problem. Two psychosocial studies reported that an average of 17% of patients refused assignment to a treatment. Similarly, Foa et al. (1991) noted that approximately one-half of patients scheduled for initial evaluation did not come to their appointments.

A number of factors affecting the conclusions that can be drawn from our effect size analysis should be noted. For example, in two psychosocial treatment studies (Cooper & Clum, 1989; Keane et al., 1989), some patients received medications during the study period. Patients in several pharmacotherapy trials were also receiving medications other than those under study. For example, several subjects in the J. B. Frank et al. (1988), Kosten et al. (1991), and van der Kolk et al. (1994) studies were taking benzodiazepines. The vast majority of patients in pharmacologic trials were also receiving some sort of supportive psychotherapy, which may have contributed to the effect size (on the order of 0.18). Likewise, in several psychosocial studies using inpatients as subjects, patients tended to receive milieu therapy in addition to the interventions under study.

Studies also differed in terms of their gender ratios; type, severity, and duration of the patients' traumas; and comorbid disorders. These are potentially important differences, as Davidson et al. (1993) found that low combat exposure, good social/interpersonal adjustment, low depression scores, low PTSD symptom scores, low autonomic arousal, low anxiety scores, and low avoidance of trauma cues were each associated with a better outcome. Also, van der Kolk et al. (1994) reported much stronger effects for fluoxetine among their civilian patient sample from a trauma clinic than among their VA patient sample.

It is important to note that all pharmacologic studies were of single agents, and that few agents have shown efficacy across all three symptom dimensions in PTSD. Consequently, combination pharmacologic treatments (e.g., antidepressants and benzodiazepine treatment) may target a broader range of PTSD symptoms. Likewise, outcome for both pharmacologic and exposure-based programs was examined following a very brief course of treatment; prolonged treatment (allowing for additional psychosocial interventions) may substantially improve outcome.

NOVEL TECHNIQUES: THE CURRENT STATUS OF EYE MOVEMENT DESENSITIZATION AND REPROCESSING

Eye movement desensitization and reprocessing (EMDR) is a new therapeutic technique that combines imaginal exposure with a procedure involving rapid eye movements. EMDR is especially noteworthy for three reasons: (1) the introduction of a novel and interesting exposure procedure, (2) the potential for effective treatment, and (3) its rapid dissemination and the attention it has captured in the popular and professional media. In professional publications, much of this attention has been devoted to the lack of empirical validation for the procedure, including three reviews of the methodologic shortcomings of early trials and the absence of empirical support in controlled studies (Acierno, Hersen, Van Hasselt, Tremont, & Meuser, 1994; Herbert & Meuser, 1992; Lohr, Kleinknecht, Conley, & dal Cerro, 1992). These concerns have not precluded EMDR from emerging into the national spotlight, including attention in a recent television newsmagazine.

The genesis for the EMDR procedure was Shapiro's (1989) discovery that her negative emotional responses to disturbing memories and thoughts were attenuated by rapid back-and-forth eye movements. Excitement about this discovery led her to combine eye movement techniques and imaginal exposure in the treatment of several of her patients. She found that their trauma-related anxiety appeared to be rapidly reduced by these procedures. The eye movement techniques were further standardized with preparatory experiences and debriefing procedures, and the full EMDR protocol is now available in a comprehensive training program. However, this training has been limited to expensive workshops with restrictive pledges for nondissemination—a procedure that has drawn criticism from clinical researchers (Baer et al., 1992; Marifiote, 1992). Nonetheless, general information on the EMDR procedure is provided in a report of an early open trial of the procedure (Shapiro, 1989).

According to this report, the imaginal exposure component of EMDR appears to correspond well with other exposure-based treatment. An affect-laden image of the traumatic experience or phobic event is constructed, along with a summary statement that best characterizes the memory (e.g., "I may be killed"); subjective distress is rated; and an alternative, positive characterizing statement is then formulated (e.g., "I am going to live"). The eye movement procedure is then initiated, with the patient attending to the image of the trauma and the negative statement. The patient is asked to visually track the therapist's finger as it is moved rhythmically from side to side across the patient's field of vision, approximately 12 to 14 inches from the patient's face. At the end of 12 to 24 repetitions, patients are instructed to note and report on their current emotional state, as well as other thoughts and emotions that may have emerged. The procedure is repeated until a significant reduction in distress is achieved (often 3 to 15 sets of the eye movements), with a final review of the original image and cognitive summary statements.

In a review of many of the EMDR studies published to date, Acierno et al. (1994) identified eight uncontrolled case studies describing over 100 patients treated with EMDR. Although the results generally support the efficacy of EMDR, serious methodologic shortcomings characterize all of these reports: the absence of validated assessment instruments, lack of control for random treatment factors, the potential for unintentional experimenter bias and/or experimenter demand effects, and the uncontrolled inclusion of other cognitive-behavioral interventions.

In contrast to the open trials, controlled studies have provided little evidence for the efficacy of EMDR over other exposure methods. For example, Boudewyns, Stwertka, Hyer, Albrecht, and Sperr (1993) found that significant differences between EMDR and a control treatment (imaginal exposure and milieu therapy) for combat veterans were limited to in-session distress ratings made by the patients or therapists, whereas no treatment differences were evident on physiologic measures or standardized assessment instruments. Jensen (1994) found that EMDR was effective for reducing in-session subjective anxiety but not for improving PTSD symptoms in combat veterans. Results such as these led Acierno et al. (1994) to conclude that although the earlier trials of EMDR encourage further study, the current dissemination of EMDR is not in accordance with standards in the field for validation of behavioral techniques.

What then is the lure of EMDR, given its unimpressive showing in well-controlled studies? Exposure treatment for PTSD is an emotionally difficult process for both patients and therapists, because of the significant negative affect induced during therapy. As such, any procedure that offers a means to shorten the treatment process affords both therapists and patients the hope of escaping from some of the aversive aspects of exposure treatment. The interest in EMDR may reflect this hope, and one potential benefit is that EMDR may encourage nonbehavioral clinicians to embark on an exposure-based treatment for trauma-related disorders and phobias (see Litz, Blake, Gerardi, & Keane, 1990, regarding the low rates for the use of exposure). Of course, this benefit may be outweighed if clinicians seek training only in EMDR, rather than learning much more strongly validated cognitive-behavioral interventions (Acierno et al., 1994).

Although there is not yet evidence that EMDR techniques should replace other programs of exposure and cognitive restructuring for PTSD, eye movement procedures may still have a place in a clinician's armamentarium of exposure techniques. In our clinical application of an eye movement procedure similar to EMDR (we have not had the benefit of formal training in EMDR), we have observed an acute decrease in the severity of anxiety and dissociation induced by imaginal exposure. That is, patients report that their traumatic images disappear and/or that feelings of dissociation decrease as they attend to the eye movement procedure. This observation coincides with the finding in a controlled study that EMDR decreased in-session anxiety associated with imaginal exposure to traumatic memories (Jensen, 1994). We believe that these effects may be the result of the attentional demands of the eye movement procedure; tracking the therapist's rapidly moving finger appears to require enough attention that other ongoing information processing is disrupted. This occurs in the absence of instructions for the patient to terminate the aversive image. As such, the procedure allows temporary escape from the aversive image without efforts at avoidance. Any other act requiring concentration may lead to similar benefit. Consistent with this hypothesis, there is preliminary evidence that alternative procedures requiring rapid shifting of attention (e.g., an auditory attention procedure) may also benefit the exposure process (Cocco & Sharpe, 1994). There is also preliminary evidence suggesting that eye movement procedures interfere with ongoing emotional processing (Tallis & Smith, 1994). From this perspective, EMDR may have specific value in terminating activation of the trauma memory network by competing for the cognitive resources necessary to keep the image active. In some cases, the cessation of the image and of the associated emotional distress appears to provide patients with a sense of relief and control over the exposure process.

The acute reduction of anxiety within the context of exposure has the potential to provide the patient with an experience wherein the emotional response to the trauma is indeed manageable and modifiable. Similarly, Dyck (1993) has suggested that a cessation of anxiety provided by a distraction task (the EMDR procedure) helps interrupt self-perpetuating cycles of trauma-relevant thoughts and intense anxiety, thereby helping extinguish the fear response. From this perspective, Shapiro's discovery may not represent a novel exposure procedure, but rather a novel and nonverbal method of providing increased controllability of the exposure process, which may facilitate the rapidity by which exposure sessions can be utilized. These notions are consistent with the observation that the initial two sessions of EMDR provide the most benefit, with few incremental benefits as EMDR is repeated (Forbes, Creamer, & Rycroft, 1994).

Given the current state of the literature, a conservative conclusion is that EMDR appears to reduce acute anxiety associated with exposure, but may offer little clinical benefit over other exposure procedures. We have provided an alternative explanation for the EMDR effect, but this interpretation awaits additional empirical validation. Until additional supporting evidence for EDMR is found, we recommend that it be considered a simple clinical adjunct to better-supported exposure procedures.

MAXIMIZING TREATMENT EFFECTIVENESS

Although the data are limited by the paucity of controlled studies conducted to date, our review of the pharmacologic treatment literature suggests that agents with greater serotonergic relative to noradrenergic potential are associated with stronger effects on PTSD symptoms. Hence, patients failing to respond to other agents may benefit from the substitution (or in some cases the addition) of an antidepressant with stronger serotonergic action. The strongest treatment effects, however, were found to be associated with exposure-based interventions. The available evidence leads us to recommend that clinicians always include a program of exposure and cognitive restructuring in their program of treatment for PTSD.

Current research suggests that clinicians have a fairly broad degree of freedom in choosing the type of exposure and cognitive interventions to apply. There is evidence supporting the efficacy of exposure delivered in imaginal, *in vivo*, hypnotic, or structured dynamic therapy formats. Nonetheless, numerous studies with clinical and analogue populations suggest several procedures for maximizing exposure effectiveness. As discussed above, these include insuring that the exposure is of sufficient duration, includes both stimulus and response (emotional) elements, is attended to by the patient, and includes a range of emotions in addition to fear (e.g., anger and disgust) that may be associated with trauma cues. Finally, given the diversity of exposure methods available (ranging from discussions of the trauma and writing assignments to *in vivo* exposure and eye movement procedures), the clinician has a range of methods to insure full, stepwise exposure without overemphasis on a particular strategy or rate of exposure. As emphasized by Barlow (1988), there appears to be little reason to substitute intensely aversive procedures aimed at emotional abreaction for a more gradually increasing hierarchy of exposure intensity.

We join other clinical researchers (Jones & Barlow, 1990; Resnick & Newton, 1992) in emphasizing that advances in the conceptualization and treatment of panic disorder may be applied fruitfully to PTSD. In particular, we have emphasized the potential importance of interoceptive exposure in decreasing anxiogenic interpretations of symptoms of autonomic arousal and anxiety, and in aiding patients in tolerating the symptoms that may accompany initial exposure sessions. In our behavior therapy clinic, interoceptive exposure is being more generally used as an initial element of treatment for PTSD. In particular, interoceptive exposure is used to teach individuals about the nature of anxiety symptoms that may be experienced, and to offer initial training in becoming comfortable with these symptoms if they should arise. Once fears and misinterpretations of these symptoms have been minimized, treatment proceeds to exposure and cognitive restructuring around the trauma cues themselves.

Informational and cognitive restructuring interventions are other elements of cognitive-behavioral treatment of panic disorder that may play an especially important role in PTSD. We recommend devoting time in initial sessions to helping patients with PTSD understand why emotional responses to trauma persist under conditions of continued avoidance. This discussion of the nature of the enduring emotional response to trauma cues (in the absence of actual danger) sets the stage for the cognitive restructuring and exposure interventions to follow. In particular, it provides patients with a basis for discriminating memories and events (trauma cues) that *feel* dangerous from those that actually are dangerous. In addition, patients are provided with information on the types of emotional responses and associated cognitions that are likely to be evoked during exposure, in order to help prevent misinterpretations of symptoms (particularly misinterpretations of anxiety symptoms and/or flashbacks).

The value of these informational interventions has been underscored by reports from our patients. At times, patients have received years of previous treatment without having been given an understanding of the nature and varying content of flashbacks. Consequently, with each flashback these patients feared loss of control, and this fear contributed to panic and further attempts at cognitive avoidance. Informational interventions have been extremely helpful for eliminating these patterns. Cognitive restructuring interventions have then been targeted toward helping patients reestablish a sense of safety and control in their world, while exposure interventions have been used to aid this process and help decrease emotional reactivity to trauma cues.

In cases where entry into exposure treatment has been greatly delayed (as is the case with many patients who experienced childhood trauma), characteristic patterns of cognitive and behavioral avoidance may have become well entrenched. Years of rehearsal of avoidance strategies may significantly lengthen the course of treatment, requiring both patient and therapist to struggle with multiple layers of avoidance responses to trauma and other emotional cues. Well-rehearsed avoidance strategies may also dominate behavior to such an extent that they hinder the development or expression of skills in social problem solving, assertiveness, or emotional regulation. Under these conditions, treatment will necessarily require additional attention to improving these skills, particularly under conditions of fear or cue exposure (where avoidance strategies were originally learned). Skill training, and then rehearsal under conditions of trauma-related cue exposure, offer patients the opportunity to develop and strengthen these adaptive skills.

For all of these procedures, attempts to maximize or rebuild social support networks may also be of use (Barlow, 1988). As noted at the outset of this chapter, low social support has been found to be associated with the emergence of greater trauma symptoms. The inclusion of couple sessions designed to educate significant others about the range of symptoms and the nature of avoidance patterns in PTSD has the potential to improve a patient's social support. These interventions may be especially important, given that many patients have delayed entering treatment, thereby allowing patterns of avoidance of trauma cues to become solidified within their family and social lives. Instruction of significant others in the rationale for and course of treatment also has the potential to increase support for and compliance with treatment.

REFERENCES

Acierno, R., Hersen, M., Van Hasselt, V. B., Tremont, G., & Meuser, K. T. (1994). Review of the validation and dissemination of eye-movement desensitization and reprocessing: A scientific and ethical dilemma. *Clinical Psychology Review, 14,* 287–299.

American Psychiatric Association. (1987). *Diagnostic and statistical manual of mental disorders* (3rd ed., rev.). Washington, DC: Author.

American Psychiatric Association (1994). *Diagnostic and statistical manual of mental disorders* (4th ed.). Washington, DC: Author.

Anisman, H. L., Ritch, M., & Sklar, L. S. (1981). Noradrenergic and dopaminergic interaction in escape behavior. *Psychopharmacology, 74,* 263–268.

Anisman, H. L., & Sklar, L. S. (1979). Catecholamine depletion in mice upon exposure to stress: Mediation of the escape deficits reduced by inescapable shock. *Journal of Comparative and Physiological Psychology, 93,* 610–625.

Baer, L., Hurley, J. D., Minichiello, W. E., Ott, B. D., Penzel, F., & Ricciardi, J. (1992). EMDR workshop: Disturbing issues? *The Behavior Therapist, 15,* 110–111.

Ballenger, J.C., Burrows, G.D., Dupont, R.L., Lesser, I. M., Notes, R., Pecknold, J. C., Rifkin, A., & Swinson, R. P. (1988). Alprazolam in panic disorder and agoraphobia: Results from a multicenter trial. I. Efficacy in short-term treatment. *Archives of General Psychiatry, 45,* 413–422.

Barlow, D. H. (1988). *Anxiety and its disorders: The nature and treatment of anxiety and panic.* New York: Guilford Press.

Black, D. W., Wesner, R., Bowers, W., & Gabel, J. (1993). A comparison of fluvoxamine, cognitive therapy, and placebo in the treatment of panic disorder. *Archives of General Psychiatry, 50,* 44–50.

Bleich, A., Siegel, B., Garb, R., & Lerer, B. (1986). Post-traumatic stress disorder following combat exposure: Clinical features and psychopharmacological treatment. *British Journal of Psychiatry, 149,* 365–369.

Birkhimer, L., DeVane, C., & Muniz, C. (1985). Posttraumatic stress disorder: Characteristics and pharmacological response in the veteran population. *Comprehensive Psychiatry, 26,* 304–310.

Boehnlein, J., Kinzie, J., Ben, R., & Flech, J. (1985). One year follow-up study of posttraumatic stress disorder among survivors of Cambodian concentration camps. *American Journal of Psychiatry, 142,* 956–959.

Boudewyns, P. A., & Hyer, L. (1990). Physiological response to combat memories and preliminary treatment outcome in Vietnam veteran PTSD patients treated with direct therapeutic exposure. *Behavior Therapy, 21,* 63–87.

Boudewyns, P. A., Hyer, L., Woods, M. G., Harrison, W. R., & McCranie, E. (1990). PTSD among Vietnam veterans: An early look at treatment outcome using direct therapeutic exposure. *Journal of Traumatic Stress, 3,* 359–368.

Boudewyns, P. A., Stwertka, S. A., Hyer, L. A., Albrecht, J. W., & Sperr, E. V. (1993). Eye movement desensitization for PTSD of combat: A treatment outcome pilot study. *The Behavior Therapist, 16,* 29–33.

Braun, P., Greenberg, D., Dasberg, H., & Lerer, B. (1990). Core symptoms of posttraumatic stress disorder unimproved by alprazolam treatment. *Journal of Clinical Psychiatry, 51,* 236–238.

Breslau, N., Davis, G. C., Andreski, P., & Peterson, E. (1991). Traumatic events and post-traumatic stress disorder in an urban population of young adults. *Archives of General Psychiatry, 48,* 216–222.

Brom, D., Kleber, R. J., & Defares, P. B. (1989). Brief psychotherapy for posttraumatic stress disorders. *Journal of Consulting and Clinical Psychology, 57,* 607–612.

Burnam, M. A., Stein, J. A., Golding, J. M., Siegel, J. M., Sorenson, S. B., Forsythe, A. B., & Telles, C. A. (1988). Sexual assault and mental disorders in a community population. *Journal of Consulting and Clinical Psychology, 56,* 843–850.

Burstein, A. (1984). Treatment of post-traumatic stress disorder with imipramine. *Psychosomatics, 25,* 681–686.

Cahil, L., Prins, B., Weber, M., & McGaugh, J. L. (1994). β-Adrenergic activation and memory for emotional events. *Nature, 371,* 702–704.

Calhoun, K. S., & Resick, P. A. (1993). Post-traumatic stress disorder. In D. H. Barlow (Ed.), *Clinical handbook of psychological disorders: A step-by-step treatment manual* (2nd ed., pp. 48–98). New York: Guilford Press.

Chen, C.-J. (1991). The obsessive quality and clomipramine treatment in PTSD. *American Journal of Psychiatry, 148,* 1087–1088.

Clark, D. M. (1986). A cognitive approach to panic. *Behaviour Research and Therapy, 24,* 461–470.

Cocco, N., & Sharpe, L. (1994). An auditory variant of eye movement desensitization in a case of childhood post-traumatic stress disorder. *Journal of Behavior Therapy and Experimental Psychiatry, 24,* 373–377.

Cooper, N. A., & Clum, G. A. (1989). Imaginal flooding as a supplementary treatment for PTSD in combat veterans: A controlled study. *Behavior Therapy, 20,* 381–391.

Davidson, J. R. T., & Foa, E. B. (1991). Diagnostic issues in posttraumatic stress disorder: Considerations for the DSM-IV. *Journal of Abnormal Psychology, 100,* 346–355.

Davidson, J. R. T., Hughes, D., Blazer, D. G., & George, L. K. (1991a). Posttraumatic stress disorder in the community: An epidemiological study. *Psychological Medicine, 21,* 713–721.

Davidson, J. R. T., Kudler, H. S., Saunders, W. B., Erickson, L., Smith, R. D., Stein, R. M., Lipper, S., Hammett, E. B., Mahorney, S. L., & Cavenar, J. O., Jr. (1993). Predicting response to amitriptyline in posttraumatic stress disorder. *American Journal of Psychiatry, 150,* 1024–1029.

Davidson, J. R. T., Kudler, H., Smith, R., Mahorney, S. L., Lipper, S., Hammett, E., Saunders, W. B., & Cavenar, J. O., Jr. (1990). Treatment of posttraumatic stress disorder with amitriptyline and placebo. *Archives of General Psychiatry, 47,* 259–266.

Davidson, J. R. T., Roth, S., & Newman, E. (1991b). Fluoxetine in post-traumatic stress disorder. *Journal of Traumatic Stress, 4,* 419–423.

Davidson, J. R. T., Walker, J. I., & Kilts, C. D. (1987). A pilot study of phenelzine in post-traumatic stress disorder. *British Journal of Psychiatry, 130,* 252–255.

Dyck, M. J. (1993). A proposal for a conditioning model of eye movement desensitization treatment for posttraumatic stress disorder. *Journal of Behavior Therapy and Experimental Psychiatry, 24,* 201–210.

Fairbank, J. A., Gross, R. T., & Keane, T. M. (1983). Treatment of posttraumatic stress disorder: Evaluating outcome with a behavioral code. *Behavior Modification, 7,* 557–568.

Falcon, S., Ryan, C., Chamberlain, K., & Curtis, G. (1985). Tricyclics: Possible treatment for posttraumatic stress disorder. *Journal of Clinical Psychiatry, 46,* 385–388.

Fava, M., Bless, E., Otto, M. W., Pava, J. A., & Rosenbaum, J. F. (1994). Dysfunctional attitudes in major depression: Changes with pharmacotherapy. *Journal of Nervous and Mental Disease, 182,* 45–49.

Fava, M., Rosenbaum, J. F., Pava, J. A., McCarthy, M. K, Steingard, R. J., & Bouffides, M. A. (1993). Anger attacks in unipolar depression: Part 1. Clinical correlates and response to fluoxetine treatment. *American Journal of Psychiatry, 150,* 1158–1163.

Fesler, F. A. (1991). Valproate in combat-related posttraumatic stress disorder. *Journal of Clinical Psychiatry, 52,* 361–364.

Foa, E. B., Freund, B., Hembree, E., Dancu, C. V., Franklin, M. E., Perry, K. J., Riggs, D. S., & Molnar, C. (1994, November). *Efficacy of short-term behavioral treatment of PTSD in sexual and nonsexual assault victims.* Paper presented at the 28th Annual Convention of the Association for Advancement of Behavior Therapy, San Diego, CA.

Foa, E. B., & Kozak, M. J. (1986). Emotional processing of fear: Exposure to corrective information. *Psychological Bulletin, 99,* 20–35.

Foa, E. B., Rothbaum, B. O., Riggs, D. S., & Murdock, T. B. (1991). Treatment of posttraumatic stress disorder in rape victims: A comparison between cognitive-behavioral procedures and counseling. *Journal of Consulting and Clinical Psychology, 59,* 715–723.

Foa, E. B., Steketee, G., & Rothbaum, B. O. (1989). Behavioral/cognitive conceptualizations of post-traumatic stress disorder. *Behavior Therapy, 20,* 155–176.

Fontaine, R., & Chouinard, G. (1985). Antiobsessive effect of fluoxetine. *American Journal of Psychiatry, 142,* 989.

Forbes, D., Creamer, M., & Rycroft, P. (1994). Eye movement desensitization and reprocessing in posttraumatic stress disorder: A pilot study using assessment measures. *Journal of Behavior Therapy and Experimental Psychiatry, 25,* 113–120.

Foy, D. W., Carroll, E. M., & Donahoe, C. P., Jr. (1987). Etiological factors in the development of PTSD in clinical samples of Vietnam combat veterans. *Journal of Clinical Psychology, 43,* 17–27.

Frank, E., Anderson, B., Stewart, B. D., Dancu, C., Hughes, C., & West, D. (1988). Efficacy of cognitive behavior therapy and systematic desensitization in the treatment of rape trauma. *Behavior Therapy, 19,* 403–420.

Frank, J. B., Kosten, T. R., Giller, E. L., & Dan, E. (1988). A randomized clinical trial of phenelzine and imipramine for post traumatic stress disorder. *American Journal of Psychiatry, 145,* 1289–1291.

Friedman, M. J. (1988). Toward rational pharmacotherapy for posttraumatic stress disorder: An interim report. *American Journal of Psychiatry, 145,* 281–285.

Glass, G. V., McGaw, B., & Smith, M. L. (1981). *Meta-analysis in social research.* Beverly Hills, CA: Sage.

Greendyke, R. M., Kanter, D. R., Schuster, D. B., Verstreate, S., & Wooton, J. (1986). Propranolol treatment of assaultive patients with organic brain disease. *Journal of Nervous and Mental Disease, 174,* 290–294.

Helzer, J. E., Robins, L. N., & McEvoy, L. (1987). Post-traumatic stress disorder in the general population: Findings of the Epidemiologic Catchment Area survey. *New England Journal of Medicine, 317,* 1630–1634.

Herbert, J. D., & Meuser, K. T. (1992). Eye movement desensitization: A critique of the evidence. *Journal of Behavior Therapy and Experimental Psychiatry, 23,* 169–174.

Hogben, G., & Cornfield, R. (1981). Treatment of traumatic war neuroses with phenelzine. *Archives of General Psychiatry, 38,* 440–445.

Horowitz, M. (1986). *Stress response syndromes* (2nd ed.) New York: Jason Aronson.

Hyman, S. E., & Nestler, E. J. (1993). *The molecular foundations of psychiatry.* Washington, DC: American Psychiatric Press.

Jenike, M. A., Hyman, S., Baer, L., Holland, A., Minichiello, W. E., Buttolph, L., Summergrad, P., Seymour, R., & Ricciardi, J. (1990). A controlled trial of fluvoxamine in obsessive–compulsive disorder: Implications for a serotonergic theory. *American Journal of Psychiatry, 147,* 1209–1215.

Jensen, J. A. (1994). An investigation of eye movement desensitization and reprocessing (EMD/R) as a treatment for posttraumatic stress disorder (PTSD) symptoms of Vietnam combat veterans. *Behavior Therapy, 25,* 311–325.

Jones, J. C., & Barlow, D. H. (1990). The etiology of posttraumatic stress disorder. *Clinical Psychology Review, 10,* 299–328.

Keane, T. M., Fairbank, J. A., Caddell, J. M., & Zimering, R. T. (1989). Implosive (flooding) therapy reduces symptoms of PTSD in Vietnam combat veterans. *Behavior Therapy, 20,* 245–260.

Keane, T. M., Fairbank, J. A., Caddell, J. M., Zimering, R. T., & Bender, M. E. (1985). A behavioral approach to assessing and treating posttraumatic stress disorder in Vietnam veterans. In C. R. Figley (Ed.), *Trauma and its wake: The study and treatment of post-traumatic stress disorder* (pp. 257–294). New York: Brunner/Mazel.

Keane, T. M., & Kaloupek, D. G. (1982). Imaginal flooding in the treatment of posttraumatic stress disorder. *Journal of Consulting and Clinical Psychology, 50,* 138–140.

Keane, T. M., Litz, B. T., & Blake, D. D. (1990). Post-traumatic stress disorder in adulthood. In M. Hersen & C. G. Last (Eds.), *Handbook of child and adult psychopathology: A longitudinal perspective* (pp. 275–291). Elmsford, NY: Pergamon Press.

Keane, T. M., & Wolfe, J. (1990). Comorbidity in post-traumatic stress disorder: An analysis of community and clinical studies. *Journal of Applied Social Psychology, 20,* 1776–1788.

Kilpatrick, D. G., & Calhoun, K. S. (1988). Early behavioral treatment for rape trauma: Efficacy or artifact? *Behavior Therapy, 19,* 421–427.

Kilpatrick, D. G., Saunders, B. E., Amick-McMullan, A., Best, C. L., Veronen, L. J., & Resnick, H. S. (1989). Victim and crime factors associated with the development of crime-related post-traumatic stress disorder. *Behavior Therapy, 20,* 199–214.

Kilpatrick, D. G., Saunders, B. E., Veronen, L. J., Best, C. L., & Von, J. M. (1987). Criminal victimization: Lifetime prevalence, reporting to police, and psychological impact. *Crime and Delinquency, 33,* 479–489.

Kinzie, J. D., & Leung, P. (1989). Clonidine in Cambodian patients with post-traumatic stress disorder. *Journal of Nervous and Mental Disease, 177,* 546–550.

Kline, N. A., Dow, B. M., Brown, S. A., & Matloff, J. L. (1994). Sertraline efficacy in depressed combat veterans with posttraumatic stress disorder. *American Journal of Psychiatry, 151,* 621.

Kolb, L. C. (1987). A neuropsychological hypothesis explaining posttraumatic stress disorder. *American Journal of Psychiatry, 144,* 989–995.

Kolb, L. C., Burris, B., & Griffiths, S. (1984). Propranolol and clonidine in the treatment of post-traumatic stress disorders of war. In B. van der Kolk (Ed.), *Post-traumatic stress disorder: Psychological and biological sequelae* (pp. 97–105). Washington, DC: American Psychiatric Press.

Kosten, T. R., Frank, J. B., Dan, E., McDougle, C. J., & Giller, E. L. (1991). Pharmacotherapy for posttraumatic stress disorder using phenelzine or imipramine. *Journal of Nervous and Mental Disease, 179,* 366–370.

Kulka, R. A., Schlenger, W. E., Fairbank, J. A., Jordan, B. K., Hough, R. L., Marmar, C. R., & Weiss, D. S. (1991). Assessment of posttraumatic stress disorder in the community: Prospects and pitfalls from recent studies of Vietnam veterans. *Psychological Assessment, 3,* 547–560.

Kushner, M. G., Riggs, D. S., Foa, E. B., & Miller, S. M. (1992). Perceived controllability and the development of posttraumatic stress disorder (PTSD) in crime victims. *Behaviour Research and Therapy, 31,* 105–110.

Lang, P. J. (1977). Imagery in therapy: An information processing analysis of fear. *Behavior Therapy, 8,* 862–886.

LeDoux, J. E., Romanski, L., & Xagoraris, A. (1989). Indelibility of subcortical emotional memories. *Journal of Cognitive Neuroscience, 1,* 238–243.

Liebowitz, M. R., Gorman, J. M., Fyer, A. J., & Klein, D. F. (1985). Social phobia: Review of a neglected anxiety disorder. *Archives of General Psychiatry, 42,* 729–736.

Lipper, S., Davidson, J. R. T., Grady, T. A., Tana, A., Edinger, J. D., Hammett, E. B., Mahorney, S. L., & Cavenar, J. O. (1986). Preliminary study of carbamazepine in post-traumatic stress disorder. *Psychosomatics, 27,* 849–853.

Litz, B. T., Blake, D. D., Gerardi, R. G., & Keane, T. M. (1990). Decision making guidelines for the the use of direct therapeutic exposure in the treatment of post-traumatic stress disorder. *The Behavior Therapist, 13,* 91–93.

Lohr, J. M., Kleinknecht, R. A., Conley, A. T., & dal Cerro, S. (1992). A methodological critique of the current status of eye movement desensitization (EMD). *Journal of Behavior Therapy and Experimental Psychiatry, 23,* 159–167.

Long, N., Chamberlain, K., & Vincent, C. (1994). Effect of the Gulf War on reactivation of adverse combat-related memories in Vietnam veterans. *Journal of Clinical Psychology, 50,* 138–144.

Marafiote, R. (1992). On EMDR and controlled outcome studies. *The Behavior Therapist, 17,* 22–24.

March, J. (1992). Fluoxetine and fluvoxamine in PTSD. *American Journal of Psychiatry, 149,* 413.

McDougle, C. J., Southwick, S. M., Charney, D. S., & St. James, R. L. (1991). An open trial of fluoxetine in the treatment of posttraumatic stress disorder. *Journal of Clinical Psychopharmacology, 11,* 325–327.

Miller, P. P., Brown, T. A., DiNardo, P. A., & Barlow, D. H. (1994). The experimental induction of depersonalization and derealization in panic disorder and nonanxious subjects. *Behaviour Research and Therapy, 32,* 511–519.

Mowrer, O. H. (1960). *Learning theory and behavior.* New York: Wiley.

Otto, M. W., Pollack, M. H., Fava, M., Uccello, R., & Rosenbaum, J. F. (1995). Elevated Anxiety Sensitivity Index scores in patients with major depression: Correlates and changes with antidepressant treatment. *Journal of Anxiety Disorders, 9,* 117–123.

Peniston, E. G. (1986). EMG biofeedback-assisted desensitization treatment for Vietnam combat veterans post-traumatic stress disorder. *Clinical Biofeedback and Health, 9,* 35–41.

Perls, F. S. (1969). *Gestalt therapy verbatim.* Moab, UT: Real People Press.

Peterson, R. A., & Reiss, S. (1992). *Anxiety Sensitivity Index revised test manual.* Worthington, OH: International Diagnostic Systems.

Pitman, R. K., Orr, S. P., Forgue, D. F., de Jong, J. B., & Claiborn, J. M. (1987). Psychophysiologic assessment of posttraumatic stress disorder imagery in Vietnam combat veterans. *Archives of General Psychiatry, 44,* 970–975.

Post, R. M., Rubinow, D. R., & Ballenger, J. C. (1984). Conditioning, sensitization and kindling: Implications for the course of affective illness. In R. M. Post & J. C. Ballenger (Eds.), *Neurobiology of mood disorders* (pp. 432–466). Baltimore: Williams & Wilkins.

Post, R. M., & Weiss, S. R. B. (1989). Sensitization, kindling and anticonvulsants in mania. *Journal of Clinical Psychiatry, 50*(12, Suppl.), 23–30.

Rainey, J. M., Aleem, A., Ortiz, A., Yragani, V., Pohl, R., & Berchou, R. (1987). A laboratory procedure for the induction of flashbacks. *American Journal of Psychiatry, 144,* 1317–1319.

Ratey, J. J., Sorgi, P., O'Driscoll, G. A., Sands, S., Daehler, M. L., Fletcher, J.R., Kadish, W., Spruiell, G., Polakoff, S., Lindem, K.J., Bemporad, J.R., Richardson, L., & Rosenfeld, B. (1992). Nadolol to treat aggression and psychiatric symptomatology in chronic psychiatric inpatients: A double-blind, placebo-controlled study. *Journal of Clinical Psychiatry, 53,* 41–46.

Reist, C., Kauffman, C. D., & Haier, R. J. (1989). A controlled trial of desipramine in 18 men with post-traumatic stress disorder. *American Journal of Psychiatry, 146,* 513–516.

Resick, P. A., Jordan, C. G., Girelli, S. A., Hutter, C. K., & Marhoefer-Dvorak, S. (1988). A comparative outcome study of behavioral group therapy for sexual assault victims. *Behavior Therapy, 19,* 385–401.

Resick, P. A., & Schnicke, M. K. (1992). Cognitive processing therapy for sexual assault victims. *Journal of Consulting and Clinical Psychology, 60,* 748–756.

Resick, P. A., & Schnicke, M. K. (1993). *Cognitive processing therapy for rape victims: A treatment manual.* Newbury Park, CA: Sage.

Resnick, H. S., & Newton, T. (1992). Assessment and treatment of post-traumatic stress disorder in adult survivors of sexual assault. In D. W. Foy (Ed.), *Treating PTSD: Cognitive-behavioral strategies* (pp. 99–126). New York: Guilford Press.

Rickels, K., Downing, R., Schweizer, E., & Hassman, H. (1993). Antidepressants for the treatment of generalized anxiety disorder: A placebo-controlled comparison of imipramine, trazodone, and diazepam. *Archives of General Psychiatry, 50,* 884–895.

Risse, S. C., Whitters, A., Burke, J., Chen, S., Scurfield, R. M., & Raskind, M. A. (1990). Severe withdrawal symptoms after discontinuation of alprazolam in eight patients with combat-induced posttraumatic stress disorder. *Journal of Clinical Psychiatry, 51,* 206–209.

Rosenbaum, J. F., & Pollack, M. H. (1994). Anxiety. In N. H. Cassem (Ed.), *Massachusetts General Hospital handbook of general hospital psychiatry* (3rd ed., pp. 159–190). St. Louis, MO: Mosby/Year Book.

Rothbaum, B. O., Foa, E. B., Riggs, D. S., Murdock, T., & Walsh, W. (1992). A prospective examination of post-traumatic stress disorder in rape victims. *Journal of Traumatic Stress, 5,* 455–475.

Saigh, P. A. (1987). *In vitro* flooding of childhood post-traumatic stress disorders: A systematic replication. *Professional School Psychology, 2,* 133–144.

Salkovskis, P. M., & Campbell, P. (1994). Thought suppression induces intrusion in naturally occurring negative intrusive thoughts. *Behaviour Research and Therapy, 32,* 1–8.

Salkovskis, P. M., & Mills, I. (1994). Induced mood, phobic responding and the return of fear. *Behaviour Research and Therapy, 32,* 430–445.

Saxe, G. N., van der Kolk, B. A., Berkowitz, R., Chinman, G., Hall, K., Lieberg, G., & Schwartz, J. (1993). Dissociative disorders in psychiatric inpatients. *American Journal of Psychiatry, 150,* 1037–1042.

Schepple, K. L., & Bart, P. B. (1983). Through women's eyes: Defining danger in the wake of sexual assault. *Journal of Social Issues, 39*, 63–81.

Schweizer, E., Rickels, K., Case, W. G., & Greenblatt, D. J. (1990). Long-term use of benzodiazepines: II. Effects of gradual taper. *Archives of General Psychiatry, 47*, 908–915.

Shalev, A. Y., Rogel-Fuchs, Y., & Pitman, R. K. (1992). Conditioned fear and psychological trauma. *Biological Psychiatry, 31*, 863–865.

Shapiro, F. (1989). Eye movement desensitization: A new treatment for posttraumatic stress disorder. *Journal of Behavior Therapy and Experimental Psychiatry, 20*, 211–217.

Shay, J. (1992). Fluoxetine reduces explosiveness and elevates mood of Vietnam combat vets with PTSD. *Journal of Traumatic Stress, 5*, 97–101.

Shestatzky, M., Greenberg, D., & Lerer, B. (1988). A controlled trial of phenelzine in posttraumatic stress disorder. *Psychiatry Research, 24*, 149–155.

Smucker, M. R., & Niederee, J. (1995). Treating incest-related PTSD and pathogenic schemas through imaginal exposure and rescripting. *Cognitive and Behavioral Practice, 2*, 63–93.

Solomon, S. D., Gerrity, E. T., & Muff, A. M. (1992). Efficacy of treatments for posttraumatic stress disorder: An empirical review. *Journal of the American Medical Association, 268*, 633–638.

Southwick, S. M., Krystal, J. H., Morgan, C. A., Johnson, D., Nagy, L. M., Nicolaou, A., Heninger, G. R., & Charney, D. S. (1993). Abnormal noradrenergic function in post traumatic stress disorder. *Archives of General Psychiatry, 50*, 266–274.

Steketee, G., & Foa, E. B. (1987). Rape victims: Post-traumatic stress responses and their treatment. A review of the literature. *Journal of Anxiety Disorders, 1*, 69–86.

Sutherland, S. M., & Davidson, J. (1994). Pharmacotherapy for posttraumatic stress disorder. *Psychiatric Clinics of North America, 17*, 409–423.

Tallis, F., & Smith, E. (1994). Does rapid eye movement desensitization facilitate emotional processing? *Behaviour Research and Therapy, 32*, 459–461.

Taylor, S., Koch, W. J., & McNally, R. J. (1992). How does anxiety sensitivity vary across the anxiety disorders? *Journal of Anxiety Disorders, 6*, 249–259.

Telch, M. J., Agras, W. S., Taylor, C. B., Roth, W. T., & Gallen, C. (1985). Combined pharmacological and behavioural treatment for agoraphobia. *Behaviour Research and Therapy, 23*, 325–335.

Tesar, G. E., Rosenbaum, J. F., Pollack, M. H., Otto, M. W., Sachs, G. S., Herman, J. B., Cohen, L. S., & Spier, S. A. (1991). Double-blind placebo-controlled comparison of clonazepam and alprazolam for panic disorder. *Journal of Clinical Psychiatry, 52*, 69–76.

Turchan, S. J., Holmes, V. F., & Wasserman, C. S. (1992). Do tricyclic antidepressants have a protective effect in post-traumatic stress disorder? *New York State Journal of Medicine, 92*, 400–402.

van der Kolk, B. A. (1983). Psychopharmacological issues in posttraumatic stress disorder. *Hospital and Community Psychiatry, 34*, 683–691.

van der Kolk, B. A. (1987). The drug treatment of post-traumatic stress disorder. *Journal of Affective Disorders, 13*, 203–213.

van der Kolk, B. A. (1994). The body keeps the score: Memory and the evolving psychobiology of posttraumatic stress. *Harvard Review of Psychiatry, 1*, 253–265.

van der Kolk, B. A., Dreyfuss, D., Michaels, M., Shera, D., Berkowitz, R., Fisler,

R., & Saxe, G. (1994). Fluoxetine in post traumatic stress disorder. *Journal of Clinical Psychiatry, 55,* 517–522.

van der Kolk, B. A., Greenberg, M. S., Boyd, H., & Krystal, J. H. (1985). Inescapable shock, neurotransmitters and addiction to trauma: Towards a psychobiology of post traumatic stress. *Biological Psychiatry, 20,* 314–325.

Veronen, L. J., & Kilpatrick, D. G. (1983). Stress management for rape victims. In D. Meichenbaum & M. E. Jaremko (Eds.), *Stress reduction and prevention* (pp. 341–374). New York: Plenum Press.

Wirtz, P. W., & Harrell, A. V. (1987). Effects of postassault exposure to attack-similar stimuli on long-term recovery victims. *Journal of Consulting and Clinical Psychology, 55,* 10–16.

Wolf, M. E., Alavi, A., & Mosnaim, A. D. (1988). Posttraumatic stress disorder in Vietnam veterans: Clinical and EEG findings; possible therapeutic effects of carbamazepine. *Biological Psychiatry, 23,* 642–644.

Zarate, R., Rapee, R. M., Craske, M. G., & Barlow, D. H. (1988). *The effectiveness of interoceptive exposure in the treatment of simple phobia.* Paper presented at the 22nd Annual Convention of the Association for Advancement of Behavior Therapy, New York.

III

EATING DISORDERS

10

Treatment Resistance in Eating Disorders: Psychodynamic and Pharmacologic Perspectives

PAUL HAMBURG
DAVID B. HERZOG
ANDREW BROTMAN

Anorexia nervosa (AN) is an eating disorder primarily affecting adolescent women; it is characterized by willful weight loss to the point of extreme starvation, a malignant fear of becoming fat, and a severely distorted image of one's own body shape and size. By its very definition, AN is a "treatment-resistant" disorder. The hallmark of AN is denial, and an anorectic does not typically initiate treatment without some subtle or overt coercion. Therefore, all patients with AN are resistant to some degree, and this makes even the normal course of treatment very difficult. For most patients with AN, self-starvation is to a large degree ego-syntonic; it feels better not to eat. There is no magic bullet that can be a rapid cure for most patients with AN. We discuss the consultation requests we get from clinicians and family members concerning patients who refuse to enter or are "not responding to treatment," and we present our concept of the "therapeutic envelope" designed to contain the damage during the difficult process of treating AN.

Bulimia nervosa (BN) is another eating disorder primarily affecting young women; it is characterized by episodes of rapacious and excessive binge eating, followed by purging behavior or extreme food restriction. BN is generally considered a less treatment-resistant condition than AN, because bulimics are distressed by their behavior and more readily seek treatment. Although several shorter-term treatment modalities have been effective for some patients, the bulimic patients evaluated in our outpatient unit have had the disorder for an average of 6 years by the time they seek treatment. Many fail to respond to short-term treatment or relapse after an initial good response; this suggests that for some patients BN may be chronic, requiring multiple therapeutic interventions over the long term. We discuss a variety of treatment modalities for BN, including some promising pharmacotherapeutic strategies.

RESISTANCE TO ENTERING TREATMENT

For many patients with eating disorders, treatment resistance begins as a prolonged reluctance to come for evaluation or enter treatment. For the anorectic, this resistance to seeking treatment is often a manifestation of the denial and egocentricity of the disorder. For the bulimic, the initial resistance to treatment is often a manifestation of the shame and embarrassment she feels about her eating disorder, and frequently about other pathologic behaviors as well. (Note that in this chapter we use the feminine pronoun to refer to a patient with AN or BN, for the sake of simplicity; of course, we recognize that these conditions occur in males as well as females.) Knowledge about the patient's family, social system, and previous experience with medical/mental health professionals is essential in order to make an adequate differential diagnosis of the resistance and plan a strategy for intervention.

A patient's parents may have strong misgivings about psychiatry for a variety of reasons, including family culture, a previous frustrating experience with the mental health field, or a family secret that they fear will be revealed. Family secrets can include sexual misuse or abuse, marital discord (e.g., potential parental separation), parental alcoholism, or a psychotic relative. Sometimes the parents want someone else to assume the responsibility for their "sick child" without having to participate in the treatment process themselves; the child, fearful of being extruded from the family, refuses the evaluation. In our Eating Disorders Unit, we routinely ask to see the family as part of the evaluation process.

The social system may exacerbate the resistance to treatment. The bulimic patient has often hidden her symptoms from family, friends, spouse, coworkers, and even her therapist. She is apprehensive about revealing her secret or having it revealed to these various parties. The male eating-disordered patient wonders why he has a disorder that is primarily manifested in women, and is concerned that others will question his masculinity if they become aware of his problem.

Eating-disordered individuals seeking treatment have typically been symptomatic for a year or more. They have frequently had contact with professionals, including pediatricians, internists, gynecologists, family practitioners and/or mental health professionals. At times the interactions with these caregivers have been harmful. A gynecologist may quickly prescribe estrogen hormone replacement to an amenorrheic woman with AN who is ambivalent, if not terrified, about the prospect of menses. A pediatrician or internist may make an off-the-cuff remark about a patient's body that is frightening or humiliating: A preadolescent may be told that she is looking "chunky"; a 14-year-old may hear that she is looking "very sexy"; or a bulimic may be informed that her behaviors are "just plain disgusting." The eating-disordered patient in psychotherapy may fear that if she informs her psychotherapist about her behaviors, the psychotherapist will be repelled and even ask her to leave the therapy.

Patients present in different ways, and the initial goal is often to decrease their resistance to entering treatment. For example, a parent calls to say her daughter is anorectic and won't come to the unit. We advise the whole family to come for an evaluation to "take the heat off" the child; if the parents cannot convince the patient to accompany them, we meet with the parents first to help empower them to bring in the entire family for assessment.

A college girl may call about her bulimic roommate who won't seek help. Often this caller is actually calling for herself. We try to provide information about the disorder; we discuss confidentiality issues; and we may ask the caller to accompany her roommate. If the roommate is too fearful to come in, then we suggest contacting the local self-help organization for AN and BN as a way of entering the health care system.

A bulimic may call, but may be unsure that she wants to come in for an evaluation or ambivalent about treatment. Again, we clarify confidentiality concerns and show the respect for her that she desperately needs, by listening to her descriptions without judgment or anxiety. We explore "family business" by asking about current conflicts and issues in the family, review the caller's previous experience with health care professionals, and present various treatment options.

Some eating-disordered individuals do not want any psychiatric help at the time they present for evaluation, and we may refer them to a nutritionist and/or an internist. Often over time, such patients feel safer with the institution or the professionals providing care, and are then ready to use psychiatric help. Some will consider self-help groups. In our unit we provide psychoeducational groups, consisting of 10-week sessions that give patients information about their disorder and treatment options; at the end of the 10 weeks, they are better able to make decisions about further treatment. We also may prescribe "extended evaluations" for 8 or 10 sessions, so that a patient can get a chance to see what psychotherapy is like and determine whether it could be useful for her.

TREATMENT RESISTANCE IN ANOREXIA NERVOSA

Much of psychiatric practice, like medical practice in general, depends upon the shared commitment of patient and physician to promoting recovery from illness. No such shared commitment exists with the anorectic patient, even once she has been prevailed upon to begin treatment. Forming a treatment alliance is therefore a difficult, slow task, which must be based on a search for shared perceptions and goals. For example, the patient and physician may not agree at first that maintaining a minimum safe weight is desirable, but they *can* agree on the perception that the patient experiences pain when asked to gain weight. They cannot agree that the emaciated patient "looks fat," but they can agree that to *feel* fat while everybody else is challenging this self-perception is a painful, confusing predicament. The alliance is gradually created from such shared perceptions and acknowledgments of affect.

If treatment resistance is assumed to be an inevitable aspect of the care of an anorectic patient, how is the clinician to achieve a balance between the requirements of medical safety and the goal of creating an alliance with a suspicious, reluctant patient? This difficult balancing act is made somewhat easier if the treater(s) can create a "safety envelope" to contain the medical and nutritional damage while the therapeutic effort proceeds. For the more difficult cases, treatment by a team including an internist/family practitioner/pediatrician, a nutritionist, and a clinician offers the most effective therapy; in other cases, the clinician may assume several of these roles. Simply stated, the goal is to keep the patient alive and relatively free of medical harm while the treatment remains in a period of intense resistance to change.

In order to accomplish this goal, clear guidelines concerning weight, vital signs, and hospitalization must be established and communicated early in the treatment to the patient and the patient's family. Ideally, these guidelines should be discussed and agreed to by all members of the treatment team, and formalized in a treatment contract between the team and the patient. The patient must understand that continuing treatment outside the hospital depends upon the maintenance of medical safety. A minimum safe weight should be established on the basis of the patient's height and body build; for example, a patient with average build whose ideal body weight is 110 pounds and who presents at 82 pounds (75% of her ideal body weight) will need to gain 5 pounds to reach 80% of ideal body weight, a minimally safe plateau. Should her vital signs change, her weight fall below the agreed-upon minimum, or her electrolytes fall into an unsafe range, then she should be hospitalized and outpatient treatment suspended until she is medically stable.

It is essential that the patient and her family understand the rationale for this contingency plan, even if they cannot believe it is necessary. The patient needs to hear that the specific messages her body is communicating make emergent medical intervention necessary. This is far easier to explain to the patient if the treatment team refrains from struggles about weight gain at times when she is able to maintain the established minimum safe weight. Weight gain should be an appropriate, critical concern when medical safety is compromised, and at other times should be subordinated to the task of fostering an alliance with the patient concerning common concerns and issues. Weight should be monitored during regular meetings with the professional who is responsible for medical management. The frequency of these visits should depend upon the margin of safety that the patient can establish between current weight and minimum safe weight, and should be increased at times of weight loss.

Because AN is characterized by periods of remission and relapse, vigilance is prudent even when a patient seems to begin moving along the road to recovery. Anorectic patients have an uncanny ability to fool those around them into complacency; it is not unusual to make the painful discovery that a patient who comes twice weekly for psychotherapy and who seems to be doing just fine has actually lost critical amounts of weight over a period when she has not been followed by an internist or pediatrician, or weighed by the clinician. During crises, visits to the physician may be scheduled several times each week to monitor weight and vital signs. Should hospitalization for medical stabilization be necessary, we have found that a brief stay in a medical–psychiatric unit is the treatment of choice. The hospitalization should focus on the goal of weight gain, using strict protocols that limit activity on the basis of caloric balance.

Some patients test the safety envelope several times by allowing their weight to fall below the established minimum. The clinician's response must be firm, explicitly justified on the basis of medical necessity, and nonpunitive. He or she should keep in mind that the patient is not being "bad," manipulative, or obstinate; she simply cannot give up a practice of self-starvation that she finds essential to her psychologic survival. Although the patient may be furious with the clinician who hospitalizes her, their alliance is more likely to survive if the response is one of empathy for the patient's predicament, rather than one of disappointment, rage, or recrimination. Most patients are able to maintain a minimum safe weight after a few tests of the safety envelope. Sometimes a patient will insist on hovering at the precipice, just barely maintaining a minimum safe weight without an additional margin of safety. This behavior can tax the patience of the treatment team to the limit.

If the absence of a safety margin results in recurrent hospitalization, it is reasonable to insist on renegotiating the minimum safe weight upward to provide an additional buffer. If, on the other hand, the patient successfully stops losing weight while hovering at the edge of her minimum weight, and is making good progress in therapy with respect to issues other than weight gain, then it may be helpful to accept this precarious balance as a necessary temporary condition to permit continued therapeutic work. When there is an impasse between the therapist's discomfort with persistent marginal weight and the patient's discomfort with any further weight gain, consultation may be useful. A more neutral observer—someone who has not been a party to the struggles about weight—can often provide clarification for the patient and treatment team, permitting treatment to continue.

Many anorectic patients who have successfully stabilized their weight at low but medically safe levels need months and even years of psychotherapy before they can allow themselves to gain weight. In AN, some of the perceived risks of gaining weight include fear of becoming fat; fear of bingeing; fear of taking on more feminine, less girlish bodily proportions; fear of becoming sexually attractive; and fear of resuming menstruation and fertility. Often the patient who begins to gain weight and encounters one of these risks suddenly begins to lose weight once more. Some patients simply avoid any risk by refusing to gain more weight.

In general, it is not helpful to struggle with the patient whose weight is medically safe but still very low. Whereas most patients can reluctantly accept the rationale for drastic intervention when their lives are threatened by malnutrition and medically unsafe low weight, they are unlikely to accept a coercive approach to reentering the world of nonanorectic life. The involvement of a skilled dietician is of definite benefit throughout the course of treatment. The nutritionist should accept the slow pace of weight gain that these patients tolerate, and must be resourceful in discovering and encouraging incremental changes in eating behavior that fit the patient's own style and idiosyncrasies. For example, one patient may be willing to eat an egg as part of her breakfast if she can exercise during the morning, while another may only tolerate additional calories in the form of a bedtime snack. Another patient may need permission to continue obsessive food rituals (e.g., cutting portions into tiny morsels before consuming them) in order to facilitate gradual increases in intake and weight. Patience, flexibility, and ingenuity are essential in the treatment of AN.

Some anorectic patients begin to eat more, only to find themselves overwhelmed by urges to binge. Although some of these patients respond to support and reassurance, others will go on to develop BN. It is important for the treater(s) to help these patients accept that this may be part of the natural history of the eating disorder, and may in fact be a step toward recovery. BN, when not severe, is a less dangerous disorder than AN and can be more compatible with medical and psychologic well-being.

Whether treatment resistance occurs at the time of initial diagnosis of AN or later in the course of treatment, the approach to resolving impasses is essentially the same. First, a thorough evaluation is necessary, including a medical, nutritional, psychologic, and psychopharmacologic assessment. A treatment plan encompassing an envelope of safety needs to be designed by the treatment team, presented to the patient and the family, set down in a formal contract, and then carefully monitored and enforced with firm flexibility. At each crisis point in the treatment, additional interventions should be considered, including family treatment, group therapy, pharmacologic intervention, and therapy consultation. Family therapy is often a vital aspect of the treatment plan, particularly with younger patients living at home, or with patients for whom family members pose obstacles to recovery. Involvement of grandparents, siblings, boyfriend or spouse, and others who are important to the patient may sometimes provide the additional support and leverage necessary for the patient to make progress in treatment. Group therapy can be of considerable benefit to patients with AN, once they have progressed to the point where dangerous weight loss is not an issue. If anorectic patients are placed together in groups before their low weight is dystonic, there is a significant risk that the group members will simply compete to see who can be the "best" anorectic and lose weight the fastest. When these patients are further along the road to recovery, a group supports and encourages them to improve their nutritional state and expand the range of their personal and interpersonal lives, which have also been restricted to starvation levels. The group helps to bind the enormous anxiety anorectic patients inevitably feel about giving up their symptoms.

Psychotherapy consultation is a valuable option at any point during the treatment when either the patient or the therapist feels that progress is inadequate or that they have reached an impasse. Rarely, it will become clear that a new therapist could provide more effective treatment; more often, some misunderstanding can be discovered and resolved, allowing the existing therapy to proceed. Such misunderstandings may stem from unrecognized transference feelings, including the patient's guilt about keeping secrets, fear of disappointing the therapist, concern that getting better may deprive her of the advantages of her symptoms, or a sense that the therapist cannot understand her experience. They may also reflect countertransference problems that may arise in the therapist, such as impatience, despair, and a need to control.

PHARMACOTHERAPY FOR ANOREXIA NERVOSA

Anorectic patients often refuse pharmacotherapy because they fear loss of control, believe that taking medication means they are crazy, or are misinformed about the side effects or addictive potential of medication. Families in denial may collude with the patients in their refusal to take medication. Patients may also be exquisitely sensitive to side effects; they frequently report excessive sedation, insomnia, or dizziness even at very low doses. It is important to inform a patient and family about the purpose of medication and its potential side effects, in order to enhance the therapeutic alliance and prevent premature abandonment of treatment.

Various medications have been tried in the treatment of AN, including antidepressants, neuroleptics, antihistamines, and opiate antagonists. None have demonstrated consistent or robust effectiveness, and most were short-term, inpatient-based trials in which forms of nonpharmacologic therapy were the primary modalities. Controlled studies using amitriptyline (Biederman, Herzog, & Rivinus, 1985), clomipramine (Lacey & Crisp, 1981), and lithium carbonate (Gross et al., 1981) have demonstrated no or limited efficacy in treating AN. A controlled study of cyproheptadine (up to 32 mg/day) in an inpatient setting found it moderately effective for inducing weight gain and decreasing depressive symptoms when used as part of a comprehensive treatment program (Halmi, Eckert, & Falk, 1982). We conclude that pharmacotherapy should not be employed as the sole treatment modality for an anorectic; rather, it should be used in the context of an ongoing psychotherapeutic relationship.

We recommend the use of an antidepressant as a first choice for the anorectic with concomitant major depressive disorder, significant neurovegetative signs, or recent preoccupations with obsessions or rituals. The choice of a specific agent involves several factors. Although amitriptyline is the best-studied tricyclic antidepressant (TCA) in AN, it frequently produces uncomfortable side effects, particularly excessive sedation and anticholinergic effects. Imipramine and desipramine have not been well studied in AN but are generally better tolerated. Monoamine oxidase inhibitors (MAOIs) in low to moderate doses may be helpful for some patients, though the dietary proscriptions associated with them can exacerbate the patients' focus on diet.

Some investigators have been interested in the possible therapeutic effects of selective serotonin reuptake inhibitors (SSRIs), including fluoxetine, sertraline, paroxetine, and fluvoxamine, in AN. Two open studies have demonstrated some efficacy for fluoxetine in the treatment of AN (Gwirtsman, Guze, Yager, & Gainsley, 1990; Kaye, Welzin, Hsu, & Bulik, 1991). Both of these studies showed that mood and obsessional features improved, as opposed to a direct treatment effect on AN per se. Although SSRIs may cause weight loss in some overweight individuals treated for depression, they do not have this effect in individuals with AN. They may be useful in some anorectic patients because of a more favorable side effect profile, allowing more of such patients to complete a therapeutic trial.

Anorectic patients may present with medical complications. Therefore, before antidepressant or any other pharmacotherapy is initiated, laboratory tests (including a complete blood count, serum electrolytes, liver function tests, blood urea nitrogen, creatinine, thyroid functions, and an electrocardiogram) should be routinely performed. The patient should be metabolically stabilized prior to the initiation of a medication trial. Medication should be started at a low dose (e.g., 5–10 mg/day of fluoxetine or its equivalent), and this should be slowly titrated upward. Plasma blood levels of TCAs should be drawn, to assess compliance and adequacy of dose. Successful outcome is measured by weight gain, increased interest in eating, fewer obsessional thoughts and compulsive rituals, reduced depressive symptomatology, decreased anxiety, and willingness to participate in a treatment program. Like patients with other disorders, patients with AN should generally be kept on antidepressant medication for 6 months to a year before tapering is initiated.

Other medications to be considered if a patient does not respond to antidepressants include cyproheptadine (see above). Some interesting preliminary work has been done with opiate antagonists, but they remain experimental agents for AN. There have been a few case reports on both intravenous naloxone and oral naltrexone (the oral dose was 50 mg/day) for the treatment of AN with modestly positive results (Mitchell, 1987). The endogenous opiate system may be hyperactive in AN, causing an autoaddictive syndrome, which may be broken by the opiate antagonists (Halmi, 1995). Antianxiety agents (e.g., alprazolam, 0.5 mg; lorazepam, 1 mg) have not been well studied but can be useful, especially around mealtime, to reduce food-related anxiety and enhance eating. Chlorpromazine and higher-potency antipsychotics are rarely used today, except transiently and in low doses, for anorectic patients who have concomitant psychotic illness or overwhelming anxiety not relieved by minor tranquilizers.

In summary, although no medication has been shown to control AN specifically, various medications may be useful to treat associated depressive, obsessive, and anxiety symptomatology.

TREATMENT RESISTANCE IN BULIMIA NERVOSA

Patients with BN may resist treatment in ways similar to those of patients with AN. However, a bulimic patient is more likely to establish a therapeutic alliance, with treatment goals agreed upon by therapist and patient. Bulimic patients generally experience their symptoms as shameful and ego-dystonic, even if they also recognize that the symptoms are difficult to give up and may serve a purpose in their psychologic economy (i.e., they may alleviate emptiness, anxiety, anger, or loneliness). Although it often takes years for a bulimic patient to overcome her shame and seek professional help, she may be strongly motivated once treatment begins. Often the bulimic symptoms have abated during the weeks prior to seeking help, and there may be a dramatic improvement during the first several months of treatment. For some patients this improvement is sustained. For those patients with more severe psychopathology and entrenched bulimic symptoms, relapse is common and a source of great disappointment. Some patients break off treatment at this point. It is helpful to warn all patients that an initial remission may not last, and that a return of symptoms is an expectable part of their recovery process, not the equivalent of "failure."

Reassessment of the treatment plan is appropriate when a relapse occurs. The reassessment may reveal the need for changes in the psychotherapy (e.g., increased frequency of visits) or further psychopharmacologic interventions (e.g., increase in dose or change in medication). Comorbid conditions such as alcohol abuse, major depression, or psychosis may require additional psychiatric intervention. Often there is evidence of more personality pathology than was suspected at the beginning of treatment, suggesting the need for a more intensive and lengthier psychotherapy. Family issues may have surfaced, preventing the patient from making necessary changes in her life, and requiring family intervention. At times nutritional counseling is needed to help restructure eating habits that promote binges, such as prolonged fasting in an attempt to "be good." The most important principle in approaching the patient who has relapsed after an initial response to treatment is to be flexible in tailoring a treatment plan to the patient's current needs. Bulimic patients exhibit a surprising diversity of psychodynamic and biologic phenomenology, despite their common eating symptoms. There is little place, given the current lack of a universally effective treatment, for dogmatic or rigid prescriptions that fail to consider the full range of psychodynamic, psychopharmacologic, and cognitive-behavioral techniques of potential benefit for these patients.

Some bulimic patients have severe symptomatology that puts them at medical risk, including ipecac abuse, which may cause irreversible cardiac muscle damage; binges and purges and use of laxatives or diuretics, which can compromise electrolyte balance; and suicidal acts or threats. The patient and clinician need to establish a therapeutic envelope to insure medical safety, analogous to the one dealing with maintenance of weight for an anorectic. Our experience suggests that with respect to potassium homeostasis and ipecac abuse, the best approach is to establish and maintain clear limits that place the burden of safety on the patient. Most patients can contract to avoid all use of ipecac and to maintain a minimum potassium level, if failure to do so will result in hospitalization. The use of potassium supplements on an outpatient basis should be avoided, because it may give a false sense of reassurance to both patient and clinician, and in fact permits the patient to continue a level of purging that is incompatible with fluid and electrolyte balance. It is important for the patient and clinician to establish clear contractual limits on behavior that compromises medical safety; useless attempts to ban binges or purges that do not threaten survival, like struggles with anorectic patients over weight gain, should be avoided.

PHARMACOTHERAPY FOR BULIMIA NERVOSA

Bulimic patients are often resistant to accepting medication. They may express a number of concerns, including fears that they will get "hooked" on the medicine, that drugs are an "artificial" way to treat the problem, that they may "get fat" from medication, or that taking medication means that they are extremely disturbed. These concerns can be dealt with by properly explaining medications and their side effects. The issue of whether this is an "artificial" means of control is most difficult. Our usual technique is to explain that many individuals have a biologic predisposition to eating disorders, which may be expressed when environmental circumstances or intrapsychic conflict causes a threshold to be crossed. Therefore, by attacking the problems on both fronts—the biologic and the environmental/psychologic—we can make most progress. Furthermore, the medication, if successful, can be tapered after about 6 months in order to determine whether it remains necessary.

We recommend pharmacotherapy for the bulimic who has concomitant major depressive disorder, substantial depressive or anxiety symptomatology, significant obsessive–compulsive symptomatology, or bulimic behavior that has not responded to the usual psychotherapeutic interventions. Pharmacotherapy in the outpatient setting with bulimics who are unreliable, are suicidal, abuse drugs, or have severe character pathology should be administered cautiously, with frequent contact and the prescription of modest quantities of medication. Particularly for these patients, antidepressants and psychotherapy in conjunction are more effective than either modality alone. We usually do not recommend pharmacotherapy as the sole intervention in BN, except under close supervision in selected patients who either are not appropriate for therapy or do not require psychologic interventions.

Antidepressants have been the most widely studied class of agents for BN; results of these studies are much more encouraging than studies conducted for AN. Several placebo-controlled, double-blind studies with antidepressants have been completed. In these, positive results were obtained for desipramine (Hughes, Wells, Cunningham, & Ilstrup, 1985), imipramine (Pope, Hudson, Jonas, & Yurgelun-Todd, 1983), phenelzine (Walsh, Stewart, Roose, Gladis, & Glassman, 1984; Walsh et al., 1988) and fluoxetine (Fluoxetine Bulimia Nervosa Collaborative Study Group, 1992); and marginally positive findings were obtained for amitriptyline (Mitchell & Grout, 1984) and trazodone (Pope, Keck, McElroy, & Hudson, 1989). In therapeutic doses, antidepressants can decrease bingeing and purging over the short term, even when there is no concomitant depression.

Antidepressant treatment for BN should be initiated with agents with favorable side effect profiles, such as desipramine, SSRIs, or imipramine. Excessive weight gain and carbohydrate craving are not common side effects among bulimics treated with antidepressants. Weight gain can be expected in underweight bulimics who are not absorbing many calories because of chronic vomiting or laxative abuse, but we have not found excessive weight gain to be a common problem, above and beyond that accounted for by nutritional improvement. Treatment should be initiated with low doses (e.g., 10–25 mg/day of imipramine or its equivalent, or 20 mg/day of fluoxetine), and these should gradually be increased to about 3.5 mg/kg/day of body weight for TCAs by the third week. There is evidence that 60 mg of fluoxetine is more effective in decreasing binge–purge activity than 20 mg. TCAs should be taken at bedtime to minimize medication loss through purging. Plasma levels of TCAs are recommended to help monitor compliance and the adequacy of the dose. Evidence of a successful therapeutic trial includes a decrease in bingeing and purging behaviors and in depressive or anxiety symptoms.

In patients who do not respond to an adequate trial of a TCA or an SSRI, another class of antidepressant, such as trazodone or an MAOI, should be administered. MAOIs should be used with caution for bulimics, because impulsive bingeing on tyramine-containing foods can be life-threatening. These risks must be fully explored and evaluated with each patient. We have found that most bulimics can accurately assess their ability (or inability) to abstain from tyramine-containing foods.

In some depressed bulimics, both the affective symptoms and the eating disorder respond to medication; for others, only one or the other syndrome may improve. Most patients show at least a 50% improvement in their eating disorder, although fewer than a third will experience a sustained remission. Follow-up studies have suggested that many patients may require successive trials of medication in order to sustain improvement or improve further (Pope & Hudson, 1986). Patients failing to respond adequately to antidepressant therapy may respond to augmentation with lithium. In addition, preliminary results from an open trial of naltrexone in doses up to 250 mg/day, which are much higher doses than usually seen to treat the opiate addict, were encouraging (Jonas & Gold, 1986); by contrast, a double-blind study using 50 mg/day showed no superiority of naltrexone over placebo (Mitchell et al., 1989). A placebo-controlled, double-blind study of mianserin, an antihistamine with serotonin-inhibiting qualities, obtained negative results (Sabine, Yonnaie, Forringten, Barrett, & Wakeling, 1983). However, fenfluramine, a serotonin-enhancing agent that promotes satiety via central serotonergic mechanisms, may be effective in BN at doses of 20 mg three times a day (Blouin et al., 1988). This observation is consistent with the hypothesis that an abnormality in serotonin metabolism may be an etiologic factor in bulimia (Halmi, 1995).

REFERENCES

Biederman, J., Herzog, D. B., & Rivinus, T. (1985). Amitriptyline in anorexia nervosa: A double blind study. Journal of Clinical Psychopharmacology, 591, 10–16.

Blouin, A. G., Blouin, J. H., Perez, E. L., Bushnik, T., Zuro, C., & Mulder, E. (1988). Treatment of bulimia with fenfluramine and desipramine. Journal of Clinical Psychopharmacology, 8, 261–269.

Fluoxetine Bulimia Nervosa Collaborative Study Group. (1982). Fluoxetine and the treatment of bulimia nervosa: A multi-center placebo double-blind trial. Archives of General Psychiatry, 39, 139–147.

Gross, H. A., Ebert, M. H., Faden, V. B., Goldberg, N. C., Nee, L. C., & Kaye, W. H. (1981). A double blind controlled trial of lithium carbonate in primary anorexia nervosa. Journal of Clinical Psychopharmacology, 1, 376–381.

Gwirtsman, H. E., Guze, B. H., Yager, J., & Gainsley, B. (1990). Fluoxetine treatment of anorexia nervosa: An open clinical trial. Journal of Clinical Psychiatry, 51, 378–382.

Halmi, K. A. (1995). Basic biological overview of eating disorders. In F. E. Bloom & D. J. Kupfer (Eds.), Psychopharmacology: The fourth generation of progress (pp. 200–220). New York: Raven Press.

Halmi, K. A., Eckert, E., & Falk, J. R. (1982). Cyproheptadine for anorexia nervosa. *Lancet, i,* 1376–1378.

Hughes, P. L., Wells, L. A., Cunningham, L. J., & Ilstrup, D. M. (1985). Treating bulimia with desipramine: A placebo-controlled double-blind study. *Archives of General Psychiatry, 43,* 182–186.

Jonas, J. M., & Gold, M. S. (1986). Treatment of antidepressant resistant bulimia with naltrexone. *International Journal of Psychiatric Medicine, 16*(4), 305–310.

Kaye, W. H., Welzin, T. E., Hsu, L. K., & Bulik, C. M. (1991). An open trial of fluoxetine in patients with anorexia nervosa. *Journal of Clinical Psychiatry, 52,* 464–471.

Lacey, J. H., & Crisp, A. H. (1981). Hunger, food intake and weight: The impact of clomipramine on a refeeding anorexia nervosa population. *Postgraduate Medical Journal, 56,* 79–85.

Mitchell, J. E. (1987). Psychopharmacology of anorexia nervosa. In H Y. Meltzer (Ed.), *Psychopharmacology: The third generation of progress* (pp. 1273–1276). New York: Raven Press.

Mitchell, J. E., Christenson, G., Jennings, J., Huber, M., Thomas, B., Pomeroy, C., & Morley, J. (1989). A placebo controlled double blind crossover study of naltrexone hydrochloride in outpatients with normal weight bulimia. *Journal of Clinical Psychopharmacology, 9*(2), 94–97.

Mitchell, J. E., & Grout, R. (1984). A placebo controlled double-blind trial of amitriptyline in bulimia. *Journal of Clinical Psychopharmacology, 4,* 186–193.

Pope, H. G., & Hudson, J. I. (1986). Antidepressant drug therapy for bulimia: Current status. *Journal of Clinical Psychiatry, 47,* 339–345.

Pope, H. G., Hudson, J. I., Jonas, J. M., & Yurgelun-Todd, D. (1983). Bulimia treated with imipramine: A placebo-controlled double-blind study. *American Journal of Psychiatry, 140,* 554–558.

Pope, H. G., Keck, P. E., McElroy, I. S., & Hudson, J. I. (1989). A placebo-controlled study of trazodone in bulimia nervosa. *Journal of Clinical Psychopharmacology, 9,* 254–259.

Sabine, E. T., Yonaie, A., Forringten, A. T., Barratt, K. H., & Wakeling, A. (1983). Bulimia nervosa: A placebo controlled, double-blind, therapeutic trial of mianserin. *Journal of Clinical Pharmacology, 16,* 1955–2025.

Walsh, B. T., Gladis, M., Roose, S. P., Stewart, J. W., Stetner, F., & Glassman, A. H. (1988). Phenelzine vs. placebo in 50 patients with bulimia. *Archives of General Psychiatry, 45,* 471–475.

Walsh, B. T., Stewart, J. W., Roose, S. P., Gladis, M., & Glassman, A. H. (1984). Treatment of bulimia with phenelzine: A double-blind placebo-controlled study. *Archives of General Psychiatry, 41,* 1105–1109.

11

Cognitive-Behavioral Strategies for the Treatment of Eating Disorders

MAUREEN L. WHITTAL
ARI ZARETSKY

Bulimia nervosa (BN) is characterized by episodic bingeing and subsequent use of inappropriate methods to prevent weight gain. Also central to the diagnosis of BN is an overreliance on body image (shape and/or weight) as an index of self-worth. In the fourth edition of the *Diagnostic and Statistical Manual of Mental Disorders* (DSM-IV; American Psychiatric Association, 1994), BN is divided into purging and nonpurging subtypes. Individuals diagnosed with the purging subtype engage in behaviors that include self-induced vomiting, abuse of laxatives or diuretics, or overuse of enemas to prevent weight gain. Bulimics who engage in nonpurging behaviors typically restrict their food intake or exercise excessively after a binge episode.

The fundamental difference between anorexia nervosa (AN) and BN is the refusal of anorectics to eat a sufficient quantity of food to maintain an adequate level of nourishment and normal body weight. AN can result in physical impoverishment and is fatal in 20% of patients, secondary to suicide or cardiac arrest (Theander, 1985). The DSM-IV (American Psychiatric Association, 1994) diagnostic criteria for AN stipulate that individuals must either weigh 15% below what is expected compared to age and height norms, or fail to make expected developmental gains. Intense fear of fatness and of weight gain are hallmark characteristics. This fear of fatness can lead to problematic behaviors, including excessive weighing of self, rituals surrounding the preparation and/or intake of food, or impulse control disorders such as alcohol or drug abuse (Anderson, 1987).

Like bulimics, anorectics have a distorted view of body image and rely excessively on that body image for self-evaluation. Anorectic women who have passed the menarche frequently have amenorrhea and will typically menstruate only after the administration of exogenous hormone. AN subtypes reflect the primary method used to control weight and shape and include restricting and binge eating-purging type.

For both BN and AN, a number of dysfunctional behaviors are obvious targets for treatment: the binge–purge cycle, rituals surrounding food, excessive or phobic avoidance of weighing, distorted body image and the inappropriate attention body image receives in self-evaluation. Also implicit in treatment, but typically not part of formal protocols, is the attempt to reduce the focus on food in the patients' lives. Patients often report that they spend the majority of their waking hours thinking about food and have no pleasurable activities in their lives besides dieting or other food-related situations. The goal of decreasing patients' focus on food is typically accomplished by increasing enjoyable aspects of life that are unrelated and/or incompatible with a focus on food.

Current epidemiologic data as reported in DSM-IV (American Psychiatric Association, 1994) indicate that the prevalences of BN and AN are 1–3% and 0.5–1%, respectively. These disorders primarily affect adolescent girls and young women, who account for approximately 90% of the diagnosed eating disorder population (American Psychiatric Association, 1994). (Because of these prevalence rates, we refer to patients as female for the sake of simplicity, despite the fact that small percentages of BN and AN patients are men.)

The purpose of this chapter is to describe cognitive-behavioral conceptualizations of eating disorders and to review the treatment outcome literature. Detailed treatment manuals and outcome data are available for BN (e.g., Fairburn et al., 1991; Fairburn, Marcus, & Wilson, 1993c). In contrast, cognitive-behavioral treatment (CBT) of AN has lagged behind and in some cases has remained in the pilot stage (e.g., Treasure et al., 1995). Consequently, relatively greater emphasis is placed here on conceptual models of AN, whereas the review of BN stresses treatment outcome.

BULIMIA NERVOSA

Prevailing Viewpoints Regarding Maintenance of the Disorder

Until recently, the cognitive-behavioral literature on BN was dominated by two competing theories regarding the maintenance of the disorder: the cognitive model (Fairburn, 1981) and the anxiety model (Rosen & Leitenburg, 1982). The main distinction between the two theories is the proposed mechanism that maintains the disorder and, correspondingly, determines the target(s) of treatment.

In the cognitive approach (also referred to in the literature as the cognitive-behavioral approach) described by Fairburn (1981), treatment has two aims: (1) control of binge eating, and (2) identification and challenge of distorted beliefs regarding food, body shape, and weight. Vomiting is not a target for direct modification, but is conceptualized as epiphenomenal to binge eating; if binge eating can be controlled, vomiting should cease to be an issue. The treatment approach that follows from this theoretical position emphasizes cognitive restructuring similar to that originally utilized with depressed patients (Beck, Rush, Shaw, & Emery, 1979). The cognitive approach emphasizes identification of dysfunctional cognitive processes (e.g., "black-and-white" thinking), distorted beliefs (e.g., "I must be thin to be happy"), and the relationship between emotion and behavior. By challenging and altering the dysfunctional cognitions, the treatment targets maladaptive patterns of emotion and behavior, ultimately decreasing or eliminating the inappropriate binge–purge cycles.

In contrast, the anxiety model suggests that BN is maintained to a greater extent by vomiting than by bingeing (Rosen & Leitenburg, 1982). Rosen and Leitenburg (1982) suggest that vomiting is maintained by negative reinforcement: Vomiting decreases the fear of fatness and associated anxiety that escalate during and after a binge. This decrease in anxiety is hypothesized to strengthen the tendency to binge. Therefore, if vomiting can be controlled, then bingeing should decrease. Accordingly, in the anxiety model, treatment for BN focuses attention on (1) eliminating vomiting as a response to anxiety arising from eating, and (2) decreasing the anxiety response to eating through exposure plus response prevention (ERP). In ERP, bulimics are encouraged to eat until they reach the point at which they would typically vomit, and then are prevented from doing so. Theoretically, with repeated applications of ERP, the association between the anxiety produced by eating and its relief by vomiting will be broken.

Treatment Outcome

Currently, some authors (Fairburn, Agras, & Wilson, 1992; Wilson & Fairburn, 1993) consider CBT the treatment of choice for BN, and CBT was strongly endorsed at a recent conference sponsored by the National Institute of Mental Health (D. B. Herzog, personal communication, January 27, 1995). In the most recent well-controlled studies of CBT for BN, the reductions in bingeing from pre- to posttreatment (typically 19 or 20 weeks) ranged from 73% to 93%. Posttreatment decreases in purging ranged from 77% to 94%. According to a recent review of studies, 51–71% of subjects cease bingeing and 36–56% cease purging (Wilson & Fairburn, 1993). Gains made during treatment have been found to remain essentially stable for up to 1 year (Fairburn, Jones, Peveler, Hope, & O'Connor, 1993b). For patients who fail to respond to a course of standard CBT, utilization of ERP techniques or interpersonal therapy may be helpful (Agras, 1993; Smith, Marcus, & Eldredge, 1994).

Active Components of CBT for BN

The vast majority of BN patients can be treated on an outpatient basis. Exceptions to this general rule include patients with significant medical complications, suicidal patients, or those who fail an adequate trial of CBT. Treatment is problem-focused and semistructured, and directs attention to the factors that maintain rather than cause the eating disorder. Table 11.1 provides an overview of specific interventions.

Current treatment manuals for CBT (e.g., Fairburn et al., 1993c) advocate 19 sessions of treatment (50 minutes each in duration) over 20 weeks. Fairburn et al. (1993c) recommend that clinicians contract with patients for a specified number of sessions, because these authors believe that a clear termination date helps both patients and therapists approach each session with high motivation. Within sessions a therapist is initially more active than a patient in treatment, but the responsibility shifts to the patient as treatment progresses. Because patients are not typically "cured" (i.e., they retain residual problems secondary to the eating disorder) during treatment, the ultimate goal is to have patients become their own therapists as they continue to work to reduce their symptoms after formal treatment is terminated.

In the Fairburn et al. (1993c) protocol, treatment is conducted in three distinct stages or phases. In the first phase (sessions 1–8), emphasis is placed on elucidating the cognitive-behavioral model of BN and normalizing eating patterns through the scheduling of regular meals and healthy snacks. The second stage of treatment (sessions 9–16) emphasizes cognitive restructuring, focusing on the distorted perceptions of shape and weight and the rigid rules that govern eating. The third phase of treatment (sessions 17–19) is concerned primarily with maintenance of treatment gains and relapse prevention.

First Stage of Treatment (Sessions 1–8)

The cognitive-behavioral model of BN takes into account the relationship among bingeing, purging, dietary restraint, concerns about shape and weight, and low self-esteem. Explanation of the model usually begins with the presenting complaint of binge eating and its relationship to purging. Patients typically have no problem in understanding that purging maintains binge eating, particularly if they believe that purging is an effective means of weight control. However, the relationship between strict dieting and binge eating may be less clear initially. Episodes of binge eating encourage dieting, but dieting also promotes binge eating. In the latter case, rigid food rules (i.e., rules about "forbidden" foods) are usually established as a consequence of dieting. Patients typically attempt to restrain themselves from these foods or reduce their food intake, which results in a state of deprivation (Polivy & Herman, 1993). Because the forbidden foods are typically enjoyable (e.g., chocolate, ice cream), and deprivation

TABLE 11.1. Cognitive-Behavioral Treatment Strategies for BN

Intervention	Specific steps in the intervention and the point at which they are introduced in therapy	Function of the intervention
Introduction of the cognitive model of BN	Occurs in session 1 and is referred to throughout the course of treatment. Therapist introduces the relationship between bingeing and purging, and describes how it is maintained by extreme dieting, concerns about shape and weight, and low self-esteem.	To inform patients that treatment will involve more than decreasing bingeing–purging, but will also target modification of dietary restraint, and distorted attitudes toward shape and weight.
Self-monitoring	Begins in session 1 and continues throughout treatment. Patients monitor all food and liquid intake, record subjective binges and any purges attempted, and make a general comment on concomitant emotional state.	To identify antecedents and consequences of binge eating, and to begin to normalize eating patterns.
Psychoeducation	Occurs in the first stage of treatment (sessions 1–8). Patients are given information on body weight (a specific weight vs. a weight range; a 5- to 6-lb. fluctuation in weight is considered normal), physical consequences of bingeing–purging, ineffectiveness of purging to control weight, and impact of dieting on mood.	To help patients become better informed about the negative consequences and ineffectiveness of their behavior.
Scheduling meals	Begins in session 1 or 2 and continues throughout treatment. Patients are encouraged to eat three planned meals plus two or three snacks.	To decrease dietary restraint (i.e., fasting) and to normalize eating patterns.
Stimulus control of eating	Occurs in the first stage of treatment. Includes a variety of techniques, including eating in one room of the house, eating slowly and chewing food thoroughly, sitting down to eat, eating off a plate, not engaging in other behaviors while eating, ridding the pantry of tempting foods, shopping with a list, shopping when not hungry, and purchasing foods that require preparation.	To assist in preventing a binge.

TABLE 11.1. (cont.)

Intervention	Specific steps in the intervention and the point at which they are introduced in therapy	Function of the intervention
Decreasing dietary restraint	Occurs in the second stage of treatment (sessions 9–16). Involves gradual introduction of avoided foods over a 4-week period and increase in energy intake to a range of 1500–1800 calories/day.	To modify strict dieting and deprivation.
Problem solving	Occurs in the second stage of treatment. Involves a series of steps: writing down a problem (work-related, social, relationship-related, etc.), listing and evaluating potential solutions, identifying the best solution and the steps involved in carrying it out, and evaluating its success.	To isolate and prevent the remaining intermittent binge episodes.
Cognitive restructuring	Occurs in the second stage of treatment. Patients are taught to identify and challenge dysfunctional thoughts and to look for errors in reasoning (e.g., dichotomous ["black-and-white"] reasoning).	To alter distorted beliefs regarding shape and weight.
Behavioral experiments	Occurs in the second stage of treatment. Examples include standing in front of a full-length mirror, wearing form-fitting clothing (particularly when feeling fat), comparing body shape and weight to other women's, and comparing subjective feeling of fatness with weight according to a scale.	To assist patients in practicing cognitive restructuring and gaining evidence that does not support their beliefs.
Maintenance plan	Occurs in the third stage of treatment (sessions 17–19). Patients prepare a written list of interventions that were helpful and the appropriate times to put them into place. Therapist differentiates a lapse from a relapse and educates patients that they will be vulnerable to bingeing during times of stress.	To prevent relapses.

(continued)

TABLE 11.1. (cont.)

Intervention	Specific steps in the intervention and the point at which they are introduced in therapy	Function of the intervention
Broadening patients' experience past a food focus	Occurs early in treatment (session 2 or 3) and continues throughout treatment. Therapist gives patients Adult Pleasant Events Schedule from Linehan (1993) and instructs them to engage in one pleasurable event each week that has nothing to do with food and is not dependent upon success/progress with CBT.	To prevent relapses and decrease patients' focus on food.

Note. Data from Fairburn et al. (1993c).

heightens awareness of food, these foods are eventually eaten; this initiates a binge that might have been prevented if the food had not been forbidden.

Likewise, overzealous concerns about shape and weight promote dieting and increase the risk of future binge episodes. The binges elicit concern about shape and weight and potentiate renewed efforts at dieting. Moreover, poor self-concept or low self-esteem can foster concerns about shape and weight. Shame centering around binge eating may have a negative impact on self-esteem and may subsequently heighten concerns about shape and weight, renewing efforts at dieting. Review of the model with patients is designed to inform them of treatment targets and the rationale of targeting each element of the cycle: binge eating, dietary restraint, body image, and self-esteem.

Patients are asked to self-monitor food intake and binge episodes, in order to highlight aspects of the model, help them identify antecedents and consequences to binge eating, and help them begin to normalize eating patterns. Fairburn et al. (1993c) suggest that self-monitoring should begin in session 1 and continue throughout treatment. Subsequent sessions begin with a review of monitoring forms and a collaborative effort to identify antecedents to binge episodes. When higher-risk situations or times of day are identified, the therapist's goal is to aid patients in developing alternate and pleasurable incompatible behaviors to reduce slips during these high-risk times. Examples include such activities as visiting friends and talking on the telephone.

Various behavioral techniques are also used to decrease the potential to binge. These techniques include restricting eating to one room of the house, eating slowly, sitting down to eat, putting all food on a plate, not engaging in other activities while eating (e.g., watching television), temporarily ridding the house of tempting foods, shopping with a list and while not hungry, and buying foods that require preparation. These behavioral techniques are utilized to bring eating under stimulus control (i.e., eating only if the appropriate conditions are in place). Once eating is under stimulus control, patients are asked to throw away laxatives and/or diuretics. According to Fairburn et al. (1993c), many patients can do so without further instruction. Tapering rather then abruptly discontinuing laxatives can be helpful for patients who find this task difficult.

Additional goals in the first phase of treatment involve weekly weighing and education regarding body weight, physical consequences of bingeing and purging, the ineffectiveness of purging to control weight, and the negative effects of dieting. Establishing normal eating patterns (i.e., three planned meals and two or three snacks) is an important behavioral technique to decrease binge episodes. Many patients have been eating intermittently throughout the day and/or at inappropriate times (e.g., late in the evening). If patients can eat at regularly scheduled intervals, they may prevent a binge that is initiated because of excessive hunger. Patients should be instructed not to vomit after eating and to engage in distracting activities (e.g., talking on the telephone or running an errand) until the urge to vomit declines. Hence this treatment approach does include elements of ERP, but the exposure is strictly to normal eating patterns and amounts.

Typically, the majority of patients will have decreased their episodes of binge eating at the end of stage 1 (Fairburn et al., 1993c). However, for patients who have not decreased their bingeing, progress to stage 2 is not recommended. Either a few more sessions at stage 1 or inpatient treatment may be indicated. If treatment is still not successful in decreasing bingeing frequency, the CBT approach may have to consider other potential controlling variables or adjunctive pharmacologic treatments (see Hamburg, Herzog, & Brotman, Chapter 10, this volume).

Second Stage of Treatment (Sessions 9–16)

Aims of the second stage of treatment include decreasing dietary restraint and breaking rigid rules surrounding food. Dietary restraint can manifest itself in three ways: fasting for long periods, avoiding "dangerous" foods, and eating foods that have a low caloric value. Negation of fasting is achieved in the first phase of treatment by eating regular meals and scheduling snacks. Avoided foods are introduced gradually over four sessions. Patients are asked to make a list of foods that are avoided because of their potential impact on shape and weight. Fairburn et al. (1993c) recommend that patients go to the grocery store to make their list of avoided foods. The list is then divided into a four-step hierarchy, with each step reflecting foods that are more dangerous because of their potential effects on shape and weight. Subjects are instructed each week for 4 weeks to introduce the foods within the corresponding hierarchy step. Patients are instructed not to vomit after eating, and thus exposure to the feared foods (i.e., eating the forbidden foods) should be completed when the patients' control is intact. In-session exposure guided by the therapist may be necessary for patients who cannot complete the homework assignments. Increasing caloric intake, a response to the third form of dietary restraint, is initiated following review of self-monitoring. Daily food diaries will reveal whether patients are not eating enough. If not, patients are instructed to increase their intake gradually until it is between 1500 and 1800 calories/day.

At this point in treatment, most patients have decreased the frequency of their binge–purge episodes (Fairburn et al., 1993c). Instruction in problem solving may assist patients in preventing the intermittent binges that may remain. Patients are taught a series of steps: identifying a potential problem (e.g., an interpersonal issue) in written form as soon as it occurs, listing and evaluating the potential solutions, identifying the best solution (or combination of solutions) and the steps involved in carrying them out, and subsequently evaluating the success of the strategy.

The remaining sessions in the second phase of treatment are devoted to altering the maladaptive cognitions and belief systems that maintain the eating disorder. This goal is accomplished through the use of cognitive restructuring, adapted from its use with depressed patients (Beck et al., 1979). Cognitive restructuring is used to identify and challenge distortions in thinking. After identifying the dysfunctional cognition (e.g., "I'm getting fat" after a 2 pound increase) and writing it down, patients are taught to evaluate the evidence for and against the thought and to generate alternative explanations (e.g., "Is the weight gain due to fluid retention?" "Is it normal for weight to fluctuate?"). Patients are also taught to look for errors in their reasoning about eating and food. Dichotomous thinking (also referred to as "black-and-white"/"all-or-nothing thinking") is one of the most common types of unproductive cognitive styles. (See Beck et al., 1979, or Burns, 1989, for a discussion and list of errors in thinking.) Finally, patients should be taught to examine the difference between subjective feeling and objective reality (e.g., the feeling of getting fat vs. body mass index, a statistical indicator of height-to-weight ratio).

Exposure can be used to elicit dysfunctional thoughts between sessions. Examples include standing in front of a full-length mirror, wearing form-fitting clothing, and engaging in activities such as aerobics where comparison of shape and weight is likely to occur. Patients are instructed to write down their thoughts that occur during exposure, and then to practice their techniques of disputing and challenging the thoughts. Other behavioral experiments can be used to test the dysfunctional thoughts. Fairburn et al. (1993c) suggest that patients ask trusted friends for an unbiased opinion of the patients' shape and weight, or that the patients decide each morning whether they are fat and determine whether the decision coincides with the weight on the scale (probably it does not).

Dysfunctional attitudes regarding shape and weight include such beliefs as these: "If I were skinny, all my problems would be gone," "Thin people are happy and successful," and "I would be more valuable as a person if I were thin." Dysfunctional attitudes are best conceptualized as conditional assumptions or rules that patients use to govern their behavior. The process of altering dysfunctional attitudes is generally accomplished with repeated practice at challenging dysfunctional cognitive processes and examining the advantages and disadvantages of the attitudes. Behavioral experiments can also be used in conjunction with challenging dysfunctional attitudes. For example, patients may be asked to identify an attractive woman and compare her shape and weight to their own. These exposure exercises will invariably elicit dysfunctional thoughts, which can be used to sharpen skills of disputing problematic thoughts and should be discussed at the following session.

Third Stage of Treatment (Sessions 17–19)

The third phase of treatment involves maintenance of treatment gains and relapse prevention. A maintenance plan should be written down with the help of the therapist; it should contain the active components of treatment that the patient found helpful, and behavioral indicators of when the plan would be appropriately instituted. The difference between a lapse and a relapse should be discussed. Patients should understand that they will be vulnerable to bingeing at times of stress, and should be encouraged to examine life events and the possible relationship between the events and their bingeing behavior. However, a "lapse" (one or two episodes of bingeing–purging) does not indicate a full-blown relapse of the eating disorder.

Broadening patients' experience to include pleasurable activities that are incompatible with a food focus is not specifically discussed by Fairburn et al. (1993c), but may be helpful in preventing a relapse. At the beginning of treatment, many patients with eating disorders report that they spend the majority of their waking hours thinking about food, planning what and when to eat, or worrying about the consequences of eating. When given a list of pleasurable activities (e.g., see Linehan, 1993), patients tend to focus on items such as losing weight, exercising, or staying on a diet. Patients often report that they don't know how to have fun because the eating disorder has taken over their lives. Thus, in conjunction with the procedures outlined above, patients should be encouraged to include more activities in their lives that do not involve food. These changes should be introduced early in treatment, with the recommendation that patients engage in one pleasurable activity each week. Completing these activities should be independent of success with other treatment goals. Pleasurable activities should not be used as a reward if patients are successful in scheduling meals or completing a week with no binges. The introduction of pleasurable activities will expand patients' experience and leave them less time to think about food, thereby decreasing the probability of a relapse.

Treatment Outcome Studies of Behavioral and Cognitive-Behavioral Treatment of BN

Treatment outcome studies for BN have demonstrated that a behavior therapy (BT), CBT, and interpersonal psychotherapy (IPT) can reduce the frequency of bingeing and purging (Fairburn, Kirk, O'Connor, & Cooper, 1986; Fairburn et al., 1991, 1993b, 1995), sometimes in as little as 8 weeks of treatment (Thackwray, Smith, Bodfish, & Meyers, 1993), and that all three are clearly superior to waiting-list controls (Freeman, Barry, Dunkeld-Turnbull, & Henderson, 1988; Lee & Rush, 1986; Leitenburg, Rosen, Gross, Nudelman, & Vara, 1988; Ordman & Kirshenbaum, 1985).

A full course of CBT (i.e., 19-session treatment as described by Fairburn et al., 1993c) may not be necessary for some patients. Olmsted et al. (1991) reported that subjects who were treated with a brief educational package (five 90-minute sessions) had a 61% decrease in bingeing and a 55% decrease in vomiting from pre- to posttreatment. A purely educational intervention was particularly effective for subjects who reported relatively infrequent episodes of vomiting. From the four controlled studies that have investigated the efficacy of adding ERP to CBT, it appears that ERP techniques add little to the comprehensive CBT packages currently available. Although early studies were promising (Wilson, Rossiter, Kleifield, & Lindhom, 1986), more recent studies have found no advantage for adding ERP to CBT (Leitenberg et al., 1988; Wilson, Eldredge, Smith, & Niles, 1991), and one investigation reported a deleterious outcome (Agras, Schneider, Arnow, Raeburn, & Telch, 1989). It is currently recommended that ERP not be utilized routinely in CBT packages, but rather that it be reserved for patients who remain symptomatic after standard CBT (Agras, 1991).

The efficacy of CBT packages is further supported by dismantling studies designed to investigate the relative efficacy of CBT versus BT. CBT and BT appear to be equivocal in reducing the dysfunctional behavior of bingeing–purging associated with BN when assessed at posttreatment. However, CBT is superior to BT in reducing core psychopathology of distorted weight and shape (Fairburn et al., 1991) and in maintaining treatment gains regarding binge–purge frequency (Fairburn et al., 1993b; Thackwray et al., 1993). Overall, in the studies completed to date, there appears to be an advantage for complex CBT techniques over simpler BT approaches (i.e., self-monitoring, stimulus control of eating, and normalizing eating patterns) at posttreatment (Fairburn et al., 1991), at 1-year follow-up (Fairburn et al., 1993b) and at 6-year follow-up (Fairburn et al., 1995).

When compared to nonspecific treatments, CBT techniques are superior in decreasing binge–purge frequency and improving, distorted attitudes toward shape and weight (Kirkley, Schneider, Agras, & Bachman, 1985), as well as in maintaining treatment gains during follow-up (Fairburn et al., 1986; Thackwray et al., 1991). However, equivocal results have been obtained in one controlled study (Fairburn et al., 1993b) that compared CBT with IPT, a treatment that does not share CBT components but is matched for nonspecific factors, including credibility of treatment and therapist contact. IPT, originally developed for outpatient treatment of depression, is an active, structured treatment that focuses on current interpersonal functioning (Klerman, Weissman, Rounsaville, & Chevron, 1984). It does not target dysfunctional attitudes regarding shape and weight or the disturbed eating pattern and purging (Fairburn, in press). Fairburn et al. (1991) reported at posttreatment that CBT was more effective than IPT in reducing dietary restraint, improving attitudes regarding weight, and decreasing the frequency of vomiting episodes, but not in altering the core psychopathology of disturbed weight and shape, general psychiatric symptoms, self-reported depression, or social adjustment.

However, after 1 year of follow-up, the differences between CBT and IPT were attenuated (Fairburn et al., 1993b). In a recent article comparing long-term follow-up of subjects receiving CBT, IPT, and BT, Fairburn et al. (1995) reported that compared to BT subjects, IPT subjects were twice as likely and CBT subjects three times as likely to be in remission at 6-year follow-up. There was no significant difference between IPT and CBT subjects. Given that CBT and IPT were equivocal at short- and long-term follow-up, but not at posttreatment, suggests different mechanisms of action and perhaps different mediating variables (Fairburn et al., 1993b).

In an analysis of behavior change, Jones, Peveler, Hope, and Fairburn (1993) reported that IPT and CBT resulted in equivocal declines in binge eating and purging in the initial weeks of treatment, but that CBT subjects continued to demonstrate further declines at posttreatment, whereas IPT subjects plateaued. These data provide further support that different mechanisms of action are responsible for the treatment gains ascribed to CBT and IPT.

Wilson and Fairburn (1993) have put forward six speculative hypotheses regarding possible mechanisms of action of CBT for BN: (1) altering beliefs about shape and weight, (2) reducing dietary restraint, (3) bringing about changes in information processing associated with identifying antecedents for a binge, (4) extinguishing the classically conditioned associations between internal/external cues and eating, (5) increasing self-efficacy to solve problems and control behavior, and (6) weakening the link between anxiety reduction and vomiting. All of these explanations appear plausible, with the exception of the fact that current data fail to support anxiety reduction through vomiting. It is unlikely that a single mechanism of action is responsible for the effects of CBT; more likely, CBT operates through a combination of these mechanisms (Wilson & Fairburn, 1993). Future research will determine the relative importance of each hypothesized mechanism.

ANOREXIA NERVOSA

Biopsychosocial Model of the Disorder

At present, no single overriding etiologic theory for AN can claim universal appeal. Although some attractive biologic theories exist, encompassing genetic vulnerability, hypothalamic dysfunction, mood disorder variant, and autoaddiction models, most authorities accept that developmental factors and social learning contribute substantially to the appearance of all eating disorders. In addition, given the lack of specificity of currently available psychopharmacologic treatments for AN, psychologic treatment approaches remain the most effective intervention methods for AN (American Psychiatric Association, 1994; Yates, 1989).

A more useful perspective than the traditional biologic–psychologic dichotomy is to conceptualize AN as a multiply determined disorder with complex biologic, psychologic, and psychosocial predisposing, precipitating, and perpetuating factors. This perspective is illustrated in Table 11.2.

The table lists distal (genetic and familial) and proximal (personality and sociocultural) predisposing factors; the proximal factors also include the precipitating stressors hypothesized to be etiologically significant in the development of pathologic beliefs and behaviors in AN. Symptomatology and maintaining factors are likewise listed. In the following pages, we describe predisposing and maintaining factors in more detail and clarify how they function in the etiology and maintenance of AN. In our elaboration of the biopsychosocial model of AN, we focus particularly on the role of personality characteristics, sociocultural issues, positive and negative reinforcement contingencies, cognitive processes, and the effects of starvation. Later, we outline CBT strategies for AN and provide specific examples where possible.

One cautionary note we should sound prior to discussing psychologic factors associated with AN, is the difficulty in separating cause from consequence. For instance, investigators who observe that anorectics score low on self-esteem questionnaires can only speculate as to whether low self-esteem is etiologically significant in the development of AN or whether it is the result of becoming anorectic. Likewise, investigators who observe the persistence of self-esteem deficits after AN is in remission cannot conclusively determine whether what is being measured is a durable trait or residual "scarring" from the disorder itself. However, there is some reassurance, in that the character traits described below exhibit unusually high interobserver and cross-theoretical reliability (Vitousek & Ewald, 1993).

Predisposing Factors

Personality Characteristics. Examination of personality variables has revealed three clusters—a sense of worthlessness, perfectionism, and a ten-

TABLE 11.2. Biopsychosocial Model of AN

Distal predisposing factors	Proximal predisposing factors	Symptomatology	Maintaining factors
Genetic vulnerability	Associated personality features	Anorectic belief	Positive reinforcement
	Low self-esteem	Thinness is the solution to personal distress	Feelings of success, virtue, pride, and superiority
Family environment	Overcompliance with authority		
	Helplessness	Anorectic behaviors	Increased sense of control
	Hypersensitivity to rejection	Dieting	Attention/concern from others
	Perfectionism	Exercise	
	Preference for simplicity and certainty	Bingeing	Negative reinforcement
		Purging	Avoidance of fatness
		Eating rituals	Relief from anxiety
	Sociocultural variables		Schematic processing
	Environment that equates thinness with beauty and personal worth		Mental filter
			Resistance to disconfirmation
	Precipitating factors		Effects of starvation
	Experience of loss		Concrete thinking
	Failure		Selective attention
	Change		Isolation
	Disappointment		Loss of responsiveness
	Onset of puberty		Depression

Note. Adapted from Vitousek and Ewald (1993). Copyright 1993 by The Guilford Press. Adapted by permission.

dency to become overwhelmed—that are hypothesized to interact in AN (Vitousek & Ewald, 1993). Low self-esteem, feelings of hopelessness and ineffectiveness, a poorly developed sense of identity, a tendency to seek external verification, extreme sensitivity to criticism, and conflict over autonomy and dependency all contribute to a sense of worthlessness (Bruch, 1973, 1978; Casper, 1983; Crisp, 1980; Garner & Bemis, 1985; Goodsitt, 1985; Guidano & Liotti, 1983; Lerner, 1986; Strober, 1991). Perfectionism may partially represent a compensatory strategy for anorectic individuals; that is, they may preserve their self-esteem by adopting harsh standards to feel special and superior. Regardless of its function in AN, "obsessive–compulsive traits or perfectionistic tendencies are [among] the most commonly endorsed and most evident premorbid, predisposing factors reported in the literature" (Slade, 1982, p. 171). The last cluster of personality traits is characterized by a preference for simplicity and certainty (i.e., a desire for predictability, clear task demands, and a high degree of personal control), as well as a tendency to retreat from complex or intense social environments. Perhaps to cope with this aversive overwhelmed state, preanorectics develop a longing for simplicity, clarity, certainty, and predictability (Vitousek & Hollon, 1990).

Sociocultural Factors. Cultural factors are hypothesized to play a central role in the etiology of eating disorders (Brumberg, 1988; Dolan, 1991; Polivy, Garner, & Garfinkel, 1986; Striegel-Moore, Silberstein, & Rodin, 1986b). Exemplars of female beauty (e.g., models and beauty contestants) have become thinner over the years, so that the ideal physique is below the actuarial norm (Garner, Garfinkel, Schwartz, & Thompson, 1980). Not surprisingly, the majority of U.S. women are dissatisfied with their weight, and 56% diet on a regular basis (Schlundt & Johnson, 1990). In Western culture, thinness has come to symbolize competence, control, success, and sexuality (Bennett & Gurin, 1982). Correspondingly, the prevalence of body image disturbance, as well as of clinical and subclinical eating disorders, has increased (Cash & Pruzinsky, 1990). Given society's linkage of personal worth with weight and shape, AN should be conceptualized as both an ego-syntonic and a culturally syntonic disorder.

Third World immigrants to industrialized countries have higher rates of eating disorders, compared to people of the same nationalities who remain in their own countries (Nasser, 1988). Furthermore, studies conducted in the United States and United Kingdom suggest a racial difference in body size preference. When socioeconomic class was controlled for, more black females than white females reported satisfaction with their size and were not attempting to reduce their weight (Furnham & Baguma, 1994; Gray, Ford, & Kelly, 1987; Harris, 1994; Rosen & Gross, 1987; Stevens, Kumanyika, & Keil, 1994). Two additional studies (Gray et al., 1987; Gross & Rosen, 1988) found lower rates of BN in black women, which suggests that racial differences in body image may play an important role in explaining the discrepant prevalence rates. Despite these suggestive data, the true relationship between race or culture and eating disorders remains uncertain, given that epidemiologic studies of eating disorders across time and cultures have been nonstandard and inconsistent (Rosen, 1990).

Precipitating Stressors. Precipitating stressors for AN typically consist of developmental milestones, such as puberty, changing schools, and moving away from home (Levine & Smolak, 1989). The shifts from childhood to adolescence and from adolescence to young adulthood correlate with the modal peaks for age of onset of AN.

One explanation for the onset of AN during the transition from childhood to adolescence is that the perfectionistic and compliant individual experiences adolescence, with its lack of clear rules and guidelines for behavior, as extremely ambiguous and confusing. At this stage, the preanorectic may feel disoriented in an environment where social skills and autonomy are valued more than compliance. Because puberty is usually characterized by an increase in fat deposition, a maturing young woman may experience a painful dissonance between her actual body shape and current cultural ideals for feminine attractiveness. She may experience teasing and critical comments at a developmental stage where concerns over popularity and appearance are paramount. In addition, the amount of food intake may be one of the few aspects of life where it is possible for her to achieve absolute control. The choice of dieting may also be reinforced by the preanorectic's equating of self-control with self-deprivation. It is hypothesized that these critical experiences may lead the pre-anorexic to believe that fatness is the cause of all misfortune and therefore must be corrected (Garner & Bemis, 1982).

Unlike the psychoanalytic perspective, which emphasizes the fear of emerging sexuality (Crisp, 1980), the cognitive model of AN stresses the underlying fears of the cognitive and social consequences of sexual maturation. Most objective comparisons of anorectics with normal or psychiatric controls have not found unusual patterns of sexual attitudes, behaviors, or experiences (Scott, 1987). Comparisons of anorectics with normals demonstrated no significant differences in sexual fears, desire to menstruate or to have children, fear of pregnancy, frequency of masturbation, or the percentage of subjects who had romantic partners and were sexually active (Haimes & Katz, 1988). Although there have been a number of case reports linking eating disorders with sexual abuse (Fairburn, Hay, & Welch, 1993a), controlled studies have failed to confirm any specific association. For example, Finn, Hartman, Leon, and Lawson (1986) compared samples of sexually abused and nonabused women and reported a high prevalence of eating disorders, but no group differences. A recent survey of college women (Smolak, Levine, & Sullins, 1990) found no differences between abused and nonabused groups on the subscales of the Eating Disorder Inventory. Moreover, Pope and Hudson (1992) found no difference between the rates of sexual abuse in bulimic patients and reported rates for general psychiatric populations; they also noted that a substantial number of the patients reported experiencing the sexual abuse after the onset of their eating disorder.

Maintaining Factors

Table 11.2 lists four types of consequences that both result from and maintain anorectic beliefs: positive reinforcement, negative reinforcement, schematic processing, and the effects of starvation. Anorectics are hypothesized to receive positive reinforcement in a number of different ways. Initially, they may experience praise for their slenderness and dietary restraint. Subsequently, as praise from family and friends changes to concern and criticism, they may experience positive reinforcement in the form of attention and concern from friends and family.

Negative reinforcement is hypothesized to play an even larger role in maintaining anorectic symptoms (Bemis, 1983, 1986; Garner & Bemis, 1985; Slade, 1982). The intense fear of gaining weight or "weight phobia" functions as the aversive stimulus (Crisp, 1980). Individuals with AN, BN, agoraphobia, and specifc phobias describe feeling intense fear during imaginal exposure to relevant feared situations, and also describe feeling a strong sense of relief and enhanced security after the successful avoidance of feared stimuli (Vitousek & Ewald, 1993). By continuing to avoid anxiety-provoking stimuli such as food and weight gain, anorectics insulate themselves from the opportunity to disconfirm their beliefs (e.g., their conviction that any exposure to food will lead to a complete loss of control, massive weight gain, and social rejection).

According to the cognitive model (Beck et al., 1979), "schemas" are cognitive structures based on life experiences that organize how people process incoming information about their world and subsequent experiences. Vitousek and Hollon (1990) have suggested that individuals with AN develop organized cognitive structures or schemas around the issues of weight (e.g., a view of weight as being the most central aspect of their existence), and that these profoundly influence their perceptions, thoughts, feelings, and behavior. Once weight-related schemas have developed, they begin to function to distort the way that anorectic patients perceive and interpret their experiences. Other individuals are evaluated not on the basis of personal qualities, but in terms of being thinner or fatter than anorectic individuals. All activities are assessed according to their effects on weight control. Any situation that leads to self-evaluation also results in an intensified focus on weight and shape, and any weight fluctuation has a profound effect on thoughts and feelings (Striegel-Moore, McAvay, & Rodin, 1986a).

Starvation results from anorectic behavior and is also hypothesized to play a critical role in perpetuating the symptoms of AN. Commonly observed effects of starvation include poor concentration, concrete thinking, rigidity, withdrawal, obsessive–compulsive behavior, and depression. Recently, empirical studies have linked starvation effects to cognitive perseveration (Demitrack et al., 1990), impairments in information-processing capacity, and problems with executive planning (Laessle, Bossert, Hank, Hahlweg, & Pirke, 1989). Thus, starvation may produce a positive feedback loop, in which anorectics become more vulnerable to the effects of their own distorted perceptions, and this in turn may lead to still more anorectic behavior.

Treatment

All elements specified in the biopsychosocial model of AN (see Table 11.2) are targets for treatment. Restoration of weight and of normal eating is the first priority, followed by challenging distorted thoughts and beliefs secondary to schematic processing, and finally by examination of sociocultural influences and underlying self-esteem deficits.

BT with anorectic patients predominantly involves the application of learning principles to eliminate the maladaptive eating and weight control patterns of behavior. BT has been recognized as being most effective in the acute phase of illness, where stabilization and normalization of weight and eating may be critical (Cinciripini, Kornblith, Turner, & Hersen, 1983; Halmi, 1982, 1985; McFarlane, Bellissimo, & Upton, 1982). Interventions generally aim to alleviate symptoms by altering the external social and environmental factors that maintain the pathologic eating and dieting behaviors. Functional analyses are completed to identify the antecedent events and consequences associated with a reduction of food intake. A treatment paradigm is then designed to reward desirable behaviors and discourage undesirable behaviors (Edgette & Prout, 1989).

Controlled studies examining the specific reinforcers that work most effectively to establish weight gain in AN suggest that weight gain can be facilitated by a variety of positive and negative reinforcers (Agras, Barlow, Chapin, Abel, & Leitenberg, 1974; Blinder, Freeman, & Stunkard, 1970; Eckert, Goldberg, Halmi, Casper, & Davis, 1979; Leitenberg et al., 1988; Neuman & Gaoni, 1975; Scrignar, 1971). Positive reinforcers, such as increased social privileges, access to visitors, and exercise privileges, are made contingent on weight gain and the demonstration of healthier eating behaviors. Punishment for restrictive eating, weight loss, or vomiting after meals include delayed discharge, isolation, enforced bed rest, and (in extreme cases) tube feedings (Cinciripini et al., 1983; Halmi, 1982).

Agras (1987) reported promising results for a combination of positive and negative reinforcement with large meals and informational feedback regarding weight gain and calories consumed. Even without complex behavioral programs, many patients will gain weight in a milieu where they receive good nursing care combined with simple negative reinforcers, such as hospitalization and separation from family members (Halmi, 1985; Fairburn & Cooper, 1989).

Weight restoration should be a central early treatment for the seriously underweight patient; this intervention alone will frequently result in an improvement in obsessional thinking, mood, and personality disturbance. The ultimate weight target should be a return to a weight at which normal reproductive function resumes (Frisch, 1990) and dieting is not necessary to maintain the weight (Fairburn & Cooper, 1989). Given the tendency of weight to fluctuate from day to day, a weight range of about 5–6 pounds is advocated by most experts (Fairburn & Cooper, 1989). Many eating disorder specialists today prefer to use the body mass index. Healthy ranges for this index are related to the age and height of the patient, and appropriate tables can be consulted (Beaumont, Al-Alami, & Touyz, 1988).

Although some AN patients who are less than 20% below average weight for height can be successfully treated outside the hospital, such treatment usually requires a highly motivated patient, a cooperative family, and a brief duration of symptoms. Such patients may be treated in outpatient programs with close monitoring of treatment response (American Psychiatric Association, 1993; Anderson, 1985). Partial hospitalization or day programs are being increasingly utilized to decrease the length of inpatient stays, but such programs cannot always replace hospitalization, especially for those patients who are at less than 70% of average weight for height or for those with suicidal ideation, rapid weight loss, or physiologic instability (Kaplan, 1991; Pirin & Kaplan, 1990).

Pertschuk (1977) completed an in-depth 5-year follow-up study of 27 AN patients, the majority of whom received BT with supplemental family therapy. Antidepressant medication was given to those suffering from severe depression. Treatment for weight gain was successful for a striking 25 of these patients, and as a group they continued to gain weight after discharge. However, only 2 of the 27 were reported as completely recovered with no residual adjustment or eating problems. Rehospitalization was required for 6 of the patients who had attempted suicide or were severely depressed. An additional 4 patients required rehospitalization to gain weight.

Review studies provide evidence for dramatic short-term efficacy of CBT (Hsu, 1980; Schwartz & Thompson, 1981). For example, Schwartz and Thompson (1981) reported that 50–65% of patients returned to normal weight, whereas 20% did not receive significant benefit. However, approximately 50% of patients reported significant psychiatric impairment or poor marital and social adjustment at 12-month follow-up.

A Program of CBT for AN

Unlike the cognitive models of anxiety and depression, the cognitive model of eating disorders (Bemis, 1983; Fairburn & Garner, 1988; Garner & Bemis, 1985; Vitousek & Hollon, 1990) explicitly addresses motivational factors and attends to the function of the symptomatic behaviors for patients (Bruch, 1973, 1978; Goodsitt, 1985).

CBT for AN offers powerful strategies for modifying the distorted beliefs associated with eating and body shape and for addressing the developmental themes, interpersonal themes, and central beliefs underpinning the disorder. One particular advantage of this treatment approach is its compatibility with other psychologic treatments, especially more traditional psychotherapy, where developmental deficits are seen as central pathognomonic factors. CBT with anorectic patients needs to address the following:

1. Idiosyncratic beliefs about weight and shape.
2. The interaction between physical and psychologic components of the disorder.
3. The patients' desire to retain certain focal symptoms.
4. The development of motivation for treatment, with an emphasis on the gradual evolution of a trusting therapeutic relationship.
5. Fundamental self-esteem deficits.

A longer duration of therapy than is typical of depression or anxiety disorders may be required for AN. Garner and Bemis (1985) have developed a comprehensive CBT approach for AN modeled after the work of Beck and other cognitive-behavioral theorists (Beck et al., 1979; Ellis, 1962; Goldfried, 1971; Mahoney, 1974; Meichenbaum, 1974). Like CBT for depression, CBT for AN is highly structured, with the therapist taking a very active role in conducting the sessions.

Citing Hollon and Beck (1979), Garner and Bemis (1985) describe the essence of CBT as teaching patients to analyze the utility and validity of their food- and weight-related beliefs on a moment-to-moment basis. The main focus of treatment is on identifying and modifying the dysfunctional beliefs and assumptions that govern patients' behavior. Garner and Bemis (1985) postulate that anorectics share a number of characteristic beliefs, including the belief that body weight or shape can serve as the sole criterion for self-worth, that complete control over their bodies is necessary, and that there is a perfect balance between hunger and satiety without any need for readjustment.

Most importantly, therapy should not degenerate into logical disputation of the validity of anorectic beliefs, as patients are likely to experience this confrontation as a personal attack. The first step in treatment is to recognize how patients' weight control strategies are intended to fulfill important functions for the patients, and to appreciate that these strategies have been partially successful. The next step is for the therapist to ask whether the weight control measures can provide everything that patients had intended, and to evaluate the emotional and physical costs of the extreme dieting. Much of the first few sessions of therapy are devoted to helping patients construct an exhaustive list of both the pros and cons of their eating disorder, and to begin the process of exploring the implications of these. Behavioral exercises (e.g., role playing or rehearsal) can then be used in conjunction with various cognitive techniques to help patients articulate previously unspoken premises (e.g., "My worth as a person depends on how thin I look"). Honest recognition of these silent beliefs can help to weaken their power over the patients. Behavioral techniques are also used to help patients gather data regarding how events influence their feelings and thoughts, and to offer opportunities to practice different ways of interpreting the environment.

Although there is some evidence that exposure therapy may benefit some anorectics (Mavissakalian, 1982), Garner and Bemis (1985) discourage the use of ERP involving food, since they identify the core fear in AN as pertaining not to food but to viewing the self at a higher weight. The behavioral techniques used in their model include rehearsal of patients' reactions to weight gain and the scheduling of pleasant activities unassociated with weight control to expand the patients' repertoire of rewarding behaviors. The supplementary use of desensitization and social skills training is also encouraged, to help insure that patients experience success and pleasure in their social interactions and other activities.

Once the therapist helps patients become motivated to gain weight, cognitive interventions can then be used to modify the patients' dysfunctional belief systems (e.g., the basing of self-esteem solely on weight, and the importance of extreme dieting to accomplish this goal). Examples of cognitive techniques include operationalizing and articulating beliefs, challenging arbitrary personal rules, decentering, decatastrophizing, gathering data, and reattribution of events.

Operationalizing distorted beliefs helps patients to analyze their validity. For example, a patient who believes that thinness equals popularity can be asked to operationalize popularity in concrete terms, using a list of specific criteria that one would use to assess another person's popularity. The patient can then be asked to evaluate whether popularity diminishes with weight gain. Articulating beliefs also facilitates cognitive change by allowing the beliefs or thoughts to be analyzed more critically. Anorectic patients frequently make errors in information processing, such as dichotomous thinking ("If I eat one cookie I'll eat the box"), magnification ("If I gain more than 5 pounds I'll have to kill myself"), and mind reading ("That woman who stared at me must have been thinking how fat I've become"). Again, having patients articulate their beliefs provides an opportunity to evaluate their validity.

Decentering is a process through which patients learn how to become more objective by stepping back from their experience to evaluate it from alternative perspectives. For example, a patient who is exquisitely concerned about how others perceive her weight can be asked to establish some criteria to decide when her appearance and behavior are actually eliciting responses from others in her environment. Such a patient may predict that weight gain will result in strangers' staring at her legs. By counting the number of times that staring at her legs occurs before and after the behavioral change, the patient may come to accept the fact that she is not being scrutinized by others as much as she initially predicted.

Decatastrophizing is a technique used to help patients cope with anxiety associated with weight gain. When patients are forced to focus on specific fears rather than making global predictions of catastrophe, they can reality test the actual degree of threat posed by an event. Specific problem-solving techniques can be used to increase the patients' perception of having available resources to cope with the danger. An example of this is to have a patient imagine being told by her boyfriend that she is no longer attractive to him because she has gained weight. By having the patient anticipate the painful feelings and thoughts associated with this scenario, the therapist can "inoculate" the patient and help her become desensitized enough to cope. The patient can also be asked how she would help a friend cope in a similar situation, and can be asked to develop a list of the things she can tell herself to feel better.

"Challenging the shoulds" is a technique intended to help patients evaluate the reasonableness of some of their arbitrary self-expectations and personal rules of living, such as "I should always diet" or "I should always exercise." The emphasis is on having the patients recognize how their harsh, unattainable personal expectations lead to extreme stress and diminished self-esteem.

Gathering data is a technique used to help patients empirically evaluate the accuracy and validity of their dysfunctional beliefs. For example, if a patient has a belief that no man will ever talk to her if she gains 5 pounds, she can be asked to make a list of the number of male friends she had before she began her dieting and the number of male friends she has made since her extreme weight loss began.

Reattribution techniques are used to assist patients in altering their interpretations of their perceptions. Garner and Bemis (1985) conceptualize the body image disturbance of anorectics as being essentially a cognitive rather than a perceptual phenomenon. The therapeutic strategy they advocate is to alter the anorectics' *interpretations* of what they see, rather than modifying their *misperceptions*. For example, a cachectic patient is encouraged to view her obese self-perception as a manifestation of her illness. This approach avoids any unnecessary conflicts that might arise out of attempts to contradict the patient's subjective perception.

Empirical Research Utilizing the Cognitive Model

Although an elegant cognitive model for AN has been constructed, its elements have not been adequately empirically tested, and research in this area clearly lags behind the research devoted to BN (Fairburn, 1990). Anorectics are usually more acutely ill than bulimics and need to be followed for a longer period of time to detect changes in eating-related cognitions. Because of their lack of insight and investment in preserving their symptomatology, their tendency to be overcompliant, and their poor introspective skills, anorectics present a formidable challenge to clinicians who want to empirically study their subjective experience (Vitousek, Garner, & Hollon, 1991). The studies that do exist have serious methodologic limitations, such as the lack of psychiatric and restrained-eating control groups, overuse of college subjects, and use of nonstandardized assessment devices (Vitousek & Ewald, 1993).

Despite these drawbacks, a few cross-sectional studies that support the cognitive model of AN have demonstrated important differences between anorectic and normal populations. Anorectic and bulimic subjects demonstrate lower levels of self-esteem (Casper, Offer, & Ostrov, 1981; Dykens

& Gerrard, 1986; Weinreich, Doherty, & Harris, 1985) and obtain higher scores on indices of perfectionism (Garner, Olmsted, Polivy, & Garfinkel, 1984; Slade & Dewey, 1986). AN and BN patients are also more likely to exhibit dysfunctional attitudes than are normal individuals (Ruderman, 1986; Steiger, Fraenkel, & Leichner, 1989; Steiger, Goldstein, Mongrain, & Van der Feen, 1990), and are more likely than control groups to display cognitive distortions when eating- and weight-related concerns are controlled for (Fremouw & Heyneman, 1983; Strauss & Ryan, 1988).

The CBT approach advocated by Garner and Bemis (1985) targets not only anorectic patients' individual cognitive distortions surrounding food- and weight-related concerns, but ultimately addresses the patients' broader belief systems, such as the importance of thinness as a life goal relative to other goals. The specificity with which Garner and Bemis have described their treatment for AN has been intended to encourage replication and evaluation by other investigators. However, to date there have been virtually no controlled studies of psychotherapy of any kind for AN. This may be partially explained by a number of factors, including attrition during the long course of therapy that must follow short-term weight restoration.

The only controlled study of CBT yielded equivocal results for its efficacy compared to that of BT alone (Channon, deSilva, Hemsley, & Perkins, 1989). At the end of treatment and at 6- and 12-month follow-ups, most patients showed improvement, but there were few detectable differences between CBT and pure BT. However, the CBT approach appeared to be more acceptable to patients and was associated with a higher rate of compliance, which may be clinically relevant, given the difficulty of engaging anorectic patients in treatment.

THE ROLE OF BODY IMAGE IN EATING DISORDERS

Body image is a complex construct that has been conceptualized, described, and measured from many points of view. At the present time there is controversy in the eating disorder literature regarding the role of body image disturbance in the etiology and maintenance of AN and BN symptoms. A problematic issue is the multiple meanings associated with the term "body image," including the neural representations determining body experience, the mental image, and the feelings that individuals have about their bodies (Garner & Garfinkel, 1981).

Despite widespread clinical agreement that patients with eating disorders are remarkable for their belief that they are too fat, the measurement of these perceptions through standardized tests of size perception (e.g., the movable-caliper technique, the image-marking method, and the distorting-photograph technique) has yielded inconsistent results. The equivocal results have cast doubt on the validity of perceptual distortion as a fundamental characteristic of eating disorders (Cash & Brown, 1987;

Cooper & Taylor, 1987), and have led some experts to contend that perceptual body image disturbance should not be a criterion for eating disorders (Hsu, 1982).

Although current research suggests that body image distortion is neither necessary nor sufficient in the etiology of eating disorder symptomatology, disturbances in body and weight *attitudes* have been more convincingly linked to a variety of eating disorder variables. Body dissatisfaction is significantly correlated with feelings of ineffectiveness and perfectionism in AN patients (Garner et al., 1984) and with severity of eating and dieting symptoms in BN patients (Post & Crowther, 1987).

Although there have been some methodologic limitations in the prospective studies that have followed high-risk populations over time, there is consistent evidence that negative body image predicts severity of eating and dieting pathology. For example, body size overestimation predicted weight loss relapse among patients who restored their weight during hospitalization (Button, 1986). Those patients with more extreme body size overestimation prior to inpatient treatment gained less weight at discharge (Button, 1986; Leon, Lucas, Colligan, Ferdinande, & Kamp, 1985). Anorectics who were pleased with their emaciated appearance as shown to them on videotape gained less weight during treatment and were more likely to relapse after discharge (Vandereycken, Probst, & Meermann, 1988).

Many of the data on body image after treatment have come from BN treatment trials. For example, Conners, Johnson, and Stuckey (1984) reported a correlation between improved body satisfaction and a decrease in bingeing and purging. Freeman, Beach, Davis, and Solyom (1985) found that ongoing body dissatisfaction was one of the two best predictors of relapse within 6 months in a group of bulimics who were abstinent from bingeing–purging at posttreatment. Studies of CBT for body image in BN patients have demonstrated that treated bulimics were significantly more satisfied with their appearance (Ordman & Kirshenbaum, 1985) and more accurate in their size estimation (Leitenberg et al., 1988). These results confirm other uncontrolled studies of CBT that also found significant reductions in body dissatisfaction and size distortion after treatment and during follow-up (Birtchell, Lacey, & Harte, 1985; Wilson et al., 1986).

The effectiveness of CBT packages in decreasing body dissatisfaction suggests that therapy targeting eating behavior alone is not sufficient to produce attitudinal change, and that body dissatisfaction may be improved by therapies dealing with more global self-evaluations rather than core eating disorder cognitions.

CONCLUSIONS

The numerous etiologic and maintaining factors in AN and BN make conceptualizations of these disorders inherently complex. Nevertheless, current outcome studies suggest that acute treatment is efficacious but that residual pathology does persist. We have outlined the central concepts to be addressed in CBT with BN patients; we hope that continued refinement of these strategies and better understanding of the mechanisms of action will allow for continued improvement in both acute and long-term treatment effects. As alternative treatments are replicated and validated, matching patients to treatment is perhaps the next step in improving treatment outcomes.

We have also attempted to provide a succinct cognitive-behavioral conceptualization of AN that encompasses personality features, sociocultural variables, information processing, and contingencies of reinforcement. There appears to be an increasing awareness that ultimate goals in the treatment of anorectic patients must include not only the maintenance of healthy weights and eating habits, but also associated improvements in psychologic, sexual, and social adjustment. It is in these latter areas that CBT may make a unique contribution. The treatment of anorectic patients from a cognitive-behavioral perspective has not received a great deal of systematic attention, but utilization of the principles of CBT promises to be useful in helping patients gain weight, alter their dysfunctional belief systems, and maintain these gains at follow-up.

REFERENCES

Agras, W. S. (1987). Eating disorders: Management of obesity, bulimia, and anorexia. Elmsford, NY: Pergamon Press.

Agras, W. S. (1991). Nonpharmacologic treatments of bulimia nervosa. Journal of Clinical Psychiatry, 52(Suppl.), 29–33.

Agras, W. S. (1993). Short-term psychological treatments for binge eating. In C. G. Fairburn & G. T. Wilson (Eds.), Binge eating: Nature, assessment, and treatment (pp. 270–286). New York: Guilford Press.

Agras, W. S., Barlow, D. H., Chapin, H. N., Abel, G. G., & Leitenberg, H. (1974). Behavior modification of anorexia nervosa. Archives of General Psychiatry, 30, 279–286.

Agras, W. S., Schneider, J. A., Arnow, B., Raeburn, S. D., & Telch, C. F. (1989). Cognitive-behavioral and response-prevention treatment for bulimia nervosa. Journal of Consulting and Clinical Psychology, 57, 215–221.

American Psychiatric Association. (1993). APA practice guidelines for eating disorders. American Journal of Psychiatry, 150, 207–225.

American Psychiatric Association. (1994). Diagnostic and statistical manual of mental disorders (4th ed.). Washington, DC: Author.

Anderson, A. E. (1985). Practical comprehensive treatment of anorexia nervosa and bulimia. Baltimore: John Hopkins University Press.

Anderson, A. E. (1987). Contrast and comparison of behavioral, cognitive-behavioral, and comprehensive treatment methods for anorexia nervosa and bulimia nervosa. Behavior Modification, 11, 522–543.

Beaumont, P., Al-Alami, M., & Touyz, S. (1988). Relevance of a standard measurement of undernutrition to the diagnosis of anorexia nervosa: Use of Quetelet's body mass index (BMI). *International Journal of Eating Disorders, 7,* 399–405.

Beck, A. T., Rush, A. J., Shaw, B. F., & Emery, G. (1979). *Cognitive therapy of depression.* New York: Guilford Press.

Bemis, K. M. (1983). A comparison of functional relationships in anorexia nervosa and phobia. In P. L. Darby, P. E. Garfinkel, D. M. Garner, & D. V. Coscina (Eds.), *Anorexia nervosa: Recent developments in research* (pp. 403–415). New York: Alan R. Liss.

Bemis, K. M. (1986). *A comparison of the subjective experience of individuals with eating disorders and phobic disorders.* Unpublished doctoral dissertation, University of Minnesota.

Bennett, W., & Gurin, J. (1982). *The dieter's dilemma.* New York: Basic Books.

Birtchell, S. A., Lacey, J. H., & Harte, A. (1985). Body image distortion in bulimia nervosa. *British Journal of Psychiatry, 147,* 408–412.

Blinder, B. J., Freeman, D. M. A., & Stunkard, A. J. (1970). Behavior therapy of anorexia nervosa: Effectiveness of activity as a reinforcer of weight gain. *American Journal of Psychiatry, 128,* 77–82.

Bruch, H. (1973). *Eating disorders: Obesity, anorexia nervosa, and the person within.* New York: Basic Books.

Bruch, H. (1978). *The golden cage: The enigma of anorexia nervosa.* Cambridge MA: Harvard University Press.

Brumberg, J. J. (1988). *Fasting girls: The emergence of anorexia nervosa as a modern disease.* Cambridge, MA: Harvard University Press.

Burns, D. D. (1989). *The feeling good handbook.* New York: Morrow.

Button, E. (1986). Body size perception and response to in-patient treatment in anorexia nervosa. *International Journal of Eating Disorders, 5,* 617–629.

Cash, T. F., & Brown, T. A. (1987). Body image in anorexia nervosa and bulimia nervosa: A review of the literature. *Behavior Modification, 11,* 487–521.

Cash, T. F., & Pruzinsky, T. (Eds.). (1990). *Body images: Development, deviance, and change.* New York: Guilford Press.

Casper, R. C. (1983). Some provisional ideas concerning the psychologic structure in anorexia nervosa and bulimia. In P. L. Darby, P. E. Garfinkel, D. M. Garner, & D. V. Coscina (Eds.), *Anorexia nervosa: Recent developments in research* (pp. 387-392). New York: Alan R. Liss.

Casper, R. C., Offer, D., & Ostrov, E. (1981). The self-image of adolescents with acute anorexia nervosa. *Journal of Pediatrics, 98,* 656–661.

Channon, S., deSilva, P., Hemsley, D., & Perkins, R. (1989). A controlled trial of cognitive-behavioural and behavioural treatments of anorexia nervosa. *Behaviour Research and Therapy, 27,* 529–535.

Cinciripini, P. M., Kornblith, S. J., Turner, S. M., & Hersen, M. (1983). A behavioral program for the management of anorexia and bulimia. *Journal of Nervous and Mental Disease, 171,* 186–189.

Conners, M., Johnson, C. L., & Stuckey, M. K. (1984). Treatment of bulimia with brief psychoeducational group therapy. *American Journal of Psychiatry, 141,* 1512–1516.

Cooper, P. J., & Taylor, M. A. E. (1987). Body image disturbance in bulimia nervosa. *British Journal of Psychiatry, 151*(Suppl. 2), 34–38.

Crisp, A. H. (1980). *Anorexia nervosa: Let me be.* London: Academic Press.

Demitrack, M. A., Lesem, M. D., Listwak, S. J., Brandt, H. A., Jimerson, D. C., & Gold, P. W. (1990). CSF oxytocin in anorexia nervosa and bulimia nervosa: Clinical and pathophysiologic considerations. *American Journal of Psychiatry, 147,* 882–886.

Dolan, B. (1991). Cross cultural aspects of anorexia and bulimia: A review. *International Journal of Eating Disorders, 10,* 67–80.

Dykens, E. M., & Gerrard, M. (1986). Psychological profiles of purging bulimics, repeat dieters, and controls. *Journal of Consulting and Clinical Psychology, 54,* 283–288.

Eckert, E. D., Goldberg, S. C., Halmi, K. A., Casper, R. C., & Davis, J. M. (1979). Behavior therapy in anorexia nervosa. *British Journal of Psychiatry, 139,* 533–539.

Edgette, J. S., & Prout, M. F. (1989). Cognitive and behavioral approaches to the treatment of anorexia nervosa. In A. Freeman, K. M. Simon, L. E. Beutler, & H. Arkowitz (Eds.), *Comprehensive handbook of cognitive therapy* (pp. 367–384). New York: Plenum Press.

Ellis, A. (1962). *Reason and emotion in psychotherapy.* Secaucus, NJ: Lyle Stuart.

Fairburn, C. G. (1981). A cognitive behavioural approach to the treatment of bulimia. *Psychological Medicine, 11,* 707–711.

Fairburn, C. G. (1990). Bulimia nervosa. *British Medical Journal, 300,* 485–486.

Fairburn, C. G. (in press). Interpersonal psychotherapy for bulimia nervosa. In G. L. Klerman & M. M. Weissman (Eds.), *New Applications of Interpersonal Psychotherapy.* Washington, DC: American Psychiatric Press.

Fairburn, C. G., Agras, W. S., & Wilson, G. T. (1992). The research on the treatment of bulimia nervosa: Practical and theoretical implications. In G. H. Anderson & S. H. Kennedy (Eds.), *The biology of feast and famine: Relevance to eating disorders* (pp. 317–340). San Diego, CA: Academic Press.

Fairburn, C. G., & Cooper, P. J. (1989). Eating disorders. In K. Hawton, P. M. Salkovskis, J. Kirk, & D. M. Clark (Eds.), *Cognitive behavior therapy for psychiatric disorders* (pp. 304–314). New York: Oxford University Press.

Fairburn, C. G., & Garner, D. M. (1988). Diagnostic criteria for anorexia nervosa and bulimia nervosa: The importance of attitude to shape and weight. In D. M. Garner & P. E. Garfinkel (Eds.), *Diagnostic issues in anorexia nervosa and bulimia nervosa* (pp. 36–55). New York: Brunner/Mazel.

Fairburn, C. G., Hay, P. J., & Welch, S. L. (1993a). Binge eating and bulimia nervosa: Distribution and determinants. In C. G. Fairburn & G. T. Wilson (Eds.), *Binge eating: Nature, assessment, and treatment* (pp. 123–143). New York: Guilford Press.

Fairburn, C. G., Jones, R., Peveler, R. C., Carr, S. J., Solomon, R. A., O'Connor, M. E., Burton, J., & Hope, R. A. (1991). Three psychological treatments for bulimia nervosa: A comparative trial. *Archives of General Psychiatry, 48,* 463–469.

Fairburn, C. G., Jones, R., Peveler, R. C., Hope, R. A., & O'Connor, M. (1993b). Psychotherapy and bulimia nervosa: The longer-term effects of interpersonal psychotherapy, behavior therapy and cognitive behavior therapy. *Archives of General Psychiatry, 50,* 419–428.

Fairburn, C. G., Kirk, J., O'Connor, M., & Cooper, P. J. (1986). A comparison of two psychological treatments for bulimia nervosa. *Behaviour Research and Therapy, 24,* 629–643.

Fairburn, C. G., Marcus, M. D., & Wilson, G. T. (1993c). Cognitive-behavioral therapy for binge eating and bulimia nervosa: A comprehensive treatment manual. In C. G. Fairburn & G. T. Wilson (Eds.), *Binge eating: Nature, assessment, and treatment* (pp. 361–404). New York: Guilford Press.

Fairburn, C. G., Norman, P. A., Welch, S., O'Connor, M. E., Doll, H. A., & Peveler, R. C. (1995). A prospective study of outcome in bulimia nervosa and the long-term effects of three psychological treatments. *Archives of General Psychiatry, 52,* 304–312.

Finn, S., Hartman, M., Leon, G. R., & Lawson, L. (1986). Eating disorders and sexual abuse: Lack of confirmation for a clinical hypothesis. *International Journal of Eating Disorders, 5,* 1051–1060.

Freeman, C. P. L., Barry, F., Dunkeld-Turnbull, J., & Henderson, A. (1988). Controlled trial of psychotherapy for bulimia nervosa. *British Medical Journal, 296,* 521–525.

Freeman, R. J., Beach, B., Davis, R., & Solyom, L. (1985). Prediction of relapse in bulimia nervosa. *Journal of Psychiatric Research, 19,* 349–353.

Fremouw, W. J., & Heyneman, N. E. (1983). Cognitive styles and bulimia. *The Behavior Therapist, 6,* 143–144.

Frisch, R. E. (1990). The right weight: Body fat, menarche and ovulation. *Baillière's Clinical Obstetrics and Gynecology, 4,* 419–439.

Furnham, A., & Baguma, P. (1994). Cross-cultural differences in the evaluation of male and female body shapes. *International Journal of Eating Disorders, 15,* 81–89.

Garner, D. M., & Bemis, K. M. (1982). A cognitive-behavioral approach to anorexia nervosa. *Cognitive Therapy and Research, 6,* 123–150.

Garner, D. M., & Bemis, K. M. (1985). Cognitive therapy for anorexia nervosa. In D. M. Garner & P. E. Garfinkel (Eds.), *Handbook of psychotherapy for anorexia nervosa and bulimia* (pp. 107–146). New York: Guilford Press.

Garner, D. M., & Garfinkel, P. E. (1981). Body image in anorexia nervosa: Measurement theory and clinical implications. *International Journal of Psychiatry in Medicine, 11,* 263–284.

Garner, D. M., Garfinkel, P. E., Schwartz, D., & Thompson, M. (1980). Cultural expectations of thinness in women. *Psychological Reports, 47,* 483–491.

Garner, D. M., Olmsted, M. P., Polivy, J., & Garfinkel, P. E. (1984). Comparison between weight preoccupied women and anorexia nervosa. *Psychosomatic Medicine, 46,* 255–266.

Goldfried, M. R. (1971). Systematic desensitization as training in self-control. *Journal of Consulting and Clinical Psychology, 37,* 228–234.

Goodsitt, A. (1985). Self psychology and the treatment of anorexia nervosa. In D. M. Garner & P. E. Garfinkel (Eds.), *Handbook of psychotherapy for anorexia nervosa and bulimia* (pp. 55–82). New York: Guilford Press.

Gray, J. J., Ford, K., & Kelly, L. M. (1987). The prevalence of bulimia in a black college population. *International Journal of Eating Disorders, 6,* 733–740.

Gross, J., & Rosen, J. C. (1988). Bulimia in adolescents: Prevalence and psychosocial correlates. *International Journal of Eating Disorders, 7,* 51–61.

Guidano, V. F., & Liotti, G. (1983). *Cognitive processes and emotional disorders: A structural approach to psychotherapy.* New York: Guilford Press.

Haimes, A. L., & Katz, J. K. (1988). Sexual and social maturity versus social conformity in restricting anorectic, bulimic and borderline women. *International Journal of Eating Disorders, 7,* 331–341.

Halmi, K. A. (1982). Pragmatic information on the eating disorders. *Psychiatric Clinics of North America, 5,* 371–377.

Halmi, K. A. (1985). Behavioral management for anorexia nervosa. In D. M. Garner & P. E. Garfinkel (Eds.), *Handbook of psychotherapy for anorexia nervosa and bulimia* (pp. 147–159). New York: Guilford Press.

Harris, S. M. (1994). Racial differences in the predictors of college women's body image attitudes. *Women and Health, 21,* 89–104.

Hollon, S. D., & Beck, A. T. (1979). Cognitive therapy of depression. In P. C. Kendall & S. D. Hollon (Eds.), *Cognitive-behavioral interventions: Theory, research, and procedures* (pp. 153–203). New York: Academic Press.

Hsu, L. K. G. (1980). Outcome of anorexia nervosa: A review of the literature (1954 to 1978). *Archives of General Psychiatry, 37,* 1041–1043.

Hsu, L. K. G. (1982). Is there a disturbance of body image in anorexia nervosa? *Journal of Nervous and Mental Disease, 82,* 305–306.

Jones, R., Peveler, R. C., Hope, R. A., & Fairburn, C. G. (1993). Changes during treatment for bulimia nervosa: A comparison of three psychological treatments. *Behaviour Research and Therapy, 31,* 479–485.

Kaplan, A. S. (1991). Day hospital treatment for anorexia and bulimia nervosa. *Eating Disorders Review, 2,* 1–3.

Kirkley, B. G., Schneider, J. A., Agras, W. S., & Bachman, J. A. (1985). Comparison of two group treatments for bulimia. *Journal of Consulting and Clinical Psychology, 53,* 43–48.

Klerman, G. L., Weissman, M. M., Rounsaville, B. J., & Chevron, E. S. (1984). *Interpersonal psychotherapy of depression.* New York: Basic Books.

Laessle, R. G., Bossert, S., Hank, G., Hahlweg, G., & Pirke, K. M. (1989). Cognitive processing in bulimia nervosa: Preliminary observations. *Annals of the New York Academy of Sciences, 575,* 543–544.

Lee, N. F., & Rush, A. J. (1986). Cognitive-behavioral group therapy for bulimia. *International Journal of Eating Disorders, 5,* 599–615.

Leitenberg, H., Rosen, J. C., Gross, J., Nudelman, S., & Vara, L. S. (1988). Exposure plus response-prevention treatment of bulimia nervosa. *Journal of Consulting and Clinical Psychology, 56,* 535–541.

Leon, G. R., Lucas, A. R., Colligan, R. C., Ferdinande, R. J., & Kamp, J. (1985). Sexual, body-image, and personality attitudes in anorexia nervosa. *Journal of Abnormal Child Psychology, 13,* 245–258.

Lerner, H. D. (1986). Current developments in psychoanalytic psychotherapy of anorexia nervosa and bulimia nervosa. *The Clinical Psychologist, 39,* 39–43.

Levine, M. P., & Smolak, L. (1989). *Toward a developmental psychopathology of eating disorders: The example of the middle school transition.* Paper presented at the Eighth National Conference of the National Anorexic Aid Society, Columbus, OH.

Linehan, M. M. (1993). *Skills training manual for treating borderline personality disorder.* New York: Guilford Press.

Mahoney, M. J. (1974). *Cognition and behavior modification.* Cambridge, MA: Ballinger.

Mavissakalian, M. (1982). Anorexia nervosa treated with response prevention and prolonged exposure. *Behaviour Research and Therapy, 20,* 27–31.

McFarlane, A. H., Bellissimo, A., & Upton, E. (1982). Atypical anorexia nervosa: Treatment and management on a behavioural medicine unit. *The Psychiatric Journal of the University of Ottawa, 7,* 158–162.

Meichenbaum, D. (1974). *Therapist manual for cognitive behavior modification.* Waterloo, Ontario, Canada: University of Waterloo Press.

Nasser, M. (1988). Culture and weight consciousness. *Journal of Psychosomatic Research, 32,* 573–577.

Neuman, M., & Gaoni, B. (1975). Preferred food as the reinforcing agent in a case of anorexia nervosa. *Journal of Behavior Therapy and Experimental Psychiatry, 6,* 331–333.

Olmsted, M. P., Davis, R., Rockert, W., Irvine, M. J., Eagle, M., & Garner, D. M. (1991). Efficacy of a brief group psychoeducational intervention for bulimia nervosa. *Behaviour Research and Therapy, 29,* 71–83.

Ordman, A. M., & Kirshenbaum, D. S. (1985). Cognitive-behavioral therapy for bulimia: An initial outcome study. *Journal of Consulting and Clinical Psychology, 53,* 305–313.

Pertschuk, M. J. (1977). Behavior therapy: Extended follow-up. In R. A. Vigersky (Ed.), *Anorexia nervosa* (pp. 305–314). New York: Raven Press.

Pirin, A., & Kaplan, A. S. (1990). *A day hospital treatment program for anorexia nervosa and bulimia nervosa.* New York: Brunner/Mazel.

Polivy, J., Garner, D. M., & Garfinkel, P. E. (1986). Causes and consequences of the current preference for thin female physiques. In C. P. Herman, M. P. Zanna, & E. T. Higgins (Eds.), *The Ontario Symposium: Vol. 3. Physical appearance, stigma and social behavior* (pp. 173–206). Hillsdale, NJ: Erlbaum.

Polivy, J., & Herman, C. P. (1993). Etiology of binge eating: Psychological mechanisms. In C. G. Fairburn & G. T. Wilson (Eds.), *Binge eating: Nature, assessment, and treatment* (pp. 173–205). New York: Guilford Press.

Pope, H. G., Jr., & Hudson, J. I. (1992). Is childhood sexual abuse a risk factor for bulimia nervosa? *American Journal of Psychiatry, 149,* 455–463.

Post, G., & Crowther, J. H. (1987). Restricter–purger differences in bulimic adolescent females. *International Journal of Eating Disorders, 6,* 757–761.

Rosen, J. C. (1990). Body-image disturbances in eating disorders. In T. F. Cash & T. Pruzinsky (Eds.), *Body images: Development, deviance, and change* (pp. 190–214). New York: Guilford Press.

Rosen, J. C., & Gross, J. (1987). Prevalence of weight reducing and weight gaining in adolescent girls and boys. *Health Psychology, 6,* 131–147.

Rosen, J. C., & Leitenburg, H. (1982). Bulimia nervosa: Treatment with exposure and response prevention. *Behavior Therapy, 13,* 117–124.

Ruderman, S. (1986). Bulimia and irrational beliefs. *Behaviour Research and Therapy, 24,* 193–197.

Schlundt, D. G., & Johnson, W. G. (1990). *Eating disorders: Assessment and treatment.* Boston: Allyn & Bacon.

Schwartz, D. M., & Thompson, M. G. (1981). Do anorexics get well? Current research and future needs. *American Journal of Psychiatry, 138,* 319–323.

Scott, D. W. (1987). The involvement of psychosexual factors in the causation of eating disorders: Time for reappraisal. *International Journal of Eating Disorders, 6,* 199–213.

Scrignar, C. B. (1971). Food as the reinforcer in the outpatient treatment of anorexia nervosa. *Journal of Behavior Therapy and Experimental Psychiatry, 2,* 31–36.

Slade, P. (1982). Towards a functional analysis of anorexia nervosa and bulimia nervosa. *British Journal of Clinical Psychology, 21,* 167–179.

Slade, P., & Dewey, M. E. (1986). Development and preliminary validation of SCANS: A screening instrument for identifying individuals at risk of developing anorexia and bulimia nervosa. *International Journal of Eating Disorders, 5,* 117–138.

Smith, D. E., Marcus, M. D., & Eldredge, K. L. (1994). Binge eating syndromes: A review of assessment and treatment with an emphasis on clinical application. *Behavior Therapy, 25,* 635–658.

Smolak, L., Levine, M. P., & Sullins, E. (1990). Are child sexual experiences related to a college sample? *International Journal of Eating Disorders, 9,* 167–178.

Steiger, H., Fraenkel, L., & Leichner, P. P. (1989). Relationship of body image distortion to sex-role identifications, irrational cognitions, and body weight in eating-disordered females. *Journal of Clinical Psychology, 45,* 61–65.

Steiger, H., Goldstein, C., Mongrain, M., & Van der Feen, J. (1990). Description of eating-disordered, psychiatric, and normal women along cognitive and psychodynamic dimensions. *International Journal of Eating Disorders, 9,* 129–140.

Stevens, J., Kumanyika, S. K., & Keil, J. E. (1994). Attitudes toward body size and dieting differences between elderly black and white women. *American Journal of Public Health, 84,* 1322–1325.

Strauss, J., & Ryan, R. M. (1988). Cognitive dysfunction in eating disorders. *International Journal of Eating Disorders, 7,* 19–27.

Striegel-Moore, R. H., McAvay, G., & Rodin, J. (1986a). Psychological and behavioral correlates of feeling fat in women. *International Journal of Eating Disorders, 5,* 935–947.

Striegel-Moore, R. H., Silberstein, L. R., & Rodin, J. (1986b). Toward an understanding of risk factors for bulimia. *American Psychologist, 41,* 246–263.

Strober, M. (1991). Disorders of the self in anorexia nervosa: An organismic–developmental paradigm. In C. L. Johnson (Ed.), *Psychodynamic treatment of anorexia nervosa and bulimia* (pp. 354–373). New York: Guilford Press.

Thackwray, D. E., Smith, M. C., Bodfish, J. W., & Meyers, A. W. (1993). A comparison of behavioral and cognitive-behavioral interventions for bulimia nervosa. *Journal of Consulting and Clinical Psychology, 61,* 639–645.

Theander, S. (1985). Outcome and prognosis in anorexia and bulimia: Some results of previous investigations, compared with those of a Swedish long-term study. *Journal of Psychiatric Research, 19,* 493–508.

Treasure, J., Todd, G., Brolly, M., Tiller, J., Nehmed, A., & Denman, F. (1995). A pilot study of a randomised trial of cognitive analytical therapy vs. educational behavioural therapy for adult anorexia nervosa. *Behaviour Research and Therapy, 33,* 363–368.

Vandereycken, W., Probst, M., & Meermann, R. (1988). An experimental video-confrontation procedure as a therapeutic technique and research tool in the treatment of eating disorders. In K. M. Pirke, W. Vandereycken, & D. Ploog (Eds.), *The psychobiology of bulimia nervosa* (pp. 172–178). Heidelberg: Springer-Verlag.

Vitousek, K. B., & Ewald, L. S. (1993). Self-representation in eating disorders: A cognitive perspective. In Z. V. Segal & S. J. Blatt (Eds.), *The self in emotional distress: Cognitive and psychodynamic perspectives* (pp. 221–257). New York: Guilford Press.

Vitousek, K., Garner, D. M., & Hollon, S. D. (1991). *The assessment of cognitive processes in eating disorders.* Unpublished manuscript, University of Hawaii.

Vitousek, K., & Hollon, S. D. (1990). The investigation of schematic content and processing in eating disorders. *Cognitive Therapy and Research, 14,* 191–214.

Weinreich, P., Doherty, J., & Harris, P. (1985). Empirical assessment of identity in anorexia nervosa. *Journal of Psychiatric Research, 19,* 297–302.

Wilson, G. T., Eldredge, K. L., Smith, D., & Niles, B. (1991). Cognitive-behavioural treatment with and without response prevention for bulimia. *Behaviour Research and Therapy, 29,* 575–583.

Wilson, G. T., & Fairburn, C. G. (1993). Cognitive treatments for eating disorders. *Journal of Consulting and Clinical Psychology, 61,* 261–269.

Wilson, G. T., Rossiter, E., Kleifield, E. I., & Lindholm, L. (1986). Cognitive-behavioural treatment of bulimia nervosa: A controlled evaluation. *Behaviour Research and Therapy, 24,* 277–288.

Yates, A. (1989). Current perspectives on eating disorders: I. History, psychological, and biological aspects. *Journal of the American Academy of Child and Adolescent Psychiatry, 28,* 813–828.

IV

OTHER DISORDERS

12

Treatment-Resistant Schizophrenia and Psychotic Disorders

DONALD C. GOFF
DAVID C. HENDERSON

Schizophrenia is a chronic syndrome that typically follows a deteriorating course over time. With the exception of about 10% of patients who may achieve relative remission, schizophrenia rarely responds fully to treatment, and so "treatment resistance" tends to be the rule rather than the exception (Breier, Schreiber, Dyer, & Pickar, 1991). In fact, about 30% of patients with schizophrenia derive little or no benefit from conventional antipsychotic agents. The term "Kraepelinian schizophrenia" is used by some investigators to refer to patients who have failed to achieve a remission and to live independently for a period of 5 years. In one study, patients fitting this description showed no deterioration when their conventional neuroleptics were discontinued, and subsequently failed to improve when medication was reinstituted (Harvey et al., 1991).

The wide variability in response and the generally poor long-term treatment outcome have led to several different definitions of "treatment resistance" for schizophrenic patients. An international study group convened for this purpose recently defined treatment-resistant schizophrenia as the presence of continuing psychotic symptoms with substantial functional disability for at least 2 years, despite adequate pharmacologic and psychologic treatment (Brenner et al., 1990). In contrast, Meltzer (1992b) has argued for a more inclusive clinical definition, suggesting that any patient who does not return to his or her premorbid level of functioning should be considered treatment-resistant. For the purposes of this chapter, "treatment resistance" refers to the persistence of clinically significant symptoms of schizophrenia, despite an adequate trial of a conventional antipsychotic agent. A related topic, "treatment intolerance," is also discussed, since side effects prevent as many as 20% of patients from achieving an adequate trial of pharmacotherapy. Because psychotic symptoms and negative symptoms of schizophrenia may differ in their patterns of response to treatment, these two components of schizophrenic pathology are addressed separately.

DIAGNOSTIC ASSESSMENT

The first step in approaching a patient with persistent symptoms of schizophrenia is to reassess the diagnosis and degree of compliance with treatment. It should be emphasized that the diagnosis of schizophrenia is not made solely on the basis of a cross-sectional view of active symptoms; rather, it requires careful review of the duration and course of illness, as well as exclusionary criteria. Smith, MacEwan, Ancill, Honer, and Ehman (1992) examined 50 consecutive admissions with treatment-resistant psychosis and concluded that 46% were incorrectly diagnosed. In most of the cases in which the diagnosis was changed, patients previously diagnosed with schizophrenia were rediagnosed with bipolar disorder or psychotic depression. These patients were given mood-stabilizing agents and tended to show more improvement than patients whose diagnosis was not changed. It should be noted, however, that schizophrenic patients frequently present with superimposed depressive episodes, which may not always benefit from the addition of tricyclic antidepressants (Knights & Hirsch, 1981; Green, Nuechterlein, Ventura, & Mintz, 1990). Kramer et al. (1989) found that addition of amitriptyline or desipramine during the early stages of treatment of a psychotic exacerbation did not improve depressive symptoms and appeared to delay response of psychotic symptoms. However, addition of an antidepressant to an antipsychotic agent in depressed schizophrenic patients with stable psychotic symptoms may be helpful for depressive symptoms (Siris, Mason, Bermanzohn, Alvir, & McCorry, 1990).

In addition to assessment for an underlying psychotic mood disorder, patients should be carefully evaluated for the presence of substance abuse. Approximately 40–60% of schizophrenic patients actively abuse substances, most commonly alcohol and stimulants (Cuffel, 1992). The abuse may produce persistent psychotic symptoms and will further impair functioning (Bartels et al., 1993; Bowers, Mazure, Nelson, & Jatlow, 1990). Wilkins, Shaner, Patterson, Setoda, and Gorelick (1991) found that schizophrenic patients are less likely than other psychiatric patients to acknowledge substance abuse, so direct questioning may not adequately assess this important factor. When possible, interviews with family and residential staff may be helpful, as well as urine and blood screens. In some cases, evaluation in a restricted setting free of access to drugs and alcohol may be necessary to determine the role that substances play in relation to treatment resistance.

Tobacco is also widely used by schizophrenic patients, possibly in part to self-medicate neuroleptic side effects, dysphoric mood, and attentional deficits (Goff, Henderson, & Amico, 1992). Because tobacco smoking may significantly lower neuroleptic blood levels (Jann et al., 1986), assessment of patients in a smoke-free environment may further complicate decisions about the adequacy of neuroleptic dose and the presence of drug side effects. It is not clear whether the effects of cigarette smoking on drug levels and medication effects result from a pharmacokinetic interaction with nicotine (which could be replaced by a nicotine dermal patch) or from one of the more than 1000 other constituents of cigarette smoke.

In addition, patients should be assessed for other potential causes of psychosis, as listed in Table 12.1. Most can be ruled out by history, physical examination, and routine laboratory screening. Although the yield from brain imaging tends to be quite low in the absence of any focal neurologic signs, it is generally recommended that a brain scan (computed tomography or magnetic resonance imaging) be performed at least once in any patient with atypical or nonresponsive psychotic symptoms (Weinberger, 1984).

ASSESSING COMPLIANCE WITH TREATMENT

An equally important step in the assessment of treatment-resistant patients is to determine the level of compliance with pharmacotherapy. It has been estimated that 30–50% of schizophrenic patients do not take their medication as prescribed (Buchanan, 1992; Van Putten, 1974). Side effects are a major reason for this very high rate of noncompliance and need to be carefully assessed and managed. Finn, Bailey, Schultz, and Faber (1990) found that when patients were asked to compare the therapeutic benefit of antipsychotic medication with the burden of side effects, the burden of side effects substantially outweighed the therapeutic benefit from all perspectives except those of family and society. Compliance can be ruled out as a factor in treatment resistance either by switching the patient to haloperidol and monitoring plasma haloperidol concentrations, or by switching the patient to a depot preparation. In addition to removing the question of compliance, depot neuroleptics also reduce interindividual variability in steady-state plasma drug concentrations, because first-pass hepatic metabolism is bypassed (Marder, Hubbard, Van Putten, & Midha, 1989).

A final step in the reassessment of treatment resistance is to identify psychosocial stressors. It is well established that elevated levels of "expressed emotion" in families are associated with higher rates of relapse (Kavanagh, 1992). "Expressed emotion" refers to several factors, including critical attitudes expressed by family members toward the patient and overinvolve-

TABLE 12.1. Differential Diagnosis of Schizophrenia-Like Symptoms

Drug-induced psychosis
Amphetamines
Alcohol
Barbiturates (withdrawal)
Cocaine
Hallucinogens
Phencyclidine (PCP)
L-Dopa
Steroids

Drug-induced delirium
Anticholinergic agents
Disulfiram
Digitalis
Alcohol and benzodiazepines (withdrawal)
Nonsteroidal anti-inflammatory drugs

Other medical or neurologic disorders
Hypoglycemia
Acute intermittent porphyria
Cushing's syndrome or Addison's disease
Hypo- and hypercalcemia
Hypo- and hyperthyroidism
Korsakoff's psychosis (due to thiamine deficiency)
Pellagra (due to niacin deficiency)
Vitamin B_{12} deficiency
Tumors
Complex partial seizures
Central nervous system infections
Alzheimer's disease
Heavy-metal poisoning
Huntington's disease
Wilson's disease
Systemic lupus erythematosus

Psychiatric disorders
Autistic disorder
Brief reactive psychosis
Mood disorder
Delusional disorder
Malingering
Factitious psychosis
Personality disorder
Obsessive–compulsive disorder
Posttraumatic stress disorder

ment on the part of family members, both of which can be moderated through appropriate interventions. Other stressors may similarly destabilize patients and contribute to treatment resistance.

OPTIMIZING THE ANTIPSYCHOTIC DOSE

After the diagnosis has been reassessed, along with issues of compliance and psychosocial stressors, the next step is to optimize the dose of a conventional neuroleptic. Studies utilizing position emission tomography indicated that approximately 60–75% occupancy of dopamine (D_2) receptors is necessary for antipsychotic efficacy, regardless of which conventional agent is used (Farde, Wiesel, Nordstrom, & Sedvall, 1989). Once antipsychotic effect is achieved, the dose–response curve tends to plateau, meaning that further increases in plasma drug concentrations generally do not produce substantial increases in efficacy (Perry, Pfohl, & Kelly, 1988). Extrapyramidal symptoms, particularly parkinsonism, are associated with D_2 receptor blockade of approximately 80% or greater (Farde et al., 1992). In most cases, inadequate dosing is not the primary cause of treatment resistance, although adjustment of dose may minimize side effects while optimizing therapeutic response.

The decision whether to increase or decrease the dose of neuroleptic can usually be based on clinical assessment, although use of neuroleptic blood levels may be helpful, particularly in cases of potential drug–drug interactions (e.g., when the antipsychotic agent is combined with carbamazepine) (Goff & Baldessarini, 1993). Unfortunately, attempts to correlate clinical response with plasma drug concentrations have been complicated by the great interpatient variability in potential drug responsiveness that is characteristic of schizophrenia. The degree of symptomatic response is probably determined to a greater degree by poorly understood physiologic characteristics of individual patients than by more subtle factors such as plasma drug level. In addition, it is unclear to what extent plasma drug levels reflect concentrations in the brain. There is some evidence, (although not entirely consistent) of a "therapeutic window" for haloperidol, suggesting that some patients may experience clinical worsening if plasma concentrations fall above or below an optimal range. Patients have been described who develop agitation or worsening of psychotic symptoms at high plasma concentrations, which then improve with dose reduction (Van Putten, Marder, Wirshing, Aravagiri, & Chabert, 1991). A list of proposed therapeutic plasma concentrations is provided in Table 12.2. Among blood levels of all antipsychotic agents, haloperidol blood levels are best studied, are most commonly available, and probably are most clinically relevant because haloperidol is the drug least complicated by active metabolites.

The decision whether to increase or decrease the dose of a conventional neuroleptic should be based on the patient's history of previous

TABLE 12.2. Typical Clinical Plasma Concentrations of Antipsychotic Drugs

Drug	Plasma concentration (ng/ml)
Chlorpromazine	30–100
Clozapine	350
Haloperidol	5–15
Perphenazine	0.8–2.4
Fluphenazine decanoate	>1.0

response and on an assessment of neuroleptic side effects. The presence of akathisia (a sensation of lower-extremity motor restlessness) or of parkinsonism (rigidity, tremor, stooped posture, slowed gait, and reduced affective display) suggests that the dose should be gradually tapered downward. The absence of extrapyramidal symptoms should lead to an upward titration of dose in partial responders or nonresponders. This process of dose titration is intended to identify the most effective antipsychotic dose with the lowest level of side effects. Additional agents, such as beta-adrenergic blockers for akathisia and anticholinergics for parkinsonism, may be added if antipsychotic efficacy continues to improve along with the emergence of side effects as the dose is increased. Occasionally, the overlap of an optimal antipsychotic dose with extrapyramidal side effects may necessitate switching to a lower-potency agent or to an atypical antipsychotic agent. If increasing the antipsychotic dose does not result in clear clinical benefit within 4–6 weeks, the clinician should return to the lowest effective dose. Again, this process should be guided by clinical response and an appreciation of the wide variability among patients in degree of potential response and range of optimal doses. For example, some patients exhibit complete remission of psychotic symptoms at 1–2 mg/day of haloperidol, whereas others improve when the daily dose is raised to 40–60 mg of haloperidol.

AFTER A FIRST ANTIPSYCHOTIC DRUG TRIAL FAILS

If symptoms persist after the dose of a first antipsychotic agent is optimized, the next step involves either a switch to a second agent or the addition of an adjuvant. To meet the current definition of treatment resistance required for eligibility for clozapine, patients must complete at least two trials of antipsychotic agents lasting a minimum of 6 weeks. Although there are anecdotal accounts of patients responding dramatically to a second conventional agent after failing to respond to a first, this is probably an infrequent occurrence. In theory, all conventional agents act by the same mechanism (blockade of D_2 receptors), so that the optimal doses of such agents should have roughly comparable therapeutic effects. A few conventional agents, notably thioridazine and mesoridazine, have less typical profiles with respect to activity at other receptors and so may be more likely to produce a response when a patient has failed to respond to a more selective high-potency agent, although data from controlled trials are not available to support this observation (Vital-Herne, Gerbino, Kay, Katz, & Opler, 1986; Osser et al., 1991). In the Clozapine Collaborative Trial, only 4% of patients responded to chlorpromazine after failing to respond to a trial of high-dose haloperidol (Kane, Honigfeld, Singer, & Meltzer, 1988).

Risperidone

Risperidone is the first of a family of atypical agents that combine D_2 and serotonin (5-HT_2) antagonism. Five controlled studies of risperidone involving 2070 schizophrenic inpatients have provided compelling evidence of a reduced risk for neurologic side effects and, compared to high-dose haloperidol, better efficacy for negative symptoms (Borison, Pathiriraja, Diamond, & Meibach, 1992; Claus et al., 1992; Muller-Spahn & Group, 1992; Hoyberg et al., 1993; Chouinard et al., 1993; Marder & Meibach, 1994). Several of these studies have also suggested that risperidone may be more effective than conventional neuroleptics for psychotic symptoms in certain patients. Risperidone has not yet been studied in rigorously defined treatment-resistant patients, nor has its antipsychotic efficacy been directly compared to clozapine. In the North American Risperidone Trial, patients were randomly assigned to one of four doses of risperidone ranging from 2 to 16 mg/day, or to haloperidol at 20 mg/day. Only the group receiving 6 mg/day of risperidone displayed significantly greater therapeutic effects than the haloperidol group (Chouinard et al., 1993).

Whereas the evidence for efficacy of clozapine in treatment-resistant schizophrenic patients is quite compelling, and preliminary evidence for risperidone is encouraging, evidence supporting the use of other agents in combination with conventional neuroleptics is scant and generally inconsistent. Christison, Kirch, and Wyatt (1981) have recently provided a comprehensive review of this literature.

Lithium Augmentation

Addition of lithium to a conventional antipsychotic in treatment-resistant schizophrenic and schizoaffective patients has been studied in three small controlled trials (Carmen, Bigelow, & Wyatt, 1981; Growe, Crayton, Klass, Evans, & Stizich, 1979; Small, Kellams, Milstein, & Moore, 1975). The results have been modestly encouraging, and suggest that one-third to one-half of patients will exhibit some improvement within 4 weeks. Augmentation of antipsychotic efficacy has been associated with lithium blood levels in the range of 0.8–1.2 mEq/liter. Although patients with an affective component to their clinical presentation may be most likely to benefit from addition of lithium, the literature indicates that response may also occur in the absence of affective symptoms, and may include improvement of psychotic symptoms and negative symptoms as well. It remains uncertain whether the addition of lithium to a neuroleptic places a patient at greater risk for neurotoxic reactions, including neuroleptic malignant syndrome (Goff & Baldessarini, 1993). Clinicians should monitor patients carefully for extrapyramidal symptoms, confusion, or fever when this combination is employed.

Benzodiazepines and Buspirone

Addition of benzodiazepines may improve agitation, psychotic symptoms, and social withdrawal in a subgroup of treatment-resistant schizophrenic patients, although controlled trials have produced inconsistent results (Christison et al., 1991; Arana et al., 1986b). Benzodiazepines are probably most effective for patients with high levels of psychotic symptoms and anxiety. Because abuse and disinhibition may develop, benzodiazepines should be tapered and discontinued if no benefit is apparent after 2–3 weeks. Some patients may even display worsening of psychosis following addition of benzodiazepines (Dixon, Wieden, Frances, & Sweeney, 1989). Withdrawal of the short-acting benzodiazepine alprazolam has been associated with worsening of psychotic symptoms in some patients (Wolkowitz et al., 1988). Although controlled trials have not been conducted, we have observed encouraging results with the atypical anxiolytic buspirone at doses ranging from 15 to 40 mg/day, particularly in agitated patients (Goff et al., 1991).

Electroconvulsive Therapy

Electroconvulsive therapy (ECT) has not been well studied in neuroleptic-resistant schizophrenic patients, although uncontrolled trials suggest that some patients may experience symptomatic improvement lasting up to 6 months. ECT has generally been considered to be most effective early in the course of schizophrenia and most appropriate for patients with affective symptoms. However, a naturalistic study of 110 schizophrenic and schizoaffective patients treated with ECT challenges these guidelines. Milstein, Small, Miller, Sharpley, and Small (1990) reported an overall 54% response rate, with paranoid schizophrenics showing the greatest response (67%). Neither age nor presence of affective symptoms predicted response. Although the number of treatments ranged from 12–20 in this series, the authors noted that six of the seven patients who stopped treatment prematurely (fewer than six treatments) were classified as responders. Maintenance treatment following ECT remains problematic for treatment-resistant schizophrenic patients, although use of atypical antipsychotics or monthly ECT treatments may be appropriate.

Anticonvulsants

Carbamazepine is the best-studied anticonvulsant for augmentation of conventional antipsychotics. At doses producing typical anticonvulsant plasma levels, carbamazepine has produced moderate improvement of tension, excitement, manic symptoms, and suspiciousness in a series of small trials (Christison et al., 1991). Carbamazepine may be most effective for patients with electroencephalographic abnormalities, manic symptoms, or episodic violence, although cases have been reported of clinical improvement in the absence of any of these characteristics (Neppe, 1983; Sramek et al., 1988). Addition of carbamazepine to neuroleptic agents is complicated by a potential pharmacokinetic interaction, since carbamazepine increases hepatic microsomal enzyme metabolism and so can substantially lower plasma concentrations of antipsychotic agents (Goff & Baldessarini, 1993). When carbamazepine is added to low-dose haloperidol, this drug–drug interaction may produce clinical deterioration (Arana et al., 1986a). For this reason, clinicians should be prepared to increase the dose of neuroleptic, or possibly switch to haloperidol so that plasma concentrations can be monitored. Carbamazepine should not be added to clozapine because of the risk that bone marrow suppression will complicate clozapine's adverse hematologic effects.

Valproate has also been reported to improve treatment-resistant psychosis when added to conventional neuroleptics, although not all trials have not produced positive results and controlled trials have not been conducted (Wassef & Waston, 1989). Although valproate may produce modest elevations in blood levels, it is generally recommended as the most appropriate anticonvulsant for combination therapy with clozapine.

Beta-Adrenergic Blockers

The beta-adrenergic blockers, particularly propranolol, previously received considerable attention as adjuncts to conventional neuroleptics (Yorkston et al., 1977; Donaldson, Gelenberg, & Baldessarini, 1986). Used at high doses (up to 1200 mg/day), propranolol is reported to decrease agitation, psychotic symptoms, and violence in some treatment-resistant patients, but results from controlled trials have generally been disappointing. It has been suggested that the inconsistent therapeutic effect of propranolol may result in some cases from either its potential to elevate plasma concentrations of antipsychotic agents, or its beneficial effect on akathisia (Adler et al., 1986). Because the evidence for efficacy remains unconvincing, and the potential adverse effects upon cardiovascular and pulmonary function are considerable, high-dose propranolol augmentation should be utilized only when other approaches fail.

Clozapine

Currently, the most effective intervention for treatment-resistant or treatment-intolerant patients is the atypical agent clozapine. When rigorously defined treatment resistant patients were treated with clozapine for 6 weeks in the Clozapine Collaborative Trial, 30% exhibited a clinically significant improvement, defined by a reduction of at least 20% in the Brief Psychiatric Rating Scale (BPRS) score (Kane et al., 1988). Cloza-pine response was superior to chlorpromazine response on most items of the BPRS, including psychotic symptoms, negative symptoms, depression, anxiety, and hostility. Subsequently, open trials have suggested that the response rate may reach 50–60% if trials are extended to 6 months (Melt-zer, Burnett, Bastani, & Ramierz, 1990). Few predictors of response have been identifed. Pickar et al. (1992) found that patients exhibiting extrapy-ramidal symptoms from conventional antipsychotic agents may be more likely to respond. One survey reported higher rates of response among pa-tients with affective symptoms, particularly those meeting criteria for schizoaffective disorder (McElroy et al., 1991). In general, since it is not possible to predict response to clozapine with any reasonable degree of specificity, a trial of clozapine should be attempted in all seriously ill pa-tients who have failed to respond to at least two trials of antipsychotic agents. Risperidone is the most appropriate intermediate step prior to proceeding to a clozapine trial in patients who have failed to respond to an adequate trial of a conventional agent or who are unable to tolerate a conventional agent.

The considerable expense of clozapine has limited its availability to many patients. However, several studies have indicated that clozapine can be quite cost-effective as a result of its reduction in hospitalization (Franken-burg, Zanarini, Cole, & McElroy, 1992). The 1–2% risk of agranulocyto-sis has also limited clozapine's use and has greatly complicated its administration because of the mandatory weekly hematologic monitoring system. This monitoring system has successfully reduced mortality from agranulocytosis; at this writing, there have been 7 deaths in the United States out of more than 40,000 patients treated.

Guidelines for Clozapine Use

Several experts have recommended that conventional antipsychotic agents be discontinued prior to starting a patient on clozapine. This policy is based in part on the belief that adding clozapine to a conventional antipsychot-ic will diminish the efficacy of clozapine by altering the ratio of $5\text{-}HT_2$ blockade to D_2 blockade. In our experience, this is an unnecessary precaution that adds the expense of hospitalization and that subjects pa-tients to the risk of clinical worsening associated with stopping medica-tion. Some patients may revoke their consent to take clozapine if they are allowed to decompensate off neuroleptics. There is no evidence that combining conventional high-potency neuroleptics with clozapine impairs therapeutic efficacy; in fact, some patients may experience improved an-tipsychotic efficacy at the cost of some extrapyramidal side effects (Naber, Holzbach, Perro, & Hippius, 1992). We routinely start clozapine by gradually adding it to conventional high-potency neuroleptics on an outpatient basis. Once the clozapine dose has reached 100 mg/day, the conventional neuroleptic can be gradually tapered and discontinued as the clozapine dose is increased. Combining clozapine with low-potency agents, such as thioridazine, should be avoided, since cardiovascular and sedative side effects of the two drugs can be additive. The gradual transition from conventional antipsychotic to an optimal dose of clozapine may require up to 2 months to achieve under outpatient conditions, but we have found that over 80% of outpatients tolerate this procedure. Early experience suggests that patients can similarly make the transition from risperidone to clozapine if the two agents are combined during a process of gradual dose titration.

There are no clear guidelines for determining the optimal dose of clozapine. European clinicians have tended to use clozapine in a range of 200–300 mg/day, whereas average doses in the United States generally run in the range of 400–600 mg, with a maximum allowed dose of 900 mg/day. In a clinician-determined dose optimization study, Pickar et al. (1992) reported a mean optimal clozapine dose of 550 mg/day. Titration of clozapine is often complicated by a considerable delay in the emergence of therapeutic effects. As many as 50% of potential responders do not exhibit therapeutic improvement until after 4–6 months of treatment, thus necessitating a six-month trial to identify potential responders (Meltzer et al., 1990). The rate and ultimate level of upward titration of clozapine are usually determined by side effects, particularly sedation, orthostatic hypotension, and sialorrhea. If it can be tolerated, a dose of 500 mg/day is probably adequate for most patients. The dose can be kept at this level while evidence of clinical effect is awaited. If a patient has not responded by 4 months, the dose can be gradually increased to 900 mg/day. Because seizure risk is related to both the absolute dose and the rate of dose increase, dose titration should be performed gradually, and prophylactic treatment with valproic acid should be considered for doses above 600 mg/day (Baldessarini & Frankenburg, 1991). Although the therapeutic effect of dosage increase may follow considerable delay, in our experience clinical worsening usually follows within 1–2 weeks of dose reduction, thereby making downward titration a much easier process. Once an adequate response has been achieved, the dose can be decreased gradually, particularly if side effects are present. Preliminary work with clozapine blood levels has suggested that plasma concentrations above 350 ng/ml are associated with better outcome, although further research is needed before clozapine blood levels become a standard clinical tool (Perry, Miller, Arndt, & Cadoret, 1991).

Options for Clozapine Nonresponders

No data from systematic research are available to guide treatment options for the 40–60% of patients who fail to respond to clozapine. If psychotic symptoms persist despite a dose increase to 900 mg/day, it may be useful to try lowering the dose. Preliminary data suggest a possible "therapeutic window" for clozapine in some patients (Perry et al., 1991; Owen, Delva, & Lawson, 1992). Addition of a high-potency neuroleptic may also improve antipsychotic response, although patients should be carefully monitored for emergence of extrapyramidal symptoms. We have found buspirone (10–40 mg/day) helpful for anxiety and agitation in combination with clozapine. Some clozapine-resistant patients also appear to benefit from addition of valproic acid or the selective serotonin reuptake inhibitors. Sertraline is less likely to affect hepatic metabolism of clozapine than is fluoxetine, and in our experience may improve negative symptoms as well as psychotic symptoms in some patients. We have found that some patients benefit from the careful addition of risperidone to clozapine, particularly those patients who cannot tolerate a full therapeutic dose of clozapine because of side effects.

NEGATIVE SYMPTOMS

Negative symptoms of schizophrenia tend to receive less attention than psychotic symptoms, but can be just as disabling. Negative symptoms include apathy, social withdrawal, poverty of thought and speech, neglect of "activities of daily living" (including hygiene), flattened affect, and anhedonia (Carpenter, Heinrichs, & Alphs, 1985). Negative symptoms tend to respond less completely to conventional antipsychotic agents than psychotic symptoms do; in a review of data from six trials, Kay and Singh (1989) found a mean 35% reduction of negative symptom severity, as opposed to a 52% reduction of psychotic symptoms. Response of negative symptoms may occur independently of psychotic symptom response and may follow a different time course (Breier et al., 1987). The assessment of negative symptoms is seriously complicated by the fact that neuroleptic-induced akinesia can be indistinguishable from negative symptoms. Although a trial of an anticholinergic agent may improve neuroleptic-induced akinesia (Van Putten & May, 1978), it remains unclear whether this constitutes a diagnostic test, as Tandon and Greden (1989) have reported evidence that anticholinergic agents may directly improve negative symptoms while worsening psychotic symptoms. This finding has led to a theory of cholinergic overactivity as a mechanism underlying negative symptoms (Tandon, Dutchak, & Greden, 1989). Substantial evidence suggests that agents that act at $5\text{-}HT_2$ receptors, such as clozapine and risperidone, are more effective than conventional antipsychotics for the treatment of negative symptoms (Meltzer, 1992a). Preliminary evidence also indicates that agents acting at other serotonergic sites may also improve negative symptoms when added to conventional antipsychotics; most encouraging at present are results from studies of selective serotonin reuptake inhibitors (Silver & Nassar, 1992). Finally, negative symptoms may result in part from dopamine hypoactivity in frontal cortex. This model has led to trials of dopamine agonists, such as methylphenidate, with inconsistent results. Because of the risk of exacerbating psychotic symptoms in a subgroup of patients, psychostimulants and other dopamine agonists are generally not recommended for the treatment of negative symptoms (Chiarello & Cole, 1987).

Assessment of patients with negative symptoms should begin with a differential diagnosis of negative symptoms, including depression, parkinsonism, hypothyroidism, and substance abuse. Although behavioral manifestations may be quite similar, depression and negative symptoms can usually be distinguished on the basis of the patient's report of mood state (Newcomer, Faustman, Yeh, & Csernansky, 1989). A brief trial of an antiparkinsonism medication, such as benztropine or amantadine, may help distinguish neuroleptic side effects from negative symptoms. Since anticholinergic agents can substantially impair cognitive functioning, it is best to treat neuroleptic-induced parkinsonism with dose reduction of the neuroleptic or with amantadine, particularly in elderly patients (Baker, Cheng, & Amara, 1983; McEvoy et al., 1987).

No data are available regarding dose–response relationships for antipsychotic treatment of negative symptoms, but clinical titration of dose remains the best approach to optimizing the response to conventional agents. If negative symptoms persist, preliminary evidence supports either switching to an atypical "$5\text{-}HT_2D_2$" agent such as risperidone (Chouinard et al., 1993), or adding a selective serotonin reuptake inhibitor such as fluoxetine or sertraline (Goff, Midha, Sarid-Segal, Hubbard, & Amico, 1990; Silver & Nassar, 1992). If negative symptoms remain sufficiently disabling, a trial of clozapine should be considered.

CONCLUSION

In summary, treatment resistance in schizophrenic patients should prompt a careful review of diagnosis, compliance, and psychosocial stressors. The dose of a conventional antipsychotic can be optimized by titrating antipsychotic efficacy versus the emergence of extrapyramidal symptoms. Preliminary evidence suggests that the atypical agent risperidone may represent a reasonable second step; risperidone may be particularly useful in the presence of negative symptoms. Although some patients may benefit from augmentation of conventional antipsychotic agents with lithium, benzodiazepines, or buspirone, the data supporting these approaches remain somewhat sparse and inconsistent. Similarly, ECT may produce short-term improvement in some patients. Without question, the alternative most likely to produce substantial improvement in patients who are resistant to or intolerant of conventional antipsychotic agents is clozapine. After adequate trials of a conventional antipsychotic and a serotonin–dopamine antagonist (e.g., risperidone) have been completed, a clozapine trial lasting at least 6 months should be offered to patients who remain seriously impaired by their illness.

REFERENCES

Adler, L., Angrist, B., Peselow, E., Corwin, J., Maslansky, R., & Rotrosen, J. (1986). A controlled assessment of propranolol in the treatment of neuroleptic-induced akathisia. *British Journal of Psychiatry, 149,* 42–45.

Arana, G. W., Goff, D. C., Friedman, H., Ornsteen, M., Greenblatt, D. J., Black, B., & Shader, R. I. (1986a). Does carbamazepine-induced reduction of plasma haloperidol levels worsen psychotic symptoms? *American Journal of Psychiatry, 143,* 650–651.

Arana, G. W., Ornsteen, M. L., Kanter, F., Friedman, H. L., Greenblatt, D. J., & Shader, R. I. (1986b). The use of benzodiazepines for psychiatric disorders: A literature review and preliminary findings. *Psychopharmacology Bulletin, 22,* 77–87.

Baker, L. A., Cheng, L. Y., & Amara, I. B. (1983). The withdrawal of benztropine mesylate in chronic schizophrenic patients. *British Journal of Psychiatry, 143,* 584–590.

Baldessarini, R. J., & Frankenburg, R. (1991). Clozapine: A novel antipsychotic agent. *New England Journal of Medicine, 324,* 746–754.

Bartels, S. J., Teague, G. B., Drake, R. E., Clark, R. E., Bush, P. W., & Noordsy, D. L. (1993). Substance abuse in schizophrenia: Service utilization and cost. *Journal of Nervous and Mental Disease, 181,* 227–232.

Borison, R., Pathiriraja, A., Diamond, B., & Meibach, R. (1992). Risperidone: Clinical safety and efficacy in schizophrenia. *Psychopharmacology Bulletin, 28,* 213–218.

Bowers, M. B. J., Mazure, C. M., Nelson, J. C., & Jatlow, P. I. (1990). Psychotogenic drug use and neuroleptic response. *Schizophrenia Bulletin, 16,* 81–85.

Breier, A., Schreiber, J., Dyer, J., & Pickar, D. (1991). National Institute of Mental Health longitudinal study of chronic schizophrenia: Prognosis and predictors of outcome. *Archives of General Psychiatry, 48,* 239–246.

Breier, A., Wolkowitz, O. M., Doran, A. R., Roy, A., Boronow, J., Hommer, D. W., & Pickar, D. (1987). Neuroleptic responsivity of negative and positive symptoms in schizophrenia. *American Journal of Psychiatry, 144,* 1549–1555.

Brenner, H. D., Sven, D. J., Goldstein, M. J., Hubbard, J. W., Keegan, D. L., Kruger, G., Kulhanek, F., Liberman, R. P., Malm, U., & Midha, K. K. (1990). Defining treatment refractoriness in schizophrenia. *Schizophrenia Bulletin, 16,* 551–561.

Buchanan, A. (1992). A two-year prospective study of treatment compliance in patients with schizophrenia. *Psychological Medicine, 22,* 787–797.

Carmen, J. S., Bigelow, L. B., & Wyatt, R. J. (1981). Lithium combined with neuroleptics in chronic schizophrenic and schizoaffective patients. *Journal of Clinical Psychiatry, 42,* 124–128.

Carpenter, W. T., Heinrichs, D. W., & Alphs, L. D. (1985). Treatment of negative symptoms. *Schizophrenia Bulletin, 11,* 440–452.

Chiarello, R. J., & Cole, M. O. (1987). The use of psychostimulants in general psychiatry. *Archives of General Psychiatry, 44,* 286–295.

Chouinard, G., Jones, B., Remington, G., Bloom, D., Addington, D., MacEwan, G. W., Labelle, A., Beauclair, L., & Arnott, W. (1993). A Canadian multicenter placebo-controlled study of fixed doses of risperidone and haloperidol in the treatment of chronic schizophrenic patients. *Journal of Clinical Psychopharmacology, 13*, 25–40.

Christison, G., Kirch, D., & Wyatt, R. (1991). When symptoms persist: Choosing among alternative somatic treatments. *Schizophrenia Bulletin, 17*, 217–245.

Claus, A., Bollen, J., De Cuyer, H., Eneman, M., Malfroid, M., Peuskens, J., & Heylen, S. (1992). Risperidone versus haloperidol in the treatment of chronic schizophrenia inpatients: A multicentre double-blind comparative study. *Acta Psychiatrica Scandinavica, 85*, 295–305.

Cuffel, B. J. (1992). Prevalence estimates of substance abuse in schizophrenia and their correlates. *Journal of Nervous and Mental Disease, 180*, 589–592.

Dixon, L., Weiden, P. J., Frances, A. J., & Sweeney, J. (1989). Alprazolam intolerance in stable schizophrenic outpatients. *Psychopharmacology Bulletin, 25*, 213–214.

Donaldson, S. R., Gelenberg, A. J., & Baldessarini, R. J. (1986). Alternative treatments for schizophrenic psychoses. In S. Arieti (Ed.), *American handbook of psychiatry* (Vol. 8, pp. 513–535). New York: Basic Books.

Farde, L., Nordstrom, A. L., Wiesel, F. A., Pauli, S., Halldin, C., & Sedvall, G. (1992). Positron emission tomographic analysis of central D1 and D2 dopamine receptor occupancy in patients treated with classical neuroleptics and clozapine: Relation to extrapyramidal side effects. *Archives of General Psychiatry, 49*, 538–544.

Farde, L., Wiesel, F., Nordstrom, A.-L., & Sedvall, G. (1989). D1- and D2-dopamine receptor occupancy during treatment with conventional and atypical neuroleptics. *Psychopharmacology, 99*, S28–S31.

Finn, S. E., Bailey, J. M., Schultz, R. T., & Faber, R. (1990). Subjective utility ratings of neuroleptics in treating schizophrenia. *Psychological Medicine, 20*, 843–848.

Frankenburg, F. R., Zanarini, M. C., Cole, J. O., & McElroy, S. I. (1992). Hospitalization rates among clozapine-treated patients: A prospective cost–benefit analysis. *Annals of Clinical Psychiatry, 4*, 247–250.

Goff, D. C., & Baldessarini, R. (1993). Drug interactions with antipsychotic agents. *Journal of Clinical Psychopharmacology, 13*, 57–67.

Goff, D. C., Henderson, D. C., & Amico, E. (1992). Cigarette smoking in schizophrenia: Relationship to psychopathology and medication side effects. *American Journal of Psychiatry, 149*, 1189–1194.

Goff, D. C., Midha, K., Brotman, A., McCormick, S., Waites, M., & Amico, E. (1991). An open trial of buspirone added to neuroleptics in schizophrenic patients. *Journal of Clinical Psychopharmacology, 11*, 193–197.

Goff, D. C., Midha, K. K., Sarid-Segal, O., Hubbard, J. W., & Amico, E. (1995). A placebo-controlled trial of fluoxetine added to neuroleptic inpatients with schizophrenia. *Psychopharmacology, 117*, 417–473.

Green, M. F., Nuechterlein, K. H., Ventura, J., & Mintz, J. (1990). The temporal relationship between depressive and psychotic symptoms in recent-onset schizophrenia. *American Journal of Psychiatry, 147*, 179–182.

Growe, G. A., Crayton, J. W., Klass, D. B., Evans, H., & Stizich, M. (1979). Lithium in chronic schizophrenia. *American Journal of Psychiatry, 136*, 454–455.

Harvey, P. D., Putnam, K. M., Davidson, M., Kahn, R. S., Powchik, P., McQueeney, R., Keefe, R. S. E., & Davis, K. L. (1991). Brief neuroleptic discontinuation and clinical symptoms in Kraepelinian and non-Kraepelinian chronic schizophrenic patients. *Psychiatry Research, 38*, 285–292.

Hoyberg, O., Fensbo, C., Remvig, J., Lingiaerde, O., Sloth-Nielsen, M., & Salvesen, I. (1993). Risperidone versus perphenazine in the treatment of chronic schizophrenic patients with acute exacerbations. *Acta Psychiatrica Scandinavica, 88*, 395–402.

Jann, M. W., Saklad, S. R., Ereshefsky, L., Richards, A. L., Harrington, C. A., & Davis, C. M. (1986). Effects of smoking on haloperidol and reduced haloperidol plasma concentrations and haloperidol clearance. *Psychopharmacology, 90*, 468–470.

Kane, J., Honigfeld, G., Singer, J., & Meltzer, H. (1988). Clozapine for the treatment-resistant schizophrenic: A double-blind comparison with chlorpromazine. *Archives of General Psychiatry, 45*, 789–796.

Kavanagh, D. J. (1992). Recent developments in expressed emotion and schizophrenia. *British Journal of Psychiatry, 160*, 601–620.

Kay, S. R., & Singh, M. M. (1989). The positive–negative distinction in drug-free schizophrenic patients: Stability, response to neuroleptics, and prognostic significance. *Archives of General Psychiatry, 46*, 711–718.

Knights, A., & Hirsch, S. R. (1981). "Revealed" depression and drug treatment for schizophrenia. *Archives of General Psychiatry, 38*, 806–811.

Kramer, M., Vogel, W., DiJohnson, C., Dewey, D., Sheves, P., Cavicchia, S., Litle, P., Schmidt, R., & Kimes, I. (1989). Antidepressants in "depressed" schizophrenic inpatients: A controlled trial. *Archives of General Psychiatry, 46*, 922–928.

Marder, S. R., Hubbard, J. W., Van Putten, T., & Midha, K. K. (1989). Pharmacokinetics of long-acting injectable neuroleptic drugs: Clinical implications. *Psychopharmacology, 98*, 433–439.

Marder, S. R., & Meibach, R. C. (1994). Risperidone in the treatment of schizophrenia. *American Journal of Psychiatry, 151*, 825–835.

McElroy, S. L., Dessain, E. C., Pope, H. G., Cole, J. O., Keck, P. E., Frankenberg, F. R., Aizley, H. G., & O'Brien, S. (1991). Clozapine in the treatment of psychotic mood disorders, schizoaffective disorder, and schizophrenia. *Journal of Clinical Psychiatry, 52*, 411–414.

McEvoy, J., McCue, M., Spring, B., Mohs, R., Lavori, P., & Farr, R. (1987). Effects of amantadine and trihexyphenidyl on memory in elderly normal volunteers. *American Journal of Psychiatry, 144*, 573–577.

Meltzer, H. Y. (1992a). The importance of serotonin–dopamine interactions in the action of clozapine. *British Journal of Psychiatry, 160*(Suppl. 17), 22–29.

Meltzer, H. Y. (1992b). Treatment of the neuroleptic-nonresponsive patient. *Schizophrenia Bulletin, 18*, 515–542.

Meltzer, H. Y., Burnett, S., Bastani, B., & Ramierz, L. F. (1990). Effect of six months of clozapine treatment on the quality of life of chronic schizophrenic patients. *Hospital and Community Psychiatry, 41*, 892–897.

Milstein, V., Small, J. G., Miller, M. J., Sharpley, P. H., & Small, I. F. (1990). Mechanisms of action of ECT: Schizophrenia and schizoaffective disorder. *Biological Psychiatry, 27*, 1282–1292.

Muller-Spahn, F., & International Risperidone Research Group. (1992). Risperidone in the treatment of chronic schizophrenic patients: An international double-blind parallel-group study versus haloperidol. *Clinician*, 15, 90A–101A.

Naber, D., Holzbach, R., Perro, C., & Hippius, H. (1992). Clinical management of clozapine patients in relation to efficacy and side-effects. *British Journal of Psychiatry*, 160(Suppl. 17), 54–59.

Neppe, V. M. (1983). Carbamazepine as adjunctive treatment in nonepileptic chronic inpatients with EEG temporal lobe abnormalities. *Journal of Clinical Psychiatry*, 44, 326–331.

Newcomer, J. W., Faustman, W. O., Yeh, W., & Csernansky, J. G. (1989). Distinguishing depression and negative symptoms in unmediated patients with schizophrenia. *Psychiatry Research*, 31, 243–250.

Osser, D. N., Albert, L. G., Figueiredo, S., O'Connor, H., Barden, Y., & Carmichael, W. G. (1991). Mesoridazine in neuroleptic-resistant psychoses. *Journal of Clinical Psychopharmacology*, 11, 328–330.

Owen, J. A., Delva, N. J., & Lawson, J. S. (1992). Clozapine concentrations and response in schizophrenia. *American Journal of Psychiatry*, 149, 1120–1121.

Perry, P. J., Miller, D., Arndt, S. V., & Cadoret, R. (1991). Clozapine and norclozapine plasma concentrations and clinical response of treatment refractory schizophrenic patients. *American Journal of Psychiatry*, 148, 231–235.

Perry, P. J., Pfohl, B. M., & Kelly, M. W. (1988). The relationship of haloperidol concentrations to therapeutic response. *Journal of Clinical Psychopharmacology*, 8, 38–43.

Pickar, D., Owen, R. R., Litman, R. E., Konicki, P. E., Guitierrez, R., & Rapaport, M. H. (1992). Clinical and biological response to clozapine in patients with schizophrenia. *Archives of General Psychiatry*, 49, 345–353.

Silver, H., & Nassar, A. (1992). Fluvoxamine improves negative symptoms in treated chronic schizophrenia: An add-on double-blind, placebo-controlled study. *Biological Psychiatry*, 31, 698–704.

Siris, S. G., Mason, S. E., Bermanzohn, P. C., Alvir, J. J., & McCorry, T. A. (1990). Adjunctive imipramine maintenance in post-psychotic depression/negative symptoms. *Schizophrenia Bulletin*, 26, 91–94.

Small, J. G., Kellams, J. J., Milstein, V., & Moore, J. (1975). A placebo-controlled study of lithium combined with neuroleptics in chronic schizophrenic patients. *American Journal of Psychiatry*, 132, 1315–1317.

Smith, G. N., MacEwan, G. W., Ancill, R. J., Honer, W. G., & Ehmann, T. S. (1992). Diagnostic confusion in treatment-refractory psychotic patients. *Journal of Clinical Psychiatry*, 53, 197–200.

Sramek, J., Herrera, J., Costa, J., Heh, C., Tran-Johnson, T., & Simpson, G. (1988). A carbamazepine trial in chronic treatment-refractory schizophrenia. *American Journal of Psychiatry*, 145, 748–750.

Tandon, R., Dutchak, D., & Greden, J. F. (1989). Cholinergic syndrome following anticholinergic withdrawal in a schizophrenic patient abusing marijuana. *British Journal of Psychiatry*, 154, 712–714.

Tandon, R., & Greden, J. F. (1989). Cholinergic hyperactivity and negative schizophrenic symptoms. *Archives of General Psychiatry*, 46, 745–753.

Van Putten, T. (1974). Why do schizophrenic patients refuse to take their drugs? *Archives of General Psychiatry*, 31, 67–72.

Van Putten, T., Marder, S., Wirshing, W., Aravagiri, M., & Chabert, N. (1991). Neuroleptic plasma levels. *Schizophrenia Bulletin*, 17, 197–216.

Van Putten, T., & May, P. R. A. (1978). 'Akinetic depression' in schizophrenia. *Archives of General Psychiatry, 35,* 1101–1107.

Vital-Herne, J., Gerbino, L., Kay, S. R., Katz, I. R., & Opler, L. A. (1986). Mesoridazine and thioridazine: Clinical effects and blood levels in refractory schizophrenics. *Journal of Clinical Psychiatry, 47,* 375–379.

Wassef, A., & Waston, D. J. (1989). Neuroleptic–valproic acid combination in the treatment of psychotic symptoms: A three-case report. *Journal of Clinical Psychopharmacology, 9,* 45–48.

Weinberger, D. R. (1984). Brain disease and psychiatric illness: When should a psychiatrist order a CAT scan? *American Journal of Psychiatry, 141,* 1521–1527.

Wilkins, J. N., Shaner, A. L., Patterson, C. M., Setoda, D., & Gorelick, D. (1991). Discrepancies between patient report, clinical assessment, and urine analysis in psychiatric patients during inpatient admission. *Psychopharmacology Bulletin, 27,* 149–154.

Wolkowitz, O. M., Breier, A., Doran, A., Kelsoe, J., Lucas, P., Paul, S. M., & Pickar, D. (1988). Alprazolam augmentation of the antipsychotic effects of fluphenazine in schizophrenic patients. *Archives of General Psychiatry, 143,* 664–671.

Yorkston, N. J., Zaki, S. A., Pitcher, D. R., Gruzelier, J. H., Hollander, D., & Sergeant, H. G. S. (1977). Propranolol as an adjunct to the treatment of schizophrenia. *Lancet, ii,* 575–578.

13

When a Substance Use Disorder Is the Cause of Treatment Resistance

DAVID R. GASTFRIEND

Patients with substance abuse or dependence often seem treatment-resistant as if by definition: Because these disorders tend to distort the patients' awareness of what is pathologic use, they produce resistance to treatment. This resistance may be manifested through open denial, treatment rejection, failure to follow through with longitudinal care, or relapse that occurs despite what seems to be solid treatment efforts. Treatment resistance may therefore be manifested in multiple ways, which require flexible and creative solutions. These problems and solutions are summarized in Table 13.1 and discussed in detail in this chapter. First, however, a brief discussion of recent U.S. statistics on substance use may be revealing.

PREVALENCE AND TRENDS IN SUBSTANCE USE

Overall, the impact of substance abuse/dependence on U.S. society is enormous and has grown rapidly, with government estimates of the total cost increasing from $117 billion in 1984 (Harwood, Napolitano, Kristiannsen, & Collins, 1984) to $238 billion in 1993 (Institute for Health Policy, Brandeis University, 1993). A 10% annual increase in drug-related hospital emergencies occurred at the beginning of the 1990s, with 433,000 visits reported in 1992 (National Institute on Drug Abuse [NIDA], 1993). The substance most commonly involved in emergencies is alcohol, followed, in order of decreasing magnitude, by cocaine, combinations of alcohol and other substances, and (at substantially lower incidence) narcotics and benzodiazepines (NIDA, 1986b). Nevertheless, heroin emergencies increased by a third at the beginning of the 1990s, with every age group affected (NIDA, 1993). Also, phencyclidine- and marijuana-related emergencies increased by approximately 50% between 1991 and 1992 (NIDA, 1993).

Alcoholic beverage use is normative in the United States; however, 55% of Americans report drinking fewer than three drinks per week, and 35% report abstaining. Only 11% acknowledge consuming more than 1 ounce daily (NIDA, 1986a). The National Institute of Mental Health Epidemiologic Catchment Area study reported a prevalence of alcohol abuse or dependence of 13% (Regier et al., 1990). Social policies have had a positive impact on reducing social drinking and limiting alcohol-related automobile deaths, which decreased by 25% between 1989 and 1993 (NIDA, 1993).

Cocaine use has been the most rapidly changing psychoactive substance use in recent years, quadrupling between the years of 1974 and 1982: The number of Americans acknowledging one-time use rose from 5.4 to 21.6 million (NIDA, 1986a). Cocaine deaths tripled from 1983 to 1986 (NIDA, 1986b), and cocaine-related hospital emergency visits grew from 1% in 1978 to 28% in 1992 (NIDA, 1993). Despite a 50% decrease in the incidence of cocaine use between 1985 and 1992, the trend in danger continues to worsen, with an 18% increase in cocaine emergencies from 1991 to 1992 (NIDA, 1993). By 1992, cocaine was thought to be covertly responsible for a high proportion of inner-city general hospital psychiatric admissions (Galanter, Egelko, DeLeon, Rohrs, & Franko, 1992).

Benzodiazepines remain the most commonly used psychoactive prescription drugs, having replaced the more dangerous barbiturates and other sedative/hypnotics in the 1960s and 1970s. By the 1980s, 15% of the adult U.S. population received prescriptions for benzodiazepines annually (Rickels, 1981), and 16% of this group continued to take them for 1 year or more (Rickels, 1983). By the 1990s, clinician awareness was bringing benzodiazepine prescribing trends downward; however, coercive influences such as the New York State triplicate reporting system produced a 50% decrease in benzodiazepine use but a 115% increase in prescriptions of other sedative/hypnotics (Weintraub, Singh, Byrne, Maharaj, & Guttmacher, 1991). Among patients who reported to hospitals with drug emergencies, between 25% and 35% were using benzodiazepines and other sedative/hypnotics as their primary drugs (NIDA, 1986b). Opiate addicts appear to be at substantial risk for benzodiazepine dependence, as multiple methadone and nonmethadone treatment centers have reported high rates of benzodiazepine-positive urine samples (Iguchi et al., 1990; San, Torrens, Castillo, Porta, & De La Torre, 1993), and heroin dependence is estimated to afflict 500,000 Americans (General Accounting Office, 1990).

COVERT SUBSTANCE ABUSE/DEPENDENCE

Whenever any psychiatric patient fails to respond to conventional thera-pies, the clinician needs to reconsider in the differential diagnosis that covert substance abuse or dependence may masquerade in myriad ways. Unfortunately, most clinicians are less than adequately prepared to recog-nize and treat this important group of psychiatric syndromes (GAP Com-mittee, 1991). Substance abuse and dependence syndromes mimic the symptoms of all major psychiatric illnesses and produce a host of compli-cations (American Psychiatric Association, 1994; Galanter et al., 1992; Hall, Stickney, Gardner, Perl, & LeCann, 1979; Hasin & Grant, 1987; Lehman, Meyers, & Corty, 1989). Conversely, one of the most impor-tant predictors of treatment resistance in addiction is severity of psychiatric illness (McLellan, Luborsky, Woody, O'Brien, & Druley, 1983).

In the early stages of substance abuse, patients may manifest no symp-toms or only subtle problems, such as reporting vague medical or psycho-logic symptoms that are difficult to target with pharmacotherapy, unauthorized modification of medication regimen, and lateness or absence at follow-up visits. At later stages of addiction, the course of treatment often becomes chaotic, with social and vocational disorganization, medi-cal sequelae, impulsivity, and high risk for accidents and suicide.

Treatment resistance may be iatrogenic, through nonspecific prescribing or failure to recognize and treat the substance abuse/dependence. This may result in protracted dysfunction, relapse, or serious medical morbidity and mortality, including the use of prescribed agents in suicide. Treatment may result in "mere" abstinence (i.e., no use of illicit drugs), though with con-tinued psychiatric symptoms and compliance problems; the preferable result, of course, is more comprehensive recovery from addictive and psychiatric disorders. Recovery is associated with progressively improving compliance and character symptomatology. It is helpful to emphasize nonpharmacologic strategies for addiction and to use a formal treatment contract to increase the likelihood of resolving treatment resistance (Gastfriend, 1993).

Detecting Evidence of Covert Substance Misuse

It can be very difficult to detect covert substance misuse, particularly in the presence of other psychiatric disorders. One psychiatric unit reported that despite a screening evaluation intended to exclude substance abuse patients, 58% of inpatients had a concurrent substance abuse diagnosis (Hall et al., 1979). Even subsequent observation on an inpatient unit may fail to detect substance misuse. At a Veterans Administration (VA) hospital, 60% of general psychiatric patients continued to use alcohol or drugs while on the hospital grounds, and 25% of those who later were found to have substance use problems acknowledged that their problems had worsened while they were in the hospital (McLellan, Druley, & Carson, 1978).

TABLE 13.1. Treatment Resistance in Substance Abuse/Dependence: Problems and Solutions

Problem	Solutions
Covert substance abuse/dependence (patient denies, minimizes use)	Review signs and symptoms for quality (e.g., vagueness) and pattern (e.g., binge). Obtain alternate data sources.
Resistance to acute treatment (patient admits problem but expects to overcome it without efforts)	Develop "readiness" by persistently confronting with evidence of substance use problems, without rejecting patient. Facilitate family intervention.
Resistance to continuing care (patient fails to follow through with sustained recovery efforts)	Help patient anticipate longer-term risks; have others in recovery relate their efforts (e.g., through group counseling). Propose contingency plan if patient begins to show signs of behavioral progression toward relapse.
High problem severity	Refer to setting/treatment with adequate intensity:
• Medical problems (e.g., high seizure risk, brittle diabetes)	• Refer to general hospital inpatient rehabilitation unit.
• Cognitive impairment (e.g., subclinical dementia or poor planning capacity)	• Use highly structured, repetitive, concrete, and sustained teaching techniques.
• Psychiatric illness (e.g., dual diagnosis)	• Refer to dual-disorders program and employ specific therapies for each disorder.
• Social problems (e.g., family sabotages recovery or environment is highly provocative)	• Provide family therapy and/or seek alternate residence (e.g., halfway or sober house).
High risk for late relapse (patient makes good recovery efforts but repeatedly relapses)	Review history of treatments and circumstances surrounding relapses. Consider what new modalities may help (e.g., dynamic or behavioral therapies). Increase intensity of prior treatments.

Another problem is that covert substance abuse or dependence may lead to manifest psychiatric symptomatology and misdiagnosis (Hall et al., 1979). In one sample, substance-abusing patients were twice as likely as nonabusers to present with a major psychotic episode (Hall et al., 1979). Drugs of abuse are known to precipitate mania; depressed mood; delusions, hallucinations, and other manifestations of thought disorder; panic attacks and generalized anxiety; and organic syndromes (including amnesia, delirium, and dementia). The chart of diagnoses that can be caused by psychoactive substances has been revised in DSM-IV (American Psychiatric

Association, 1994), and a version of this chart is presented in Table 13.2. Proper diagnosis is essential in treatment planning, as patients with substance abuse have 10% longer lengths of stay and are three times more likely to leave psychiatric inpatient units against medical advice (Hall, 1979). In one VA hospital study, only 7% of patients with alcohol abuse and none of the patients with drug abuse received any specific therapy for their substance abuse problems (O'Farrell, Connors, & Upper, 1983).

Counterproductive Myths about Patient Management

Some counterproductive myths about the management of substance abuse/dependence patients are particularly pertinent to the issues of denial or minimization of use.

The most common myth is that "useful screening or diagnostic information is obtained by asking how much a patient drinks or uses drugs." In fact, quantity is not really of consequence in making a diagnosis, and it invites the patient to negotiate the diagnosis by minimizing the amount he or she reports consuming. Furthermore, there is tremendous interindividual variance in the amount of consumption that causes brain and other tissue damage, particularly when men are compared to women (Becker & Jaffe, 1984).

A second myth is as follows: "Always maintain a neutral stance, even with a patient who has a substance use disorder." This myth has held that the preservation of neutrality is paramount in any treatment relationship. This has the effect of inhibiting care providers from confronting covert substance misuse, on the grounds that the provider may appear untrusting, unempathic, or rejecting. The reality is that when evidence points to substance abuse or dependence, it behooves both patient and provider to adopt a distrust *of the addictive disorder.* Patients often complain, "You mean you don't trust me any more!" To this, the clinician must respond, "I trust you to work with me, but neither of us should trust the illness of addiction."

Persistent confrontation of the destructiveness of substance abuse/dependence is most empathic with the patient's desire for health. After a treatment relationship has been established, therapeutic rejection is actually of pivotal importance. However, the effective clinician rejects not the patient, but rather the patient's denial of the addiction. This entails openly rejecting the fantasy that nonspecific treatments will be effective or safe. The patient is not rejected from treatment, but is told that until abstinence has been safely established, other pharmacotherapies must be withheld and various psychotherapeutic issues must be held in abeyance. This frustrating but supportive stance is often catalytic.

A third myth is this: "If only the patient can obtain relief from psychiatric symptoms, then the substance misuse will abate." Pharmacotherapies require stable and predictable pharmacokinetic and pharmacodynamic states (e.g., steady-state levels of medication) in order to be effective. As

TABLE 13.2. Psychiatric Disorders That Can Be Caused by Psychoactive Substances

Disorder	Substance	Temporal state
Delirium	Alcohol and sedatives[a]	Intoxication and withdrawal
	Amphetamines and cocaine	Intoxication
	Cannabis	Intoxication
	Hallucinogens and phencyclidine	Intoxication
	Inhalants	Intoxication
	Opioids	Intoxication
Psychotic disorders	Alcohol and sedatives	Intoxication and withdrawal
	Amphetamines and cocaine	Intoxication
	Cannabis	Intoxication
	Hallucinogens	Intoxication and flashbacks
	Phencyclidine	Intoxication
	Inhalants	Intoxication
	Opioids	Intoxication
Amnestic disorder/dementia	Alcohol and sedatives	Persisting
	Inhalants	Persisting (dementia only)
Mood disorders	Alcohol and sedatives	Intoxication and withdrawal
	Amphetamines and cocaine	Intoxication and withdrawal
	Hallucinogens and phencyclidine	Intoxication
	Inhalants	Intoxication
	Opioids	Intoxication
Anxiety disorders	Alcohol	Intoxication and withdrawal
	Sedatives	Withdrawal
	Amphetamines	Intoxication
	Cocaine	Intoxication and withdrawal
	Caffeine	Intoxication
	Cannabis	Intoxication
	Hallucinogens and phencyclidine	Intoxication
	Inhalants	Intoxication
Sexual dysfunctions	Alcohol and sedatives	Intoxication
	Amphetamines and cocaine	Intoxication
	Opioids	Intoxication
Sleep disorders	Alcohol and sedatives	Intoxication and withdrawal
	Amphetamines and cocaine	Intoxication and withdrawal
	Caffeine	Intoxication
	Opioids	Intoxication and withdrawal

Note. Adapted with permission from the *Diagnostic and Statistical Manual of Mental Disorders,* Fourth Edition. Copyright 1994 American Psychiatric Association.
[a]"Sedatives" in this table is shorthand for "sedatives, hypnotics, or anxiolytics" in DSM-IV.

a general principle, pharmacotherapy alone is ineffective in the treatment of addicted patients. Most therapeutic tools will generally remain ineffective for psychiatric disorders as long as psychoactive substance abuse or dependence persists. Two classes of agents may be exceptions to this general rule. Disulfiram (Fuller et al., 1986) and the mu-opiate antagonist naltrexone have been shown to decrease drinking in alcoholics (Volpicelli, Alterman, Hayashida, & O'Brien, 1992). Recent studies also suggest that the serotonin uptake inhibitors fluoxetine (Cornelius et al., 1993), citalopram (Naranjo, Poulos, Bremner, & Lanctot, 1992; Naranjo et al., 1987), sertraline (Brands, Sellers, & Kaplan, 1990), and others (Naranjo & Sellers, 1989) may reduce excessive alcohol consumption. Long-term studies are not yet available, however, and it is unclear to what extent "anticraving" pharmacotherapies will be effective in patients with severe substance dependence.

All psychotherapies require a stable capacity for learning. Dynamic psychotherapies, in particular, require the capacity to access internal dysphoria in order to succeed. All forms of substance abuse/dependence can sharply disrupt neurophysiologic states, learning states, and the ability to access and tolerate psychologic discomfort. Thus, reduction or elimination of substance use is critical to the success of all therapeutic interventions.

Engaging the Patient When Addiction Becomes Evident

The point at which treatment failure occurs can be the most crucial time to intervene with a firm revision of the entire treatment plan. At this point, a patient presents as "sick, sad, and sorry" (Royce, 1989). Even if the patient's sudden acknowledgment of an addiction comes as a surprise to the clinician, the need for immediate intervention—with a direct referral for addiction-specific treatment—is critical. The revision of the treatment plan should include at least reconsideration (and usually cessation) of previous pharmacotherapies and modification of previous psychotherapies, which may have been erroneously directed at, for example, primary depression or anxiety.

When it is clear that a patient has a substance use disorder, it is critical that the clinician and patient return to a basic historical review of the patient's specific psychoactive substance use profile. This review must objectively characterize the setting in which misuse usually occurs (time, place, and occasion); social network; quantity, frequency, and rate of consumption; perceived pressures and precipitants; and subjective responses. The pursuit of this profile convinces the patient that the psychiatric clinician is interested, skilled, and objective. It helps to confront the patient's denial, to restore confidence in the care provider, and to educate the patient about the risks and complications in his or her life. When the examiner is curious, straightforward, and nonjudgmental about the individual (not the behavior), the patient's defenses are not provoked, and a refreshing dialogue may ensue.

RESISTANCE TO ACUTE TREATMENT

Engaging a patient with substance abuse/dependence in acute treatment is a daunting challenge. For example, most clinicians' early training experiences with "skid row" alcoholics in emergency rooms have left the indelible impression that all substance-misusing patients are unmotivated (Clark, 1981). Clinicians may be reluctant to provide motivational counseling, but this role is obligatory in dealing with these patients (Gastfriend, 1986). When a clinician assertively elicits the elements of a substance use crisis and reframes the evidence that alcohol or drug use is the common theme underlying loss of stamina, organ function, cognitive function, job performance, and social relationships, most patients will feel that the concern is sincere (Miller, Benefield, & Tonigan, 1993).

Many sober patients, particularly those in Alcoholics Anonymous (AA), have described the onset of their recovery after reaching a "bottom" or crisis (Royce, 1989). For a patient who refuses to acknowledge the need for acute treatment, the clinician can catalyze such a crisis by facilitating a confrontation between the patient and family members, employers, and/or a probation officer. The Johnson Institute in Minneapolis has conceptualized a process known as the "family conference" or "family intervention." In this, family members and friends are gathered to prepare a factual list of problems, to anticipate the patient's denial and anger, to maintain a united front, to model a nonjudgmental but resolute attitude favoring the disease model of addiction, and to anticipate a failure in initial treatment with a contract to accept more vigorous treatment in that contingency (Bien, Miller, & Tonigan, 1993).

In subsequent treatment, however, it must be noted that confidentiality is vital to maintaining the therapeutic relationship with an addicted patient. In fact, it is even more important in cases of substance abuse or dependence than in other psychiatric disorders, because of the greater stigma of addiction. When a substance use disorder is diagnosed, it is particularly helpful to review how the patient's privacy will be protected, and to inquire whether family members, primary care physicians, employers, and legal contacts are aware of the substance use issues. Regulations protecting addicted patients require that whenever a release of information is made or requested, if substance use information is involved, it must be specifically mentioned in the consent.

Sometimes a patient objects to all appropriate treatment options on the basis of expense, lack of coverage, an undesirable "climate," or a program's clientele. This response is a common manifestation of resistance and must be interpreted as such. This patient may need to be advised that no further effective treatment is available. Rather than a complete disruption of care, however, a "readiness" model is preferable, in which the clinician meets with the patient over subsequent weeks so that both parties can observe how the patient's condition is proceeding. Often, this supportive but clear plan retains the clinical rapport and permits the patient to come to a realization that he or she must choose to enter addictions treatment if any progress is to be made (Rollnick, Heather, Gold, & Hall, 1992).

Other patients will reject inpatient treatment or day treatment as too restrictive. The clinician should recommend the optimal treatment, but if a patient will not budge in his or her consideration, it is helpful to compromise on a less restrictive initial treatment if the patient will agree to the optimal recommendation after a time-limited period in the event of a treatment failure. It is most helpful if the clinician will write out this agreement in the chart and obtain the patient's signature on it.

RESISTANCE TO CONTINUING CARE

Most substance abuse/dependence patients are highly ambivalent about treatment, and need to be persuaded to pursue healthy changes over the extended time frame that is required for success. Motivational counseling is a vital and continuing role of the provider (Miller & Rollnick, 1991). Instruments exist for measuring motivation (Gastfriend, Filstead, Reif, Najavits, & Parrella, 1995; Mee-Lee, Hoffman, & Smith, 1992; Miller & Rollnick, 1991; Prochaska & DeClemente, 1992) and can be used for "tracking" a patient's motivational progress. Examples of motivational questions include "To what extent do you think that now that you have acknowledged your alcohol/drug problem, your problems will be over?" and "What is the likelihood that you will be in treatment for your substance dependence in 90 days?"

Even the most treatment-refractory patient may be influenced through specific approaches that address resistance (Miller et al., 1993). Patients in crisis can often be helped by anticipating further potential negative consequences of their substance misuse, such as divorce, restraining orders, job loss, or incarceration. Interestingly, forced treatment (as in court-mandated sentencing) has empirically been found effective (Rosenberg & Liftik, 1976), as has the contingency contract for adverse consequences in the event of relapse or treatment noncompliance (Crowley, 1984; Rosenberg & Liftik, 1976). Contingency contracting can be utilized in the outpatient setting and is a proactive readiness tool. The clinician and patient jointly identify an adverse action item (e.g., sending a letter reporting ongoing substance use to the patient's spouse or employer) that will be executed if ongoing use or relapse occurs within some specified time (e.g., 6 weeks or 6 months). The patient is asked to write the letter and seal it in an addressed envelope, which remains in the therapist's possession, to be mailed only if necessary; at the end of the specified time, it is given to the patient to be destroyed. A contingency plan is another tool, in which the patient who rejects a recommended treatment (e.g., hospital rehabilitation) in favor of a less intensive one (e.g., day treatment) signs a statement in which he or she agrees to enter the more intensive treatment if relapse occurs over a specified period (e.g., 6 weeks to 6 months).

This is also the time to induce a significant other to accept treatment for codependency, independently of the identified patient. The most treatment-resistant patient may ultimately be persuaded into a longitudinal commitment to recovery if treatment of the spouse is initiated at this point.

RESISTANCE BECAUSE OF HIGH PROBLEM SEVERITY

Two general rules of thumb are that (1) the sicker a patient is, the more restrictive and intensive the treatment should be; and (2) it is better to overtreat than to undertreat. According to placement criteria published by the American Society of Addiction Medicine, patients should receive residential treatment to initiate treatment when there is (1) a history of treatment resistance in a less intensive setting, (2) a high risk for dangerous relapse, or (3) serious psychiatric or medical concurrent conditions or complications (Hoffman, Halikas, Mee-Lee, & Weedman, 1991; Millman, 1986). Managed-care approval of hospitalization is increasingly dependent on these criteria. A high-quality treatment facility is one that rises above treatment biases, offers multimodal care, and individualizes a program to patients' specific needs.

This section discusses such factors in high problem severity as intravenous heroin use, cognitive impairment, and dual diagnoses (substance abuse/dependence plus other psychiatric disorders). The risk of relapse is discussed in a later section.

High-Severity Addiction: Intravenous Heroin Use

Intravenous heroin use is a particularly serious source of treatment resistance (Ball & Ross, 1991). Covert addiction is a common problem, as these patients often present to clinicians, emergency rooms, and crisis units with requests for anxiolytics but without identifying themselves as opiate users. Resistance to acute treatment is also common, as only 100,000 intravenous heroin addicts receive methadone treatment in the United States out of an estimated 600,000 with the disorder. Methadone treatment provides the best likelihood for continuing care; however, many patients remain symptomatic despite enrollment in methadone treatment. Most heroin addicts have been initiated into the drug culture in early adolescence, have developed highly specialized skills for maintaining drug access, and have an extensive network of drug-using supports. Conversely, these patients have lost years of opportunity for healthy character development, are isolated from mainstream society and non-drug-dependent supports, and have developed an intense mistrust of the health care system and care providers.

Nevertheless, almost one-fifth of addicts cease intravenous drug use rapidly upon entering a methadone program (Ball & Ross, 1991).

The high severity of addiction in this group is often manifested in concurrent substance abuse/dependence, which is also a critical source of treatment resistance. At least half of methadone recipients also use other drugs and alcohol (Kolar, Brown, Weddington, & Ball, 1990; Nurco, Kinlock, Hanlon, & Ball, 1988), and specialized treatment guidelines have been published by the federal government to address this problem (Barthwell & Gastfriend, 1991). Not surprisingly, it has been shown that methadone treatment either does not significantly reduce other concurrent substance abuse/dependence (Millman, 1986) or does so only indirectly (Fairbank, Dunteman, & Condelli, 1993). Methadone treatment programs are often thought of as a "black box," but evaluation of the internal treatment components has shown that the programs that closely individualize methadone doses and services are most successful at retention (McLellan, Arndt, Metzger, Woody, & O'Brien, 1993; Millman, 1986). The key to helping the treatment-resistant opiate addict is to examine the past and potential present barriers to long-term retention. Ideally, the patient should receive the range of needed services within the walls of the methadone program (McLellan et al., 1993). If the methadone program lacks individualized services that are indicated for a particular patient (e.g., services for psychiatric, family, medical, vocational, and other needs), then external resources should be vigorously sought. These other resources need to be coordinated carefully, with (1) the patient's consent and (2) frequent telephone communication among service providers.

Cognitive Impairment

Cognitive impairment is often overlooked as a source of treatment resistance in patients with substance use disorders. Chronic use of alcohol and inhalants produces lasting effects on short-term memory, learning, attention, and abstraction (Brandt, Butters, Ryan, & Bayog, 1983; Tarter & Edwards, 1985). These impairments make it difficult for patients to learn from past adverse consequences and may render rehabilitation efforts ineffective (Becker & Jaffe, 1984). These impairments may also be subclinical and may go unrecognized without formal testing, because verbal skills are often intact in these patients. In patients with primary dependence on drugs, such as cocaine, subclinical cognitive impairments may be overlooked because concurrent dependence on alcohol may be ignored.

The keys to addressing treatment resistance secondary to cognitive impairment are (1) routine screening for cognitive impairment (e.g., with the Mini-Mental State Examination—Crum, Anthony, Bassett, & Folstein, 1993); (2) formal characterization of the nature of impairments (e.g., with neuropsychologic testing); and (3) specific structures and learning aids to compensate for the impairments. A patient with mild dementia may require a structured living setting, such as a halfway house. A patient with

mild concreteness may benefit from repetitive, written learning aids or
the simple, straightforward messages commonly issued at AA meetings:
"One day at a time," "Keep on coming," and the mnemonic for warning
of relapse conditions, "HALT," which stands for "hungry, angry, lonely,
or tired."

Dual Diagnoses: Comorbid Substance Abuse/Dependence and Psychiatric Pathology

Clinicians may neglect to consider substance abuse or dependence in the
differential diagnosis, once another psychiatric disorder has been established as the primary treatment objective. This may be a critical source
of treatment resistance. A prior diagnosis of another major psychiatric disorder in no way protects a patient against vulnerability to a substance use
disorder. In fact, the population with psychoactive substance use syndromes
is at greater risk of having other psychiatric disorders than is the general
population. Figure 13.1 illustrates the percentages of Americans with psychiatric syndromes who report comorbid substance abuse or dependence
(Regier et al., 1990).

The symptoms of many psychiatric disorders are thought to predispose
patients toward substance misuse in attempts to self-medicate. Khantzian
(1990) has proposed that individuals select a drug on the basis of its selec-

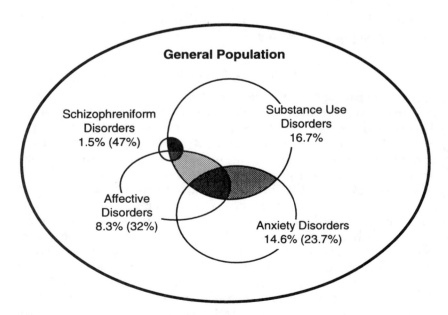

FIGURE 13.1. Comorbidity of psychiatric disorders with substance use disorders. Lifetime prevalence of each disorder in the general population, followed by percentage within
each disorder of comorbid substance abuse or dependence (in parentheses). Data from
Epidemiologic Catchment Area Study (Regier et al., 1990).

TABLE 13.3. The Theory of Selective Self-Medication

Class of agent	Principal effect on:	Relieves distress associated with:
Stimulants	Energy state	Boredom, depression, hypomania, hyperactivity, frustration intolerance, low self-esteem
Opiates	Sense of well-being	Disorganization, rage, aggression
Alcohol and CNS depressants	Inhibition	Closeness, dependency, self-assertion, "alexithymia"

Note. Adapted from Khantzian (1990). Copyright 1990 by Plenum Publishing Corporation. Adapted by permission.

tivity for relieving or augmenting emotions that they cannot achieve or maintain on their own (see Table 13.3). This phenomenon often confounds the care provider. Patients may conceal substance use problems because of denial or the perception that addiction is an even greater stigma than mental illness. Relapse may be triggered repeatedly, as a patient who is newly abstinent is unprepared to encounter intolerable feelings such as anhedonia, rage, or dependency that were previously masked by the substance abuse.

Incidence of Dual Diagnoses

Psychiatric patients are two to five times more likely to misuse substances than the general population (Crowley, Chesluk, Dilts, & Hart, 1974). Some of the variation in these figures results from measurements across different treatment settings. For instance, VA inpatient psychiatric units have reported from 32.8% to 58% of patients admitted for psychiatric diagnoses to be concurrently suffering from substance use problems (Hall et al., 1979; McLellan et al., 1978; O'Farrell et al., 1983). In a study from a non-VA psychiatry hospital, 31% of patients reported abuse of one or more drugs during their lifetime, and 15% were currently using those drugs (Fisher, Mason, Keeley, & Fisher, 1975).

Different psychiatric disorders have different propensities for association with substance misuse. Twenty-eight percent of panic patients in one study were reported to suffer from alcoholism (Reich, Winokur, & Mullaney, 1975). In a recent VA study, over one-third of hospitalized schizophrenic patients were found to use cocaine (Shaner et al., 1993). Individuals with psychiatric disorders and comorbid substance use disorders are at a high risk for suicide (Marzuk & Mann, 1988), and adolescents seem to be at particularly high risk (Crumley, 1990). The highest incidence of concurrent substance use diagnoses may occur with personality-disordered patients, particularly those with Cluster B ("impulsive") disorders, including borderline, narcissistic, and antisocial personality. Samples of patients with antisocial personality have been found to have a high prevalence of serious alcohol abuse. This is not surprising, since antisocial and borderline personality disorders both formerly included substance abuse among their criteria (Dulit, Fyer, Haas, Sullivan, & Frances, 1990).

Prognosis and Treatment Approaches

Patients with personality disorders and substance misuse are often particularly difficult to treat. Patients with personality disorders experience earlier onset of substance abuse and dependence than the general population, as well as increased severity of substance misuse, increased rates of polysubstance use, and more relationship problems (fewer marriages, more divorces). Individuals with borderline personality disorder report that psychotic episodes worsen with substance misuse, including increased frequency and severity of transient illusions, depersonalization and derealization, and greater likelihood of permanent delusions following use of psychotomimetic agents (LSD, mescaline). In fact, Gunderson and Zanarini (1989) have proposed that any new, abrupt onset of persistent psychosis following alcohol or cannabis use supports the diagnosis of borderline personality disorder.

However, the prognosis is not always worse when addiction occurs in personality disorder patients (Kosten, Kosten, & Rounsaville, 1989; Nace, Saxon, & Shore, 1986). Paradoxically, multiple disorders may confer some unique prognostic optimism in some patients. In one study, opiate addicts with both antisocial personality disorder and depression had better outcomes than those without depression (Woody, McLellan, Luborsky, & O'Brien, 1987), possibly because the provision of antidepressant pharmacotherapy may increase treatment retention. Specialized dual-diagnosis treatment programs have been reported to produce optimal outcomes even in severely ill patients (Hoffman, DiRito, & McGill, 1993; Wilens, O'Keefe, O'Connell, Springer, & Renner, 1993). Dual-diagnosis patients seem to do better when a comprehensive review of their problems is made and a full range of treatment services is provided to match their individual needs (Alterman, McLellan, & Shifman, 1993; Kosten et al., 1989).

For a patient with a diverse range of problems, it is critical that a single provider coordinate the patient's care. This includes making certain that complete physical and psychiatric examinations are completed, as well as providing the patient with thorough information on the diagnosis, risk factors, potential consequences of future substance use, and available resources. It is important that treatment providers be aware of the psychosocial factors that reinforce continued abuse/dependence and intervene when possible. Family therapy (Bowen, 1974), family loop mapping (Liepman, Silvia, & Nirenberg, 1989), and network therapy (Galanter, 1993) are systems approaches that have been reported to benefit recidivist substance misusers with diverse family and social problems, by enhancing patients' awareness of environmental impediments to recovery and promoting patients' healthy involvement with supportive others.

Inpatient Treatment. Inpatient rehabilitation programs that last 10–14 days are still considered by expert consensus panels to be optimal for middle- to late-stage abuse, even if a patient shows no physical dependence (Mee-Lee, 1993). There is convincing evidence that these inpatient programs are more effective than referral to self-help groups alone, even with careful monitoring (Walsh et al., 1991). Inpatient programs provide a strong educational component, reorient the patient to a peer group with a common interest in maintaining sobriety, and introduce the patient to self-help groups such as AA. Most, however, have limited resources for treating patients with psychiatric dual diagnoses.

Outpatient Treatment. Outpatient treatment can be effective with dual-diagnosis and other treatment-resistant substance-misusing patients (Kofoed, Kania, Walsh, & Atkinson, 1986). Outpatient treatment is appropriate if a patient is not very ill, has not reached late stages of dependence, has sufficient motivation to participate in active outpatient care and is not immediately vulnerable to relapse because of rampant availability in the current living situation. Many patients are initially suited to outpatient treatment alone, but all patients will need it following discharge from inpatient detoxification and rehabilitation units. This initial phase of aftercare should have a psychoeducational approach and should reinforce participation in self-help groups for most patients. Many specialists believe that a period of cognitive and behavioral compensation is necessary before dynamically oriented psychotherapy can even be considered. There is, however, some evidence that such psychotherapy (and cognitive therapy) can benefit more severely psychiatrically ill substance-misusing patients (Winokur & Coryell, 1991).

RESISTANCE BECAUSE OF LATE RELAPSE

Initial treatment should engender an alliance with the therapist or group, in a highly interactive approach involving frequent contacts. The goal of this is to prepare the patient for the likely risk of relapse, which is a natural feature of addiction. It should educate the patient about the disease model of addiction. It should support the tendency for a growing dependence on the therapist and outside supports such as self-help groups. It must focus on abstinence *a priori* and help the patient establish new adaptive behaviors; these should include a schedule of daily routines, a healthy diet, exercise, and meeting new sober friends. Finally, it should help the patient to anticipate risk factors for relapse. These highly diverse and patient-specific factors include retention of negative affects; passive responding to interpersonal challenges; social withdrawal; and engaging in compulsive substitutes for addiction that are themselves risk-prone, such as gambling or promiscuity (Marlatt & Gordon, 1985).

In the early phase of treatment, psychodynamic techniques such as interpretation of transference are likely to be useful only when the alliance is threatened. This stage is fertile ground for the development of a positive transference, on the other hand, and this can usefully be fostered (Blane, 1977). The patient needs help in cognitively labeling anxious and depressed feelings, as well as in verbally expressing anger. Previously, these emotions may have been the cues for drug or alcohol craving (Galanter, 1983). Insight-oriented dynamic psychotherapy may become appropriate later, but the therapist must be familiar with the unique risks of previously addicted patients, in whom this treatment may induce strong dysphoric affects that may cue cravings for alcohol or drugs and provoke relapse (Childress, McLellan, Natale, & O'Brien, 1987).

The most widely used and readily available supports for recovery are AA and similar peer self-help groups, such as Narcotics Anonymous, Cocaine Anonymous, and newer groups such, as Saving Our Sobriety (SOS) and Rational Recovery (RR). More recovering substance misusers attribute their success to these groups than to any other form of treatment, yet these approaches have not been subjected to scientific trials. Clinically, extroverted and socially competent patients do better than introverted ones; psychotic and paranoid patients may do particularly poorly. Patients with dual diagnoses may do well, however, at meetings in community mental health centers, which tend to tolerate psychotic behavior and approve of physician-prescribed psychotropic medication. One needs to consider whether a given patient may have particular difficulties with AA and orient the patient before sending him or her to a meeting. A simple recommendation to attend mutual-help groups may be inadequate for most patients. Patients often need explanation about the value of AA, the range of meeting formats and audiences, purpose of sponsors, and the utility of the program's concept of spirituality. Therefore, any mental health professional should become acquainted with AA by attending meetings and reading some of its basic literature.

PHARMACOTHERAPY OF TREATMENT-RESISTANT PATIENTS WITH DUAL DIAGNOSES

Specific comorbid disorders that account for treatment resistance sometimes require unique pharmacotherapy considerations. Perhaps the most critical factors in effective pharmacotherapy of patients are painstaking psychoeducation and a treatment contract (Gastfriend, 1993). Key components of such a contract are presented in Table 13.4. The essential principles are that pharmacotherapy targets specific symptoms, is time-limited, is modified only one step at a time, is monitored for compliance, and is provided only in the context of a comprehensive psychosocial treatment plan.

TABLE 13.4. Key Components of a Pharmacotherapy Contract for the Dual-Diagnosis Patient

1. Medication is part of a rational psychosocial treatment "package," and will be discontinued if key psychosocial components are neglected.

2. Urine or blood testing may be required at any time to provide an independent source of data about the course of the chemical dependence, or to determine if prescribed medication is reaching adequate levels in the blood.

3. Medication will be used only as prescribed. Any need for changes will first be discussed with the physician. A unilateral change in medication by the patient often is an early sign of relapse.

4. Changes in medication will be prescribed one at a time (e.g., two agents will not be initiated simultaneously).

5. When used, the purpose of medication is to treat predetermined target symptoms. If medication proves ineffective for these, it will be discontinued.

6. Once target symptoms remit, a process of dose tapering may be initiated to determine the minimum dose necessary to maintain healthy function. Periodically, the medication strategy will include a period of discontinuation, or "drug holiday." Medication may not be necessary on a long-term basis.

Note. From Gastfriend (1993). Copyright 1993 by The Haworth Press. Reprinted by permission.

Schizophrenia

Schizophrenia may be the comorbid condition most difficult to treat, and the young chronic schizophrenic group with a dual diagnosis is twice as likely as non-substance-misusing schizophrenics to require rehospitalization (Caton, Gralnick, Bender, & Simon, 1989). Covert benzodiazepine dependence is a concern, given that in one sample 41% of schizophrenic patients were receiving both neuroleptics and benzodiazepines (Pecknold, 1993). Since the first priority is to achieve abstinence and then to initiate antipsychotic pharmacotherapy, inpatient hospitalization is usually essential. Since dopamine blockers do not block cocaine or amphetamine craving or euphoria in humans, antipsychotics should be reserved for use in clear comorbid psychotic syndromes. In most cases, standard antipsychotic doses are indicated; however, occasional drug–drug interactions may warrant higher-than-usual doses. Barbiturates, for example, may reduce chlorpromazine levels through induction of hepatic microsomal enzymes. Some agents may aggravate psychosis and counteract effects of antipsychotics; for instance, disulfiram inhibits dopamine beta-hydroxylase, and bromocriptine and amantadine are dopamine agonists. Problems may be minimized if the patient is first stabilized on an antipsychotic dose, prior to initiation of other pharmacotherapy.

The combination of opiate dependence and chronic Axis I disorders, especially psychotic disorders, warrants serious consideration of methadone maintenance for initial treatment as opposed to detoxification and abstinence. Aside from the benefit of the stabilizing routine of daily outpatient methadone administration, methadone treatment personnel tend to be more supportive and reinforcing of pharmacotherapy compliance, compared to staff members at abstinence-oriented treatment programs (McLellan et al., 1983).

Affective Disorders

Depressed patients with substance use disorders may fail to improve with abstinence alone. Antidepressant pharmacotherapy serves multiple purposes, including restoration of the euthymic state, treatment retention, and relapse prevention. Standard therapeutic levels for antidepressants and lithium remain the pharmacologic objectives. Selective serotonin reuptake inhibitors show great promise for reducing both alcohol consumption and affective symptoms in alcoholics, even those who resist psychosocial treatments (Brands et al., 1990; Cornelius et al., 1993; Naranjo & Sellers, 1989; Naranjo et al., 1987, 1992).

In treatment-resistant cocaine dependence, recent data, primarily from open trials, suggest that postwithdrawal craving and depressive symptoms such as anhedonia may respond to dopamine agonists (e.g., bromocriptine, amantadine) and antidepressants (Gawin et al., 1989; Kosten et al., 1992a). Unfortunately, other trials have produced contradictory results (Kosten, Morgan, Falcione, & Schottenfeld, 1992b). The effects of these agents for patients who do not meet full criteria for major depression are probably modest at best for normalizing mood, enhancing treatment activity, improving treatment retention, and preventing early relapse (Vaughan, 1990). Conversely, desipramine has been reported to provoke relapse in three cocaine addicts who experienced jitteriness as the agent was initiated (Weiss, 1988). Newer agents with specificity for both serotonin and norepinephrine reuptake blockade (e.g., venlafaxine) may achieve more consistent benefits.

Some authors have reported lithium to promote cocaine abstinence in bipolar and cyclothymic patients; however, this finding has not been replicated (Lemere, 1991; Nunes, McGrath, Wager, & Quitkin, 1990). There is no evidence that lithium is useful for treatment in cocaine or other substance abuse/dependence in patients without comorbid bipolar disorder.

Comorbid psychiatric illness is a major cause of treatment unresponsiveness in opiate addicts and is associated with continued illicit drug use and increased high-risk behavior for HIV transmission. Depressive symptoms occur often in opiate addicts; however, antidepressants may yield no better response than placebo (Kleber, Weissman, & Rounsaville, 1983), because most depression in opiate-dependent patients (even those in methadone treatment) is transient and may be situational or related to withdrawal (Rounsaville, Kosten, & Kleber, 1986). Antidepressants are more likely to be useful in refractory methadone maintenance patients with a discrete major depressive disorder (Nunes et al., 1990). Another cause of treatment resistance in opiate addicts is concurrent cocaine dependence. There is evidence that this population may respond from the mixed opiate agonist buprenorphine (Gastfriend, Mendelson, Mello, Teoh, & Reif, 1993; Schottenfeld, Pakes, Ziedonis, & Kosten, 1993). Buprenorphine is a long-acting, sublingually administered agent, recently submitted for Food and Drug Administration review, that has been shown to reduce opiate use in a manner that is similar to methadone, and may also reduce craving for and use of cocaine in individuals with combined opiate and cocaine dependence.

Anxiety Disorders

Anxiolytic therapy with reinforcing agents (e.g., benzodiazepines) is a common contributing source of treatment resistance and poses a serious iatrogenic risk; however, alternatives are available to minimize this problem. Since withdrawal from central nervous system depressants may produce symptoms of generalized anxiety and agoraphobia over 3 to 6 months and remit over time, pharmacotherapy may be unnecessary in this context (Schuckit, Irwin, & Brown, 1990). Other causes of anxiety symptoms should be considered, such as use of caffeine, over-the-counter diet pills, and androgenic steroids. Alcohol, stimulants, marijuana, and hallucinogens may provoke the onset of an anxiety disorder. Patients often discontinue marijuana and hallucinogen use when these are associated with increased anxiety, whereas alcohol dependence may persist or be replaced by anxiolytic dependence.

Stabilization of an anxiety disorder may be extremely difficult without initial detoxification and benefit of a period of drug-free observation. However, agoraphobic patients may object to hospitalization for chemical abuse/dependence citing a fear of confinement. It may be helpful to contract with the patient for intensive outpatient treatment or an extended outpatient evaluation over several weeks, after which the patient will agree to reconsider hospitalization if he or she is still not abstinent.

After detoxification, substance-dependent patients with anxiety require exceptional efforts to engage in behavior therapy, because of their substance-induced preoccupation with immediate (i.e., pharmacologic) gratification. This effort is essential, as behavior therapy can address both anxiety and substance dependence with relaxation, cognitive restructuring, *in vivo* or other exposure techniques, and addiction relapse prevention training.

Persistent, specific symptoms of panic attacks, compulsions, and generalized anxiety usually respond to appropriate conventional therapies, with the caveat that benzodiazepines are usually contraindicated in the dual-diagnosis patient (Schuckit et al., 1990). When necessary, pharmacotherapy should therefore always begin with antidepressants. The strategy should include a contract in which the patient makes a commitment to an adequate dose for an adequate duration (usually 1 month), and indicates an

understanding that side effects are not uncommon and may require management. Monitoring plasma levels of some tricyclics (e.g., nortriptyline,
desipramine) may be necessary, both because of altered rates of elimination in substance-dependent individuals and because of concerns about
compliance. Some newly abstinent anxious patients may be noncompliant with antidepressants in an attempt to receive benzodiazepines.

Benzodiazepines, despite their efficacy and safety as anxiolytics, place
the anxious chemically dependent patient at risk via pharmacologic tolerance (Greenblatt & Shader, 1978) and physiologic dependence (Busto et
al., 1986; Greenblatt & Shader, 1978). Treatment resistance may evolve
because the patient has an iatrogenically induced addiction to benzodiazepines as a substitute for alcohol, or because the patient may relapse
as a result of the reinforcing psychologic and physical dependence on benzodiazepines.

The goal of overcoming treatment resistance is to achieve not just
abstinence, but recovery. Recovery from chemical abuse/dependence is the
process of restoring intrapsychic well-being and psychosocial function. In
the patient with dual substance use and anxiety disorders, recovery includes compliance with the full range of psychiatric treatments. Benzodiazepines, particularly those with rapid onset (e.g., alprazolam, diazepam,
and lorazepam), offer a degree of immediate gratification that appears to
impede initiation of this effort and retention of gains. In severe conditions that prove refractory to behavioral and antidepressant approaches,
a slow-onset, long-acting agent such as clonazepam may be the safest of
this class (Herman, Rosenbaum, & Brotman, 1987). Yet even clonazepam
has addictive potential in severe substance dependence. In contrast, buspirone appears safe, may be combined with antidepressants, and is effective
for generalized anxiety if the patient and family are vigorously educated
and reminded about the slow onset and subtle perceptibility of its unique
response (Gastfriend & Rosenbaum, 1989). Thus, the use of benzodiazepines should be reserved for patients with well-documented failure on antidepressants or other agents, who have demonstrated continued distress
and a commitment to treatment.

ACKNOWLEDGMENT

The writing of this chapter was supported by Grant Nos. DA 06116, DA 07693,
and DA 08781 from the National Institute on Drug Abuse, and by the U.S. Center
for Substance Abuse Treatment.

REFERENCES

Alterman, A. I., McLellan, A. T., & Shifman, R. B. (1993). Do substance abuse
    patients with more psychopathology receive more treatment? Journal of Ner-
    vous and Mental Disease, 181, 576–582.

American Psychiatric Association. (1994). *Diagnostic and statistical manual of mental disorders* (4th ed.). Washington, DC: Author.

Ball, J., & Ross, A. (1991). *The effectiveness of methadone maintenance treatment.* New York: Springer-Verlag.

Barthwell, A., & Gastfriend, D. (1991). Treating multiple substance abuse. In M. Parrino (Ed.), *State methadone maintenance treatment guidelines* (pp. 151–171). Rockville, MD: U.S. Department of Health and Human Services.

Becker, J. T. , & Jaffe, J. H. (1984). Impaired memory for treatment-relevant information in inpatient men alcoholics. *Journal of Studies on Alcohol, 45,* 339–343.

Bien, T., Miller, W., & Tonigan, S. (1993). Brief interventions for alcohol problems: A review. *Addictions, 88,* 315–336.

Blane, H. (1977). Psychotherapeutic approach. In B. Kissen & H. Begleiter (Eds.), *The biology of alcoholism* (Vol. 5, pp. 105–160). New York: Plenum Press.

Bowen, M. (1974). Alcoholism as viewed through family systems theory and family psychotherapy. *Annals of the New York Academy of Sciences, 233,* 115–122.

Brands, B., Sellers, E., & Kaplan, H. (1990). The effects of the 5-HT uptake inhibitor, sertraline, on ethanol, water and food consumption. *Alcoholism: Clinical and Experimental Research, 14,* 273.

Brandt, J., Butters, N., Ryan, C., & Bayog, R. (1983). Cognitive loss and recovery in long-term alcohol abusers. *Archives of General Psychiatry, 40,* 435–442.

Busto, U., Sellers, E. M., Naranjo, C. A., Cappell, H., Sanchez, C. M., & Sykora, K. (1986). Withdrawal reaction after long-term therapeutic use of benzodiazepines. *New England Journal of Medicine, 315,* 854–859.

Caton, C., Gralnick, A., Bender, S., & Simon, R. (1989). Young chronic patients and substance abuse. *Hospital and Community Psychiatry, 40,* 1037–1040.

Childress, A. R., McLellan, A. T., Natale, M., & O'Brien, C. P. (1987). Mood states can elicit conditioned withdrawal and craving in opiate abuse patients. In R. M. Brown, D. M. Clove, & D. P. Friedman (Eds.), *Opiate receptor subtypes and brain function* (NIDA Research Monograph No. 76, pp. 137–144). Washington, DC: U.S. Government Printing Office.

Clark, W. (1981). Alcoholism: blocks to diagnosis and treatment. *American Journal of Medicine, 71,* 275–286.

Cornelius, J. R., Salloum, I. M., Cornelius, M. D., Perel, J. M., Thase, M. E., Ehler, J. G., & Mann, J. J. (1993). Fluoxetine trial in suicidal depressed alcoholics. *Psychopharmacology Bulletin, 29,* 195–199.

Crowley, T. J. (1984). Contingency contracting treatment of drug-abusing physicians, nurses, and dentists (NIDA Research Monograph No. 46, pp. 68–83). Washington, DC: U.S. Government Printing Office.

Crowley, T. J., Chesluk, D., Dilts, S., & Hart, R. (1974). Drug and alcohol abuse among psychiatric admissions: A multidrug clinical-toxicologic study. *Archives of General Psychiatry, 30,* 13–20.

Crum, R., Anthony, J., Bassett, S., & Folstein, M. (1993). Population-based norms for the Mini-Mental State Examination by age and educational level. *Journal of the American Medical Association, 269,* 2386–2391.

Crumley, F. (1990). Substance abuse and adolescent suicidal behavior. *Journal of the American Medical Association, 263,* 3051–3056.

Dulit, R. A., Fyer, M. R., Haas, G. L., Sullivan, T., & Frances, A. J. (1990). Substance use in borderline personality disorder. *American Journal of Psychiatry, 147,* 1002–1007.

Fairbank, J. A., Dunteman, G. H., & Condelli, W. S. (1993). Do methadone patients substitute other drugs for heroin? Predicting substance abuse at 1-year follow-up. *American Journal of Drug and Alcohol Abuse*, 19(4), 465–474.

Fisher, J., Mason, R., Keeley, K., & Fisher, J. (1975). Physicians and alcoholics: The effect of medical training on attitudes toward alcoholics. *Journal of Studies on Alcohol*, 36, 948–955.

Fuller, R., Branchey, L., Brightwell, D., Derman, R. M., Emrick, C. D., Iber, F. L., James, K. E., Lacoursiere, R. B., Lee, K. K., Lowenstam, I., Maany, I., Neiderhiser, D., Nocks, J. J., & Shaw, S. (1986). Disulfiram treatment of alcoholism. *Journal of the American Medical Association*, 256, 1449–1455.

Galanter, M. (1983). Psychotherapy for alcohol and drug abuse: An approach based on learning theory. *Journal of Psychiatric Treatment and Evaluation*, 5, 551–556.

Galanter, M. (1993). Network therapy for addiction: A model for office practice. *American Journal of Psychiatry*, 150, 28–36.

Galanter, M., Egelko, S., DeLeon, G., Rohrs, C., & Franco, H. (1992). Crack/cocaine abusers in the general hospital: Assessment and initiation of care. *American Journal of Psychiatry*, 149, 810–815.

Group for the Advancement of Psychiatry Committee. (1991). Substance abuse disorders: A psychiatric priority. *American Journal of Psychiatry*, 148, 1291–1299.

Gastfriend, D. R. (1986). Going the distance with alcoholic patients. *New Physician*, 35, 7–50.

Gastfriend, D. R. (1993). Pharmacotherapy of psychiatric syndromes with comorbid chemical dependency. *Journal of Addictive Disorders*, 12, 155–170.

Gastfriend, D. R., Filstead, W. J., Reif, S., Najavits, L. M., & Parrella, D. P. (1995). Validity of assessing treatment readiness in patients with substance use disorders. *American Journal on Addictions*, 4(3), 254–260.

Gastfriend, D. R., Mendelson, J., Mello, N., Teoh, S., & Reif, S. (1993). Buprenorphine pharmacotherapy for concurrent heroin and cocaine dependence. *American Journal of Addictions*, 2, 269–278.

Gastfriend, D. R., & Rosenbaum, J. (1989). Adjunctive buspirone in benzodiazepine treatment of four patients with panic disorder. *American Journal of Psychiatry*, 146, 914–916.

Gawin, F., Kleber, H., Bych, R., Rounsaville, B. J., Kosten, T. R., Jatlow, P. I., & Morgan, C. (1989). Desipramine facilitation of initial cocaine abstinence. *Archives of General Psychiatry*, 46, 117–121.

General Accounting Office. (1990). *Methadone maintenance—Some treatment programs are not effective; greater federal oversight needed*. Washington, DC: U.S. Government Printing Office.

Greenblatt, D., & Shader, R. (1978). Dependence, tolerance, and addiction to benzodiazepines: Clinical and pharmacokinetic considerations. *Drug Metabolism Reviews*, 8, 13–28.

Gunderson, J. G., & Zanarini M. C. (1989). Pathogenesis of borderline personality. In A. Tasman, R. E. Hales, & A. J. Frances (Eds.), *Review of psychiatry* (Vol. 8, pp. 25–48). Washington, DC: American Psychiatric Press.

Hall, R., Stickney, S., Gardner, E., Perl, M., & LeCann, A. (1979). Relationship of psychiatric illness to drug abuse. *Journal of Psychedelic Drugs*, 11, 337–342.

Harwood, H., Napolitano, D., Kristiannsen, P., & Collins, J. (1984). *Economic costs to society of alcohol and drug abuse and mental illness.* Research Triangle Park, NC: Research Triangle Institute.

Hasin, D., & Grant, B. (1987). Psychiatric diagnosis of patients with substance abuse problems: A comparison of two procedures, DIS and the SADS-L. *Journal of Psychiatric Research, 21,* 7–22.

Herman, J. B., Rosenbaum, J. F., & Brotman, A. W. (1987). The alprazolam to clonazepam switch for the treatment of panic disorder. *Journal of Clinical Psychopharmacology, 7,* 175–178.

Hoffman, G., Jr., DiRito, D., & McGill, E. (1993). Three-month follow-up of 28 dual diagnosis inpatients. *American Journal of Drug and Alcohol Abuse, 19,* 79–88.

Hoffman, N., Halikas, J., Mee-Lee, D., & Weedman, R. (1991). *ASAM patient placement criteria for the treatment of psychoactive substance use disorders* (2nd ed.). Washington, DC: American Society of Addiction Medicine.

Iguchi, M., Griffiths, R., Bickel, W., Handelsman, L., Childress, A., & McLellan, A. (1990). Relative abuse liability of benzodiazepines in methadone maintained populations in three cities. In L. Harris (Ed.), *Problems of drug dependence 1989* (NIDA Research Monograph No. 95, pp. 364–365). Washington, DC: U.S. Government Printing Office.

Institute for Health Policy, Brandeis University. (1993). *Substance abuse: The nation's number one health problem. Key indicators for policy.* Waltham, MA: Robert Wood Johnson Foundation.

Khantzian, E. J. (1990). Self-regulation and self-medication factors in alcoholism and the addictions: Similarities and differences. *Recent Developments in Alcoholism, 8,* 255–271.

Kleber, H., Weissman, M., & Rounsaville, B. (1983). Imipramine as treatment for depression in addicts. *Archives of General Psychiatry, 40,* 649–653.

Kofoed, L., Kania, J., Walsh, T., & Atkinson, R. (1986). Outpatient treatment of patients with substance abuse and coexisting psychiatric disorders. *American Journal of Psychiatry, 143,* 867–872.

Kolar, A. F., Brown, B. S., Weddington, W. W., & Ball, J. C. (1990). A treatment crisis: Cocaine use by clients in methadone maintenance programs. *Journal of Substance Abuse Treatment, 7,* 101–107.

Kosten, T., Gawin, F. H., Kosten, T., Morgan, C., Rounsaville, B. J., Schottenfeld, R., & Kleber, H. D. (1992a). Six-month follow-up of short-term pharmacotherapy for cocaine dependence. *American Journal on Addictions, 1,* 40–49.

Kosten, T. A., Kosten, T. R., & Rounsaville, B. J. (1989). Personality disorders in opiate addicts show prognostic specificity. *Journal of Substance Abuse Treatment, 6,* 163–168.

Kosten, T., Morgan, C., Falcione, J., & Schottenfeld, R. (1992b). Pharmacotherapy for cocaine-abusing methadone-maintained patients using amantadine or desipramine. *Archives of General Psychiatry, 49,* 894–899.

Lehman, A., Meyers, C., & Corty, E. (1989). Assessment and classification of patients with psychiatric and substance abuse syndromes. *Hospital and Community Psychiatry, 40,* 1019–1025.

Lemere, F. (1991). Lithium treatment of cocaine addiction. *American Journal of Psychiatry, 148,* 276.

Liepman, M., Silvia, L., & Nirenberg, T. (1989). The use of family behavior loop mapping for substance abuse. *Family Relations, 38,* 282–287.

Marlatt, A. G., & Gordon, J. R. (Eds.). (1985). *Relapse prevention: Maintenance strategies in the treatment of addictive behaviors*. New York: Guilford Press.

Marzuk, P., & Mann, J. (1988). Suicide and substance abuse. *Psychiatric Annals, 18*, 639–645.

McLellan, A. T., Arndt, I. O., Metzger, D. S., Woody, G. E., & O'Brien, C. P. (1993). The effects of psychosocial services in substance abuse treatment. *Journal of the American Medical Association, 269*, 1953–1959.

McLellan, A., Druley, K., & Carson, J. (1978). Evaluation of substance abuse problems in a psychiatric hospital. *Journal of Clinical Psychiatry, 39*, 425–430.

McLellan, A., Luborsky, L., Woody, G., O'Brien, C., & Druley, K. (1983). Predicting response to alcohol and drug abuse treatments. *Archives of General Psychiatry, 40*, 620–625.

Mee-Lee, D. (1993, March/April). Patient placement criteria for chemical dependency: Progress towards validation. *Behavioral Healthcare, 28*–31.

Mee-Lee, D., Hoffman, N., & Smith, M. (1992). *Recovery Attitude and Treatment Evaluator (RAATE) manual* (2nd ed.). St. Paul, MN: CATOR/New Standards.

Miller, W. R., Benefield, R. G., & Tonigan, J. S. (1993). Enhancing motivation for change in problem drinking: A controlled comparison of two therapist styles. *Journal of Consulting and Clinical Psychology, 61*, 455–461.

Miller, W. R., & Rollnick, S. (1991). *Motivational interviewing: Preparing people to change addictive behavior*. New York: Guilford Press.

Millman, R. (1986). General principles of diagnosis and treatment. In A. Frances & R. Hales (Eds.), *Psychiatry update* (Vol. 5, pp. 122–136). Washington. DC: American Psychiatric Press.

Nace, E., Saxon, J., & Shore, N. (1986). Borderline personality disorder and alcoholism treatment: A one-year follow-up study. *Journal of Studies on Alcohol, 47*, 196–200.

National Institute on Drug Abuse (NIDA). (1986a). *Capsules—1986 U.S. Department HHS–PHS–ADAMHA: Overview of its 1985 National Household Survey*. Washington, DC: U.S. Government Printing Office.

National Institute on Drug Abuse (NIDA). (1986b). *Statistical series: Annual data 1985; data from the Drug Abuse Warning Network (DAWN)* (Series 1, No. 5). Washington, DC: U.S. Government Printing Office.

National Institute on Drug Abuse (NIDA). (1993). *Estimates from the Drug Abuse Warning Network* (Advance Report No. 4). Washington, DC: U.S. Government Printing Office.

Naranjo, C. A., Poulos, C. X., Bremner, K. E., & Lanctot, K. L. (1992). Citalopram decreases desirability, liking, and consumption of alcohol in alcohol-dependent drinkers. *Clinical Pharmacology and Therapeutics, 51*, 729–739.

Naranjo, C. A., & Sellers, E. M. (1989). Serotonin uptake inhibitors attenuate ethanol intake in problem drinkers. *Recent Developments in Alcoholism, 7*, 255–266.

Naranjo, C. A., Sellers, E. M., Sullivan, J. T., Woodley, D. V., Kadlec, K., & Sykora, K. (1987). The serotonin uptake inhibitor citalopram attenuates ethanol intake. *Clinical Pharmacology and Therapeutics, 41*, 266–274.

Nunes, E., McGrath, P., Wager, S., & Quitkin, F. (1990). Lithium treatment for cocaine abusers with bipolar spectrum disorders. *American Journal of Psychiatry, 147*, 655–657.

Nurco, D. N., Kinlock, T. W., Hanlon, T. E., & Ball, J. C. (1988). Non-narcotic drug use over an addiction career: A study of heroin addicts in Baltimore and New York City. *Comprehensive Psychiatry, 29,* 450–459.

O'Farrell, T., Connors, G., & Upper, D. (1983). Addictive behaviors among hospitalized psychiatric patients. *Addictive Behavior, 8,* 329–333.

Pecknold, J. C. (1993). Survey of the adjuvant use of benzodiazepines for treating outpatients with schizophrenia. *Journal of Psychiatry and Neuroscience, 18,* 82–84.

Prochaska, J. O., & DiClemente, C. C. (1992). Stages of change in the modification of problem behaviors. In M. Hersen, R. M. Eisler, & P. M. Miller (Eds.), *Progress in behavior modification* (Vol. 28, pp. 183–218). Sycamore, IL: Sycamore.

Regier, D. A., Farmer, M. E., Rae, D. S., Locke, B. Z., Keith, S. J., Judd, L. L., & Goodwin, F. K. (1990). Comorbidity of mental disorders with alcohol and other drug abuse: Results from the Epidemiologic Catchment Area (ECA) study. *Journal of the American Medical Association, 264,* 2511–8.

Reich, T., Winokur, G., & Mullaney, J. (1975). The transmission of alcoholism. *Proceedings of the Annual Meeting of the American Psychopathology Association, 63,* 259–271.

Rickels, K. (1981). Are benzodiazepines overused and abused? *British Journal of Clinical Pharmacology, 11,* 71S–83S.

Rickels, K. (1983). Benzodiazepines in emotional disorders. *Journal of Psychoactive Drugs, 15,* 49–54.

Rollnick, S., Heather, N., Gold, R., & Hall, W. (1992). Development of a short 'readiness to change' questionnaire for use in brief, opportunistic interventions among excessive drinkers. *British Journal of Addiction, 87,* 743–754.

Rosenberg, C., & Liftik, J. (1976). Use of coercion in the outpatient treatment of alcoholism. *Journal of Studies on Alcohol, 37,* 58–65.

Rounsaville, B., Kosten, T., & Kleber, H. (1986). Long term changes in current psychiatric diagnoses of treated opiate addicts. *Comprehensive Psychiatry, 27,* 480–498.

Royce, J. (1989). *Alcohol problems and alcoholism: A comprehensive survey.* New York: Free Press.

San, L., Torrens, M., Castillo, C., Porta, M., & De La Torre, R. (1993). Consumption of buprenorphine and other drugs among heroin addicts under ambulatory treatment: Results from cross-sectional studies in 1988 and 1990. *Addictions, 88,* 1343–1351.

Schottenfeld, R., Pakes, J., Ziedonis, D., & Kosten, T. (1993). Buprenorphine: Dose related effects on cocaine and opioid use in cocaine abusing opioid dependent humans. *Biological Psychiatry, 3,* 66–74.

Schuckit, M., Irwin, M., & Brown, S. (1990). The history of anxiety symptoms among 171 primary alcoholics. *Journal of Studies on Alcohol, 51,* 34–41.

Shaner, A., Khalsa, M., Roberts, L., Wilkins, J., Anglin, D., & Hsien, S. (1993). Unrecognized cocaine use among schizophrenic patients. *American Journal of Psychiatry, 150,* 758–762.

Tarter, R., & Edwards, K. (1985). Neuropsychology of alcoholism. In R. Tarter & D. Van Thiel (Eds.), *Alcohol and the brain: Chronic effects* (pp. 217–242). New York: Plenum Press.

Vaughan, D. (1990). Frontiers in pharmacologic treatment of alcohol, cocaine, and nicotine dependence. *Psychiatric Annals, 20,* 695–708.

Volpicelli, J., Alterman, A., Hayashida, M., & O'Brien, C. (1992). Naltrexone in the treatment of alcohol dependence. *Archives of General Psychiatry, 49,* 876–880.

Walsh, D. C., Hingson, R. W., Merrigan, D. M., Levenson, S. M., Cupples, L. A., Heeren, T., Coffman, G. A., Becher, C. A., Barker, T. A., & Hamilton, S. K. (1991). A randomized trial of treatment options for alcohol-abusing workers. *New England Journal of Medicine, 325,* 775–782.

Weintraub, M., Singh, S., Byrne, L., Maharaj, K., & Guttmacher, L. (1991). Consequences of the 1989 New York State triplicate benzodiazepine prescription regulations. *Journal of the American Medical Association, 266,* 2392–2397.

Weiss, R. (1988). Relapse to cocaine abuse after initiating desipramine treatment. *Journal of the American Medical Association, 260,* 2545–2546.

Wilens, T. E., O'Keefe, J., O'Connell, J. J., Springer, R., & Renner, J. A. (1993). A public dual diagnosis detoxification unit: Part I. Organization and structure. *American Journal on Addiction, 2,* 91–98.

Winokur, G., & Coryell, W. (1991). Familial alcoholism in primary unipolar major depressive disorder. *American Journal of Psychiatry, 148,* 184–188.

Woody, G., McLellan, T., Luborsky, L., & O'Brien, C. (1987). Twelve-month follow-up of psychotherapy for opiate dependence. *American Journal of Psychiatry, 144,* 590–596.

14

The Recalcitrant Patient: Treating Disorders of Personality

SCOTT E. EWING
WILLIAM E. FALK
MICHAEL W. OTTO

Personality *disorders* should be distinguished from personality *traits*. Personality traits characterize a person's style of interacting with and relating to others; these traits influence the person's perception of self and others. Only when personality traits become maladaptive, resulting in significant social and occupational impairment or subjective distress, are they considered disorders. Personality disorders are coded on Axis II in the multiaxial system of classification of the *Diagnostic and Statistical Manual of Mental Disorders*, fourth edition (DSM-IV; American Psychiatric Association, 1994).

DIAGNOSTIC CONSIDERATIONS

Diagnosis of a personality disorder does not preclude an Axis I diagnosis; indeed, mood and anxiety disorders are not uncommon in personality-disordered patients. Most personality disorders appear to increase susceptibility to depression (Widiger & Hyler, 1987). Among depressed patients, the presence of a personality disorder tends to be associated with more life stressors (including marital separation and divorce), an earlier onset and more episodes of depression, greater suicidal potential, and a poorer response to pharmacologic treatment (Pfohl, Stangl, & Zimmerman, 1984;

Shea, Glass, Pilkonis, Watkins, & Docherty, 1987). Depression is especially frequent in borderline patients, with rates of 24–74% for major depression, 4–20% for bipolar depression, and 3–14% for dysthymia (Docherty, Fiester, & Shea, 1986). Moreover, despite psychoanalytic constructs to the contrary, patients with antisocial personalities may also suffer from depression (Reich, 1985).

Although the relationship between anxiety disorders and personality disorders has not been as thoroughly investigated as that between depression and personality disorders, anxiety disorders are common among personality-disordered patients. Individuals with avoidant, dependent, borderline, obsessive–compulsive, schizotypal, paranoid, and possibly antisocial personality disorders are at increased risk for anxiety disorders (Widiger & Hyler, 1987). Posttraumatic stress disorder is particularly common among borderline patients, as is social phobia in avoidant patients. The poor impulse control and self-destructive nature of borderline patients may be manifested in the Axis I disorders of bulimia nervosa and substance abuse; indeed, as many as 25% of bulimics are comorbid for borderline personality disorder (Levin & Hyler, 1986). Abuse of alcohol and other intoxicants is common among borderlines, and the alert clinician will always inquire about the use of such substances.

Despite these admonitions, one also must be careful not to overdiagnose personality disorders in patients with Axis I disorders. A patient's symptoms must be both chronic and pervasive to qualify as a personality disorder. If there is a history of episodic symptoms, a diagnosis on Axis II should generally not be made. Consider this example:

> A 32-year-old married mother of two young children had been in psychotherapy for several years to cope with her long-standing low self-esteem, emotional lability, and marital discord. Her therapist was not supportive of an evaluation for psychotropic medication, feeling that the patient's diagnosis of borderline personality disorder resulted from a difficult childhood with an alcoholic father. Significantly, the father was himself later diagnosed as suffering from depression that responded to antidepressant therapy.
>
> On careful assessment, it was found that this woman's symptoms had an episodic quality and that they fulfilled the criteria for major depression. Nortriptyline (gradually increased to 100 mg/day) provided marked benefit not only in her mood and neurovegetative symptoms, but also in her labile affect and anger. As a result, the patient's relationships with her husband and children improved dramatically. On follow-up 2 years later, she remained free of symptoms.

The presence of one personality disorder does not preclude diagnosing another. In fact, most patients who meet the criteria for one personality disorder will satisfy the criteria for another (Widiger & Rogers, 1989). This phenomenon is probably a result of the poor specificity of the diagnostic criteria for personality disorders in the past: The same or similar items have often been highly associated with a number of Axis II disorders (Morey, 1988). Changes in the DSM-IV criteria may improve diagnostic specificity, and preliminary evidence suggests that this is indeed the case (Blais & Hillsenroth, 1995). Although certain criteria have been eliminated or replaced, the DSM-IV retains its predecessors' organization of personality disorders into three clusters. Cluster A, the so-called "odd or eccentric" cluster, includes paranoid, schizoid, and schizotypal personality disorders; Cluster B, known as the "dramatic, emotional, or erratic" cluster, consists of histrionic, narcissistic, antisocial, and borderline personalities; Cluster C is the "anxious or fearful" cluster and includes avoidant, dependent, and obsessive–compulsive personality disorders.

Before the introduction of the DSM III (American Psychiatric Association, 1980), clinicians rarely agreed when diagnosing patients with personality disorders. Studies from that era demonstrated a mean interrater reliability (the kappa statistic) of only .32 (Perry, 1992). Since 1980, reliability in diagnosing personality disorders has improved, but we are still in need of studies that address the validity of these diagnoses. Because no entirely adequate criterion of validity or "gold standard" exists for personality disorders, Spitzer (1983) has proposed the "LEAD standard," an acronym referring to diagnoses based on "Longitudinal Expert evaluation using All available Data." Such data should include information about current and prior treatments, as well as input from family and friends where appropriate.

ETIOLOGY AND EPIDEMIOLOGY

The etiology of personality disorders is multifactorial. A common misconception is that these disorders are less biologic and more psychosocial in their origin than Axis I disorders. In fact, like other psychiatric disorders, personality disorders exhibit both biologic and psychosocial components. Evidence supporting a strong biologic contribution to personality disorders includes several twin studies (Goldsmith, 1983; Nichols, 1978). These studies suggest a heritability for personality traits of at least .50; the other half of the variance—that is, the variability in observed personality traits—is accounted for by environmental influences, measurement error, and temporal instability.

Contrary to popular notions that one's family profoundly influences development and expression of personality, almost none of the variability in personality traits attributable to environment is a result of sharing a common family environment (Loehlin & Nichols, 1976). Tellegen et al. (1988) administered the Multidimensional Personality Questionnaire (MPQ) to 217 monozygotic and 114 dizygotic twins reared together and to 44 monozygotic and 27 dizygotic twins reared apart. Heritabilities of the 14 personality traits measured by the MPQ ranged from .39 to .58. Only two of the measured traits, social closeness and positive emotionality, were significantly influenced by a shared family environment. Interestingly, the traditionalism scale of the MPQ, which measures endorsement of traditional moral and family values, was not influenced by family environment.

Personality disorders generally become evident by late adolescence and persist throughout adulthood. The overall lifetime rates of personality disorders range from 10% to 13.5% (Weissman, 1993). Although men and women are probably equally likely to suffer from a personality disorder, certain disorders may occur preferentially by gender. Antisocial and narcissistic personalities have traditionally been considered more common in men, whereas histrionic and borderline personalities are believed to be more commom in women. These clinical impressions, born of experience, should not be accepted uncritically. Skewed sample populations and the large number of personality-disordered patients who never present for treatment or who do so only under coercion from family members or legal authorities make reliable estimates of gender differences exceedingly difficult.

PSYCHOTHERAPY FOR PERSONALITY DISORDERS

Recommendations for Psychotherapy

Few studies of specific psychotherapies for patients with personality disorders have been undertaken; consequently, little empirical evidence exists to guide the clinician in selecting a therapy. In offering treatment recommendations, Higgitt and Fonagy (1992) reviewed various psychotherapies in the treatment of patients with borderline personality disorder, and attempted to combine the results of several follow-up and outcome studies (Akiskal, 1981; McGlashan, 1986, 1987; McGlashan & Heinssen, 1988; Paris, Brown, & Nowlis, 1987; Stone, 1987, 1990; Wallerstein, 1986). Higgit and Fonagy's suggestions are practical and remain helpful to clinicians embarking on psychotherapy with this difficult group of patients. A modified version of these recommendations is offered here, which may be extended to personality-disordered patients in general:

1. Some patients with personality disorders are treatable with psychotherapy, but these individuals probably fall into a higher-order, less ill group.
2. The aim of psychotherapy may as frequently be the reduction of suicide risk as the alleviation of symptoms (especially for patients under 30 years of age).
3. Patients with chronic dysphoria, high motivation, and low impulsivity who are also psychologically minded and who reside in a supportive environment may be the most appropriate subgroup for expressive and interpretive therapies.
4. Patients with impulse control disorders (e.g., substance-related or

eating disorders) may benefit from a limit-setting group or a therapist who is supportive of their attempts to struggle with uncontrollable impulses.

5. If interpretive or expressive therapy is used, the focus should be placed upon unconscious aspects of *current* relationships—particularly the relationship between patient and therapist—rather than past relationships.

6. Commitment and enthusiasm by the therapist may be of special significance, and subjective aspects of patient–therapist "fit" (complementarity) are particularly important for this group of patients.

7. Patients whose problems include substance-related disorders require these disorders to be addressed before psychotherapy is begun.

Combining Psychotherapy and Medication

Despite its only recently receiving attention from researchers, combining medication with psychotherapy has long been a practice among clinicians who deal with personality-disordered patients. A survey of 40 clinicians who treat borderline patients (Waldinger & Frank, 1989), revealed that 90% of them commonly prescribed medication. Often a medication was prescribed in response to a perceived lack of progress in therapy or the patient's demand for rapid relief. The risk of prescribing medication to personality-disordered patients was also evident in this survey: 87% of the clinicians reported that their patients abused medication at one time or another.

Frequently, pharmacologically treated patients may complain of severe side effects or lack of benefit early during the course of treatment. Clinical experience suggests that personality-disordered individuals are often exquisitely sensitive to the side effects of medication, and some may actually do worse when prescribed a drug (Cowdry & Gardner, 1988; Soloff, Anselm, Nathan, Schulz, & Perel, 1986a). Side effects may be diminished by starting with low doses and slowly titrating these upward to therapeutic levels. An inadequate trial of medication yields little if any useful information and only frustrates both patient and clinician. Prudent clinicians will encourage their patients to stay the course of treatment; frequent changes in medications prevent a patient from receiving an adequate trial of any of them. In the following section, pharmacologic treatment of personality disorders is discussed in greater detail.

PHARMACOTHERAPY FOR PERSONALITY DISORDERS

Borderline Personality Disorder

The term "borderline" was first used nearly 60 years ago, when Stern (1938) described a group of patients suffering from what he called the "borderline group of neuroses." Since then, "borderline" has been used to define various entities, including a schizophrenic subtype, a syndrome, a state, a personality organization, and a personality disorder. Akiskal, Chen, and Davis (1985) captured the elusive nature of "borderline" when they characterized it as an "adjective in search of a noun." Indeed, until the introduction of the DSM-III in 1980, the term seemed as polymorphous as the patients it attempted to define. Such imprecise nosology and lack of diagnostic clarity have in the past led to contradictory and confusing recommendations for treatment. Only relatively recently has pharmacotherapy been considered a reasonable option for these patients.

Although complete agreement on all the characteristics that define borderline personality disorder has still not been achieved, the criteria outlined in the DSM-IV (see Table 14.1) provide a generally reliable method of diagnosing the disorder. The diagnosis of borderline personality disorder requires five of nine interpersonal, affective, and behavioral characteristics that must be present in a persistent and pervasive manner over several years. As with other Axis II disorders, the diagnosis should not be made if the symptoms are only present episodically. As we have already emphasized, Axis I and Axis II disorders may occur together, often contributing significantly to the diagnostic challenge posed by any given patient.

Differential Diagnosis and Codiagnosis

Correct diagnosis is obviously essential for appropriate pharmacologic treatment. The following disorders can mimic or occur with borderline personality disorder:

Affective disorders
  Major depressive disorder
  Bipolar I disorder (hypomanic episode)
  Bipolar II disorder
  Hysteroid dysphoria (the DSM-IV category that encompasses symptoms of this disorder is "Major Depressive Episode with Atypical Features")
Panic disorder
Adult attention-deficit/hyperactivity disorder
Episodic behavioral dyscontrol (in DSM-IV, this is coded as "Impulse-Control Disorder Not Otherwise Specified")
Substance abuse

Certain diagnostic guidelines bear emphasis. A diagnosis on referral should never be assumed to be correct. Although such advice may seem axiomatic, clinicians are often led astray by a referring clinician's diagnosis, which may be only impressionistic or the result of frustration. Borderline personality disorder may cause, result from, coexist with, or mimic highly treatable Axis I disorders. In this regard, it is the "great imitator" of psychiatric disorders (Beresin, Falk, & Gordon, 1994). Borderline patients

TABLE 14.1. DSM-IV Criteria for Borderline Personality Disorder (301.83)

A pervasive pattern of instability of interpersonal relationships, self-image, and affects, and marked impulsivity beginning by early adulthood and present in a variety of contexts, as indicated by five (or more) of the following:

(1) frantic efforts to avoid real or imagined abandonment. **Note:** Do not include suicidal or self-mutilating behavior covered in Criterion 5.

(2) a pattern of unstable and intense interpersonal relationships characterized by alternating between extremes of idealization and devaluation

(3) identity disturbance: markedly and persistently unstable self-image or sense of self

(4) impulsivity in at least two areas that are potentially self-damaging (e.g., spending, sex, substance abuse, reckless driving, binge eating). **Note:** Do not include suicidal or self-mutilating behavior covered in Criterion 5.

(5) recurrent suicidal behavior, gestures, or threats, or self-mutilating behavior

(6) affective instability due to a marked reactivity of mood (e.g., intense episodic dysphoria, irritability, or anxiety usually lasting a few hours and only rarely more than a few days)

(7) chronic feelings of emptiness

(8) inappropriate, intense anger or difficulty controlling anger (e.g., frequent displays of temper, constant anger, recurrent physical fights)

(9) transient, stress-related paranoid ideation or severe dissociative symptoms

Note. Reprinted with permission from the *Diagnostic and Statistical Manual of Mental Disorders,* Fourth Edition. Copyright 1994 American Psychiatric Association.

in times of stress may appear agitated, intoxicated, hypomanic, depressed, psychotic, agoraphobic, panicked, or even delirious.

For example, hypomania in bipolar I or II patients may be indistinguishable from borderline personality disorder, particularly when irritability is prominent. Hypomanic episodes in bipolar patients, though, typically exhibit a waxing and waning course of weeks to months, whereas hypomanic symptoms in borderline patients may be more transient. A number of signs and symptoms of atypical depression overlap with those of borderline personality disorder in some patients. These patients, usually women, are so exquisitely sensitive to rejection that loss of a relationship may lead to depressed mood, anxiety, and the so-called reversed neurovegetative signs of hypersomnia and hyperphagia. Symptoms tend to occur in reaction to environmental and interpersonal stressors, and may improve with environmental changes such as the development of a new relationship. Monoamine oxidase inhibitors (MAOIs), bupropion, or selective serotonin reuptake inhibitors (SSRIs) may also be helpful for these patients.

Panic disorder, particularly with agoraphobia, may present with symptoms resembling those of borderline personality disorder. Terrified of being alone, a patient with panic disorder may become depressed, angry, and manipulative to avoid feeling isolated. Eliciting a clear history of panic attacks that antedate these disruptive symptoms generally suggests the correct diagnosis. Adult attention-deficit/hyperactivity disorder (ADHD) can also mimic borderline personality. Adult ADHD is a difficult diagnosis to make, particularly if the disorder was not identified in childhood. Still, for patients with a lifelong history of inattention and impulsivity—with or without hyperactivity—this diagnosis should be considered.

> A 17-year-old girl with apparent borderline personality disorder was referred after 10 psychiatric hospitalizations during the previous 3 years. Each hospitalization was necessitated by a vast array of impulsive and self-destructive behaviors associated with severe emotional lability and attacks of rage. When a careful history was taken, she was found to have been diagnosed with ADHD in childhood, but her stimulant medication was discontinued at the onset of adolescence. Pemoline was prescribed in doses up to 75 mg/day; lowered impulsivity and improved mood and attention were apparent within a week. On follow-up 5 years later, she remained free of hospitalizations, was employed, and had satisfying friendships.

Intermittent explosive disorder and other disorders of impulse control characterized by explosive outbursts and impulsivity should also be considered in the differential diagnosis of borderline personality disorder. A history of head trauma, meningitis, encephalitis, or overt epilepsy can sometimes result in symptoms resembling those of borderline personality disorder. Finally, the possibility of alcohol or other substance abuse in these patients should always be considered. Although abuse of intoxicants may be construed as a symptom of a borderline personality disorder, the benefits of treatment are invariably undermined when such abuse goes unrecognized.

When two disorders coexist, identifying the order of onset may not be as important as recognizing that comorbidity exists and targeting both entities for treatment. Clinical experience and some systematic study (Shea et al., 1987) suggest that borderline personality disorder has an adverse effect on treatment outcome in patients who also have an Axis I disorder. Soloff et al. (1986a) observed that patients with diagnoses of major depressive disorder and borderline personality disorder were more refractory to antidepressant treatment than those suffering from an affective disorder alone. In fact, some of their borderline patients with major depression experienced a paradoxical worsening of symptoms when treated with a tricyclic antidepressant.

Among the Axis II disorders, borderline personality disorder has been the most extensively studied with regard to pharmacologic management. Many of these studies have also examined the treatment of patients with schizotypal personality disorder. To date, these are the only Axis II disorders to be studied in controlled, double-blind pharmacologic research.

Pharmacologic Research with Borderline Patients

The majority of reports involving the pharmacologic treatment of personality disorders involve anecdotal cases. Interpreting these reports is complicated by the lack of consistency in defining borderline and other personality disorders. Because of this, few useful recommendations can be made from studies appearing before the publication of the DSM-III in 1980. Although the categorical definitions introduced with the DSM-III have often been criticized for lacking empirical evidence to substantiate their validity, these categories do have clinical utility and permit comparing the results of different studies. Many of the studies of borderline patients, however, give contradictory and confusing results that are difficult to reconcile.

In 1979, Brinkley, Beitman, and Friedel described five borderline patients who did not improve with psychotherapy and who were then treated with low doses of neuroleptics. Two patients responded to perphenazine (2–6 mg/day), another two responded to thiothixene (4–10 mg/day), and one benefited from thioridazine (25 mg nightly). Echoing an earlier observation by Mandell (1976), Brinkley's group cited reversal of low-grade cognitive dysfunction, including loosened associations and tangential or circumstantial speech, as the most "consistent and impressive finding."

Retrospective case studies by Soloff (1981) and Cole, Salomon, Gunderson, Sunderland, and Simmonds (1984) provided additional uncontrolled evidence of the efficacy of low-dose neuroleptics in borderline patients. Five of 11 (45%) of Soloff's subjects improved symptomatically, and 10 of 17 (58%) responded in Cole et al.'s study. Cole and colleagues observed that patients who were comorbid for depression or schizophrenia benefited the most from medication. These early studies are important, in that they were the first to suggest a role for medication in the treatment of personality-disordered patients. Nonetheless, they suffered from the methodologic limitations of an open design, a lack of placebo controls, and nonrandomized samples.

Since the mid-1980s, there have been five double-blind, placebo-controlled studies involving personality-disordered patients. In 1986, Goldberg et al. looked at the response of 50 outpatients with borderline and/or schizotypal personality disorder to the neuroleptic thiothixene. Although no drug effect was found on overall measures of borderline or schizotypal pathology, significant differences between drug and placebo were noted for certain traits, including illusions, ideas of reference, obsessive–compulsive symptoms, phobic anxiety, and psychoticism.

Soloff et al. (1986b) compared the tricyclic antidepressant amitriptyline and the neuroleptic haloperidol against placebo in 61 patients with borderline personality disorder, schizotypal personality disorder, or both. In contrast to Goldberg et al.'s study, the vast majority of patients in Soloff et al.'s study were inpatients. Haloperidol proved superior to both amitriptyline and placebo on a composite measure of general severity of symptoms. A broad spectrum of symptoms improved with haloperidol, including anxiety, hostility, paranoid ideation, and psychoticism. Depressive symptoms showed significant improvement on self-rated, but not observer-rated, scales. On the other hand, amitriptyline was only minimally effective, even against depressive symptoms. Fifteen of the patients who did not respond to amitriptyline exhibited paradoxical increases in suicidal threats, paranoid ideation, and demanding and assaultive behavior (Soloff et al., 1986a).

Cowdry and Gardner (1988), researchers at the National Institute of Mental Health, conducted a study of 16 borderline patients. Using a double-blind, crossover design, they compared four medications (trifluoperazine, tranylcypromine, carbamazepine, and alprazolam) with placebo. The patients considered themselves improved only when taking the MAOI tranylcypromine. Carbamazepine, however, significantly reduced behavioral dyscontrol, and trifluoperazine produced improvement on several objective measures. Although the patients' behavior generally deteriorated on alprazolam, perhaps as a result of benzodiazepine-induced behavioral dyscontrol, two patients actually found alprazolam of greatest benefit.

Soloff et al.'s group (1993) recently revisited the issue of efficacy for neuroleptics and MAOIs in personality-disordered patients. They were unable to replicate their own earlier finding of efficacy for haloperidol. Pairwise comparisons between phenelzine and placebo demonstrated phenelzine's efficacy against anger and hostility. Three-way comparisons between groups revealed phenelzine as the most effective in reducing borderline symptoms, depression, and anxiety, followed by placebo and haloperidol; however, when compared directly with placebo, phenelzine proved no more effective in alleviating depression and anxiety. After 5 weeks of acute treatment, medication was continued for an additional 16 weeks (Cornelius, Soloff, Perel, & Ulrich, 1993). As in the acute phase, response to medication was disappointing. Haloperidol did not diminish irritability. Similarly, little evidence of efficacy was found for continued therapy with phenelzine, other than modest improvements in depressive symptoms and irritability. The failure of Soloff's group to replicate its earlier studies may reflect differences in sample characteristics and study design. For example, earlier studies demonstrating the efficacy of neuroleptics generally involved inpatients with severe symptoms rather than outpatients.

Because of the chronic nature of borderline symptoms and the risk of developing tardive dyskinesia with prolonged exposure to neuroleptics, recent attention has focused on the SSRIs. Norden (1989) studied the effects of fluoxetine on 12 patients with borderline personality disorder who were not suffering from major depression. All of the patients improved in this open-label trial, and 75% were rated as much or very much improved. Other studies confirm that fluoxetine has efficacy in reducing both the depressive and impulsive symptoms in patients with borderline personality disorder (Cornelius, Soloff, Perel, & Ulrich, 1990, 1991; Markovitz,

Calabrese, Schulz, & Melzer, 1991). Fava et al. (1993) studied the effects of fluoxetine on a subgroup of highly irritable, depressed patients who suffered from "anger attacks." Roughly three-fourths of the patients suffering from anger attacks were also comorbid for borderline personality disorder, according to a self-report inventory. Fluoxetine significantly diminished the anger and hostility of these patients.

The first double-blind, placebo-controlled study of fluoxetine in patients with borderline personality disorder was recently completed by Salzman et al. (1995). The most striking finding in this trial was a significant decrease in anger among patients receiving fluoxetine—a decrease that was independent of antidepressant effect. Unfortunately, the small sample size and the robust response to placebo by many patients in the study limit the conclusions that may be drawn from it.

For a subgroup of patients with borderline personality disorder and pronounced psychotic symptoms who do not respond to or are unable to tolerate adequate trials of a conventional neuroleptic, clozapine may be efficacious (Frankenburg & Zanarini, 1993). Although clinical trials with risperidone in borderline patients have not yet been undertaken, risperidone's combination of serotonergic and dopaminergic antagonism, as well as its low incidence of extrapyramidal side effects, suggests promise in treating patients with borderline personality disorder.

General Considerations in Pharmacotherapy with Borderline Patients

Some general recommendations follow from these studies. First, there is no drug treatment that will effectively abolish all the core symptoms of borderline personality disorder. Until such therapy exists, clinical experience suggests targeting clusters of symptoms that resemble those of various Axis I disorders. One method for doing this involves dividing borderline personality disorder into three broad types: a mood-labile type, an impulsive/hostile type, and an identity-disordered type (Hunt et al., 1988). This clinically useful division permits the targeting of symptom clusters. Borderline patients demonstrating sensitivity to rejection and atypical depressive symptoms may respond preferentially to MAOIs, bupropion, or SSRIs. Those with prominent mood lability and behavioral dyscontrol may benefit from a mood stabilizer; lithium, carbamazepine, and valproate are all reasonable choices. Impulsive aggression, anger attacks, and depressive or obsessive–compulsive symptoms implicate dysregulation of serotonin and suggest a trial with an SSRI. Identity-disordered patients, particularly those with ideas of reference, paranoid ideation, social isolation, magical thinking, and other psychotic symptoms, warrant a course of therapy with a low-dose neuroleptic. Despite the conceptual appeal of a targeted approach to the pharmacotherapy of borderline personality disorder, few empirical data exist to support its use. Whether symptoms resembling those of Axis I disorders in borderline patients will respond as predictably to pharmacotherapy as the actual Axis I disorders themselves remains unsettled.

Initiating treatment with medications often has many pitfalls. Clinicians should not assume that a therapeutic relationship is firmly established with their borderline patients. Instead, a verbal contract with a patient may be negotiated that explicitly states the goals of pharmacotherapy, the probable and possible side effects of medication, and any reasons for terminating treatment (such as a lack of response misuse, or overdose of medications, or abuse of intoxicants). The therapeutic goals should be kept modest to avoid excessively high expectations, which, if unrealized, could lead to profound disappointment and mistrust on both sides. The collaborative creation of a realistic therapeutic contract diminishes some of the tension inherent in clinician–patient relationships with these individuals.

Schizotypal Personality Disorder

Many of the drug studies of patients with borderline personality disorder have also included patients with schizotypal personality disorder; these studies are reviewed above. One rationale for such studies is the possibility that schizotypal personality disorder represents a subtype of borderline personality disorder (Spitzer, Endicott, & Gibbon, 1979). The DSM-IV criteria for diagnosing schizotypal personality disorder are presented in Table 14.2. In their trial of low-dose thiothixene in schizotypal and borderline patients, Goldberg et al. (1986) found symptomatic improvement to be independent of diagnosis.

Hymowitz, Frances, Jacobsberg, Sickle, and Hoyt (1986) studied 17 schizotypal patients treated with low doses of haloperidol in a single-blind, 6-week trial. The mean daily dose was 3.6 mg. Because of sensitivity to side effects (sedation was the most common complaint), only eight patients were able or willing to complete the full trial. Improvement was noted on overall schizotypal symptoms measured by the Schedule for Interviewing Borderlines; scales measuring ideas of reference, odd communication, and social isolation decreased most significantly.

These early studies suggest that a trial with a neuroleptic may be warranted in patients with schizotypal personality disorder. Maintenance of these patients on neuroleptics is controversial, however, because of the long-term risk of tardive dyskinesia. In general, clear benefit—as evinced by significantly deteriorated behavior and return of prominent signs and symptoms whenever the neuroleptic is withdrawn—must be documented to justify continued treatment. The risks and benefits of maintenance therapy with a neuroleptic should be thoroughly discussed with the patient and his or her family before such a course is begun. Even in patients for whom maintenance is not indicated, episodic treatment with a neuroleptic can be useful during periods of decompensation.

The novel neuroleptic risperidone may have some advantages in treating individuals with schizotypal personality disorder. Although no placebo-controlled, double-blind studies have been attempted, clinical experience

TABLE 14.2. DSM-IV Criteria for Schizotypal Personality Disorder (301.22)

A. A pervasive pattern of social and interpersonal deficits marked by acute discomfort with, and reduced capacity for, close relationships as well as by cognitive or perceptual distortions and eccentricities of behavior, beginning by early adulthood and present in a variety of contexts, as indicated by five (or more) of the following:

   (1) ideas of reference (excluding delusions of reference)

   (2) odd beliefs or magical thinking that influences behavior and is inconsistent with subcultural norms (e.g., superstitiousness, belief in clairvoyance, telepathy, or "sixth sense"; in children and adolescents, bizarre fantasies or preoccupations)

   (3) unusual perceptual experiences, including bodily illusions

   (4) odd thinking and speech (e.g., vague, circumstantial, metaphorical, overelaborate, or stereotyped)

   (5) suspiciousness or paranoid ideation

   (6) inappropriate or constricted affect

   (7) behavior or appearance that is odd, eccentric, or peculiar

   (8) lack of close friends or confidants other than first-degree relatives

   (9) excessive social anxiety that does not diminish with familiarity and tends to be associated with paranoid fears rather than negative judgments about self

B. Does not occur exclusively during the course of Schizophrenia, a Mood Disorder with Psychotic Features, another Psychotic Disorder, or a Pervasive Developmental Disorder.

Note: If criteria are met prior to the onset of Schizophrenia, add "Premorbid," e.g., "Schizotypal Personality Disorder (Premorbid)."

Note. Reprinted with permission from the *Diagnostic and Statistical Manual of Mental Disorders*, Fourth Edition. Copyright 1994 American Psychiatric Association.

suggests that many of these patients do well on low doses of risperidone (0.5–3 mg/day), especially with regard to eccentric behaviors and social withdrawal. Risperidone's low incidence of extrapyramidal side effects further recommends it over conventional neuroleptics.

Fluoxetine and other SSRIs may also have a role in the treatment of schizotypal personality disorder (Markovitz et al., 1991); further studies are needed, though, before definitive recommendations can be made.

Antisocial Personality Disorder

Because the diagnosis of antisocial personality disorder depends on identifying overt behaviors, such as truancy, running away from home, and initiating physical fights (see Table 14.3), it is in many respects the most objectively diagnosed of the personality disorders. Despite this, and the seemingly rich array of behaviors that might be targeted pharmacologically in this disorder, relatively few drug studies have been carried out.

A number of studies suggest that lithium may ameliorate aggressive

TABLE 14.3. DSM-IV Criteria for Antisocial Personality Disorder (301.7)

A. There is a pervasive pattern of disregard for and violation of the rights of others occurring since age 15 years, as indicated by three (or more) of the following:

   (1) failure to conform to social norms with respect to lawful behaviors as indicated by repeatedly performing acts that are grounds for arrest

   (2) deceitfulness, as indicated by repeated lying, use of aliases, or conning others for personal profit or pleasure

   (3) impulsivity or failure to plan ahead

   (4) irritability and aggressiveness, as indicated by repeated physical fights or assaults

   (5) reckless disregard for safety of self or others

   (6) consistent irresponsibility, as indicated by repeated failure to sustain consistent work behavior or honor financial obligations

   (7) lack of remorse, as indicated by being indifferent to or rationalizing having hurt, mistreated, or stolen from another

B. The individual is at least age 18 years.

C. There is evidence of Conduct Disorder [see DSM-IV, p. 90] with onset before age 15 years.

D. The occurrence of antisocial behavior is not exclusively during the course of Schizophrenia or a Manic Episode.

Note. Reprinted with permission from the *Diagnostic and Statistical Manual of Mental Disorders*, Fourth Edition. Copyright 1994 American Psychiatric Association.

behavior. Sheard (1971) conducted an open trial of lithium in 12 violent delinquents from a correctional center in Connecticut. Serum lithium levels above 0.6 mmol/liter reduced the number of aggressive episodes in these individuals. Serious aggressive episodes decreased more significantly than minor antisocial acts. Three of the subjects were particularly responsive to lithium, which unduly influenced the degree of improvement in the overall sample.

In another sample of prison inmates, Sheard, Marini, Bridges, and Wagner (1976) compared the efficacy of lithium and placebo in reducing chronic aggressive behavior of an impulsive nature in 66 inmates who were not psychotic. By the end of the third month, lithium, but not placebo, completely suppressed impulsive aggression. The aggressive behavior in the inmates treated with lithium returned to baseline 1 month after being switched to placebo in this double-blind study.

The serotonin (5-HT$_{1A}$) agonist buspirone (Coccaro, Siever, Karoussi, & Davis, 1989) and SSRIs such as fluoxetine (Coccaro, Astill, Herbert, & Shut, 1990; Fava et al., 1993) may also have a role in diminishing impulsive aggression, as may the anticonvulsants carbamazepine (Gardner & Cowdry, 1986) and diphenylhydantoin (Stephens & Shaffer, 1970).

No one so far has studied these drugs in individuals who suffer from antisocial personality disorder as defined by the DSM-IV.

Other Personality Disorders

Pharmacotherapy for personality disorders other than borderline or schizotypal has not yet been investigated in systematic, controlled studies. Even case reports are rare. This may reflect the common misconception that disorders of personality are generally immutable and therefore inaccessible to pharmacotherapeutic intervention. In 1972, Dryud lamented, "If anything is impressive in the literature on the treatment of the borderline syndrome [and other disorders of personality] it is that nothing seems to work very well or for very long" (p. 165). Given the increasingly strong evidence for the genetic and biologic foundations of personality, however, there is every reason to be sanguine about pharmacologic treatments for these disorders in the years ahead.

Avoidant personality disorder (see Table 14.4) has reportedly responded to pharmacotherapy. Treatment for 2–3 months with either fluoxetine or an MAOI alleviated symptoms in patients with avoidant personality disorder, whether they were comorbid for an Axis I disorder or not (Deltito & Stam, 1989). Reich, Noyes, and Yates (1989) examined the effect of alprazolam on avoidant personality traits in 14 patients with a DSM-III-R diagnosis of social phobia. Six of nine avoidant traits improved with treatment. The results of this small uncontrolled study await replication in a more rigorously designed study.

Given the paucity of studies to date, few worthwhile recommenda-

---

TABLE 14.4. DSM-IV Criteria for Avoidant Personality Disorder (301.82)

A pervasive pattern of social inhibition, feelings of inadequacy, and hypersensitivity to negative evaluation, beginning in early adulthood and present in a variety of contexts, as indicated by four (or more) of the following:

(1) avoids occupational activities that involve significant interpersonal contact, because of fears of criticism, disapproval, or rejection

(2) is unwilling to get involved with people unless certain of being liked

(3) shows restraint within intimate relationships because of the fear of being shamed or ridiculed

(4) is preoccupied with being criticized or rejected in social situations

(5) is inhibited in new interpersonal situations because of feelings of inadequacy

(6) views self as socially inept, personally unappealing, or inferior to others

(7) is unusually reluctant to take personal risks or to engage in any new activities because they may prove embarrassing

---

Note. Reprinted with permission from the *Diagnostic and Statistical Manual of Mental Disorders,* Fourth Edition. Copyright 1994 American Psychiatric Association.

tions can be offered regarding the pharmacologic treatment of patients with avoidant personality disorder. The clinical similarity of avoidant personality disorder and social phobia, however, suggests that agents effective for social phobia (including MAOIs, SSRIs, and high-potency benzodiazepines) may also help in avoidant individuals.

Some evidence suggests a role for neuroleptics in patients with paranoid personality disorder (Munro, 1980). Similarly, low-dose neuroleptics may have a modest effect in patients with both schizotypal and obsessive–compulsive personality disorders (Schulz, 1986). Although drug studies involving patients with histrionic personality disorder have not been undertaken, individuals with this disorder share some of the characteristics of those with atypical depression (Liebowitz & Klein, 1979). MAOIs have proved useful in atypical depressives, and might therefore ameliorate similar symptoms in histrionic patients. Pharmacologic trials involving patients with narcissistic personality disorder have not been reported.

COGNITIVE-BEHAVIORAL APPROACHES TO PERSONALITY DISORDERS

Cognitive-behavioral therapy has achieved impressive results in the treatment of a variety of Axis I conditions and is among the most effective therapies for affective disorders, anxiety disorders, and eating disorders. Only recently has attention turned toward developing cognitive-behavioral treatments for Axis II conditions. Although the psychosocial treatment of personality disorders has traditionally been the domain of dynamically oriented therapists, early studies of cognitive-behavioral treatments for personality-disordered individuals suggest considerable promise.

In making this shift toward characterologic disorders, cognitive-behavioral therapists have included in their treatments methods for managing affect and increasing adaptive behavior. The empirical approach of cognitive-behavioral therapy to the treatment of Axis I conditions has worked well; however, when this approach is applied to Axis II disorders, several difficulties emerge. First, the range and type of outcome variables need to be much broader when Axis II conditions are considered, largely because of the heterogeneity of symptoms encompassed by Axis II diagnostic categories. Second, treatment trials should be significantly longer for Axis II conditions. Among the outcome studies completed to date, trials of up to a year have been utilized (Linehan, Armstrong, Suarez, Allmon, & Heard, 1991; Turner, 1989).

When cognitive-behavioral therapy is applied to personality disorders, the relationship between therapist and patient takes on increased importance. As noted by Beck, Freeman, and Associates (1990), treating conditions of acute distress such as depression helps insure that the patient is motivated to try alternative behavior patterns and is rewarded by fairly timely reductions in suffering. In contrast, changes may take place much more slowly in personality-disordered patients, and the benefits of treatment may be less perceptible. In addition, in many of these individuals, the maladaptive or self-defeating behavior patterns characterizing their disorders can have significant effects not only on their lives but on their treatment as well. Moreover, for many Axis II conditions, the patients' ability to engage in a collaborative treatment may in itself be impaired.

As a result of these factors, cognitive-behavioral treatment for personality disorders focuses on maintaining a supportive, collaborative relationship and cultivating in the patient skills for behaving adaptively both within the session and without (Beck et al., 1990; Linehan, 1993a). Consistent with this perspective, cognitive-behavioral treatments devote considerable attention to behaviors that disrupt therapy (resistance) and to identifying common cognitive-behavioral patterns that may underlie the inability to follow through with treatment recommendations (Beck et al., 1990; Newman, 1994).

A comprehensive model for treating personality disorders based on the principles of cognitive therapy has been proposed by Beck et al. (1990). Emphasis is placed on patients' core beliefs and rules ("schemas"). Personality disorders are characterized, according to Beck et al. (1990), by dominant cognitive schemas; individuals rely on their beliefs to interpret life events, and these interpretations then guide them in selecting strategies for coping with these events. In personality disorders, the belief systems are maladaptive and deeply ingrained, and must be treated in a comprehensive framework for understanding and providing alternatives to dysfunctional belief systems.

Collaborative treatment involves a process of mutual discovery and identification of dysfunctional core beliefs. Once these are identified, many different techniques can be used to help change the beliefs and the way they are substantiated in terms of dysfunctional thoughts and behaviors in individual situations. Self-monitoring, questions and answers, role playing, guided imagery, and other cognitive restructuring techniques are used throughout therapy to help patients develop alternative viewpoints from which to interpret ongoing experience. In addition, review of childhood history is used to help both patients and their therapists understand the sources of maladaptive behaviors. At times, the review of childhood experiences may take the form of exposure-based treatments, so that cognitive structures may be examined in the context of the emotions that surround traumatic memories. In addition, behavioral assignments may be used to help patients test cognitions and to help them develop new skills to end self-defeating patterns.

The cognitive therapy approach of Beck et al. (1990) provides an impressive overview of the type of cognitive distortions that may be encountered in patients with Axis II disorders and the learning histories that may accompany these disorders. At present, though, there is little empirical validation of the effectiveness of these approaches in controlled trials.

A second major approach to the cognitive-behavioral treatment of personality disorders is characterized by Linehan's "dialectical behavioral therapy" (DBT; Linehan, 1993a, 1993b). It utilizes concomitant weekly individual and group sessions that are conducted over a period of 1 year. Individual DBT includes problem-oriented, directive therapy in a balanced combination with supportive techniques. Individual goals for the treatment are set according to importance and may include behavioral skills training, contingency management, cognitive restructuring, and exposure techniques to reduce emotional sensitivity. Emphasis is placed on helping patients learn to manage emotional trauma, and topics for any individual session are determined by the events that precede the session. For example, if parasuicidal behavior has characterized the time since the previous session, problem-solving strategies will be devoted to those behaviors and the events that preceded them. A great deal of attention is devoted in DBT to helping patients with borderline personality disorder develop better skills for emotional regulation and social problem solving. The emotional instability that characterizes these patients is postulated to stem from difficulties with overall sensitivity to emotional stimuli, as well as difficulties in returning to a comfortable emotional baseline following emotional reactions.

Linehan (1993a) posits that deficits in emotional regulation, as well as maladaptive compensatory strategies, underlie the behavioral characteristics of borderline personality disorder. Chaotic interpersonal relationships are hypothesized to be a reflection of disruptions in a stable sense of self, in the capacity to tolerate and self-regulate emotions, and in the capacity for free emotional expression. Parasuicidal behavior is understood as a maladaptive emotion regulation strategy that operates in part because of an absence of more effective emotional regulation and interpersonal skills.

The treatment combines individual cognitive-behavioral therapy with group training in psychosocial skills. The emphasis in this training is placed on the development of skills in emotional regulation, interpersonal effectiveness, distress tolerance, and "mindfulness" (the ability to observe oneself and conscious experience in relation to surrounding events). Individual treatment emphasizes a collaborative approach that combines attention to well-defined goals, problem solving, monitoring of ongoing behavioral reactions and alternatives, and attention to contingencies in therapy and behaviors that interfere with therapy while providing a supportive environment.

Linehan et al. (1991) assessed the effectiveness of DBT in a controlled study of chronically parasuicidal borderline patients. These researchers conducted a randomized clinical trial of 34 patients assigned to DBT or to a control therapy. The group therapy component provided a forum for skills acquisition and included training in interpersonal skills, emotional regulation skills, and distress tolerance/reality acceptance skills. The control treatment consisted of individual psychotherapy delivered within the community; however, not all control patients accepted referral for treatment, and many of these patients (unlike the DBT patients) did not continue their treatment.

The investigators found that at the study's conclusion, patients who had received DBT had fewer episodes of parasuicidal or serious parasuicidal behavior, were more likely to stay in treatment, and had fewer inpatient days of hospitalization than patients in control treatment. The patients who received DBT had an average of 3.9 inpatient days per year, compared with 8.5 days for the control subjects. Interestingly, there were no significant differences between groups for changes in depression, hopelessness, or suicidal ideation. This study suggests that DBT is effective in diminishing parasuicidal behavior, reducing hospitalizations, and decreasing attrition in treatment among severely dysfunctional and chronically parasuicidal women with borderline personality disorder.

One characteristic of cognitive-behavioral approaches to borderline personality disorder is active training in emotional and interpersonal skills to help patients replace maladaptive and self-defeating behavior patterns with more adaptive patterns. At times, training may need to be provided in regard to the very basic skills of emotional regulation. The emotional awareness training described by Farrell and Shaw (1994) provides one example of the application of skills training to pervasive problems of emotional instability.

Like Linehan (1993a), Farrell and Shaw (1994) argue that emotional instability is a hallmark of borderline personality disorder and that it contributes to behavioral instability and disruptive interpersonal relationships. The absence of the ability to understand or describe one's emotional experience accurately is hypothesized to be a skill deficit that may underlie emotional instability in borderline patients. Correspondingly, emotional awareness training is viewed by Farrell and Shaw as a first step in helping patients acquire more adaptive information about themselves and their ongoing experiences, and as a first step in reducing emotional instability and its consequences. They posit that increased emotional awareness will lead to increased emotional stability and the ability to regulate arousal, with more effective problem solving and interpersonal functioning being the ultimate results.

Farrell and Shaw's interventions to increase emotional awareness are targeted around a series of dimensions representing a hierarchy of emotional awareness. This hierarchy ranges from simple awareness of bodily sensations, through awareness of the body in motion and arousal, awareness of extremes of emotion, and differentiation and integration of conflicting emotions, to more pervasive differentiation of emotions and combinations of emotions. Training is initiated by teaching patients to be more aware of changes in bodily and emotional sensations resulting from physical movement. In a basic procedure, the patient stands at the far end of a room and is asked to take very slow steps toward the therapist. As the patient moves, he or she is asked to describe aloud any physical sensations that are noticed. Attention is paid to gradations in the emotional experience, including taking steps backward to demonstrate better changes in the emotional experience. After completion of the slow approach, the patient and therapist return to their seats and review the patient's experience during the exercise.

As the patient progresses in repetitions of this exercise, associations may be made between the feelings during the exercise and feelings outside the session. To help patients generalize their skills, diagrams of this exercise and changes in feelings are given to patients, and homework is assigned to have patients diagram changes in feelings that occur outside the session. This basic training in labeling emotions is then combined with training in distress reduction, which may include management skills such as slow deep breathing; muscle relaxation techniques; or techniques involving kinesthetic awareness, such as the awareness of the feeling of the floor underneath one's feet or the feeling of smooth or rough objects. Patients are asked to try these techniques and rate their success outside the session.

As patients continue to progress, they are introduced to a more advanced monitoring form that asks them to monitor not only thoughts, emotions, and feelings, but the actions taken for stress reduction in response to these events. These monitoring forms provide the basis for more advanced discriminations about the nature of feelings or thoughts, including the experience of noticing more than one feeling occurring at a time. Cognitive restructuring is then used to help eliminate dichotomous thinking; patients are helped to understand that in many cases events and emotions cannot be viewed simply as good or bad, but often have a mix of desirable and undesirable characteristics. Consistent with a cognitive-behavioral focus on instruction and the use of experiences from therapy, success in discriminating emotions and in using cognitive or behavioral strategies to tolerate distressful emotions is summarized for the patient on a guide sheet for out-of-session application.

In summary, emotional awareness as described by Farrell and Shaw (1994) provides a specific method for targeting low emotional awareness in borderline patients with a step-by-step approach to acquiring new skills. All components of this treatment take place within a therapeutic relationship that is positive, supportive, and collaborative, and that includes a shared conceptualization of the patient's problems. After basic emotional awareness training has been completed, the patient may then progress to training in other skills, such as more detailed cognitive restructuring and work on maladaptive life schemas.

A multicomponent treatment approach for borderline personality disorder is also illustrated by a case study by Turner (1989). Turner utilized a year-long program that was divided into an intensive and a continuation phase. The intensive phase consisted of 12 consecutive weeks of treatment with sessions three times a week. Following this initial period of intensive treatment, psychotherapy was offered twice weekly for 9 months and emphasized supportive psychotherapy and review of cognitive-behavioral treatment components. The intensive phase of treatment was itself divided into four components.

The first component utilized pharmacologic (alprazolam) treatment at a moderate anxiolytic dose (2.5 mg/day), which was continued during the following 6 months. At 6 months, the medication was tapered slowly over the course of 10 weeks. During the second phase of intensive treatment, imaginal flooding procedures were used to help patients develop an ability to tolerate high levels of emotion. Topics for imaginal exposure included past situations in which the patients had experienced emotional dysregulation. Patients completed a total of six 90-minute sessions of imaginal exposure. Emphasis was placed on helping patients to tolerate high levels of emotion without escape.

The third phase of intensive treatment consisted of 12 scheduled sessions of cognitive restructuring over 4 weeks. Treatment components included the identification of cognitive distortions and more accurate alternatives to these distortions, and rehearsal of adaptive reactions to life problems and daily events. In part, this included imaginal rehearsal of controlled coping approaches to problem areas, and the generation of self-control techniques for better responding to negative events. Cognitive training also included exercises to help improve self-image, goal setting, and problem solving.

In the fourth phase, the remaining 4 weeks of the intensive phase of treatment were devoted to training in interpersonal skills. This included training in reflective listening skills, role playing of adaptive responses to difficult interpersonal situations, and problem solving and role playing of current interpersonal problems.

All patients in Turner's (1989) study met criteria for borderline personality disorder and were characterized by self-defeating, parasuicidal, and interpersonally disruptive behavior. Hospitalizations were frequent among this cohort. The results indicated clear reductions in the intensity of anxious and depressed mood, as well as reductions in self-injurious and other disruptive behaviors. Three of the four patients continued to have good outcomes at a 2-year follow-up, although the fourth lost her treatment gains during a 6-week period prior to the 2-year evaluation.

In summary, cognitive-behavioral approaches to psychopathology are now being expanded to include personality disorders. Empirical trials completed to date provide preliminary support for these approaches, and the training manuals and courses currently available should enable these treatments to be used by interested clinicians, as well as studied further by clinical researchers. Cognitive-behavioral therapy provides clinicians with a promising method for treating patients with personality disorders.

CONCLUSION

Patients suffering from one or more personality disorders as defined by the DSM-IV constitute a highly heterogeneous group. Conceptually and therapeutically, personality-disordered patients are among the most difficult and treatment-resistant of all psychiatric patients. Their course is often checkered and usually involves long-term treatment. Although systematic study of drug treatments for these disorders is still in its infancy, extensive clinical experience confirms the benefit of pharmacotherapy in treating comorbid Axis I disorders and in reducing symptoms that could interfere with psychotherapy. Medication may also improve certain dysregulated emotional states, thereby helping these individuals to endure with less pain and trepidation whatever life may hold for them. Finally, recent advances in cognitive-behavioral treatment hold promise for patients with Axis II disorders, particularly those with borderline personality disorder.

REFERENCES

Akiskal, H. S. (1981). Subaffective disorders: Dysthymic, cyclothymic, and bipolar II disorders in the "borderline" realm. *Psychiatric Clinics of North America, 4,* 25–36.

Akiskal, H. S., Chen, S. E., & Davis, G. C. (1985). Borderline: An adjective in search of a noun. *Journal of Clinical Psychiatry, 46,* 41–48.

American Psychiatric Association. (1980). *Diagnostic and statistical manual of mental disorders* (3rd ed.). Washington, DC: Author.

American Psychiatric Association. (1994). *Diagnostic and statistical manual of mental disorders* (4th ed). Washington, DC: Author.

Beck, A. T., Freeman, A., & Associates. (1990). *Cognitive therapy of personality disorders.* New York: Guilford Press.

Beresin, E. V., Falk, W. E., & Gordon, C. (1994). Borderline and other personality disorders. In S. E. Hyman & G. Tesar (Eds.), *Manual of emergency psychiatry.* Boston: Little, Brown.

Blais, M. A., & Hillsenroth, M. J. (1995). *The operating characteristics of the Cluster B personality disorders under DSM-III-R and DSM-IV.* Unpublished manuscript.

Brinkley, J. R., Beitman, B. D., & Friedel, R. O. (1979). Low dose neuroleptic regimes in the treatment of borderline patients. *Archives of General Psychiatry, 36,* 319–326.

Coccaro, E. F., Astill, J. L., Herbert, J. L., & Shut, A. G. (1990). Fluoxetine treatment of impulsive aggression in DSM-III personality disorder patients. *Journal of Clinical Psychopharmacology, 10,* 373–375.

Coccaro, E. F., Siever, L. J., Karoussi, R., & Davis, K. L. (1989). Impulsive aggression in personality disorder: Evidence for involvement of 5-HT1 receptors. *Biological Psychiatry, 2*(Suppl.), 57A–86A.

Cole, J. O., Salomon, M., Gunderson, J. G., Sunderland, P., & Simmonds, P. (1984). Drug therapy in borderline patients. *Comprehensive Psychiatry, 25,* 249–262.

Cornelius, J. R., Soloff, P. H., Perel, J. M., & Ulrich, R. F. (1990). Fluoxetine trial in borderline personality disorder. *Psychopharmacology Bulletin, 26,* 151–154.

Cornelius, J. R., Soloff, P. H., Perel, J. M., & Ulrich, R. F. (1991). A preliminary trial of fluoxetine in refractory borderline patients. *Journal of Clinical Psychopharmacology, 11,* 116–120.

Cornelius, J. R., Soloff, P. H., Perel, J. M., & Ulrich, R. F. (1993). Continuation pharmacotherapy of borderline personality disorder with haloperidol and phenelzine. *American Journal of Psychiatry, 150,* 1843–1848.

Cowdry, R., & Gardner, D. L. (1988). Pharmacotherapy of borderline personality disorder. *Archives of General Psychiatry, 45,* 111–119.

Deltito, J. A., & Stam, M. (1989). Psychopharmacological treatment of avoidant personality disorder. *Comprehensive Psychiatry, 30,* 498–504.

Docherty, J. P., Fiester, S. J., & Shea, T. (1986). Syndrome diagnosis and personality disorder. *Review of Psychiatry, 5,* 315–355.

Dryud, J. E. (1972). The treatment of the borderline syndrome. In E. Offer & D. X. Freedman (Eds.), *Modern psychiatry and clinical research.* New York: Basic Books.

Farrell, J. M., & Shaw, I. A. (1994). Emotional awareness training: A prerequisite to effective cognitive-behavioral treatment of borderline personality disorder. *Cognitive and Behavioral Practice, 1,* 71–91.

Fava, M., Rosenbaum, J. F., Pava, J. A., McCarthy, M. K., Steingard, R. J., & Bouffides, M. A. (1993). Anger attacks in unipolar depression: Part I. Clinical correlates and response to fluoxetine treatment. *American Journal of Psychiatry, 150,* 1158–1163.

Frankenburg, F. R., & Zanarini, M. C. (1993). Clozapine treatment of borderline patients: A preliminary study. *Comprehensive Psychiatry, 34,* 402–405.

Gardner, D. L., & Cowdry, R. W. (1986). Positive effects of carbamazepine on behavioral dyscontrol in borderline personality disorder. *American Journal of Psychiatry, 143,* 519–522.

Goldberg, S. C., Schulz, S. C., Schulz, P. M., Resnick, R. J., Harmer, R. M., & Friedel, R. O. (1986). Borderline and schizotypal personality disorders treated with low-dose thiothixene vs. placebo. *Archives of General Psychiatry, 43,* 680–686.

Goldsmith, H. H. (1983). Genetic influences on personality from infancy to adulthood. *Child Development, 54,* 331–335.

Higgitt, A., & Fonagy, P. (1992). Psychotherapy in borderline and narcissistic personality disorder. *British Journal of Psychiatry, 161,* 23–43.

Hunt, S., Clarkin, J., Widiger, T., Eyer, M., Sullivan, T., Stone, M. H., & Frances, A. (1988, August 4). *DSM-III and borderline personality disorder: Decision rules and their implications.* Paper presented at the First International Congress on Personality Disorders, Copenhagen.

Hymowitz, P., Frances, A., Jacobsberg, L. B., Sickles, M., & Hoyt, R. (1986). Neuroleptic treatment of schizotypal personality disorders. *Comprehensive Psychiatry, 27,* 267–271.

Levin, A., & Hyler, S. (1986). DSM-III personality diagnosis in bulimia. *Comprehensive Psychiatry, 19,* 448–455.

Liebowitz, M. R., & Klein, D. F. (1979). Hysteroid dysphoria. *Psychiatric Clinics of North America, 2,* 555–575.

Linehan, M. M. (1993a). *Cognitive-behavioral treatment of borderline personality disorder.* New York: Guilford Press.

Linehan, M. M. (1993b). *Skills training manual for treating borderline personality disorder.* New York: Guilford Press.

Linehan, M. M., Armstrong, H. E., Suarez, A., Allmon, D., & Heard, H. L. (1991). Cognitive behavioral treatment of chronically suicidal borderline patients. *Archives of General Psychiatry, 48,* 1060–1064.

Loehlin, J. C., & Nichols, R. C. (1976). *Heredity, environment and personality: A study of 850 sets of twins.* Austin: University of Texas Press.

Mandell, A. J. (1976). Dr. Hunter S. Thompson and the new psychiatry. *Psychiatry Digest, 37,* 12–17.

Markovitz, P. J., Calabrese, J. R., Schulz, S. C., & Meltzer, H. Y. (1991). Fluoxetine in the treatment of borderline and schizotypal personality disorders. *American Journal of Psychiatry, 148,* 1064–1067.

McGlashan, T. H. (1986). The Chestnut Lodge follow-up study: III. Long-term outcome of borderline personalities. *Archives of General Psychiatry, 43,* 20–30.

McGlashan, T. H. (1987). Borderline personality disorder and unipolar affective disorder: Long-term effects of co-morbidity. *Journal of Nervous and Mental Disease, 175,* 467–473.

McGlashan, T. H., & Heinssen, R. K. (1988). Hospital discharge status and long-term outcome for patients with schizophrenia, schizoaffective disorder, borderline personality disorder and unipolar affective disorder. *Archives of General Psychiatry, 45,* 363–368.

Morey, L. C. (1988). A psychometric analysis of the DSM-III-R personality disorder criteria. *Journal of Personality Disorders, 2,* 109–124.

Munro, A. (1980). Monosymptomatic hypochondriacal psychosis. *British Journal of Hospital Medicine, 24,* 34–38.

Newman, C. F. (1994). Understanding client resistance: Methods for enhancing motivation to change. *Cognitive and Behavioral Practice, 1,* 47–69.

Nichols, R. C. (1978). Twin studies of ability, personality, and interests. *Homo, 29,* 158–173.

Norden, M. J. (1989). Fluoxetine in borderline personality disorder. *Progress in Neuro-Psychopharmacology and Biological Psychiatry, 13,* 885–893.

Paris, J., Brown, R., & Nowlis, D. (1987). Long-term follow-up of borderline patients in a general hospital. *Comprehensive Psychiatry, 28,* 530–535.

Perry, J. C. (1992). Problems and considerations in the valid assessment of personality disorders. *American Journal of Psychiatry, 149,* 1645–1653.

Pfohl, B., Stangl, D., & Zimmerman, M. (1984). The implications of DSM-III personality disorders for patients with major depression. *Journal of Affective Disorders, 7,* 309–318.

Reich, J. (1985). The relationship between antisocial behavior and affective illness. *Comprehensive Psychiatry, 26,* 296–302.

Reich, J., Noyes, R., & Yates, W. (1989). Alprazolam treatment of avoidant personality traits in social phobic patients. *Journal of Clinical Psychiatry, 50,* 91–95.

Salzman, C., Wolfson, B. A., Schatzberg, A., Looper, J., Henke, R., Albanese, M., Schwartz, J., & Miyawaki, E. (1995). Effect of fluoxetine on anger in symptomatic volunteers with borderline personality disorder. *Journal of Clinical Psychopharmacology, 15,* 23–29.

Schulz, S. C. (1986). The use of low dose neuroleptics in the treatment of "schizo-obsessive" patients. *American Journal of Psychiatry, 143,* 1318–1319.

Shea, M. T., Glass, D. R., Pilkonis, P. A., Watkins, J., & Docherty, J. P. (1987). Frequency and implications of personality disorders in a sample of depressed outpatients. *Journal of Personality Disorders, 1,* 27–42.

Sheard, M. H. (1971). Effect of lithium on human aggression. *Nature, 230,* 113–114.

Sheard, M. H., Marini, J. L., Bridges, C. I., & Wagner, E. (1976). The effect of lithium on unipolar aggressive behavior in man. *American Journal of Psychiatry, 133,* 1409–1413.

Soloff, P. H. (1981). Pharmacotherapy of borderline disorders. *Comprehensive Psychiatry, 22,* 535–543.

Soloff, P. H., Anselm, G., Nathan, R. S., Schulz, P. M., & Perel, J. M. (1986a). Paradoxical effect of amitriptyline on borderline patients. *American Journal of Psychiatry, 143,* 1603–1605.

Soloff, P. H., Cornelius, J. R., George, A., Nathan, S., Perel, J. M., & Ulrich, R. F. (1993). Efficacy of phenelzine and haloperidol in borderline personality disorder. *Archives of General Psychiatry, 50,* 377–385.

Soloff, P. H., George, A., Nathan, R. S., Schulz, P. M., Ulrich, R. F., & Perel, J. M. (1986b). Progress in pharmacotherapy of borderline disorders: A double-blind study of amitriptyline, haloperidol and placebo. *Archives of General Psychiatry, 43,* 691–697.

Spitzer, R. L. (1983). Psychiatric diagnosis: Are clinicians still necessary? *Comprehensive Psychiatry, 24,* 398–411.

Spitzer, R. L., Endicott, J., & Gibbon, M. (1979). Crossing the border into borderline personality and borderline schizophrenia. *Archives of General Psychiatry, 365,* 17–24.

Stephens, J. H., & Schaffer, J. W. (1970). A controlled study of the effects of diphenylhydantoin on anxiety, irritability, and anger in neurotic outpatients. *Psychopharmacologia* (Berlin), *17,* 169–181.

Stern, A. (1938). Psychoanalytic investigation of and therapy in the borderline group of neuroses. *Psychiatric Quarterly, 12,* 467–489.

Stone, M. H. (1987). Psychotherapy of borderline patients in light of long-term follow-up. *Bulletin of the Menninger Clinic, 51,* 231–247.

Stone, M. H. (1990). *The fate of borderline patients: Successful outcome and psychiatric practice.* New York: Guilford Press.

Tellegen, A., Lykken, D. T., Bouchard, T. J., Wilcox, K. J., Segal, N. L., & Rich, S. (1988). Personality similarity in twins reared apart and together. *Journal of Personality and Social Psychology, 54,* 1031–1039.

Turner, R. M. (1989). Case study evaluations of a bio-cognitive-behavioral approach for the treatment of borderline personality disorder. *Behavior Therapy, 20,* 477–489.

Waldinger, R. J., & Frank, A. F. (1989). Clinicians' experiences in combining medication and psychotherapy in the treatment of borderline patients. *Hospital and Community Psychiatry, 40,* 712–718.

Wallerstein, R. S. (1986). *Forty-two lives in treatment: A study of psychoanalysis and psychotherapy.* New York: Guilford Press.

Weissman, M. M. (1993). The epidemiology of personality disorders: A 1990 update. *Journal of Personality Disorders, 7*(Suppl.), 44–62.

Widiger, T. A., & Hyler, S. E. (1987). Axis I/Axis II interactions. In J. O. Cavenar, Jr. (Ed.), *Psychiatry* (Vol. 1). Philadelphia: J. B. Lippincott.

Widiger, T. A., & Rogers, J. H. (1989). Prevalence and comorbidity of personality disorders. *Psychiatric Annals, 19,* 132–136.

15

Diagnosis and Treatment of Adult Attention-Deficit/ Hyperactivity Disorder

JOSEPH BIEDERMAN
TIMOTHY E. WILENS
THOMAS J. SPENCER
STEPHEN FARAONE
ERIC MICK
J. STUART ABLON
KATHLEEN KIELY

Attention-deficit/hyperactivity disorder (ADHD) is a disorder of unknown etiology estimated to affect 6–9% of school-age children (Anderson, Williams, McGee, & Silva, 1987; Frank, Kupfer, & Perel, 1989; Rutter, 1988; Thompson & Weissman, 1981). (The term ADHD as used here also refers to previous definitions of the disorder.) It is commonly associated with high disability affecting all aspects of life, including work and relationships. The persistent inability to concentrate, multiple failures, and resulting disapproval may also contribute to intrapsychic distress, low self-esteem, and demoralization. Although the etiology of ADHD remains unknown, family, adoption, and twin studies as well as segregation analysis have indicated that genetic risk factors may be operant in this disorder (Faraone et al., 1992).

Although ADHD was originally conceptualized as a childhood disorder, several lines of evidence suggest that it is also an adult disorder.

Follow-up studies of ADHD children show that from 10% to 50% will continue to have ADHD as adults (Barkley, 1990), and in family genetic studies (Biederman et al., 1992; Faraone et al., 1992), many parents of ADHD children report symptoms compatible with the diagnosis. Moreover, increasing numbers of adults come to clinics complaining of ADHD symptomatology. Since ADHD afflicts 6–9% of school-age children (as noted above), its adult form may be one of the most common psychiatric disorders, affecting 1–4% of adults.

However, in both adult and child clinics, adult ADHD remains an orphan diagnosis. Child clinicians do not usually follow patients into adulthood, and the possibility of adult ADHD is not often considered in adult psychiatric settings. Adult clinicians may erroneously think that ADHD remits by adolescence, and is therefore not a clinical issue in adult psychiatry. On the other hand, child psychiatrists may think that, like young children, adults cannot validly report the criteria for ADHD. Some argue that the parents of ADHD children may identify with them and therefore may be biased to endorse symptoms of ADHD (Klein & Mannuzza, 1990).

VALIDITY OF THE DIAGNOSIS

Literature Review

Although the validity of the diagnosis of adult ADHD has been questioned, we (Spencer, Biederman, Wilens, & Faraone, 1994) have systematically assessed the available literature related to ADHD in adults, and have concluded that ADHD in adults is a reliable and valid disorder. Four sources of data suggest that ADHD persists into adulthood: studies of clinically referred adults, longitudinal studies of ADHD children, family genetic studies, and psychopharmacologic studies.

A small group of studies has examined clinically referred adults who show the symptoms and characteristic impairments associated with ADHD in childhood. For example, Borland and Heckman (1976) reported that 50% of adults with childhood ADHD had a full or partial syndrome of the disorder, characterized by restlessness, impulsivity, and difficulty concentrating, compared with only 5% of their non-ADHD siblings. Furthermore, the adults with ADHD had lower socioeconomic status (SES) and shorter job tenure, in spite of normal intelligence and the same level of education. The ADHD adults attributed their work difficulties and frequent job changes to dissatisfaction, easy frustration, boredom, and impulsivity. Morrison (1980) compared outpatient adults with childhood-onset ADHD ($n = 48$) to psychiatric controls. The ADHD group had fewer years of education and lower rates of professional employment. They vividly recalled a childhood history of persistent inability to concentrate, multiple failures, social disapproval, and demoralization. These descriptions were corroborated by information provided by their parents.

Prospective, longitudinal follow-up studies provide compelling evidence for the validity of the adult ADHD syndrome. Using criterion-based instruments, comparison groups, and blind assessments, these follow-up studies clearly show that the diagnosis of ADHD can be reliably made in adults who had the diagnosis documented when they were children (Mannuzza et al., 1991b; Weiss & Hechtman, 1986). The longitudinal studies find high rates (10–60%) of persistence of ADHD symptoms into adolescence (Klein & Mannuzza, 1991; Thorley, 1984; Weiss & Hechtman, 1986) and adulthood (Mannuzza et al., 1991b; Mannuzza, Klein, Bessler, Malloy, & LaPadula, 1993). These studies also show that the persistence of ADHD into adulthood includes symptoms of inattention, disorganization, distractibility, and impulsiveness, along with academic and occupational failure.

For nearly a century, family genetic studies have provided a touchstone for validating psychiatric syndromes (Faraone & Santangelo, 1992; Faraone & Tsuang, 1995; Tsuang, Faraone, & Lyons, 1993). Although a valid syndrome need not be familial, the demonstration of familial transmission supports the hypothesis that a syndrome is a valid diagnostic entity (Tsuang, Faraone, & Lyons, 1995). As we review in detail elsewhere (Faraone et al., 1992; Faraone & Biederman, 1994; Faraone, Biederman, & Milberger, 1994), the biologic relatives of ADHD boys are at increased risk for ADHD and other psychiatric disorders (Biederman, Faraone, Keenan, Steingard, & Tsuang, 1991a; Biederman, Faraone, Keenan, & Tsuang, 1991b; Biederman et al., 1986; Cantwell, 1972; Faraone, Biederman, Keenan, & Tsuang, 1991b; Lahey et al., 1988; Mannuzza & Gittelman, 1984; Morrison, 1980; Schachar & Wachsmuth, 1990; Stewart, deBlois, & Cummings, 1980). Recently, the familiality of ADHD was also demonstrated in an epidemiologic sample (Szatmari, Boyle, & Offord, 1993). This shows that previous observations of familial transmission were not artifacts of sampling clinically referred children. Although little is known about the families of ADHD girls, one study found an excess of ADHD among relatives of afflicted girls (Faraone, Biederman, Keenan, & Tsuang, 1991a). Additional lines of evidence from twin studies (Goodman & Stevenson, 1989; Lopez, 1965), adoption studies (Cantwell, 1975; Morrison & Stewart, 1973), and segregation analysis studies (Deutsch, Matthysse, Swanson, & Farkas, 1990; Faraone et al., 1992) suggest that the familial aggregation of ADHD has a substantial genetic component. Although extant twin studies are small, and none have used *Diagnostic and Statistical Manual of Mental Disorders* (DSM-III-R) criteria, all find greater similarity for ADHD and components of the syndrome between monozygotic twins than between dizygotic twins (Gillis, Gilger, Pennington, & DeFries, 1992; Goodman & Stevenson, 1989; Lopez, 1965). Moreover, the adoptive relatives of ADHD children are less likely to have ADHD or associated disorders than are the biologic relatives of ADHD children (Cantwell, 1975; Morrison & Stewart, 1973). Thus, a growing body of evidence shows that ADHD is a familial disorder and that transmission in families is mediated, at least in part, by genetic factors.

Treatment studies of ADHD adults have noted that participating subjects reliably meet criteria for adult ADHD with childhood onset, and that adults' self-reports can be confirmed by parents or other relatives (Gualtieri, Ondrusek, & Finley, 1985; Mattes, Boswell, & Oliver, 1984; Wender, Reimherr, Wood, & Ward, 1985a; Wood, Reimherr, Wender, & Johnson, 1976). In addition to the characteristic symptoms of the disorder required for diagnosis, these adults have poor academic performance (despite adequate intellectual abilities); stubbornness; chronic conflicts in social relations with peers, spouses, and authorities; absenteeism from work and frequent job changes; and poor frustration tolerance. Moreover, psychopharmacologic studies suggest that, like childhood ADHD, adult ADHD responds to stimulant treatment (Gualtieri et al., 1985; Mattes et al., 1984; Wender et al., 1985a; Wood et al., 1976).

Findings in Clinically Referred Subjects

To help validate the diagnosis of adult ADHD, we conducted a series of studies in our clinical population of referred adults with ADHD. We reasoned that if adult ADHD is a valid diagnosis, the clinical features of these adults should mirror those of ADHD children. We did not expect all clinical features to be identical between children and adults with ADHD—for example, some data suggest that hyperactivity decreases over time (Silver, 1992)—but we did expect that some of the more reproducible correlates of childhood ADHD should persist into adulthood. Thus, we chose psychiatric comorbidity, cognitive performance, and adaptive functioning to demonstrate descriptive validity, because these are well-known correlates of ADHD among children. To this end, we studied the initial 84 referred adults with a clinical diagnosis of childhood-onset ADHD confirmed by structured interview (Biederman et al., 1993b). Findings were compared with those from a preexisting sample of referred ADHD children ($n = 140$), their nonreferred adult relatives ($n = 50$), and adult relatives of normal controls ($n = 248$) (Biederman et al., 1992).

Patients were assessed with the Structured Clinical Interview for DSM-III-R (SCID; Spitzer, Williams, Gibbon, & First, 1990), supplemented with modules from the Schedule for Affective Disorders and Schizophrenia for School-Age Children—Epidemiologic (K-SADS-E; Orvaschel, 1985) covering childhood diagnoses. As in our previous work (Biederman et al., 1992), major depression was diagnosed only when full criteria were associated with severe impairment. Also, we used two or more anxiety disorders to index the presence of a clinically meaningful anxiety syndrome (Biederman et al., 1990b). Academic achievement was assessed with the Arithmetic subtest of the Wide Range Achievement Test—Revised (WRAT-R; Jastak & Jastak, 1985) and the Gilmore Oral Reading test (Gilmore & Gilmore, 1968). Cognitive functioning was assessed with the Vocabulary, Block Design, Arithmetic, Digit Span, and Digit Symbol subtests of the Wechsler Adult Intelligence Scale—Revised (WAIS-R; Wechsler, 1981).

We used the procedure recommended by Reynolds (1984) and others (Frick et al., 1991) to define learning disabilities. Overall psychosocial functioning was assessed with the Global Assessment of Functioning (GAF) scale of the DSM-III-R (1 = worst, 90 = best) (Spitzer et al., 1990). SES was measured with the four-factor Hollingshead scale (Hollingshead, 1975). In addition, the marital status of the subjects was recorded.

Compared with normal controls, ADHD adults were more commonly males than females ($p < .01$), were more often divorced or separated ($p < .01$), had a lower SES ($p < .01$), and had significantly poorer GAF scores ($p < .01$). ADHD adults differed significantly from controls in rates of antisocial, mood, substance use, anxiety, elimination, and speech and language disorders. Significant differences between ADHD adults and controls were also detected in the rates of reading disability, repeated grades, placement in special classes, and tutoring. These findings show that ADHD adults have a pattern of demographic, psychosocial, psychiatric, and cognitive features mirroring well-documented findings among ADHD children.

The gender distribution in the adult ADHD sample was unlike that in childhood ADHD, where males and females were more equally represented. This raised additional questions as to the validity of this diagnosis in adults. Although childhood ADHD is more prevalent in boys than in girls by factors ranging from 2:1 to 9:1 (Biederman, Faraone, Keenan, Knee, & Tsuang, 1990a; Gittelman, Mannuzza, Shenker, & Bonagura, 1985; Weiss, 1985), ADHD is nevertheless a significant cause of psychiatric disability in girls (Biederman et al., 1992; Faraone et al., 1991a).

To determine whether ADHD is a valid clinical entity in adult female subjects and whether it is expressed differently in male and female adults, we reexamined the clinical, cognitive, and functional characteristics in an expanded ($n = 128$) sample of referred adults with ADHD of both sexes ($n = 78$ [61%] males; $n = 50$ [39%] females). This analysis failed to reveal meaningful demographic differences between the genders. Male and female ADHD adults had similarly impaired GAF scores, and these scores were significantly poorer than those of control adults. Gender-specific comparisons with normal controls (see Figure 15.1) revealed that ADHD adults of both sexes had significantly higher rates of major depression, oppositional disorder, various anxiety disorders, and drug dependence. ADHD females differed significantly in rates of alcohol dependence, as well as in enuresis, stuttering, and tics (not shown in Figure 15.1). ADHD males had higher rates of conduct disorder than any other subgroup, and had higher rates of antisocial personality disorder and language disorder (the latter not shown in Figure 15.1) than male controls. More male adults with ADHD had a history of repeated grades than female subjects with ADHD; nevertheless, more females with ADHD repeated grades than female controls. The rates of repeated grades and tutoring were higher in adults of both genders with ADHD than in their same-sex controls. ADHD adults of both genders had relatively low rates of learning disability. Examination of WAIS-R scores revealed overall significant differences in Digit

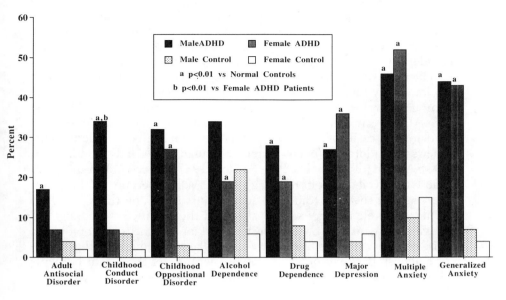

FIGURE 15.1. Patterns of psychiatric comorbidity in ADHD patients and normal controls by gender.

Symbol and Arithmetic subtests in comparisons between ADHD patients of both genders and controls.

DIAGNOSTIC ISSUES

A continuing issue for the assessment of adult ADHD is that of its diagnostic criteria. Two different approaches have been taken in making this diagnosis (Silver, 1992): one illustrated by the DSM, and the other by Wender's Utah criteria (Ward, Wender, & Reimherr, 1993). The DSM-III (American Psychiatric Association, 1980) category of residual attention deficit disorder included adults who had the full syndrome as children and a partial syndrome as adults (hence "residual type"). Although DSM-III-R (American Psychiatric Association, 1987) does not provide specific ADHD criteria for adults, there are no age limitations for this disorder, and the diagnosis of adult ADHD is made in the same way as that for children and adolescents. In contrast, the Utah criteria include (1) childhood history of ADHD with both attentional deficits and motor hyperactivity, together with at least one of the following characteristics: behavior problems in school, impulsivity, overexcitability, and temper outbursts; and (2) an adult history of persistent attentional problems and motor hyperactivity, together with two of the following five symptoms: affective lability, hot or explosive temper, stress intolerance, disorganization, and impulsivity (Ward et al., 1993). Since many of these symptoms are found in conduct, mood, and anxiety disorders and are not diagnostic criteria for ADHD as defined in DSM-III and DSM-III-R, the two sets of criteria may identify different types of patients.

The most straightforward approach to diagnosing adults with ADHD is to inquire systematically about the childhood onset of the DSM-III-R defining symptoms of the disorder, using structured interview techniques. Since ADHD is not included in any adult structured diagnostic interview, clinicians can easily use the ADHD module from available structured interviews for children. We have extensively used the ADHD module from the K-SADS-E (Orvaschel & Puig-Antich, 1987) to accomplish this goal. Because a central aspect of the diagnosis of ADHD pertains to the childhood onset of the symptoms, we query adults by asking them whether, as children in elementary school, they had the specified symptoms. If a positive response is given, we follow up by asking whether similar problems persist currently. In this fashion we can make a lifetime as well as a current diagnosis of the disorder. In patients with fewer than eight but with at least six positive symptoms, we assign the diagnosis of subthreshold ADHD.

In addition to inattention, impulsivity, and occasional hyperactivity, adults with ADHD also have clinical features commonly found in childhood ADHD. These include stubbornness, low frustration tolerance, and chronic conflicts in social relations with peers, spouses, and authorities (Biederman et al., 1993b; Spencer et al., 1995; Wood et al., 1976). These features may be responsible for the high rates of separation and divorce, as well as of poor academic and occupational achievement despite adequate intellectual abilities, in adults with ADHD (Gittelman & Mannuzza, 1988; Mannuzza et al., 1993; Weiss & Hechtman, 1986). Of particular interest is the finding that adults commonly describe their work difficulties and frequent job changes as stemming from dissatisfaction, easy frustration, boredom, and impulsiveness, as noted earlier (Borland & Heckman, 1976). Employers of these adults report that they have poor levels of work performance, impairment in task completion, lack of independent skills, and poor relationships with supervisors (Weiss & Hechtman, 1986). Hence, adults with ADHD often have a number of ADHD symptoms that they and others perceive as having a significant impact on major aspects of their lives.

COMORBIDITY

ADHD children frequently have conduct, depressive, and anxiety disorders (Biederman, Newcorn, & Sprich, 1991c; Caron & Rutter, 1991). Although spurious comorbidity can result from referral and screening artifacts (Caron & Rutter, 1991), our recent review (Biederman et al., 1991c) suggests that these artifacts cannot explain the high levels of psychiatric comorbidity observed for ADHD. For example, epidemiologic investigators find comorbidity in unselected general population samples (Anderson et al., 1987; Bird et al., 1988). Our family studies of comorbidity also dispute the notion that artifacts cause comorbidity; instead, they assign a causal role to etiologic relationships among disorders (Biederman et al., 1991a, 1991b, 1992; Faraone et al., 1991a, 1991b). Although patterns of comorbidity in ADHD adults have not been systematically evaluated, the available literature is consistent with findings reported in ADHD children. For example, follow-up studies (Mannuzza et al., 1991b) documented high rates of antisocial and substance use disorders in ADHD children followed into adulthood. Borland and Heckman (1976) reported that ADHD adults had high rates of antisocial personality, anxiety, and depressive disorders. Similarly, Morrison (1980) found elevated rates of antisocial personality disorder and alcoholism in ADHD adults. Wender et al. (1985) and Wood et al. (1976) reported high rates of mood and anxiety disorders in adults with ADHD.

We reasoned that if ADHD were a secondary disorder, it should be fairly frequent among adults with psychiatric disorders. In another sample (Biederman, 1995), we examined rates of ADHD among 25 adults who had panic disorder with agoraphobia, 20 who had major depression, and 30 who had both disorders. The 5.3% rate of ADHD among these adults was not significantly greater than the 0.0% rate observed among 40 control adults. Recently, colleagues of ours at the Massachusetts General Hospital assessed 74 adults with major depression for ADHD (M. Fava, personal communication, 1995); they found that 8.1% were positive for ADHD. Thus, the symptoms of ADHD in adulthood are not frequently observed among adults with panic disorder and major depression. This supports the divergent validity of adult ADHD.

In addition to psychiatric comorbidity, academic underachievement, placement in special classes, need for tutoring, learning disabilities, and impaired neuropsychologic performance are hallmarks of ADHD (Barkley, 1990). These problems plague ADHD children throughout childhood and adolescence, creating fertile soil for chronic psychologic and social disability in adulthood (Fischer, Barkley, Edelbrock, & Smallish, 1990; Gittelman et al., 1985; Gualtieri et al., 1985; Hechtman & Weiss, 1986; Mannuzza, Gittelman-Klein, & Addalli, 1991a). Although there is no pathognomonic neuropsychologic profile of the ADHD patient, cognitive performance measures and school dysfunction data are important validators for adult ADHD because they do not share method variance with other measures.

In a recent literature review, we (Wilens, Spencer, & Biederman, 1994) examined the evidence for an association between ADHD and psychoactive substance use disorder (PSUD). We found the following: (1) There is a consistent overlap between ADHD and PSUD in studies of both PSUD and ADHD patients; (2) prospective studies of children with persistent ADHD show them to be at high risk for PSUD as adolescents and adults;

(3) high rates of ADHD-like symptoms have been reported in longitudinal studies of children who develop PSUD; (4) elevated rates of PSUD have been found in family studies of ADHD children; and (5) elevated rates of ADHD have been reported in family studies of probands with PSUD.

Although the nature of the association between ADHD and PSUD remains unknown, two basic possibilities have been proposed: (1) ADHD alone is a risk factor for PSUD (Gittelman et al., 1985; Goodwin, Schulsinger, Hermansen, Guze, & Winokur, 1975; Tarter, McBride, Buonpane, & Schneider, 1977); and (2) the other comorbid disorders commonly associated with ADHD (i.e., conduct disorder, anxiety, depression) place an individual at elevated risk for PSUD (Biederman et al., 1990a; Biederman et al., 1992; Mannuzza et al., 1991b).

The longest follow-up studies to date have shown that ADHD children are at significant risk for PSUD as young adults (Mannuzza et al., 1993). These studies also show that PSUD is accounted for in the subgroup of children with concurrent conduct disorder and those with persistent ADHD symptoms (Barkley, DuPaul, & McMurray, 1990; Hechtman, Weiss, & Perlman, 1984; Mannuzza et al., 1991b). Similarly, in studies of PSUD adults with ADHD, there is a clear overrepresentation of conduct disorder (Wilens et al., 1994). Family genetic studies also support conduct disorder as an important variable in the relationship between ADHD and PSUD (Biederman et al., 1990a, 1992; Cantwell, 1972). Likewise, there is substantial evidence that parental PSUD with antisocial personality disorder is associated with elevated rates of ADHD and conduct disorder in the children (Biederman et al., 1990a, 1992; Earls, Reich, Jung, & Cloninger, 1988; Stewart et al., 1980), as well as early-onset PSUD in the offspring (Cloninger, 1987; Cloninger, Bohman, & Siguardsson, 1981; Irwin, Schuckit, & Smith, 1990). The risk for PSUD within subgroups of ADHD children with comorbid anxiety or depressive disorders has not been well studied, but this risk may be substantial, since pediatric and adult patients with anxiety and depressive disorders have been reported to be at higher risk for PSUD (Christie et al., 1988; Clark & Sayette, 1993; DeMilio, 1989; Deykin, Levy, & Wells, 1986; Kaminer, 1991; Kashani & Sherman, 1989; Mezzich, Tarter, Hsieh, & Fuhrman, 1992). Thus, it appears that the risk for PSUD in ADHD individuals is mediated by the other comorbid conditions frequently associated with ADHD rather than by the ADHD itself.

FORMULATING A TREATMENT PLAN

Despite the increasing recognition that children with ADHD commonly grow up to be adults with the same disorder, little is known about the treatment of this disorder in adults. This is of particular concern, given the marked impairment in multiple social and interpersonal domains associated with ADHD (Biederman et al., 1993b; Mannuzza et al., 1993). Further complicating factors in diagnosis and treatment are the facts that many adults with ADHD seeking treatment have depressive and anxiety symptoms, as well as histories of drug and alcohol dependence or abuse (Biederman et al., 1993b; Eyre, Rounsaville, & Kleber, 1982; Tarter et al., 1977; Wilens et al., 1994; Wood, Wender, & Reimherr, 1983). Thus, with the increasing recognition of the complex presentation of adults with ADHD, there is a need to develop effective pharmacotherapeutic strategies.

Pharmacotherapy should be part of a treatment plan in which consideration is given to all aspects of the patient's life. Hence, it should not be used exclusively; other interventions should be employed. The administration of medication to an adult with ADHD should be undertaken as a collaborative effort with the patient, with the physician guiding the use and management of efficacious anti-ADHD agents. The use of medication should follow a careful evaluation of the adult, including psychiatric, social, and cognitive assessments. Diagnostic information should be gathered from the patient and, whenever possible, from significant others such as partners, parents, siblings, and close friends. If ancillary data are not available, information from the adult is acceptable for diagnostic and treatment purposes, as adults with ADHD (like those with many other disorders) are appropriate reporters of their own condition. Careful attention should be paid to the childhood onset of symptoms, longitudinal history of the disorder, and differential diagnosis; medical, neurologic, and psychosocial factors contributing to the clinical presentation must all be considered.

In the ADHD adult, issues of comorbidity with learning disabilities and with other psychiatric disorders need to be addressed. Because learning disabilities do not respond to pharmacotherapy, it is important to identify these deficits to help define remedial interventions. For instance, this evaluation can assist in the design and implementation of an educational plan for the adult who may be returning to school, or can serve as an aid for structuring the current work environment. Since alcohol and drug use disorders are frequently encountered in adults with ADHD, a careful history of substance use should be completed. Patients with ongoing abuse or dependence of psychoactive substances should generally not be treated until appropriate addiction treatments have been undertaken and the patient has maintained a drug- and alcohol-free period. Other concurrent psychiatric disorders also need to be assessed, and, if possible, the relationship of the ADHD symptoms with these other disorders should be delineated. In subjects with ADHD plus bipolar disorders, for example, the risk of mania needs to be addressed and closely monitored during the treatment of the ADHD. In cases such as these, the conservative introduction of anti-ADHD medications along with mood-stabilizing agents should be considered.

PHARMACOLOGIC TREATMENT STRATEGIES

Common pharmacologic approaches for the treatment of ADHD are listed in Table 15.1. The patient needs to be familiarized with the risks and
benefits of pharmacotherapy, the availability of alternative treatments,
and the likely adverse effects. Certain adverse effects can be anticipated
on the basis of known pharmacologic properties of the drug (e.g., appetite
change, insomnia); other, more infrequent effects are unexpected (idiosyncratic) and are difficult to anticipate based on the properties of the drug.
Short-term adverse effects can be minimized by introducing the medication at a low initial dose and titrating this slowly. Idiosyncratic adverse
effects generally require drug discontinuation and selection of alternate
treatment modalities.

Patient expectations need to be explored, and realistic goals of treatment need to be clearly delineated. Likewise, the clinician should review
with the patient the various pharmacologic options available, and should
note that each will require systematic trials of the anti-ADHD medications for reasonable durations of time and at clinically meaningful doses.
The potential need for adjunctive treatment and agents should also be
explained in advance. Treatment-seeking ADHD adults who report psychologic distress related to their ADHD (i.e., self-esteem issues, self-sabo-
taging patterns, interpersonal disturbances) should be directed to appropriate
psychotherapeutic intervention with clinicians knowledgeable in ADHD
treatment. In our center, for example, we and our colleagues frequently
utilize cognitive-based therapies, with generally good patient response and
overall satisfaction (S. McDermott, personal communication, 1995).

Stimulants

The stimulant medications remain the mainstays of treatment for children, adolescents, and adults with ADHD. The effects of the stimulants
in the brain are variable. Preclinical studies have shown that the stimulants
block the reuptake of dopamine and norepinephrine into the presynaptic
neurons, and that both drugs increase the release of these monoamines
into the extraneuronal space (Elia et al., 1990). Although not entirely sufficient, alterations in dopaminergic and noradrenergic function appear necessary for clinical efficacy of the anti-ADHD medications, including the
stimulants (Zametkin & Rapoport, 1987). Stimulants reach their maximal
therapeutic effects during the absorption phase of the kinetic curve, approximately within 2 hours after ingestion. Although methylphenidate
(MPH) and amphetamines alter dopamine transmission, they appear to
have different mechanisms affecting the release of dopamine from neuronal pools (Dubovsky, 1986).

There are few pharmacokinetic studies of stimulants in humans, with
most studies limited to children and adolescents (Patrick, Mueller, & Gualtieri, 1987). Table 15.2 shows the preparations, pharmacokinetic proper-

TABLE 15.1. Medications Utilized in the Treatment of Adult ADHD

Class	Medications
Stimulants	Methylphenidate (Ritalin), dextroamphetamine (Dexedrine), pemoline (Cylert)
Tricyclic antidepressants	Desipramine (Norpramin), nortriptyline (Pamelor), and others
Atypical antidepressants	Bupropion (Wellbutrin)
Monoamine oxidase inhibitors	Tranylcypromine (Parnate), pargyline (Eutonyl), and others
Antihypertensives	Propranolol (Inderal)

ties, and dosing differences of the stimulants currently used in adults with ADHD. In adults, dextroamphetamine has a half-life of 3 to 6 hours and achieves peak plasma levels in 1 to 3 hours, with behavioral and cognitive effects usually noted between 30 minutes and 2 hours after ingestion, and dissipating by 4 hours. Administration of MPH results in a variable peak plasma concentration in 1 to 2 hours after ingestion, with an elimination half-life of 2 to 3 hours (Patrick et al., 1987; Sebrechts et al., 1986). Peak behavioral effects generally occur within 30 minutes to 2 hours and wear off by 3 to 5 hours. Pemoline has a longer half-life than that of the short-acting stimulants, reaches peak levels 1 to 4 hours after ingestion, and requires daily administration to achieve behavioral and cognitive effectiveness. Of interest is the finding that food ingestion appears to have little impact in the pharmacokinetic profile of the stimulants (Patrick et al., 1987), and may assist in reducing the occasional indigestion related to stimulant administration. Plasma stimulant levels have not been found to be clinically useful as correlates to response or toxicity (Patrick et al., 1987; Spencer et al., 1995).

Both MPH and dextroamphetamine are available in long-acting preparations (see Table 15.2). The longer-acting form of dextroamphetamine is preferable to the shorter-acting form, because the short-acting form has a very rapid onset and offset of action, as well as the potential for euphoria and addiction at higher doses. The half-life of the long-acting (sustained-release, or SR) preparation of MPH is between 2 and 6 hours, with peak behavioral effect generally occurring within 2 hours and lasting up to 8 hours after ingestion (Birmaher, Greenhill, Cooper, Fried, & Maminski, 1989; Pelham et al., 1987; Pelham, Walker, Sturges, & Hoza, 1989). In cross-comparison studies, similar efficacy has been reported for the two preparations of MPH, the sustained preparation of dextroamphetamine, and pemoline (Silver & Brunstetter, 1986). There are, however, anecdotal reports of patients who do not respond to the long-acting preparations

TABLE 15.2. Stimulant Preparations and Daily Doses

| Medication | Tablet size and preparation | | Peak levels | Half-lives | Dosing frequency |
	Short-acting	Long-acting			
Methylphenidate	5, 10, 20 mg	20 mg (SR[a])	1–2 hr (reg.) 2–3 hr (SR)	2–3 hr (reg.) 2–6 hr (SR)	1–5 times/day
Dextro-amphetamine	5 mg	5, 10, 15 mg (spansule)	1–2 hr (reg.) 1–3 hr (spansule)	3–6 hr	1–5 times/day
Pemoline		18.75, 37.5, 75 mg	1–4 hr	11–13 hr	1–2 times/day

Note. Adapted from Wilens and Biederman (1992). Copyright 1992 by W. B. Saunders Company. Adapted by permission.
[a]Sustained-release.

compared to the short-acting forms. The SR form of MPH (20 mg) is approximately equipotent to twice-daily MPH 10-mg tablets (Pelham et al., 1987).

The increasing use of psychostimulants has paralleled the increasing recognition of the persistence of childhood ADHD symptoms through adolescence and into adulthood (Wilens & Biederman, 1992). In contrast to more than 100 studies of stimulant efficacy in children and adolescents with ADHD (Wilens & Biederman, 1992), there are only six controlled studies assessing the efficacy of stimulants in adults with ADHD (Gualtieri et al., 1985; Mattes et al., 1984; Wender, Reimherr, & Wood, 1981; Wender et al., 1985a; Wood et al., 1976). In contrast to consistent robust responses to stimulants in children and adolescents of approximately 70% (Barkley, 1977; Wilens & Biederman, 1992), studies in adults have shown more equivocal responses to stimulants—ranging from 25% to 73% (mean 50%), despite moderate doses of these medications. Variability in the response rate appears to be related to the diagnostic criteria utilized to determine ADHD, low stimulant doses, and differing methods of assessing overall response.

In a recent double-blind, placebo-controlled, crossover study applying DSM-III-R criteria for adult ADHD, we (Spencer et al., 1995) found a dose-dependent improvement in symptoms. In this 7-week study in 23 adults with ADHD, a marked 78% response was noted for MPH treatment, whereas there was only a 4% response rate on placebo. This response rate was independent of gender, psychiatric comorbidity, or family history of psychiatric disorders. Interestingly, modest improvements in ADHD symptoms with MPH were noted at a total daily dose of 0.5 mg/kg/day (ca. 30–40 mg/day), whereas improvement of ADHD symptoms was far more robust when higher doses of 1.0 mg/kg/day (ca. 60–80 mg/day) were attained (see Figure 15.2), suggesting a dose-dependent response to MPH in adults with ADHD (Spencer et al., 1995). These findings are consistent with pediatric studies in which cognitive, behavioral, and academic

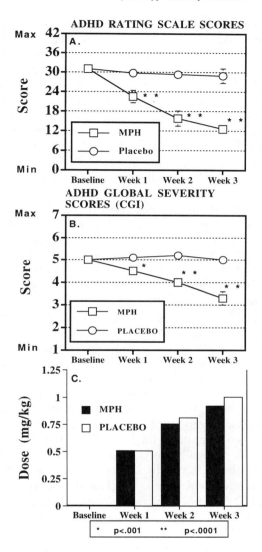

FIGURE 15.2. Response to methylphenidate versus placebo in adult ADHD. CGI, clinical general improvement.

improvements occur in a stepwise fashion with increasing doses of MPH (Rapport, DuPaul, & Kelly, 1989; Rapport et al., 1987). The results of this study strongly suggest that adults, like younger patients, may require robust dosing to attain adequate clinical response.

The half-life of the short-acting stimulants necessitates at least twice-daily dosing, with the addition of similar afternoon doses depending on breakthrough symptoms. The starting dose of both MPH and dextroamphetamine in most adults is 5 mg, with a suggested range of 0.3–1.5 mg/kg/day (approximately 20–80 mg/day in an average-sized adult) in two to four divided doses (Wilens & Biederman, 1992). Pemoline is given once or twice daily, usually at a starting dose of 37.5 mg in the morning, which is increased weekly depending on response and adverse effects. Because of its long half-life, pemoline may need up to 6 weeks for full assessment of efficacy. Once pharmacotherapy is initiated, monthly contact with the patient is necessary during the initial phase of treatment, to carefully monitor response to the intervention and adverse effects.

The side effects of the stimulants are generally mild and can be managed with an adjustment in timing of administration or dose. In studies of adult ADHD, the following side effects were reported by frequency of occurrence: insomnia, edginess, diminished appetite, weight loss, dysphoria, and headaches. No cases of stimulant-related psychosis at therapeutic doses have been reported in adults. Likewise, despite the abuse potential of the stimulants, there have been no reports of stimulant abuse in controlled or retrospective studies of adults with ADHD (Spencer et al., 1995; Wilens & Biederman, 1992; Wilens et al., 1994). The addition of low-dose beta-adrenergic blockers (e.g., propranolol at 10 mg up to three times daily) or busipirone (5–10 mg up to three times daily) may be helpful in reducing the edginess/agitation associated with stimulant administration (Ratey, Greenberg, & Lindem, 1991). "Rebound" has been described as a deterioration in behavior that exceeds baseline behavior; this usually occurs in the afternoon and evening following administration of stimulant medication. The prevalence of this effect appears to be low in adults, but rebound reactions with excitability, talkativeness, and euphoria have been described in children (Alessi & Magen, 1988). Although concerns about cardiovascular adverse effects of stimulants have been raised in children, there have been only minimal, clinically insignificant elevations of heart rate and diastolic blood pressure in controlled investigations with adults, and these were weakly correlated with stimulant dose (Biederman et al., 1993b). However, in ADHD patients with cardiac abnormalities, treatment should be carefully monitored and appropriate cardiology consultation should be obtained.

The interactions of the stimulants with other prescription and nonprescription medications are generally mild and are usually not significant sources of concern (Wilens & Biederman, 1992). Whereas coadministration of a sympathomimetic (e.g., pseudoephedrine) may potentiate both medications' effects, the antihistamines may diminish stimulant effectiveness. The coadministration of stimulants and antidepressants of the monoamine oxidase inhibitor (MAOI) type is not advised, because of the potential for hypertensive reactions with this combination. The concomitant use of stimulants and tricyclic antidepressants (TCAs) or anticonvulsants has been associated with increase in the serum levels of both medications. Thus, when combinations of stimulants with TCAs or anticonvulsants are used, it may be necessary to monitor levels of these medications more closely.

Nonstimulant Medications

Despite the increasing use of stimulants for adults with ADHD, approximately 30–50% do not respond positively to the stimulants, have untoward side effects, or have concurrent depressive and anxiety disorders that stimulant medication may exacerbate or treat ineffectively (Biederman et al., 1993b; Spencer et al., 1995; Wilens & Biederman, 1992). Hence, the need for nonstimulant pharmacotherapy continues to be an area of ongoing investigation.

Tricyclic Antidepressants

Within the past two decades, the TCAs imipramine, desipramine, and nortriptyline have been used increasingly as alternative treatments to the stimulants for ADHD in children and adolescents, regardless of psychiatric comorbidity (Biederman, Baldessarini, Wright, Keenan, & Faraone, 1993a; Biederman, Baldessarini, Wright, Knee, & Harmatz, 1989a; Rapoport, Quin, Bradbard, Riddle, & Brooks, 1974; Wilens, Biederman, Geist, Steingard, & Spencer, 1993). In part, the TCAs have been used because they have several advantages over the stimulants in the treatment of ADHD. TCAs have a long half-life, permitting flexible dosing (once daily); have little risk for abuse or dependence; and appear to be helpful in stimulant-refractory patients (Biederman et al., 1993a). TCAs have also been shown to be safe, effective, and well tolerated in adults treated for anxiety, panic, and depressive disorders (Baldessarini, 1989)—conditions that commonly co-occur with ADHD in adults (Biederman et al., 1993b). However, despite experience in children and adolescents, substantial anecdotal information (Ratey, Greenberg, Bemporad, & Lindem, 1992), and the theoretical benefits of the TCAs, these agents have not been prospectively assessed in a controlled manner for the treatment of adult ADHD.

Our clinical experience with adults indicates that TCAs may be useful for treating ADHD symptoms. A systematic chart review of 32 adults (mean age 41 years) receiving routine care at our center with TCAs for ADHD indicated a reasonably good response to desipramine and nortriptyline (Wilens, Biederman, Spencer, & Prince, 1995). The mean dose of desipramine (160 mg/day) was equipotent to that of nortriptyline (84 mg/day). The majority of patients responded favorably to treatment (72%), with 52% manifesting a marked improvement with TCA treatment. The anti-ADHD efficacy of the TCAs appeared to be sustained for an average follow-up period of 1 year. Hence, the results of this pilot investigation indicate that the secondary amines nortriptyline and desipramine may be useful agents for adult ADHD; however, more controlled investigations are necessary to evaluate this issue more fully. Currently, a controlled trial of desipramine for adult ADHD is underway at our center.

Generally, TCA daily doses of 50–250 mg are required, with a relatively rapid response to treatment (about 2 weeks) when the appropriate dose is reached. The TCAs should be initiated at 25 mg, and this should be slowly titrated upward within dosing and serum level parameters until either an acceptable response or intolerable adverse effects are reported. Common side effects of the TCAs include dry mouth, constipation, blurred vision, and sexual dysfunction. Although cardiovascular effects of reduced cardiac conduction, orthostatic hypotension, and elevated heart rates are not infrequent if monitored in healthy subjects, they rarely prevent treatment. Whereas adults commonly develop orthostatic hypotension when treated with TCAs (Tesar et al., 1987), children and adolescents tend to manifest mild elevation of diastolic blood pressure (Biederman et al., 1989b). As there is no clear relationship between serum level and response, blood level monitoring may best serve to reduce central nervous system and cardiovascular toxicity, and to check compliance.

Other Antidepressants

More recently, the atypical, stimulant-like antidepressant bupropion has been reported to be moderately helpful in reducing ADHD symptoms in children (Casat, Pleasants, & Van Wyck Fleet, 1987; Krishnan et al., 1989) and adults (Wender & Reimherr, 1990). In an open study of 19 adults treated with an average of 360 mg of bupropion for 6–8 weeks, Wender and Reimherr (1990) reported a moderate to marked response in 74% of patients, with 5 dropouts. Sustained improvement was noted in the 10 subjects remaining on the drug at a 1-year follow-up. Despite the small numbers of adults studied, bupropion may be helpful for adults with ADHD, particularly for those with comorbid mood instability or with cardiac abnormalities (Gelenberg, Bassuk, & Schoonover, 1991). The response of ADHD to bupropion appears to be rapid and sustained, with the dosing range for ADHD similar to that recommended for depression, and a suggested maximal dose of 450 mg/day divided in three daily doses. Bupropion appears to be more stimulating than other antidepressants and has no significant cardiac effects. It is associated with higher rate of drug-induced seizures than other antidepressants (Kosten, Jacobs, & Mason, 1984), which appear to be dose-related (>450 mg/day) and elevated in patients with bulimia nervosa or a previous seizure history. Bupropion has also been associated with excitement, agitation, increased motor activity, insomnia, weight loss, and tremor.

The MAOI antidepressants have also been studied for the treatment of ADHD. Moderate efficacy of MAOIs was shown in a controlled study in hyperactive children (Zametkin et al., 1985). In open studies in adult ADHD, moderate improvements were reported in 61% of subjects (Wender, Wood, & Reimherr, 1985b; Wender, Wood, Reimherr, & Ward, 1983) treated with pargyline (not available in the United States) and deprenyl. Administration of these agents was associated with numerous adverse effects and a relatively high dropout rate during the 6-week trial period (Wender et al., 1983, 1985b). The same dosing schedule of the MAOIs used for the treatment of depressive disorders appears necessary for anti-ADHD efficacy. Of interest was the authors' report of a delayed onset of action and a postdosing stimulant-like quality of the MAOIs on ADHD symptoms, lasting up to 6 hours (Wender et al., 1983). The MAOIs may have a role in the management of treatment-refractory, nonimpulsive adult ADHD subjects with comorbid depression and anxiety, who are able to comply with the stringent dietary requirements of the MAOIs. The low-tyramine dietary requirements of these agents often make compliance with treatment difficult, especially in the group of ADHD patients vulnerable to impulsivity. Other adverse effects associated with the MAOIs include agitation or lethargy, orthostatic hypotension, weight gain, sexual dysfunction, sleep disturbances, and edema, any of which may lead to treatment discontinuation (Gelenberg et al., 1991).

Selective serotonin reuptake inhibitors (SSRIs), including fluoxetine, sertraline, paroxetine, and others, have been used extensively in the past few years for the treatment of depressive and anxiety disorders. Although there are no controlled studies evaluating the efficacy of these agents for adult ADHD, fluoxetine was reported to be moderately effective for children with ADHD in one small case series (Barrickman, Noyes, Kuperman, Schumacher, & Verda, 1991). In our clinical experience with adult ADHD, the SSRIs have been invaluable in treating concurrent anxiety and depressive disorders, but not the core ADHD symptoms. This is not surprising, as the pathogenesis of ADHD appears to be related primarily to the central nervous system's dopaminergic and adrenergic systems, with little direct influence by the serotonergic systems (Zametkin & Rapoport, 1987). A novel antidepressant with both serotonergic and noradrenergic properties, venlafaxine, may be a promising new agent for adult ADHD but remains untested.

Antihypertensives

Antihypertensives have been used successfully for the treatment of childhood ADHD, especially in cases with a marked hyperactive or aggressive component. Although clonidine has been shown to be effective in the treatment of ADHD in children and adolescents (Hunt, Minderaa, & Cohen, 1985; Steingard, Biederman, Spencer, Wilens, & Gonzalez, 1993), the potential hypotensive effects of this agent may make it problematic for use in adults. Beta-adrenergic blockers may also be helpful in adult ADHD. A small open study of propranolol for adults with temper outbursts indicated some improvement in ADHD symptoms at daily doses of up to 640 mg/day (Mattes, 1986). Another report indicated that beta-adrenergic blockers may be helpful in combination with the stimulants (Ratey et al., 1991). To date, the efficacy of these agents for adult ADHD needs to be further assessed. Beta-adrenergic blockers are also associated with hypotension and bradycardia; thus, continued monitoring of this type of treatment is required.

Combined Pharmacotherapy

Combined pharmacotherapy may be useful in adults with ADHD who show an inadequate response with single agents, or who have manifest comorbid psychiatric disorders. (Whenever possible, the use of single agents is preferable, to reduce the possibility of adverse effects and to improve treatment compliance.) The administration of two agents may improve or potentiate the individual effects of both medications in ameliorating ADHD symptoms. For instance, whereas single agents may not provide acceptable control of ADHD symptoms, we have found that the addition of stimulants (e.g., MPH at 5–20 mg) often improves the anti-ADHD effectiveness of the antidepressants. Because coadministration of stimulants and TCAs has been associated with potentiation of adverse effects and TCA levels in children and adolescents, serum TCA levels should be reevaluated when other psychoactive agents are added. Coadministration of adjunctive anti-ADHD medications with the MAOIs is not recommended. In cases of partial response or adverse effects of edginess and anxiety with stimulants, the addition of low-dose beta-adrenergic blockers or busipirone may be helpful (Ratey et al., 1991).

The use of multiple agents is also helpful in treating disorders concurrent with the ADHD. For example, the combination of the stimulants or TCAs with the SSRIs may assist in the management of concurrent depressive disorders. Benzodiazepines in combination with anti-ADHD medications are useful in the management of ADHD and comorbid anxiety disorders. Likewise, for individuals with prominent mood lability, mood-stabilizing agents such as lithium carbonate or carbemazepine may assist in reducing the lability while providing the opportunity to treat the ADHD symptoms. It is important to note that whereas specific individual agents have been evaluated for safety and efficacy, the use of multiple agents simultaneously for adult ADHD remains unstudied.

Strategies for Treatment-Refractory Patients

Despite the availability of various agents for adults with ADHD, a number of individuals either do not respond to, or are intolerant of adverse effects of, medications used to treat their ADHD. In managing apparent nonresponse to medication, several therapeutic strategies are available. If psychiatric adverse effects develop concurrently with a poor medication response, alternative treatments should be pursued. Severe psychiatric symptoms that emerge during the acute phase can be problematic, regardless of the efficacy of the medications for ADHD. These symptoms may require reconsideration of the diagnosis of ADHD and careful reassessment of the presence of comorbid disorders. If a reduction of dose or a change in preparation (e.g., regular vs. SR stimulants) does not resolve the problem, consideration should again be given to alternative treatments. Concurrent nonpharmacologic interventions, such as behavioral or cognitive therapy, may assist with symptom reduction.

SUMMARY

Epidemiologic data are not available on rates of ADHD in adults; however, since 6–9% of children are estimated to have ADHD (Anderson et al., 1987; Bird et al., 1988), 1–4% of adults may have the disorder. Thus, adult ADHD may be one of the most common adult psychiatric disorders. However, despite recent mass media attention (Miller, 1993) and the possibility that adult ADHD may be a serious public health problem, diagnostic skepticism about the validity of this disorder has limited its recognition and identification. The limited recognition of adult ADHD has serious clinical implications. ADHD will not be generally accepted as a treatable adult psychiatric condition until it achieves the nosologic status of other adult disorders. Although a growing literature suggests that adult ADHD is a valid entity, full nosologic recognition of the disorder demands programmatic research aimed at establishing its descriptive, concurrent, and divergent validity.

Despite this state of affairs, an emerging literature suggests an important role for various psychopharmacologic agents in the treatment of adults with ADHD. Pharmacotherapy serves an important role in reducing the core symptoms of ADHD and other concurrent psychiatric disorders in adults. Stimulant medications continue to be the first-line drugs of choice for uncomplicated ADHD in adults, with TCAs and bupropion for nonresponders or adults with concurrent psychiatric disorders. Current clinical experience suggest that multiple agents may be necessary in the successful treatment of some complex cases of adult ADHD with poor responses to first-line agents or with psychiatric comorbidity.

REFERENCES

Alessi, N. E., & Magen, J. (1988). Panic disorder in psychiatrically hospitalized children. *American Journal of Psychiatry, 145,* 1450–1452.

American Psychiatric Association. (1980). *Diagnostic and statistical manual of mental disorders* (3rd ed.). Washington, DC: Author.

American Psychiatric Association. (1987). *Diagnostic and statistical manual of mental disorders* (3rd ed., rev.). Washington, DC: Author.

Anderson, J. C., Williams, S., McGee, R., & Silva, P. A. (1987). DSM-III disorders in preadolescent children: Prevalence in a large sample from the general population. *Archives of General Psychiatry, 44,* 69–76.

Baldessarini, R. J. (1989). Current status of antidepressants: Clinical pharmacology and therapy. *Journal of Clinical Psychiatry, 50,* 117–126.

Barkley, R. A. (1977). A review of stimulant drug research with hyperactive children. *Journal of Child Psychology and Psychiatry, 18,* 137–165.

Barkley, R. A. (1990). *Attention-deficit hyperactivity disorder: A handbook for diagnosis and treatment.* New York: Guilford Press.

Barkley, R. A., DuPaul, G. J., & McMurray, M. B. (1990). Comprehensive evaluation of attention deficit disorder with and without hyperactivity as defined by research criteria. *Journal of Consulting and Clinical Psychology, 58,* 775–798.

Barrickman, L., Noyes, R., Kuperman, S., Schumacher, E., & Verda, M. (1991). Treatment of ADHD with fluoxetine: A preliminary trial. *Journal of the American Academy of Child and Adolescent Psychiatry, 30*, 762–767.

Biederman, J. (1995). [Unpublished data.]

Biederman, J., Baldessarini, R. J., Wright, V., Keenan, K., & Faraone, S. (1993a). A double-blind placebo controlled study of desipramine in the treatment of attention deficit disorder: III. Lack of impact of comorbidity and family history factors on clinical response. *Journal of the American Academy of Child and Adolescent Psychiatry, 32*, 199–204.

Biederman, J., Baldessarini, R., Wright, V., Knee, D., & Harmatz, J. (1989a). A double-blind placebo controlled study of desipramine in the treatment of attention deficit disorder: I. Efficacy. *Journal of the American Academy of Child and Adolescent Psychiatry, 28*, 777–784.

Biederman, J., Baldessarini, R., Wright, V., Knee, D., Harmatz, J., & Goldblatt, A. (1989b). A double-blind placebo controlled study of desipramine in the treatment of attention deficit disorder: II. Serum drug levels and cardiovascular findings. *Journal of the American Academy of Child and Adolescent Psychiatry, 28*, 903–911.

Biederman, J., Faraone, S. V., Keenan, K., Benjamin, J., Krifcher, B., Moore, C., Sprich, S., Ugaglia, K., Jellinek, M. S., Steingard, R., Spencer, T., Norman, D., Kolodny, R., Kraus, I., Perrin, J., Keller, M. B., & Tsuang, M. T. (1992). Further evidence for family-genetic risk factors in attention deficit hyperactivity disorder (ADHD): Patterns of comorbidity in probands and relatives in psychiatrically and pediatrically referred samples. *Archives of General Psychiatry, 49*, 728–738.

Biederman, J., Faraone, S. V., Keenan, K., Knee, D., & Tsuang, M. T. (1990a). Family-genetic and psychosocial risk factors in DSM-III attention deficit disorder. *Journal of the American Academy of Child and Adolescent Psychiatry, 29*, 526–533.

Biederman, J., Faraone, S. V., Keenan, K., Steingard, R., & Tsuang, M. T. (1991a). Familial association between attention deficit disorder (ADD) and anxiety disorder. *American Journal of Psychiatry, 148*, 251–256.

Biederman, J., Faraone, S. V., Keenan, K., & Tsuang, M. T. (1991b). Evidence of familial association between attention deficit disorder and major affective disorders. *Archives of General Psychiatry, 48*, 633–642.

Biederman, J., Faraone, S. V., Spencer, T., Wilens, T., Norman, D., Lapey, K., Mick, E., Krifcher Lehman, B., & Doyle, A. (1993b). Patterns of psychiatric comorbidity, cognition and psychosocial functioning in adults with attention deficit hyperactivity disorder. *American Journal of Psychiatry, 150*, 1792–1798.

Biederman, J., Munir, K., Knee, D., Habelow, W., Armentano, M., Autor, S., Hoge, S. K., & Waternaux, C. (1986). A family study of patients with attention deficit disorder and normal controls. *Journal of Psychiatric Research, 20*, 263–274.

Biederman, J., Newcorn, J., & Sprich, S. (1991c). Comorbidity of attention deficit hyperactivity disorder with conduct, depressive, anxiety, and other disorders. *American Journal of Psychiatry, 148*, 564–577.

Biederman, J., Rosenbaum, J. F., Hirshfeld, D. R., Faraone, S. V., Bolduc, E. A., Gersten, M., Meminger, S. R., Kagan, J., Snidman, N., & Reznick, J.

S. (1990b). Psychiatric correlates of behavioral inhibition in young children of parents with and without psychiatric disorders. *Archives of General Psychiatry, 47,* 21–26.

Bird, H. R., Canino, G., Rubio-Stipec, M., Gould, M. S., Ribera, J., Sesman, M., Woodbury, M., Huertas-Goldman, S., Pagan, A., Sanchez-Lacay, A., & Moscoso, M. (1988). Estimates of the prevalence of childhood maladjustment in a community survey in Puerto Rico. *Archives of General Psychiatry, 45,* 1120–1126.

Birmaher, B., Greenhill, L. L., Cooper, T. B., Fried, J., & Maminski, B. (1989). Sustained release methylphenidate: Pharmacokinetic studies in ADDH males. *Journal of the American Academy of Child and Adolescent Psychiatry, 28,* 768–772.

Borland, B. L., & Heckman, H. K. (1976). Hyperactive boys and their brothers: A 25-year follow-up study. *Archives of General Psychiatry, 33,* 669–675.

Cantwell, D. P. (1972). Psychiatric illness in the families of hyperactive children. *Archives of General Psychiatry, 27,* 414–417.

Cantwell, D. P. (1975). Genetics of hyperactivity. *Journal of Child Psychology and Psychiatry, 16,* 261–264.

Caron, C., & Rutter, M. (1991). Comorbidity in child psychopathology: Concepts, issues and research strategies. *Journal of Child Psychology and Psychiatry, 32,* 1063–1080

Casat, C. D., Pleasants, D. Z., & Van Wyck Fleet, J. (1987). A double-blind trial of bupropion in children with attention deficit disorder. *Psychopharmacology Bulletin, 23,* 120–122.

Christie, K. A., Burke, J. D., Regier, D. A., Rae, D. S., Boyd, J. H., & Locke, B. Z. (1988). Epidemiologic evidence for early onset of mental disorders and higher risk of drug abuse in young adults. *American Journal of Psychiatry, 145,* 971–975.

Clark, D. B., & Sayette, M. A. (1993). Anxiety and the development of alcoholism: Clinical and scientific issues. *American Journal on Addictions, 2,* 59–76.

Cloninger, C. R. (1987). Neurogenetic adaptive mechanisms in alcoholism. *Science, 236,* 410–416.

Cloninger, C. R., Bohman, M., & Sigvardsson, S. (1981). Inheritance of alcohol abuse: Cross-fostering analysis of adopted men. *Archives of General Psychiatry, 38,* 861–867.

DeMilio, L. (1989). Psychiatric syndromes in adolescent substance abusers. *American Journal of Psychiatry, 146,* 1212–1214.

Deutsch, C. K., Matthysse, S., Swanson, J. M., & Farkas, L. G. (1990). Genetic latent structure analysis of dysmorphology in attention deficit disorder. *Journal of the American Academy of Child and Adolescent Psychiatry, 29,* 189–194.

Deykin, E. Y., Levy, J. C., & Wells, V. (1986). Adolescent depression, alcohol, and drug abuse. *American Journal of Public Health, 76,* 178–182.

Dubovsky, S. L. (1986). Coping with entitlement in medical education. *New England Journal of Medicine, 315,* 1672–1674.

Earls, F., Reich, W., Jung, K. G., & Cloninger, R. (1988). Psychopathology in children of alcoholic and antisocial parents. *Alcoholism: Clinical and Experimental Research, 12,* 481–487.

Elia, J., Borcherding, B. G., Potter, W. Z., Mefford, I. N., Rapoport, J. L., & Keysor, C. S. (1990). Stimulant drug treatment of hyperactivity: Biochemical correlates. *Clinical Pharmacology and Therapeutics, 48,* 57–66.

Eyre, S., Rounsaville, B., & Kleber, H. (1982). History of childhood hyperactivity in a clinical population of opiate addicts. *Journal of Nervous and Mental Disease, 170,* 522–529.

Faraone, S., & Biederman, J. (1994). Is attention deficit hyperactivity disorder familial? *Harvard Review of Psychiatry, 1,* 271–287.

Faraone, S., Biederman, J., Chen, W. J., Krifcher, B., Keenan, K., Moore, C., Sprich, S., & Tsuang, M. (1992). Segregation analysis of attention deficit hyperactivity disorder: Evidence for single gene transmission. *Psychiatric Genetics, 2,* 257–275.

Faraone, S. V., Biederman, J., Keenan, K., & Tsuang, M. T. (1991a). A family-genetic study of girls with DSM-III attention deficit disorder. *American Journal of Psychiatry, 148,* 112–117.

Faraone, S. V., Biederman, J., Keenan, K., & Tsuang, M. T. (1991b). Separation of DSM-III attention deficit disorder and conduct disorder: Evidence from a family-genetic study of American child psychiatric patients. *Psychological Medicine, 21,* 109–121.

Faraone, S., Biederman, J., & Milberger, S. (1994). An exploratory study of ADHD among second-degree relatives of ADHD children. *Biological Psychiatry, 35,* 398–402.

Faraone, S. V., & Santangelo, S. (1992). Methods in genetic epidemiology. In M. Fava & J. F. Rosenbaum (Eds.), *Research designs and methods in psychiatry.* Amsterdam: Elsevier.

Faraone, S. V., & Tsuang, M. T. (1995). Methods in psychiatric genetics. In M. Tohen, M. T. Tsuang, & G. E. P. Zahner (Eds.), *Textbook in psychiatric epidemiology.* New York: Wiley.

Fischer, M., Barkley, R. A., Edelbrock, C. S., & Smallish, L. (1990). The adolescent outcome of hyperactive children diagnosed by research criteria: II. Academic, attentional, and neuropsychological status. *Journal of Consulting and Clinical Psychology, 58,* 580–588.

Frank, E., Kupfer, D. J., & Perel, J. M. (1989). Early recurrence in unipolar depression. *Archives of General Psychiatry, 46,* 397–400.

Frick, P. J., Lahey, B. B., Kamphaus, R. W., Loeber, R., Christ, M. A. G., Hart, E. L., & Tannenbaum, L. E. (1991). Academic underachievement and the disruptive behavior disorders. *Journal of Consulting and Clinical Psychology, 59,* 289–294.

Gelenberg, A. J., Bassuk, E. L., & Schoonover, S. C. (1991). *The practitioner's guide to psychoactive drugs* (3rd ed.). New York: Plenum Press.

Gillis, J. J., Gilger, J. W., Pennington, B. F., & DeFries, J. C. (1992). Attention deficit disorder in reading-disabled twins: Evidence for a genetic etiology. *Journal of Abnormal Child Psychology, 20,* 303–315.

Gilmore, J. V., & Gilmore, E. C. (1968). *Gilmore Oral Reading Test.* New York: Harcourt, Brace & World.

Gittelman, R., & Mannuzza, S. (1988). Hyperactive boys almost grown up: III. Methylphenidate effects on ultimate height. *Archives of General Psychiatry, 45,* 1131–1134.

Gittelman, R., Mannuzza, S., Shenker, R., & Bonagura, N. (1985). Hyperactive boys almost grown up. *Archives of General Psychiatry, 42,* 937–947.

Goodman, R., & Stevenson, J. (1989). A twin study of hyperactivity: I. An examination of hyperactivity scores and categories derived from Rutter teacher and parent questionnaires. *Journal of Child Psychology and Psychiatry, 30,* 671–689.

Goodwin, D., Schulsinger, F., Hermansen, L., Guze, S., & Winokur, G. (1975). Alcoholism and the hyperactive child syndrome. *Journal of Nervous and Mental Disease, 160*, 349–353.

Gualtieri, C. T., Ondrusek, M. G., & Finley, C. (1985). Attention deficit disorders in adults. *Clinical Neuropharmacology, 8*, 343–356.

Hechtman, L., & Weiss, G. (1986). Controlled prospective fifteen year follow-up of hyperactives as adults: Non-medical drug and alcohol use and anti-social behaviour. *Canadian Journal of Psychiatry, 31*, 557–567.

Hechtman, L., Weiss, G., & Perlman, T. (1984). Hyperactives as young adults: Past and current substance abuse and antisocial behavior. *American Orthopsychiatric Association, 54*, 415–425.

Hollingshead, A. B. (1975). *Four factor index of social status*. New Haven, CT: Yale University, Department of Sociology.

Hunt, R. D., Minderaa, R. B., & Cohen, D. J. (1985). Clonidine benefits children with attention deficit disorder and hyperactivity: Report of a double-blind placebo–crossover therapeutic trial. *Journal of the American Academy of Child Psychiatry, 24*, 617–629.

Irwin, M., Schuckit, M., & Smith, T. L. (1990). Clinical importance of age at onset in type 1 and type 2 primary alcoholics. *Archives of General Psychiatry, 47*, 320–324.

Jastak, J. F., & Jastak, S. (1985). *The Wide Range Achievement Test—Revised*. Wilmington, DE: Jastak Associates.

Kaminer, Y. (1991). The magnitude of concurrent psychiatric disorders in hospitalized substance abusing adolescents. *Child Psychiatry and Human Development, 22*, 89–95.

Kashani, J. H., & Sherman, D. D. (1989). Mood disorders in children and adolescents. In A. Tasman, R. E. Hales, & A. J. Frances (Eds.), *Review of psychiatry* (Vol. 8). Washington, DC: American Psychiatric Press.

Klein, R., & Mannuzza, S. (1990). *Family history of psychiatric disorders in ADHD*. Paper presented at the Annual Meeting of the American Academy of Child and Adolescent Psychiatry, Chicago.

Klein, R. G., & Mannuzza, S. (1991). Long-term outcome of hyperactive children: A review. *Journal of the American Academy of Child and Adolescent Psychiatry, 30*, 383–387.

Kosten, T. R., Jacobs, S., & Mason, J. W. (1984). The dexamethasone suppression test during bereavement. *Journal of Nervous and Mental Disease, 172*, 359–360.

Krishnan, K. R., Davidson, J. R., Rayasam, K., Tanas, K. S., Shope, F. S., & Pelton, S. (1987). Diagnostic utility of the dexamethasone suppression test. *Biological Psychiatry, 22*, 618–628.

Lahey, B. B., Piacentini, J. C., McBurnett, K., Stone, P., Hartdagen, S., & Hynd, G. (1988). Psychopathology in the parents of children with conduct disorder and hyperactivity. *Journal of the American Academy of Child and Adolescent Psychiatry, 27*, 163–170.

Lopez, R. E. (1965). Hyperactivity in twins. *Canadian Psychiatric Association Journal, 10*, 421–426.

Mannuzza, S., & Gittelman, R. (1984). The adolescent outcome of hyperactive girls. *Psychiatry Research, 13*, 19–29.

Mannuzza, S., Gittelman-Klein, R., & Addalli, K. A. (1991a). Young adult mental status of hyperactive boys and their brothers: A prospective follow-up study. *Journal of the American Academy of Child and Adolescent Psychiatry,* 30, 743–751.

Mannuzza, S., Gittelman-Klein, R., Bonagura, N., Malloy, P., Giampino, T. L., & Addalli, K. A. (1991b). Hyperactive boys almost grown up: V. Replication of psychiatric status. *Archives of General Psychiatry,* 48, 77–83.

Mannuzza, S., Klein, R. G., Bessler, A., Malloy, P., & LaPadula, M. (1993). Adult outcome of hyperactive boys: Educational achievement, occupational rank and psychiatric status. *Archives of General Psychiatry,* 50, 565–576.

Mattes, J. A. (1986). Propranolol for adults with temper outbursts and residual attention deficit disorder. *Journal of Clinical Psychopharmacology,* 6, 299–302.

Mattes, J. A., Boswell, L., & Oliver, H. (1984). Methylphenidate effects on symptoms of attention deficit disorder in adults. *Archives of General Psychiatry,* 41, 1059–1063.

Mezzich, A. C., Tarter, R. E., Hsieh, Y., & Fuhrman, A. (1992). Substance abuse severity in female adolescents: Association between age at menarche and chronological age. *American Journal on Addictions,* 1, 217–221.

Miller, K. (1993, January 11). Attention deficit disorder affects adults, but some doctors question how widely. *The Wall Street Journal,* p. B1.

Morrison, J. R. (1980). Adult psychiatric disorders in parents of hyperactive children. *American Journal of Psychiatry,* 137, 825–827.

Morrison, J. R., & Stewart, M. A. (1973). The psychiatric status of the legal families of adopted hyperactive children. *Archives of General Psychiatry,* 28, 888–891.

Orvaschel, H. (1985). Psychiatric interviews suitable for use in research with children and adolescents. *Psychopharmacology Bulletin,* 21, 737–745.

Orvaschel, H., & Puig-Antich, J. (1987). *Schedule for Affective Disorders and Schizophrenia for School-Age Children—Epidemiologic* (4th version). Fort Lauderdale, FL: Nova University, Center for Psychological Study.

Patrick, K., Mueller, R., & Gualtieri, C. (1987). *Pharmacokinetics and actions of methylphenidate.* New York: Raven Press.

Pelham, W. E., Sturges, J., Hoza, J., Schmidt, C., Bjilsma, J. J., Milich, R., & Moorer, S. (1987). The effects of sustained release 20 and 10 mg Ritalin b.i.d. on cognitive and social behavior in children with attention deficit disorder. *Pediatrics,* 80, 491–501.

Pelham, W. E., Walker, J. L., Sturges, J., & Hoza, J. (1989). Comparative effects of methylphenidate on ADD girls and ADD boys. *Journal of the American Academy of Child and Adolescent Psychiatry,* 28, 773–776.

Rapoport, J. L., Quinn, P., Bradbard, G., Riddle, D., & Brooks, E. (1974). Imipramine and methylphenidate treatment of hyperactive boys: A double-blind comparison. *Archives of General Psychiatry,* 30, 789–793.

Rapport, M. D., DuPaul, G. J., & Kelly, K. L. (1989). Attention deficit hyperactivity disorder and methylphenidate: The relationship between gross body weight and drug response in children. *Psychopharmacology Bulletin,* 25, 285–290.

Rapport, M. D., Jones, J. T., DuPaul, G. J., Kelly, K. L., Gardner, M. J., Tucker, S. B., & Shea, M. S. (1987). Attention deficit disorder and methylphenidate: Group and single-subject analyses of dose effects on attention in clinic and classroom settings. *Journal of Clinical Child Psychology,* 16, 329–338.

Ratey, J., Greenberg, M., Bemporad, J., & Lindem, K. (1992). Unrecognized attention-deficit hyperactivity disorder in adults presenting for outpatient psychotherapy. *Journal of Child and Adolescent Psychopharmacology,* 2, 267–275.

Ratey, J., Greenberg, M., & Lindem, K. (1991). Combination of treatments for attention deficit disorders in adults. *Journal of Nervous and Mental Disease, 176,* 699–701.

Reynolds, C. R. (1984). Critical measurement issues in learning disabilities. *Journal of Special Education, 18,* 451–476.

Rutter, M. (1988). DSM-III-R: A postscript. In M. Rutter, A. H. Tuma, & I. S. Lann (Eds.), *Assessment and diagnosis in child psychopathology.* New York: Guilford Press.

Schachar, R., & Wachsmuth, R. (1990). Hyperactivity and parental psychopathology. *Journal of Child Psychology and Psychiatry, 31,* 381–392.

Sebrechts, M. M., Shaywitz, S. E., Shaywitz, B. A., Jatlow, P., Anderson, G. A., & Cohen, D. J. (1986). Components of attention, methylphenidate dosage, and blood levels in children with attention deficit disorder. *Pediatrics, 77,* 222–228.

Silver, L. B. (1992). Diagnosis of attention deficit-hyperactivity disorder in adult life. *Child and Adolescent Psychiatric Clinics of North America, 1,* 325–334.

Silver, L. B., & Brunstetter, R. W. (1986). Attention deficit disorder in adolescents. *Hospital and Community Psychiatry, 37,* 608–613.

Spencer, T., Biederman, J., Wilens, T., & Faraone, S. (1994). Is attention deficit hyperactivity disorder in adults a valid disorder? *Harvard Review of Psychiatry, 1,* 326–335.

Spencer, T., Wilens, T. E., Biederman, J., Faraone, S. V., Ablon, J. S., & Lapey, K. (1995). A double-blind crossover comparison of methylphenidate and placebo in adults with childhood-onset attention deficit hyperactivity. *Archives of General Psychiatry, 52,* 434–443.

Spitzer, R. L., Williams, J. B., Gibbon, M., & First, M. B. (1990). *Structured Clinical Interview for DSM-III-R, Non-Patient Edition* (Version 1.0). Washington, DC: American Psychiatric Press.

Steingard, R., Biederman, J., Spencer, T., Wilens, T., & Gonzalez, A. (1993). Comparison of clonidine response in the treatment of attention deficit hyperactivity disorder with and without comorbid tic disorders. *Journal of the American Academy of Child and Adolescent Psychiatry, 32,* 350–353.

Stewart, M. A., deBlois, C. S., & Cummings, C. (1980). Psychiatric disorder in the parents of hyperactive boys and those with conduct disorder. *Journal of Child Psychology and Psychiatry, 21,* 283–292.

Szatmari, P., Boyle, M., & Offord, D. (1993). Familial aggregation of emotional and behavioral problems of childhood in the general population. *American Journal of Psychiatry, 150,* 1398–1403.

Tarter, R., McBride, H., Buonpane, N., & Schneider, D. (1977). Differentiation of alcoholics. *Archives of General Psychiatry, 34,* 761–768.

Tesar, G. E., Rosenbaum, J. F., Biederman, J., Weilburg, J. B., Pollack, M. H., Gross, C. C., Falk, W. E., Gastfriend, D. R., Zusky, P. M., & Bouckoms, A. (1987). Orthostatic hypotension and antidepressant pharmacotherapy. *Psychopharmacology Bulletin, 23,* 182–186.

Thompson, W. D., & Weissman, M. M. (1981). Quantifying lifetime risk of psychiatric disorder. *Journal of Psychiatric Research, 16,* 113–126.

Thorley, G. (1984). Review of follow-up and follow-back studies of childhood hyperactivity. *Psychological Bulletin, 96,* 116–132.

Tsuang, M. T., Faraone, S. V., & Lyons, M. J. (1993). Recent advances in psychiatric genetics. In E. Costa, J. A. Silva, C. C. Nadelson, N. C. Andreasen,

& M. Sato (Eds.), *International review of psychiatry* (Vol. 1). Washington, DC: American Psychiatric Press.

Tsuang, M. T., Faraone, S. V., & Lyons, M. J. (1993). Identification of the phenotype in psychiatric genetics. *European Archives of Psychiatry and Clinical Neuroscience, 682,* 1–12.

Ward, M., Wender, P., & Reimherr, F. (1993). The Wender Utah Rating Scale: An aid in the retrospective diagnosis of childhood attention deficit disorder. *American Journal of Psychiatry, 150,* 885–890.

Wechsler, D. (1981). *Wechsler Adult Intelligence Scale – Revised.* New York: Psychological Corporation.

Weiss, G. (1985). Follow up studies on outcome of hyperactive children. *Psychopharmacology Bulletin, 21,* 169–177.

Weiss, G., & Hechtman, L. T. (1986). *Hyperactive children grown up.* New York: Guilford Press.

Wender, P. H., & Reimherr, F. W. (1990). Bupropion treatment of attention-deficit hyperactivity disorder in adults. *American Journal of Psychiatry, 147,* 1018–1020.

Wender, P. H., Reimherr, F. W., & Wood, D. R. (1981). Attention deficit disorder ("minimal brain dysfunction") in adults: A replication study of diagnosis and drug treatment. *Archives of General Psychiatry, 38,* 449–456.

Wender, P. H., Reimherr, F. W., Wood, D. R., & Ward, M. (1985a). A controlled study of methylphenidate in the treatment of attention deficit disorder, residual type, in adults. *American Journal of Psychiatry, 142,* 547–552.

Wender, P. H., Wood, D. R., & Reimherr, F. W. (1985b). Pharmacological treatment of attention deficit disorder, residual type (ADDRT, "minimal brain dysfunction," "hyperactivity") in adults. *Psychopharmacology Bulletin, 21,* 222–232.

Wender, P. H., Wood, D. R., Reimherr, F. W., & Ward, M. (1983). An open trial of pargyline in the treatment of attention deficit disorder, residual type. *Psychiatry Research, 9,* 329–336.

Wilens, T. E., & Biederman, J. (1992). The stimulants. *Psychiatric Clinics of North America, 15,* 191–222.

Wilens, T. E., Biederman, J., Geist, D. E., Steingard, R., & Spencer, T. (1993). Nortriptyline in the treatment of attention deficit hyperactivity disorder: A chart review of 58 cases. *Journal of the American Academy of Child and Adolescent Psychiatry, 32,* 343–349.

Wilens, T. E., Biederman, J., Spencer, T., & Prince, J. (1995). Pharmacotherapy of adult attention deficit/hyperactivity disorder: A review. *Journal of Clinical Psychopharmocology, 15,* 270–279.

Wilens, T. E., Spencer, T., & Biederman, J. (1994). Attention deficit disorder with substance abuse. In T. E. Brown (Ed.), *Subtypes of attention deficit disorders in children, adolescents, and adults.* Washington, DC: American Psychiatric Press.

Wood, D. R., Reimherr, F. W., Wender, P. H., & Johnson, G. E. (1976). Diagnosis and treatment of minimal brain dysfunction in adults: A preliminary report. *Archives of General Psychiatry, 33,* 1453–1460.

Wood, D., Wender, P. H., & Reimherr, F. W. (1983). The prevalence of attention deficit disorder, residual type, or minimal brain dysfunction, in a population of male alcoholic patients. *American Journal of Psychiatry, 140,* 95–98.

Zametkin, A. J., & Rapoport, J. L. (1987). Neurobiology of attention deficit disorder with hyperactivity: Where have we come in 50 years? *Journal of the American Academy of Child and Adolescent Psychiatry, 26,* 676–686.

Zametkin, A., Rapoport, J. L., Murphy, D. L., Linnoila, M., Karoum, F., Potter, W. Z., & Ismond, D. (1985). Treatment of hyperactive children with monoamine oxidase inhibitors: II. Plasma and urinary monoamine findings after treatment. *Archives of General Psychiatry, 42,* 969–973.

16

The Psychiatric Evaluation and Treatment of Premenstrual Dysphoric Disorder

CAROL BIRNBAUM
LEE COHEN

The term "premenstrual syndrome" (PMS) denotes the cyclic recurrence of a cluster of emotional and physical symptoms that are linked temporally to the menstrual cycle. When they are severe enough to interfere with social or occupational functioning, these symptoms characterize the emergence of a disorder, which has most recently been termed "premenstrual dysphoric disorder" (PMDD). Few unifying etiologic theories of PMS/PMDD exist that integrate factors such as preexisting psychopathology, changing female reproductive hormonal milieu, and psychosocial factors. All of these factors may contribute to the experience of premenstrual psychiatric symptoms, and investigators continue to refine both the methods used to diagnose psychiatric conditions occurring premenstrually and to develop specific treatments for them.

It is not surprising that some women who suffer premenstrual psychiatric symptoms are also described as "treatment dilemmas," given the ambiguity that exists with respect to PMS/PMDD nosology and pathophysiology. A treatment dilemma often arises from a clinician's inability to place the etiology of a given patient's complaints, which may vary from woman to woman with premenstrual psychiatric symptoms. Psychosocial as well as biologic factors must be considered. Comorbid psychiatric, gynecologic, endocrine, and neurologic disorders may exist, which may force the clinician into unfamiliar territory throughout the evaluation and treatment process.

This chapter focuses on the diagnosis and treatment of PMDD. The evolution of theories regarding pathophysiology of the disorder, and the extent to which this evolution may guide treatment decisions, are discussed. Current treatments for women suffering from PMDD are also reviewed.

PREVALENCE AND COMORBIDITY

PMS consists of a cluster of symptoms that occur in the luteal phase of the menstrual cycle, which is the phase between ovulation and the onset of menses. Early attempts to assess the lifetime prevalence of premenstrual complaints led to high and variable results, with estimates ranging from 20% to 90% (Hargrove & Abraham, 1982; Kashiwagi, McClure, & Wetzel, 1976; Kessel & Coppen, 1963). More recently, investigators have sought to refine the concept of PMS with hopes of gaining a clearer understanding of the underlying pathophysiology of the disorder and defining effective treatments. Some of the earliest efforts to define the diagnostic criteria for PMS more rigorously resulted in suggestions for prospective documentation and quantification of the level of symptom change: for example a 30% increase in symptom intensity from the follicular to the late luteal phase for at least 2 consecutive months (Hamilton, Parry, Alagna, Blumenthal, & Herz, 1984). These initial guidelines did not specify the precise symptoms to be measured. The revision to the third edition of the *Diagnostic and Statistical Manual of Mental Disorders* (DSM-III-R; American Psychiatric Association, 1987) included "late luteal phase dysphoric disorder" (LLPDD) in an appendix as a diagnosis proposed for further study. It remains in this category in DSM-IV (American Psychiatric Association, 1994), under the new title of PMDD. Criteria for PMDD include a list of symptoms (affective, behavioral, and somatic), require prospective daily self-ratings during at least two symptomatic cycles, and specify that symptoms must be present during the last week of the luteal phase and remit within a few days of the onset of the follicular phase. The diagnosis of PMDD requires the presence of an affective symptom, although somatic symptoms need not be present. Approximately 2.5–5.0% of reproductive-age women meet PMDD criteria (Mortola, 1992b). Other investigators have suggested research criteria requiring not only behavioral and affective symptoms, but evidence of identifiable dysfunction in social or economic performance as measured by given criteria (Mortola, Girton, Beck, & Yen, 1990).

Studies have shown that the prevalence of comorbid psychiatric disorders in women meeting criteria for PMDD is high, as is the lifetime prevalence of affective disorders. For example, Harrison, Endicott, Nee, Glick, and Rabkin (1989b) found the lifetime prevalence of major depression to be 70% in 86 women with prospectively confirmed LLPDD, and Stout,

Steege, Blazer, and George (1986) found the lifetime prevalence of Axis I disorders to be 81% among women presenting with a chief complaint of PMS. Pearlstein et al. found a 75% lifetime history of depressive disorders in 56 women with prospectively confirmed LLPDD. Rates of postpartum depression were also high in this study, with nearly one-third of all parous subjects reporting a history of postpartum depression. This rate is three times the reported rate for parous women in general. However, the incidence of Axis II disorders among Pearlstein et al.'s subjects was found to be approximately 10%, which is similar to rates estimated for the general population.

Fava et al. (1992) have discussed the difficulty in distinguishing between premenstrual disturbance as an exacerbation of an underlying condition and LLPDD/PMDD as a separate comorbid entity. More refined diagnostic assessment may help to clarify etiology and assess response to treatment. The DSM-IV criteria for PMDD allow for the presence of comorbid disorders, although most research criteria currently exclude women with comorbid psychopathology in an effort to eliminate heterogeneity of patients who are being evaluated (Mortola, 1992a). However, data gathered from a more homogeneous population may be less helpful to the general clinician, whose patients are likely to exhibit some comorbidity. Assessments of these patients must be geared toward identifying and treating any comorbid disorder prior to a prospective evaluation of residual premenstrual complaints.

ASSESSMENT OF PATIENTS WITH PREMENSTRUAL COMPLAINTS

Evaluation of patients presenting with premenstrual complaints should include several key elements. The assessment of reproductive endocrine function is important, as is the assessment of comorbid medical and psychiatric disorders. In addition, the prospective documentation of premenstrual symptoms will clarify symptom profile and pattern. The clinical practitioner should consider the following steps in making the diagnosis of PMDD.

Assessment of Reproductive Endocrine Status

PMDD is presumed to be a disorder of the luteal phase. Hormonal changes consistent with normal menstrual function require successful ovulation, which is the culmination of follicular maturation, extrusion of the ovum, and subsequent production of progesterone by the remaining corpus luteum. Most patients who take oral contraceptive pills have anovulatory cycles and thus are generally excluded from research in this area. Adequate evidence of ovulatory cycles may be obtained by a history of spontaneous menstrual cyclicity in a regular pattern. If there is any question about ovulation or a patient's cycles are irregular, a basal body temperature chart can be obtained, or a urine luteinizing hormone (LH) surge predictor kit can be used. Patients keeping a basal body temperature chart will find a rise in temperature just after ovulation; the LH surge detected by a simple urine dipstick occurs just prior to ovulation. There is little clinical role for obtaining serum gonadotropin or hormone levels, as these tests are quite costly.

Underlying Medical and Psychiatric Disorders

The past medical history should be taken, with careful attention to any syndromes that could mimic or suggest PMDD. For example, endometriosis can cause significant pelvic discomfort prior to and during menses; this and other physical causes of dysmenorrhea should be considered. Certain conditions (e.g., migraines, epilepsy, herpes, and allergies) can occur with a premenstrual pattern and may cause subsequent behavioral or affective symptoms that confuse the patient and the practitioner. A careful physical exam should be performed by an internist or gynecologist with this differential diagnosis in mind.

The past psychiatric history should include a careful review of responses to past pregnancies. Patients with a history of postpartum depression appear more likely to develop subsequent PMDD (Pearlstein et al., 1990). The presence of past psychiatric disorder should be reviewed carefully, as complaints of premenstrual symptoms may derive more from an exacerbation or premenstrual recrudescence of an Axis I disorder such as a mood or anxiety disorder than from circumscribed PMDD. A careful mental status exam, including questions regarding current drug or alcohol use, should be obtained twice—once in the follicular phase and once in the luteal phase—in order to maximize the likelihood of diagnosis of an Axis I disorder. Assessment across the menstrual cycle also facilitates the most accurate determination of change in severity of symptoms over time. Patients who appear quite well when initially evaluated in the follicular phase are often relieved when asked to return prior to their expected period, when their symptoms will be manifested. Axis I disorders should be treated until a patient is symptom-free in the follicular phase before the clinician and patient continue the prospective search for either comorbid PMDD or premenstrual worsening of an underlying disorder.

Prospective Daily Rating Scales

Once it is determined that the patient is not suffering from a confounding medical or psychiatric disorder (or once that disorder has been adequately treated and complaints of luteal phase symptoms persist), prospective daily rating scales should be obtained over two consecutive cycles. This allows accurate assessment of symptoms suffered, the timing of such symptoms, and level of symptom severity. Rubinow, Roy-Byrne, Hoban, Gold, and Post (1984) reported that fewer than 50% of women who present with a history of PMDD show a cycle-dependent pattern when prospective assessments are obtained. This illustrates the importance of prospective, longitudinal ratings when making the diagnosis.

The most commonly used and reliable form for prospective assessment of premenstrual symptoms is the Calendar of Premenstrual Experiences (see Figure 16.1). This instrument includes a 4-point Likert scale for each of the 10 most commonly reported physical symptoms and the 12 most commonly reported behavioral symptoms rated daily throughout the menstrual cycle (Mortola et al., 1990). Other frequently used assessments assign symptoms into clusters of most frequently reported symptoms of PMDD. Researchers are currently struggling to reach consensus regarding a single, valid, reliable daily rating instrument that will assist in interstudy comparisons (Mortola, 1992a).

For the clinician, prospective documentation can help to build a treatment alliance. Patients often value the experience of symptom charting, as it represents a tangible and careful record of their symptoms. Persistent follicular symptoms in the absence of clear worsening during the luteal phase should convince clinician and patient that PMDD is the not the primary problem, and that other causes of the discomfort need to be explored. A flowchart for the process of evaluating premenstrual symptoms is presented in Figure 16.2.

ETIOLOGY

PMDD and the Menstrual Cycle

Although precise dysregulation in the menstrual cycle associated with PMDD has yet to be clarified, it has been suggested that women with PMDD who experience premature menopause by either surgical or medical means frequently experience a dramatic resolution in their symptoms (Casper & Hearn, 1990; Hammarback & Backstrom, 1988; Helvacioglu, Yeoman, Hazelton, & Aksel, 1993; Mortola, Girton, & Fischer, 1991; Muse, Cetel, Futterman, & Yen, 1984; Shangold, 1993). It has also been noted that gonadal steroids have a major impact on central nervous system (CNS) neuronal modulation (Akwa et al., 1991; Biegon, Bercovitz, & Samuel, 1980; Biegon & McEwen, 1982; McEwen, 1988; McEwen & Parsons, 1982). A precise understanding of premenstrual symptoms must begin with an understanding of the hormonal milieu that characterizes the menstrual cycle.

Major hormonal shifts across the menstrual cycle occur during two phases: follicular and luteal. The follicular phase is characterized by ovarian follicular growth and maturation. The events of this phase, such as endometrial proliferation, are primarily responses to increasing levels of estrogen produced by a dominant follicle in response to follicle-stimulating hormone (FSH) released from the pituitary gland. The increased levels

CALENDAR OF PREMENSTRUAL EXPERIENCES

Name _____ Month/Year _____ Age _____ Unit #_____

Begin your calendar on the first day of your menstrual cycle. Enter the calendar date below the cycle day. Day 1 is your first day of bleeding. Shade the box above the cycle day if you have bleeding. ■ Put an X for spotting. ☒

If more than one symptom is listed in a category (i.e., nausea, diarrhea, constipation), you do not need to experience all of these. Rate the most disturbing symptoms on the 1–3 scale.

Weight: Weigh yourself before breakfast. Record weight in the box below date.
Symptoms: Indicate the severity of your symptoms by using the scale below. Rate each symptom at about the same time each evening.

0 = **None** (symptom not present)   2 = **Moderate** (interferes with normal activities)
1 = **Mild** (noticeable but not troublesome) 3 = **Severe** (intolerable, unable to perform normal activities)

Other symptoms: If there are other symptoms you experience, list and indicate severity.
Medications: List any medications taken. Put an X on the corresponding day(s).

	1	2	3	4	5	6	7	8	9	10	11	12	13	14	15	16	17	18	19	20	21	22	23	24	25	26	27	28	29	30	31	32	33	34	35	36	37	38	39	40
Bleeding																																								
Cycle day																																								
Date																																								
Weight																																								
SYMPTOMS																																								
Acne																																								
Bloatedness																																								
Breast tenderness																																								
Dizziness																																								
Fatigue																																								
Headache																																								
Hot flashes																																								
Nausea, diarrhea, constipation																																								
Palpitations																																								
Swelling (hands, ankles, breasts)																																								
Angry outbursts, arguments, violent tendencies																																								
Anxiety, tension, nervousness																																								
Confusion, difficulty concentrating																																								
Crying easily																																								
Depression																																								
Food cravings (sweets, salts)																																								
Forgetfulness																																								
Irritability																																								
Increased appetites																																								
Mood swings																																								
Overly sensitive																																								
Wish to be alone																																								
Other symptoms 1. _____ 2. _____																																								
Medications 1. _____ 2. _____																																								

FIGURE 16.1. Calendar of Premenstrual Experiences. Copyright 1985 by the University of California, San Diego; Department of Reproductive Medicine, H-813; Division of Reproductive Endocrinology. Reprinted by permission.

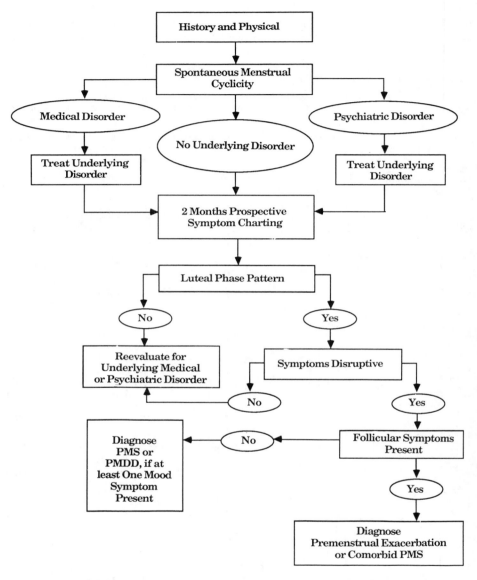

FIGURE 16.2. Flowchart for the evaluation of premenstrual symptoms.

of estrogen are thought to be the proximate stimulus for the sharp surge in pituitary release of both LH and FSH that heralds ovulation. LH stimulates follicular progesterone synthesis, which is in turn involved in the synthesis of enzymes that directly thin the follicle wall, causing extrusion of the ovum.

Following ovulation, the follicle involutes and becomes filled with luteal cells, which produce large amounts of both progesterone and estrogen. This begins the luteal phase, dominated by the effects of increased circulating progesterone. The estrogen-primed endometrium develops glycogen deposits and its glands become tortuous, preparing the uterus for a possible conceptus. Breast tenderness may also occur at this time and is thought to result from stimulation of glandular tissue by both progesterone and estrogen. The high levels of circulating progesterone and estrogen are sensed by the hypothalamus, leading to a decrease of gonadotropin-releasing hormone (GnRH) and subsequent gonadotropin production. The corpus luteum then degenerates, causing a sharp decrease in circulating estrogen and progesterone. This then causes a selective increase in FSH release, thus initiating a new wave of follicle maturation. The secretory endometrium at the same time develops hemorrhagic and degenerative changes, initiating the menstrual discharge. Figure 16.3 charts the shifts in LH, FSH, progesterone, and estrogen (estradiol) across the menstrual cycle.

Hormone Levels and PMDD

The earliest theories regarding the etiology of PMDD suggested that affected women have abnormal levels of gonadal steroids. One of the more popular of these theories was the proposal by Dalton (1984) that women with PMDD suffer from a deficiency in luteal phase progesterone. Although never confirmed in prospective scientific studies, this theory guided clinical management of PMDD in many women. These patients were treated largely with progesterone suppositories—a treatment that can be both costly and cumbersome. Subsequent prospective, double-blind studies of progesterone have noted progesterone to be no more effective than placebo in the management of PMDD (Freeman, Rickels, Sondheimer, & Polansky, 1990; Rapkin, Chang, & Reading, 1987; van der Meer, Benedek-Jaszmann, & van Loenen, 1983).

The importance of ovarian steroids in the pathophysiology of PMDD was first demonstrated by Muse et al. (1984), who administered a GnRH agonist to women with PMDD, causing cessation of ovarian stimulation and a dramatic reduction in premenstrual symptoms. Despite this significant finding, no differences in level of ovarian steroids, estrogen-to-progesterone ratio, gonadotropins, or ovarian steroid-binding globulin have been consistently detected between subjects and controls (Rubinow et al., 1986). Although some differences in LH pulsatility have been demonstrated in isolated studies, other studies demonstrate no difference in this area (Rubinow, 1992). There appears to be no consistent evidence to support earlier hypotheses that PMDD is associated with abnormal levels of circulating ovarian steroids or abnormal gonadotropin release. Women who manifest symptoms of PMDD may be more vulnerable or predisposed to an exaggerated response to normal ovarian steroid fluctuations. This is further substantiated by the finding that women with PMDD may be nearly

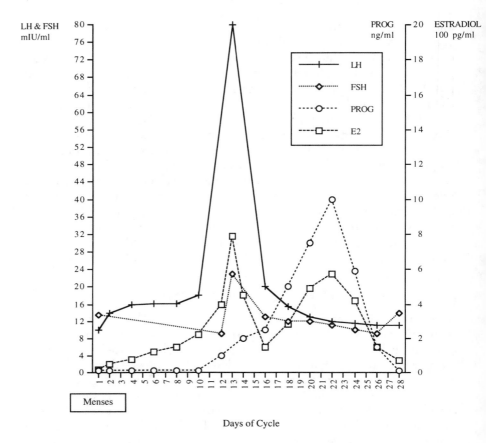

FIGURE 16.3. Hormonal shifts across the menstrual cycle.

three times as likely to develop postpartum depression as women in the general population. Both genetic and environmental origins for this predisposition have been postulated, leading some investigators to propose a multifactorial etiology, which may account for the heterogeneous presentation of the syndrome.

The nonreproductive neuroendocrine markers that have been considered in depression have also been examined in PMDD. The cortisol secretory pattern in symptomatic women appears to be the same as in asymptomatic controls (Roy-Byrne, Rubinow, Gwirtsman, Hoban, & Grover, 1986). Thyroid-stimulating hormone response to thyrotropin-releasing hormone in symptomatic women has been found to be similar to that in unaffected women in most studies; however, one study did find this response to be abnormal in symptomatic women (Rubinow et al., 1986). Another study found serum circadian melatonin profiles in PMDD women to be similar to those in depressed individuals; however, some of the women in the PMDD group also met criteria for major depression, leaving these results in question (Parry et al., 1990). Thus, results from studies of reproductive and nonreproductive hormone levels in patients with PMDD have yet to reveal consistent patterns of endocrine dysregulation.

Environmental Factors

The primary environmental factors investigated as predisposing variables for PMDD have been stress and diet. Early studies that found an association between stressful life events and PMDD have been criticized for using retrospective assessments of stressful life events (Mortola, 1992a).

A later, prospective study of women with disabling PMDD found that amount of stress experienced during a given menstrual cycle did not predict the severity of PMDD symptoms (Beck, Gevirtz, & Mortola, 1990). Dietary factors have also long been postulated as contributing to PMDD symptoms. Elimination of sweet and salty foods is frequently recommended to women suffering from PMDD, although scientific evidence to support this recommendation is sparse. Chocolate cravings have been associated with PMDD, although there has been no evidence to suggest chocolate consumption as a causal agent. In fact, one study reported that consuming a carbohydrate-rich, protein-poor evening meal during the late luteal phase improved many premenstrual mood symptoms in women with PMDD (Wurtman, Brzezinski, Wurtman, & Laferrere, 1989). The investigators suggest that consumption of carbohydrates in the absence of protein causes an insulin-driven increase in availability of the serotonin precursor tryptophan to the brain, thus ultimately enhancing serotonin levels. This is consistent with the hypothesis that serotonergic dysregulation is present in women with PMDD.

Although nutritional supplementation has been widely used as a treatment for PMDD, there has been no consistent documentation of either deficiency or excess of vitamins or minerals in affected patients as compared with controls. Studies have suggested symptom relief from treatment with a variety of substances, including vitamins A, B_6, and E; evening primrose oil; and the minerals zinc, magnesium, and calcium. However, many of these studies have been criticized for methodologic flaws, including lack of rigorous subject selection and of valid and reliable prospective rating scales to measure symptom improvement. In addition, the doses of vitamins and minerals administered in these studies often dramatically exceed recommended daily allowances for these substances. Chuong and Dawson (1992) suggest that responses to such doses may represent pharmacologic response rather than a correction of a deficiency state. They suggest that the bioavailability of vitamins and minerals in the CNS, crucial to CNS neuronal modulation, may change during the luteal phase in patients with PMDD and yet may not be reflected by measurement of peripheral levels of these substances.

Hormones and Neurotransmission

A more recent addition to the existing etiologic hypotheses for PMDD is the suggestion that ovarian sex steroid flux causes a dysregulation in central neurotransmission in susceptible individuals. Estrogen, progesterone, and their metabolites are known to alter function in the opioidergic, noradrenergic, serotonergic, and gamma-aminobutyric acid-ergic (GABA-ergic) systems. Their effects are thought to occur via three separate mechanisms: the classic genomic interaction leading to altered protein production; a direct effect on monoamine turnover and metabolism; and the direct effect of the steroid or its metabolite on the nerve cell membrane.

Progesterone metabolites are known to have both stimulatory and inhibiting effects on GABA receptors in laboratory mice (McEwen, 1988; McEwen & Parsons, 1982). Most recently, interest has turned to the effects of estrogen and progesterone on the serotonergic system, as patients have responded dramatically to the selective serotonin reuptake inhibitor (SSRI) fluoxetine as a treatment for PMDD symptoms (Biegon et al., 1980; Biegon & McEwen, 1982). Diminished whole-blood serotonin and platelet serotonin uptake have been found in the luteal phase of women with PMDD (Rapkin, 1992). Dysregulation of these CNS modulators is also implicated in the development of mood and anxiety disorders, both of which have significant symptoms in common with PMDD (Chopin & Briley, 1987; Delgado et al., 1990). Researchers are thus faced with the task of identifying subgroups of women who may be vulnerable to changes in the female reproductive hormonal milieu, and consequently may develop mood and anxiety symptoms at these vulnerable points. Still, much of the evidence supporting the hypothesis that serotonin dysregulation is associated with PMDD has not been consistently replicated, and more work is required to delineate the effects of ovarian sex steroids on this and other central neurotransmitter pathways.

Could PMDD Represent an Autonomous Mood Disorder?

Over the years, one of the most strongly supported premises regarding the pathophysiology of PMDD has been that symptoms are related to luteal phase estrogen and progesterone flux, as luteal changes in ovarian steroid levels correspond temporally to symptom manifestation. This premise was called into question by a study by Schmidt et al. (1991). In this study, women with prospectively confirmed PMDD experienced a "truncated" luteal phase because of the administration of the antiprogesterone mifepristone (RU 486). Seven days after their LH surge, the subjects were randomly administered either placebo or RU 486, which blocks progesterone receptors and subsequently causes the onset of menses within 48–72 hours. Subjects who received mifepristone also received either human chorionic gonadotropin (hCG) or placebo. Subjects receiving hCG experienced a withdrawal bleed at 48–72 hours; however, the hCG has a stimulatory effect on the corpus luteum, maintaining luteal phase progesterone levels. These patients experienced a second menses approximately 9 days later with the involution of the corpus luteum. The subjects who received RU 486 and then placebo entered the follicular phase at the time of the menses induced by RU 486.

The startling finding of this study was that these women with abbreviated luteal phases experienced their characteristic premenstrual mood state *after* the menses induced by RU 486, whereas they had peripheral endocrine profiles consistent with the follicular phase. The authors concluded that these results could support two different conclusions: Either PMDD symptoms result from hormonal events that occur before the late luteal phase, or PMDD represents an autonomous, cyclic disorder that is linked to the menstrual cycle but can become dissociated from it (Schmidt et al., 1991).

TREATMENT ISSUES

Although the etiology of PMDD remains unclear, available treatments are primarily aimed at altering potential dysregulation of hormonal factors within the menstrual cycle, dysregulation of central neurotransmission, or psychosocial and nutritional factors. Over the years, numerous treatments for PMDD have been suggested; these include dietary changes, exercise, vitamin supplementation, diuretics, hormones, and medical and surgical oophrectomy, as well as numerous psychotropic agents. Few of these have been proven effective in rigorous prospective studies. More stringent diagnostic criteria and the development of reliable prospective daily rating scales will refine the process by which a given intervention is deemed effective. The initial choice of treatment modality should be based on a careful assessment of the symptom profile and symptom severity, with an attempt to begin with the least invasive procedures available. Table 16.1 outlines current treatments for PMDD; these are discussed in more detail below.

Nonmedical Treatments

If the patient is highly motivated and symptoms are mild or of brief duration, a course of psychoeducation (in either an individual or a group format) may be appropriate. Pearlstein et al. (1992) demonstrated that women randomized to a psychoeducational group had greater symptom relief than those who received no treatment. Group sessions focused on information dissemination to the subjects and their family members, as well as prescription of lifestyle changes, including frequent small meals to prevent hypoglycemia and an enhanced exercise regimen during the luteal phase.

Preliminary studies suggest that cognitive-behavioral therapy may also be helpful in treating motivated patients with premenstrual symptoms,

TABLE 16.1 Current Treatments for Premenstrual Symptoms

Treatment	Appropriate for:	When to use:
Psychoeducation Cognitive-behavioral therapy Lifestyle changes	Patients with mild to moderate symptoms	• Initial treatment • Throughout the cycle
Calcium (1000 mg/day) Magnesium (360 mg/day)	Patients with mild to moderate symptoms	• Initial treatment • Luteal phase
Diuretics	Patients with severe bloating only	• After trying sodium restriction • Luteal phase
Bromocriptine	Patients with severe mastalgia only	• After trying a support bra, xanthine restriction • Luteal phase
Nonsteroidal anti-inflammatory drugs	Patients with arthralgias, myalgias, headache	• When symptomatic • Luteal phase

Anxiolytics
  Benzodiazepines
  Buspirone
	Patients with prominent premenstrual anxiety, panic, or irritability	• Following less invasive treatment failure, or as initial treatment if symptoms are severe
		• Luteal phase

Antidepressants
  Selective serotonin reuptake
    inhibitors
  Tricyclic antidepressants
	Patients with a prominent premenstrual mood disturbance	• Following less invasive treatment failure, or as initial treatment if symptoms are severe
		• Throughout cycle

Gonadotropin-releasing hormone analogues Danazol	Patients with severe, treatment-refractory symptoms	• Following less invasive treatment • May be used to induce amenorrhea for a maximum of 6 months unless low-dose hormones are "added back"

either alone or in conjunction with pharmacotherapy. One case report described a significant decrease in premenstrual distress and sick leave each month in a woman treated with a multicomponent behavioral approach, which included relaxation training, stress inoculation, assertiveness training, marital therapy, and prescribed exercise (Kuczmierczyk, 1989). This patient's treatment gains were maintained at a 9-month follow-up visit. The relaxation response technique was shown to significantly reduce both physical and emotional premenstrual symptoms over a 5-month period in a study that randomly assigned 46 women to one of three groups: a symptom-charting group, a reading group, and a relaxation response group (Goodale, Domar, & Benson, 1990). Another study compared cognitive-behavioral therapy with dydrogesterone therapy and a control treatment consisting of relaxation instructions (Morse, Dennerstein, Farrell, & Varnavides, 1991). The hormone treatment and relaxation groups showed initial rapid improvement, but this diminished after 2 months; there was also marked attrition in the control group. The cognitive-behavioral therapy group achieved significant symptom reduction in the first month and maintained benefits at follow-up 3 months later. Standardized therapy techniques, as well as uniform diagnostic criteria and prospective daily rating scales, are needed to fully assess the efficacy of cognitive-behavioral therapy for PMDD. Prospective comparisons of cognitive-behavioral therapy and psychotropic drug treatment alone and in combination have yet to be described.

The specific effects of dietary modifications on PMDD symptoms have not been well studied, although anecdotal reports from women who have implemented these modifications indicate some symptom improvement. The usual recommendations include increasing complex carbohydrates, decreasing intake of refined sugar, and consuming frequent small meals to avoid the effects of fasting. A decrease in salt consumption is recommended to avoid possible salt-related fluid retention. Avoidance of caffeine and chocolate is suggested and is thought to be helpful in diminishing breast tenderness. Although women with PMDD have been shown to consume more of these two xanthine-containing substances than unaffected women, these substances have not been proven to play a causative role in the mood and anxiety symptoms of PMDD. As was shown by Wurtman et al. (1989), the increased consumption of chocolate and carbohydrates in general may represent a form of self-medication of mood symptoms. However, this is best attempted through the consumption of slow-burning, low-fat complex carbohydrates taken without protein, to enhance the availability of brain tryptophan. Suggested foods include a baked potato or popped corn without butter, whole-wheat crackers, or pasta salad with a low-fat dressing.

There are also no prospective assessments of exercise as a treatment for PMDD. However, aerobic exercise may improve mood; the mechanism for this response is believed to be elevated endorphin levels (Prior & Vigna, 1987). A program of moderate, regular aerobic exercise may therefore be helpful in treating mood-related symptoms and will certainly create overall health benefits. Women who already exercise on a regular basis should be instructed to increase their activity throughout the luteal phase of their cycles.

Alterations in circadian rhythm have also been implicated in PMDD. One pilot study found that sleep deprivation, which has been shown to reduce symptoms of major depression, reduced premenstrual symptoms in 8 of 10 women with PMDD (Parry & Wehr, 1987). Another pilot study found a reduction in luteal phase depressive symptoms of six women treated with evening light therapy in the evenings (Parry et al., 1989). However, a more recent crossover study by the same investigators found bright light to be no more efficacious than placebo (Parry et al., 1993). Although additional study of these noninvasive and inexpensive treatments is required, the data suggest that they may be helpful in some cases.

Vitamins and Minerals

Optivite is a high-potency multiple vitamin preparation marketed for PMDD that has yielded beneficial results in three placebo-controlled trials. However, this preparation contains potentially unsafe levels of both vitamin B_6 and vitamin A (Johnson, 1992). Calcium and magnesium supplements have both been shown to be useful in reducing PMDD symptoms in well-designed clinical trials, although there is less scientific support for other supplements discussed above, including vitamin B_6 (Facchinetti et al., 1991; Thys-Jacobs et al., 1989). In cases of mild to moderate premenstrual symptoms, a trial of calcium (1000 mg/day) and magnesium (360 mg/day) along with dietary and exercise changes may be appropriate, prior to pursuing a more aggressive form of treatment.

Treatment of Specific Physical Symptoms

The most common physical complaints of PMDD include bloating, weight gain, and swelling. For most women these symptoms are disconcerting, but do not require treatment with prescription diuretics. A low-salt diet is frequently the initial recommendation. In the above-mentioned studies of calcium and magnesium, fluid retention symptoms improved, so these supplements are also recommended. If these recommendations fail and significant weight gain is documented during the luteal phase for more than one cycle, diuretic therapy may be initiated. Spironolactone is a reasonable choice, as it is a low-potency, potassium-sparing agent that is thought to be less likely to produce diuretic dependence or rebound cyclic edema on discontinuation than the thiazides (Johnson, 1992). When dramatic cyclic edema is uncorrelated with the menstrual cycle, the patient should be referred to an internist for the evaluation of idiopathic cyclic edema, a renal disorder that can be aggravated by improper use of diuretics.

Mastalgia, or painful breast tenderness, is a frequent somatic complaint in PMDD. Initial management should include the use of a support bra throughout the day. Anecdotal evidence also suggests that elimination of caffeine from the diet can be helpful and may be suggested. When mastalgia is severe and does not respond to these measures, bromocriptine has been shown to significantly reduce premenstrual breast tenderness; however, it may cause significant side effects, including nausea and constipation

(Blichert-Toft, Andersen, Henriksen, & Mygind, 1979; Johnson, 1992). A starting dose of 2.5 mg/day should be employed, and this should be titrated according to symptom severity and side effect tolerance.

Hormonal Treatments

For many years a popular treatment for PMDD was progesterone by vaginal suppository, usually given in doses of 200–400 mg/day during the luteal phase. Dennerstein, Spencer-Gardner, and Gotts (1985) found that oral micronized progesterone did produce a greater improvement in symptoms than placebo; however, its use is not currently approved by the Food and Drug Administration for any indication, and it is not currently marketed in the United States. Hellberg, Claesson, and Nilsson (1991) reported that medroxyprogesterone acetate was superior to placebo in relieving 10 typical PMDD symptoms, although the study has been criticized for the lack of a double-blind design. As noted earlier, several recent double-blind, placebo-controlled studies indicate that progesterone provides no better relief for PMDD symptoms than placebo (Freeman et al., 1990; Rapkin et al., 1987; van der Meer et al., 1983). Given the many treatment alternatives to both natural progesterone and progestin therapy, and the lack of solid scientific evidence suggesting their efficacy, these agents are best not used in the treatment of PMDD.

A small number of studies have suggested the potential benefit of chronic administration of estradiol for PMDD, based on the hypothesis that symptoms may be related to estrogen withdrawal in the late luteal phase (Magos, Brincat, & Studd, 1986; Watson, Studd, Savvas, & Baber, 1990; Watson, Studd, Savvas, Garnett, & Baber, 1989). These studies have generally found the chronic administration of estrogen to be more effective than placebo in the treatment of premenstrual symptoms; however, long-term treatment is complicated by PMDD-like side effects from oral progestins, which are required to prevent endometrial hyperplasia in patients who are prescribed estrogens. In addition, the long-term effects of chronic estradiol administration are not known. Increased risks for uterine cancer, breast cancer, and thromboembolic events are concerns that require exploration. Further investigation of estradiol therapy is required before this treatment can be recommended.

Oral contraceptive pills have also been tried as a potential treatment of PMDD, based on the principle that they replace endogenous menstrual cyclicity with constant levels of estrogen and progestin throughout the cycle. Oral contraceptives do seem to improve symptoms of dysmenorrhea or painful menses, but PMDD symptoms or pretreatment depression are rarely improved and can occasionally even be precipitated or made worse by use of these agents (Muse, 1992). However, most placebo-controlled studies of oral contraceptive pills in PMDD did not utilize the lower-dose pills currently available; therefore, no definitive judgment can be made about their efficacy (Morris & Udry, 1972; Silbergeld, Brast, &

Noble, 1971). This treatment should be reserved for women whose chief complaint is dysmenorrhea, and an alternative form of contraception should be utilized in women with significant premenstrual symptoms.

Psychotropic Agents

Patients with the chief complaint of PMDD may actually suffer from premenstrual worsening of depression or anxiety disorder (Glick, Harrison, Endicott, McGrath, & Quitkin, 1991; Kaspi, Otto, Pollack, Eppinger, & Rosenbaum, 1994; McMillan & Pihl, 1987; Yonkers & White, 1992). When this is the case, the treatment should be focused on the underlying condition. Women with a history of an anxiety disorder who experience premenstrual worsening of anxiety may be treated by increasing a benzodiazepine dosage or adding a benzodiazepine to the existing treatment for the last 10–14 days of the menstrual cycle. Cognitive-behavioral therapy may also be added in an effort to contain premenstrual breakthrough of symptoms. When symptoms of mania or of complex partial seizures appear to break through previously adequate treatment during the last few days of the menstrual cycle, the clinician may aim to increase levels of the mood-stabilizing agent or anticonvulsant to prevent this breakthrough. The same holds true for premenstrual worsening or recrudescence of major depression; the antidepressant dosage should be increased or augmented, as would normally be done in a case of treatment-resistant depression. The question of augmentation for only a part of the cycle is complicated by the suggestion from the study by Schmidt et al. (1991) referred to earlier—namely, that the provocative event of the hormone cycle triggering premenstrual symptoms may occur much earlier in the cycle than was previously believed. Therefore, dose increase or augmentation should probably be continuous throughout the cycle.

Only two psychotropic agents have demonstrated efficacy in double-blind studies of women with PMDD. Two controlled studies that found the high-potency benzodiazepine alprazolam to be beneficial (Harrison, Endicott, & Nee, 1990; Smith, Rinehart, Ruddock, & Schiff, 1987) have been countered by two controlled studies that found this agent no more effective than placebo (Dennerstein, Morse, Burrows, Brown, & Smith, 1986; Schmidt, Grover, & Rubinow, 1993). In one study in which alprazolam was found to be more effective than placebo (Harrison et al., 1990), a substantially higher dose (2.25 mg) was utilized than the average dose tolerated by subjects in Schmidt et al.'s (1993) study (1.4 mg), in which the drug was no more effective than placebo. The study conducted by Harrison et al. also included a greater percentage of subjects with a history of affective disorder. The discrepancy in results between these studies suggests the possible existence of a subgroup of women with PMDD who have an anxiety or depressive diathesis and may respond to and tolerate greater doses of alprazolam. However, inconsistencies in protocol and analysis of data prevent this conclusion from being firmly drawn. The obvious advantage to treatment with alprazolam is that it can be given only during the symptomatic phase, regardless of which point in the menstrual cycle any actual CNS dysregulation may occur, because of its direct anxiolytic properties. The major side effect reported was drowsiness, and in one sample withdrawal anxiety was experienced in 13% of treated subjects (Harrison et al., 1990; Smith et al., 1987). Therefore, the clinician should be alert for symptoms of withdrawal or dependence, and an adequate taper should be administered each month.

The second treatment that has been proven efficacious by prospective, double-blind studies is the SSRI fluoxetine (Stone, Pearlstein, & Brown, 1991; Wood, Mortola, Chan, Moossazadeh, & Yen, 1992; Steiner et al., 1995). Fluoxetine has been found to dramatically reduce the affective and behavioral symptoms of PMDD, with less definitive improvement in somatic symptoms. In one study, 20 women who were established prospectively to have PMDD and did not respond to a placebo wash-in were subsequently randomized to receive either 20 mg/day of fluoxetine or a placebo for two consecutive menstrual cycles. Nine of the 10 subjects receiving fluoxetine had a significant decrease in symptoms, compared to only 2 out of 10 in the placebo group. Some side effects (e.g., nausea, change in appetite, sexual dysfunction, headache, and dizziness) were reported, although all responders elected to continue on fluoxetine following the completion of the study (Stone et al., 1991).

Other studies examining serotonergic agents have also shown promising results. In one small study, five women who had severe premenstrual irritability and sadness but did not meet criteria for depression were treated with the serotonergic tricyclic antidepressant clomipramine, administered daily for five consecutive menstrual cycles. All placebo responders were screened out, and then placebo nonresponders were treated with a dose of 25–50 mg/day, which is lower than the doses normally prescribed for major depression. All five women reported a dramatic decrease in symptoms, although they also reported the anticholinergic side effects typically seen with this agent at higher doses (Eriksson et al., 1990). Studies examining the newer SSRIs, sertraline and paroxetine, are currently in progress.

A minority of patients are unable to tolerate treatment with an SSRI because of the side effects of headache, jitteriness, or nausea. When a decrease in dose is not effective in eliminating this problem, a tricyclic antidepressant may offer an effective alternative. In an open pilot study of women who did not respond to placebo or another medication, 8 out of 11 subjects who met DSM-III-R criteria for LLPDD had a good therapeutic response to a variable dose of nortriptyline (Harrison, Endicott, & Nee, 1989a). It has been our experience that women with premenstrual anxiety and irritable bowel syndrome respond better to tricyclic antidepressants than to other agents, although further research is needed in this area.

Induced Menopause

The most definitive treatment for PMDD involves stopping menses. This can be done medically with the use of a GnRH agonist, usually administered intranasally or in depot form (Hammarback & Backstrom, 1988; Helvacioglu et al., 1993; Mortola et al., 1991). Danazol has also been used successfully to suppress ovulation in PMDD treatment, but its high rate of side effects makes it a less desirable choice. The obvious drawback of ovarian suppression is that it exposes women to the known risks of menopause, such as osteoporosis and coronary artery disease. The agents themselves are also quite costly.

In patients with severe PMDD that has proven refractory to any of the treatments suggested above, a temporary suppression of ovarian function will have initial diagnostic value, as persistent symptoms in the absence of ovarian steroid function must preclude a diagnosis of PMDD. However, therapeutic ovarian suppression can only be maintained for a 6-month course because of the risk of osteoporosis, and patients should be counseled regarding calcium supplementation and appropriate exercise to minimize bone loss. One study has provided preliminary evidence that combining the GnRH agonist with postmenopausal doses of estrogen and progestin "added back" will relieve menopausal symptoms and prevent bone loss while maintaining efficacy in the treatment of PMDD (Mortola et al., 1991).

Pharmacologic Management Considerations

Patients considering pharmacologic treatment for PMDD should be informed that none of the drugs currently utilized have been approved by the Food and Drug Administration for this use (Johnson, 1992). A physician prescribing a pharmacologic treatment should also always establish that a patient is using a reliable form of contraception. If conception is desired, the physician and patient should discuss the potential teratogenic and neurobehavioral sequelae of *in utero* exposure to the given agent, and the potential risks and benefits of treatment during early conception should be outlined before contraception is eliminated. In addition, since most women require long-term treatment, both side effect profile and cost should be thoughtfully considered. Once a successful program has been established, the frequency of follow-up depends on the patient's needs. She should be counseled to expect occasional roughening of symptoms, and daily rating scales should be reinstituted whenever a treatment regimen requires alteration.

FUTURE DIRECTIONS

The constant struggle to develop more sophisticated models for the etiology of PMDD has brought us closer to understanding the multifactorial nature of the occurrence of psychiatric disorders. Future research is thus being directed toward uncovering the complex interactions among genetic predisposition toward mood and anxiety disorders, the potential triggering events of the ovulatory cycle, and the environmental factors present in women with this syndrome. Afflicted women may differ from one another as to which biologic or psychosocial factors contain the primary dysregulation. These differences need to be explored and may reveal differences in response to treatment as well. The risks for recurrent psychopathology throughout the female reproductive life cycle, including illness related to pregnancy and the postpartum as well as recurrence at the time of menopause, should also be investigated through rigorous longitudinal studies; these should further clarify the nature of the complex interrelationship between mood and female reproductive hormonal flux.

REFERENCES

Akwa, Y., Young, J., Kabbadj, K., Sancho, M. J., Zucman, D., Vourc'h, C., Jung-Testas, I., Hu, Z. Y., Le Goascogne, C., & Jo, D. H. (1991). Neurosteroids: Biosynthesis, metabolism and function of pregnenolone and dehydroepiandrosterone in the brain. *Journal of Steroid Biochemisty and Molecular Biology*, 40(1–3), 71–81.

American Psychiatric Association. (1987). *Diagnostic and statistical manual of mental disorders* (3rd ed., rev.). Washington, DC: Author.

American Psychiatric Association. (1994). *Diagnostic and statistical manual of mental disorders* (4th ed.). Washington, DC: Author.

Beck, L. E., Gevirtz, R., & Mortola, J. F. (1990). The predictive role of psychosocial stress on symptom severity in premenstrual syndrome. *Psychosomatic Medicine*, 52(5), 536–543.

Biegon, A., Bercovitz, H., & Samuel, D. (1980). Serotonin receptor concentration during estrous cycle of the rat. *Brain Research*, 187, 221–225.

Biegon, A., & McEwen, B. (1982). Modulation by estradiol of serotonin receptors in brain. *Journal of Neuroscience*, 2, 199–205.

Blichert-Toft, M., Andersen, A. N., Henriksen, O. B., & Mygind, T. (1979). Treatment of mastaglia with bromocriptine: A double-blind cross-over study. *British Medical Journal*, i(6158), 237.

Casper, R. F., & Hearn, M. T. (1990). The effect of hysterectomy and bilateral oophorectomy in women with severe premenstrual syndrome. *American Journal of Obstetrics and Gynecology*, 162(1), 105–109.

Chopin, P., & Briley, M. (1987). Animal models of anxiety: The effect of compounds that modify 5-HT neurotransmission. *Trends in Pharmacological Science*, 8, 383–388.

Chuong, C. J., & Dawson, E. B. (1992). Critical evaluation of nutritional factors in the pathophysiology and treatment of premenstrual syndrome. *Clinical Obstetrics and Gynecology*, 35(3), 679–692.

Dalton, K. (1984). *The premenstrual syndrome and progesterone therapy*. London: William Heinemann.

Delgado, P. L., Charney, D. S., Price, L. H., Aghajanian, G. K., Landis, H., &

Heninger, G. R. (1990). Serotonin function and the mechanism of antidepressant action. *Archives of General Psychiatry, 47,* 411–418.

Dennerstein, L., Morse, C., Burrows, G., Brown, J., & Smith, M. (1986). Alprazolam in the treatment of premenstrual syndrome. In L. Dennerstein & I. Fraser (Eds.), *Hormones and behavior.* New York: Elsevier.

Dennerstein, L., Spencer-Gardner, C., & Gotts, G. (1985). Progesterone and the premenstrual syndrome. *British Medical Journal, 290,* 1617–1621.

Eriksson, E., Lisjo, P., Sundblad, C., Andersson, K., Andersch, B., & Modigh, K. (1990). Effect of clomipramine on premenstrual syndrome. *Acta Psychiatrica Scandinavica, 81,* 87–88.

Facchinetti, F., Borella, P., Sances, G., Fiorini, L., Nappi, R. E., & Genazzani, A. R. (1991). Oral magnesium successfully relieves premenstrual mood changes. *Obstetrics and Gynecology, 78,* 177–181.

Fava, M., Pedrazzi, F., Guaraldi, G. P., Romano, G., Genazzani, A. R., & Facchinetti, F. (1992). Comorbid anxiety and depression among patients with late luteal phase dysphoric disorder. *Journal of Anxiety Disorders, 6,* 325–335.

Freeman, E., Rickels, K., Sondheimer, S. J., & Polansky, M. (1990). Ineffectiveness of progesterone suppository treatment for premenstrual syndrome. *Journal of the American Medical Association, 264*(3), 349–353.

Glick, R., Harrison, W., Endicott, J., McGrath, P., & Quitkin, F. (1991). Treatment of premenstrual dysphoric symptoms in depressed women. *Journal of the American Medical Women's Association, 46*(6), 182–185.

Goodale, I. L., Domar, A. D., & Benson, H. (1990). Alleviation of premenstrual syndrome symptoms with the relaxation response. *Obstetrics and Gynecology, 75*(4), 649–655.

Hamilton, J., Parry, B., Alagna, S., Blumenthal, S., & Herz, E. (1984). Premenstrual mood changes: A guide to evaluation and treatment. *Psychiatric Annals, 14,* 406–420.

Hammarback, S., & Backstrom, T. (1988). Induced anovulation as treatment of premenstrual tension syndrome: A double-blind cross-over study with GnRH-agonist versus placebo. *Acta Obstetricia et Gynecologica Scandinavica, 67,* 159–166.

Hargrove, J. T., & Abraham, G. E. (1982). The incidence of premenstrual tension in a gynecologic clinic. *Journal of Reproductive Medicine, 27,* 721–724.

Harrison, W. M., Endicott, J., & Nee, J. (1989a). Treatment of premenstrual depression with nortriptyline: A pilot study. *Journal of Clinical Psychiatry, 50,* 136–139.

Harrison, W. M., Endicott, J., & Nee, J. (1990). Treatment of premenstrual dysphoria with alprazolam: A controlled study. *Archives of General Psychiatry, 47,* 270–275.

Harrison, W. M., Endicott, J., Nee, J., Glick, H., & Rabkin, J. G. (1989b). Characteristics of women seeking treatment for premenstrual syndrome. *Psychosomatics, 30,* 405–411.

Hellberg, D., Claesson, B., & Nilsson, S. (1991). Premenstrual tension: A placebo-controlled efficacy study with spironolactone and medroxy-progesterone acetate. *International Journal of Gynaecology and Obstetrics, 34*(3), 243–248.

Helvacioglu, A., Yeoman, R. R., Hazelton, J. M., & Aksel, S. (1993). Premenstrual syndrome and related hormonal changes: Long-acting gonadotropin releasing hormone agonist treatment. *Journal of Reproductive Medicine, 38*(11), 864–870.

Johnson, S. (1992). Clinician's approach to the diagnosis and management of premenstrual syndrome. *Clinical Obstetrics and Gynecology, 35*(3), 637–657.

Kashiwagi, T., McClure, J. N. J., & Wetzel, R. D. (1976). Premenstrual affective syndrome and psychiatric disorder. *Disorders of the Nervous System, 37,* 116–119.

Kaspi, S. P., Otto, M. W., Pollack, M. H., Eppinger, S., & Rosenbaum, J. F. (1994). Premenstrual exacerbation of symptoms in women with panic disorder. *Journal of Anxiety Disorders, 8*(2), 131–138.

Kessel, N., & Coppen, A. (1963). The prevalence of common menstrual symptoms. *Lancet, ii,* 61.

Kuczmierczyk, A. R. (1989). Multi-component behavioral treatment of premenstrual syndrome: A case report. *Journal of Behavior Therapy and Experimental Psychology, 20*(3), 235–240.

Magos, A. L., Brincat, M., & Studd, J. W. W. (1986). Treatment of the premenstrual syndrome by subcutaneous oestradiol implants and cyclical oral norethisterone: Placebo controlled study. *British Medical Journal, 292*(6536), 1629–1633.

McEwen, B. S. (1988). Basic research perspective: Ovarian hormone influence on brain neurochemical functions. In L. H. Gise, N. G. Kase, & R. L. Berkowitz (Eds.), *The premenstrual syndromes.* New York: Churchill Livingstone.

McEwen, B. S., & Parsons, B. S. (1982). Gonadal steroid action on the brain: Neurochemistry and neuropharmacology. *Annual Review of Pharmacology and Toxicology, 22,* 555–598.

McMillan, M., & Pihl, R. (1987). Premenstrual depression: A distinct entity. *Journal of Abnormal Psychology, 96,* 149–154.

Morris, N. M., & Udry, F. R. (1972). Contraceptive pills and the day to day feelings of well-being. *American Journal of Obstetrics and Gynecology, 113,* 763–765.

Morse, C. A., Dennerstein, L., Farrell, E., & Varnavides, K. (1991). A comparison of hormone therapy, coping skills training, and relaxation for the relief of premenstrual syndrome. *Journal of Behavioral Medicine, 14*(5), 469–489.

Mortola, J. F. (1992a). Assessment and management of premenstrual syndrome. *Current Opinion in Obstetrics and Gynecology, 4,* 877–885.

Mortola, J. F. (1992b). Issues in the diagnosis and research of premenstrual syndrome. *Clinical Obstetrics and Gynecology, 35*(3), 587–598.

Mortola, J. F., Girton, L., Beck, L., & Yen, S. S. (1990). Diagnosis of premenstrual syndrome by a simple, prospective, and reliable instrument: The Calendar of Premenstrual Experiences. *Obstetrics and Gynecology, 76,* 302–307.

Mortola, J. F., Girton, L., & Fischer, U. (1991). Sucessful treatment of severe premenstrual syndrome by combined use of gonadotropin-releasing hormone agonist and estrogen/progestin. *Journal of Clinical Endocrinology and Metabolism, 71*(2), 252A–252F.

Muse, K. N. (1992). Hormonal manipulation in the treatment of premenstrual syndrome. *Clinical Obstetrics and Gynecology, 35*(3), 658–666.

Muse, K. N., Cetel, N. S., Futterman, L. A., & Yen, S. S. C. (1984). The premenstrual syndrome: Effects of "medical ovariectomy." *New England Journal of Medicine, 311,* 1345–1349.

Parry, B. L., Berga, S. L., Kripke, D. F., Klauber, M. R., Laughlin, G. A., Yen, S. S., & Gillin, J. C. (1990). Altered waveform of plasma nocturnal melatonin secretion in premenstrual depression. *Archives of General Psychiatry, 47,* 1139–1146.

Parry, B. L., Mahan, A. M., Mostofi, N., Klauber, M. R., Lew, G. S., & Gillin, J. C. (1989). Morning versus evening bright light treatment of late luteal phase dysphoric disorder. *American Journal of Psychiatry, 146*, 1215–1217.

Parry, B. L., Mahan, A. M., Mostofi, N., Klauber, M. R., Lew, G. S., & Gillin, J. C. (1993). Light therapy of late luteal phase dysphoric disorder: An extended study. *American Journal of Psychiatry, 150*(9), 1417–1419.

Parry, B. L., & Wehr, T. A. (1987). Therapeutic effect of sleep deprivation in patients with premenstrual syndrome. *American Journal of Psychiatry, 144*, 808–810.

Pearlstein, T. B., Frank, E., Rivera-Tovar, A., Thoft, J. S., Jacobs, E., & Mieczkowski, T. A. (1990). Prevalence of Axis I and Axis II disorders in women with late luteal phase dysphoric disorder. *Journal of Affective Disorders, 20*, 129–134.

Pearlstein, T. B., Rivera-Tovar, A., Frank, E., Thoft, J., Jacobs, E., & Mieczkowski, T. (1992). Nonmedical management of late luteal phase dysphoric disorder. *Journal of Psychotherapy Practice and Research, 1*, 49–55.

Prior, J. C., & Vigna, Y. (1987). Conditioning exercise and premenstrual symptoms. *Journal of Reproductive Medicine, 32*, 423–428.

Rapkin, A. (1992). The role of serotonin in premenstrual syndrome. *Clinical Obstetrics and Gynecology, 35*(3), 629–636.

Rapkin, A., Chang, L. H., & Reading, A. E. (1987). Premenstrual syndrome: A double-blind placebo controlled study of treatment with progesterone vaginal suppositories. *Journal of Obstetrics and Gynecology, 7*, 217–220.

Roy-Byrne, P. P., Rubinow, D. R., Gwirtsman, H., Hoban, M. C., & Grover, G. N. (1986). Cortisol response to dexamethasone in women with premenstrual syndrome. *Neuropsychobiology, 16*, 61–63.

Rubinow, D. R. (1992). The premenstrual syndrome. *Journal of the American Medical Association, 268*(14), 1908–1912.

Rubinow, D. R., Hoban, M. C., Grover, G. N., Galloway, D. S., Roy-Byrne, P., Andersen, R., & Merriam, G. R. (1986). Changes in plasma hormones across the menstrual cycle in patients with menstrually-related mood disorder and in control subjects. *American Journal of Obstetrics and Gynecology, 158*, 5–11.

Rubinow, D. R., Roy-Byrne, P., Hoban, C., Gold, P. W., & Post, R. M. (1984). Prospective assessment of menstrually related mood disorders. *American Journal of Psychiatry, 141*, 684–686.

Schmidt, P. J., Grover, G. N., & Rubinow, D. R. (1993). Alprazolam in the treatment of premenstrual syndrome: A double-blind placebo controlled trial. *Archives of General Psychiatry, 50*(6), 467–473.

Schmidt, P. J., Nieman, L. K., Grover, G. N., Muller, K. L., Merriam, G. R., & Rubinow, D. R. (1991). Lack of effect of induced menses on symptoms in women with premenstrual syndrome. *New England Journal of Medicine, 324*, 1174–1179.

Shangold, G. A. (1993). The premenstrual syndrome: Theories of etiology with relevance to the therapeutic use of GnRH agonists. *Seminars in Reproductive Endocrinology, 11*(2), 172–186.

Silbergeld, S., Brast, N., & Noble, E. P. (1971). The menstrual cycle: A double-blind study of symptoms, mood and behavior, and biochemical variables using Enovid and placebo. *Psychosomatic Medicine, 33*, 411–428.

Smith, S., Rinehart, J. S., Ruddock, V. E., & Schiff, I. (1987). Treatment of premenstrual syndrome with alprazolam: Results of a double-blind, placebo-controlled, randomized crossover clinical trial. *Obstetrics and Gynecology, 70,* 37–43.

Steiner, M., Steinberg, S., Stewart, D., Carter, D., Berger, C., Reid, R., Grover, D., & Streiner, D. (1995). Fluoxetine in the treatment of premenstrual dysphoria. *New England Journal of Medicine, 332,* 1529–1534.

Stone, A. B., Pearlstein, T. B., & Brown, W. A. (1991). Fluoxetine in the treatment of late luteal phase dysphoric disorder. *Journal of Clinical Psychiatry, 52,* 290–293.

Stout, A. L., Steege, J. F., Blazer, D. G., & George, L. K. (1986). Comparison of lifetime psychiatric diagnoses in premenstrual syndrome clinic and community samples. *Journal of Nervous and Mental Disease, 174,* 517–522.

Thys-Jacobs, S., Ceccarelli, S., Bierman, A., Weisman, H., Cohen, M. A., & Alvir, J. (1989). Calcium supplementation in premenstrual syndrome: A randomized crossover trial. *Journal of General Internal Medicine, 4,* 183–189.

van der Meer, Y. G., Benedek-Jaszmann, L. G., & van Loenen, A. C. (1983). Effect of high dose progesterone on the premenstrual syndrome: A double-blind, crossover trial. *Journal of Psychosomatics Obstetrics and Gynecology, 2*(4), 220–222.

Watson, N. R., Studd, J. W. W., Savvas, M., & Baber, R. J. (1990). The long term effect of oestradiol implant therapy for the treatment of premenstrual syndrome. *Gynecology and Endocrinology, 4,* 99–107.

Watson, N. R., Studd, J. W. W., Savvas, M., Garnett, T., & Baber, R. J. (1989). Treatment of severe premenstrual syndrome with oestradiol patches and cyclical oral norethisterone. *Lancet, ii*(8665), 730–732.

Wood, S. H., Mortola, J. F., Chan, Y. F., Moossazadeh, F., & Yen, S. S. (1992). Treatment of premenstrual syndrome with fluoxetine: A double-blind, placebo-controlled, crossover study. *Obstetrics and Gynecology, 80*(3, Part 1), 339–344.

Wurtman, J. J., Brzezinski, A., Wurtman, R. J., & Laferrere, B. (1989). Effect of nutrient intake on premenstrual depression. *American Journal of Obstetrics and Gynecology, 161,* 1228–1134.

Yonkers, K. A., & White, K. (1992). Premenstrual exacerbation of depression: One process or two? *Journal of Clinical Psychiatry,* 289–292.

17

Management of Refractory Insomnia

JEFFREY B. WEILBURG

"Insomnia" is generally defined as the complaint of persistent difficulty in falling asleep or staying asleep, or the feeling of not being rested after sleep (nonrestorative sleep), which is directly associated with daytime distress and compromised functioning (American Psychiatric Association, 1994; Diagnostic Classification Steering Committee, 1990; Erman, 1987; Gillin & Byerly, 1990; Zorick, Roth, Hartze, Piccone, & Stepanski, 1981). Typical symptoms of insomnia-related daytime distress include anergy, malaise, cognitive slowness, and irritability.

Insomnia is a common problem. Survey data reveal that from 15% to 20% of the general population complains of insomnia, and that 10% of the population reports using "sleeping pills" (Balter & Uhlenguth, 1992; Greenblatt, Harmatz, Zinny, & Shader, 1987; Mellinger, Balter, & Uhlenhuth, 1985; Zorick, 1994). Twenty percent of all adult general medical outpatients and 35% of psychiatric outpatients complain of insomnia (Coleman et al., 1982; Rosekind, 1992; Weilburg & Winkleman, in press). Higher rates are found among women, patients from lower socioeconomic groups, and the elderly. Not surprisingly, guidelines for the diagnosis and management of insomnia are extensively covered in the literature (Coleman et al., 1982; Erman, 1987; Gillin & Byerly, 1990; Mellinger et al., 1985; Mendelson, 1992; Moran, Thomson, & Nies, 1988; Reynolds, Kupfer, Buysse, Coble, & Yeager, 1991; Weilburg, 1995; Zorick, 1994).

In contrast, no definitive criteria for "treatment-resistant insomnia" (TRI) or information regarding prevalence of this problem could be found during a search of the sleep literature. The literature does, however, contain discussion of the chronicity and persistence of certain types of insomnia (Hauri & Fisher, 1986; Regestein & Reich, 1983; Reite, Buysse,

Reynolds, & Mendelson, 1995; Reynolds, Taska, & Sewitch, 1984; Scharf, Roth, & Vogel, 1994; Tan et al., 1987). For example, "primary insomnia" (sometimes called "idiopathic" or "childhood-onset") is recognized as being persistent and difficult to treat (American Psychiatric Association, 1994; Diagnostic Classification Steering Committee, 1990; Hauri, 1987, 1994; Kramer, 1982; Nino-Murcia, 1992; Reynolds et al., 1991; Spielman, Suskin, & Thorpy, 1987; Tan et al., 1987; Zorick et al., 1981). "Psychophysiologic insomnia" or "learned insomnia" can be chronic as well (Hauri & Fisher, 1986; Reynolds et al., 1984). "Delayed sleep phase syndrome" can be persistent, even though treatment is available (Czeisler et al., 1981; Schweitzer, Koshorek, Muehlback, & Morris, 1991; Weitzman, Czeisler, Coleman, Spielman, Zimmerman, & Dement, 1981). However, no category for TRI exists in the sleep disorders section of the *Diagnostic and Statistical Manual of Mental Disorders*, fourth edition (DSM-IV; American Psychiatric Association, 1994) or in the *International Classification of Sleep Disorders* (ICSD; Diagnostic Classification Steering Committee, 1990), these being the most important current classification systems for the sleep disorders. This chapter therefore begins with an attempt to define TRI as a clinical entity by offering a provisional outline for diagnostic criteria. The chapter then provides suggestions for its diagnostic evaluation and management.

DEFINING TRI:
PROVISIONAL DIAGNOSTIC CRITERIA

The following diagnostic criteria for TRI were set up to be analogous to the criteria for treatment-resistant depression (Nierenberg & Keck, 1989). They include severity and duration features, as well as attempts to clarify the diagnosis by identifying and resolving potentially treatable contributing or underlying factors (such as medical problems). An attempt to insure that past treatment was in fact adequate must also be made. Using criteria such as these allows TRI to be diagnosed only rarely.

The provisional definition of TRI includes all of the following elements: (1) persistence of insomnia for more than 6 months, despite (a) maximal treatment of any underlying medical, psychiatric, or substance use problem(s) and (b) vigorous multimodal treatment of the insomnia symptoms; and (2) objective verification with polysomnography that sleep is abnormal. The issues raised by each of these criteria are discussed in detail below.

Persistence for More Than 6 Months Despite Adequate Treatment of Underlying Problems

The majority of patients with insomnia fall into the DSM-IV categories covering insomnia secondary to psychiatric, medical, or substance use problems (Kramer, 1982; Rosekind, 1992; Walsh, Moss, & Sugarman, 1994;

Wooten, 1994; Zorick et al., 1981). In such cases, the insomnia symptoms should be considered treatment-resistant *only* when they persist despite completed treatment of the underlying disorders. This criterion may help distinguish those patients with persistent sleep disruption secondary to incomplete treatment of other disorders from those whose insomnia is a primary problem in and of itself.

The practical utility of including this criterion is that it keeps treatment efforts focused on correcting the physiologic disturbance that produces the insomnia symptoms. It recognizes that insomnia, like pain, may be the symptomatic end result of a variety of pathophysiologic processes. Proper, effective long-term treatment requires a thorough attempt at identification of the source of the symptom.

It may be of course be difficult to determine when a psychiatric condition or medical condition is fully resolved. In operational terms, if most or all the symptoms of the underlying syndrome have completely resolved with the exception of the persistent insomnia, then TRI may be diagnosed. For example, if insomnia persists despite resolution of sadness, helplessness, hopelessness, and other typical depressive symptoms, it may be reasonable to consider the insomnia as an independent problem (i.e., TRI) rather than a secondary difficulty.

Many chronic or progressive psychiatric or medical conditions never resolve fully. In such cases, when treatment efforts have been maximized and insomnia remains persistent and disruptive, TRI may be diagnosed. An exception should probably made in conditions whose basic pathophysiologic disturbances typically produce insomnia directly. For example, in senile dementia of the Alzheimer's type, disruption of normal circadian cycling often results in daytime sleepiness and nocturnal wakefulness (Prinz, Vitiello, Raskind, & Thorpy, 1990). In such cases, the insomnia should be regarded more as a dementia symptom than as TRI.

Normal variations in sleep patterns or sleep difficulties related to iatrogenic factors should not be mistaken for TRI. For example, a decreased capacity for consolidated nocturnal sleep may be a function of "normal aging" (Prinz et al., 1990; Reynolds, Kupfer, Hoch, & Sewitch, 1985a). It is therefore not sensible to consider the sleep of otherwise healthy elders who function well during the day (perhaps with a daytime nap) as reflecting "insomnia" simply because their sleep is shorter in duration than it was earlier in their lives. Hypnotics may not improve sleep in such patients and may also expose them to significant risks, such as cognitive compromise or injuries resulting from falls. It is better to address such problems as worries about changes in habits or loneliness during long hours alone at night directly, rather than trying to alter sleep itself (Monane, 1992; Moran et al., 1988; Reynolds et al., 1985b).

Some people sleep fewer than 7 hours each night but function well during the day. Such cases highlight the need to determine that daytime distress is a direct function of sleep length and quality before a diagnosis of TRI is made.

Some medications and other substances can produce trouble in falling or staying asleep (see Table 17.1). Antidepressants and antipsychotic agents can also stimulate abnormal nocturnal motor activity, leading to sleep fragmentation and secondary fatigue. When insomnia is persistent because chronic use of medications is required, it is often reasonable to treat the insomnia in order to improve patient comfort and compliance. However, insomnia of this type should not be called TRI in the sense meant in this chapter.

Examples of insomnia secondary to other psychiatric or medical conditions include the following:

1. *Insomnia secondary to an Axis II condition.* Some patients with personality disorders may attempt to focus on their insomnia complaints and ignore or refuse to attend to efforts to identify and remediate their related psychosocial difficulties. Such patients may search for the "perfect pill," continue to have insomnia despite multiple adequate trials of hypnotics, and then present with self-described "TRI." Efforts to treat such patients are often unsuccessful unless underlying Axis II and correlated situational factors are addressed (Zorick, 1994; Zorick et al., 1981; Walsh et al., 1994).

2. *Insomnia secondary to mood disorders.* Some patients with incompletely treated depression or dysthymia may have persistent anergy, irritability, and mildly fragmented sleep. Such patients may be better served by further attempts to employ antidepressant and mood-stabilizing agents (see Fava, Kaji, & Davidson, Chapter 1, this volume), because hypnotics or other methods used to improve sleep alone may not improve overall subjective outcome (Walsh et al., 1994).

Patients with a history of substance dependence or abuse (e.g., recovering alcoholics) may have insomnia that persists for many months after the start of sobriety. Since sleep disturbance in such patients may be a function of central nervous system changes related to the substance use, it should not prompt an evaluation for TRI unless it persists for > 12 months. Furthermore, it may be best to avoid using benzodiazepines or other drugs that cross-react with alcohol for such patients. Behavioral approaches are sometimes only marginally useful in such cases, but should always be tried. Patient education and support are critically important in such cases.

3. *Insomnia secondary to medical problems.* Patients with medical problems (e.g., arthritis) that produce sleep fragmentation secondary to pain may be best treated by direct management of the medical problem (e.g., inflammation and pain) (Weilburg, 1995; Wooten, 1994).

Persistence Despite Adequate Treatment of the Insomnia Symptoms

The ICSD allows the modifiers "chronic" and/or "severe" to be appended to a diagnosis of insomnia. Although not every case of chronic, severe insomnia is necessarily TRI, a basic criterion for the diagnosis of TRI should

TABLE 17.1. Substances That Can Cause Insomnia

Alcohol (long-term dependence/abuse, withdrawal)

Sedatives (long-term dependence/abuse, withdrawal)
  Barbiturates
  Benzodiazepines
  Narcotics

Stimulants
  Amphetamines
  Methylphenidate, pemoline
  Yohimbine
  Cocaine
  Caffeine and other xanthines in coffee, tea, cola, chocolate

Antidepressants (also withdrawal)
  Monoamine oxidase inhibitors (phenelzine, tranylcypromine)
  Heterocyclics (imipramine, desipramine, protriptyline)
  Selective serotonin reuptake inhibitors (fluoxetine, sertraline)
  Others (amoxapine, bupropion)

Antipsychotics (can induce periodic limb movement disorder)
  Phenothiazines
  Butyrophenones

Antiasthmatics, decongestants
  Pseudoephedrine
  Phenylephrine

Tobacco (direct stimulation, withdrawal, conditioned awakening to smoke)

Antihypertensives (can induce nightmares, periodic limb movement disorder)
  Beta-adrenergic blockers
  Alpha-methyl dopa
  Diuretics
  Reserpine, clonidine

Cimetidine

L-Dopa, baclofen, methysergide

Thyroxine, steroids, birth control pills

Tetracycline (can induce nightmares)

be that the insomnia is chronic (duration greater than 6 months) and persists despite routine treatment.

The literature offers little formal guidance as to what constitutes an adequate treatment trial for insomnia. It is generally recognized that hypnotic medications, behavioral techniques, and elimination of certain substances can all be effective in treating insomnia. The focus here is on medication, with only brief mention of the other two types of techniques. References for more information on behavioral methods are provided.

Medications

Benzodiazepine hypnotics are the drugs of first choice for the treatment of insomnia (Gelenberg, 1992; Greenblatt, Abernethy, Divoll, Harmatz, & Shader, 1983; Greenblatt, Harmatz, Engelhardt, & Shader, 1989; Nino-Murcia, 1992). No clear relative superiority in terms of efficacy has been demonstrated for any particular hypnotic. The main differences among hypnotics are pharmacokinetic: Agents vary in terms of their onset and duration of action, and in the presence or absence of active metabolites, which may accumulate with repeated dosing. Individual patients may subjectively prefer particular agents, and the benzodiazepines not marketed for use as hypnotics are sometimes more helpful for particular patients. Thus, adequate treatment probably includes trials of at least one long-acting (e.g., flurazepam, 30 mg at bedtime) and one short-acting (e.g., triazolam, 0.5 mg at bedtime) benzodiazepine hypnotic and at least one nonhypnotic benzodiazepine (e.g., clonazepam or lorazepam, both 1 mg at bedtime).

Antidepressant agents are also often very helpful for insomniac patients, especially those with anxiety or depressive symptoms, even if such symptoms do not meet criteria for a psychiatric disorder (Montgomery, Oswald, Morgan, & Adam, 1983; Scharf & Sachias, 1990; Ware, 1983). Trials of at least two different types of antidepressants (e.g., nortriptyline, 25–150 mg at bedtime; paroxetine, 5–30 mg at bedtime; trazodone, 25–150 mg at bedtime) for >8 weeks, alone or in conjunction with benzodiazepines, should be conducted unless otherwise contraindicated as part of an adequate treatment trial.

Behavioral Methods

Sleep diaries, attention to sleep hygiene, relaxation methods, deconditioning, and sleep restriction therapy are also part of basic adequate treatment. Sleep diaries may include simple self-ratings (on a scale of 1–5) of mood and anxiety, made before bed and upon arising for 2–4 weeks; estimates of time in bed and time to falling asleep; number, duration, and perceived reasons for awakenings; time out of bed in the morning; and events, food intake, and substance use during the day (Hobson, 1983; Stepanski, 1994). More information about sleep hygiene, relaxation methods, deconditioning, and sleep restriction therapy may be found in Bootzin (1977), Bootzin and Perlis (1992), Mellinger et al. (1985), Moun, Culbert, and Schwartz (1991), Spielman et al. (1987), and Stepanski (1994). TRI should not be diagnosed unless two different forms of behavioral treatment have been undertaken and have failed despite good compliance.

Elimination of Stimulating Drugs and Other Substances

Some patients are very sensitive to the sleep-disrupting effects of caffeine, chocolate, nicotine, alcohol, decongestants, or other nonmedical psychotropics. Even moderate or intermittent use of tobacco, foods with caffeine, or other substances may produce chronic insomnia in these patients. If such patients are significantly troubled by their insomnia, they can be assisted in the sometimes arduous task of total abstinence from these substances. TRI should be diagnosed only after an 8-week period of abstinence is achieved, since many otherwise refractory patients will improve after discontinuation of the offending agents.

Objective Verification of Abnormal Sleep by Polysomnography

The correlation between subjective and objective assessment of sleep is often poor in many patients who complain of insomnia. Indeed, problems with the perception of level of nocturnal alertness or arousal, as well as the perception of elapsed time, may be a critical factor in the production of chronic insomnia (Carskadon et al., 1976; Frankel, Coursey, Buchbinder, & Snyder, 1976; Standards of Practice Committee, 1995). Thus the category "sleep state misperception," in which patients complain of insomnia because they overestimate the time they spend awake in bed at night while having objectively normal or nearly normal nocturnal sleep, is included by the ICSD in the differential diagnosis of insomnia.

Patients who meet the primacy, severity, and duration criteria for TRI should have polysomnography to assess whether some objective abnormality of sleep (such as prolonged sleep latency or decreased sleep efficiency) is present. Polysomnography is also useful because it may refine the diagnosis by ruling out other primary sleep disorders, such as periodic leg movements in sleep, sleep-related respiratory abnormalities (including sleep apnea), and abnormal polysomnographic patterns (such as alpha–delta sleep) (Coleman et al., 1982; Hauri, 1983; Kramer, 1982; Mellinger et al., 1985; Nino-Murcia, 1992). If such disorders are present, treatment can be targeted at their alleviation. If no objective sleep abnormality is found, treatment efforts may be properly directed toward amelioration of problems with the *perception* of sleep, rather than toward modifying sleep itself. Polysomnography in the diagnosis of insomnia is discussed in detail by Reite et al. (1995).

APPROACH TO THE EVALUATION AND MANAGEMENT OF TRI

Reassessment of the Diagnosis

An approach to TRI begins with reassessment of the diagnosis. Several techniques may be useful in this process. First, it is often helpful to interview the patient's bed partner and family members. This will often reveal sleep-related behaviors the patient is unaware of or ignores, such as snoring, movement, or arousals. Family members or significant others may also outline behavioral or situational patterns related to sleep that the patient cannot or will not articulate. Finally, the presence of character problems, substance use, or other problems previously minimized by the patient may become clearer after discussion with other informants.

Routine laboratory screening may be useful in revealing otherwise occult hypothroidism or early renal failure. When psychiatric illness is suspected, it may be crucial to take time to conduct a systematic clinical or structured diagnostic interview, in order to make sure that no psychiatric diagnosis is overlooked (since insomnia secondary to mental disorders is so common). Finally, polysomnography may reveal the presence of other primary sleep disorders, which can then be treated (Reite et al., 1995). Table 17.2 provides a list of ICSD diagnoses that may present with insomnia symptoms.

Treatment

The literature gives little guidance regarding possible treatment algorithms for TRI. The efficiacy of using high doses of standard hypnotic agents or other sedatives, using alternative drugs, or treating patients with persistent problems over prolonged periods has not been rigorously studied. The suggestions outlined below are therefore based on clinical experience and anecdotal reports.

Use of Standard Hypnotics

All of the currently marketed hypnotics (estazolam, flurazepam, temazepam, triazolam, quazepam, and zolpidem) are equally effective in the treatment of insomnia (Jonas, Coleman, Sheridan, & Kalinske, 1992). The use of these agents for the treatment of TRI has not been studied. Most of these agents improve sleep continuity and shorten sleep latency in a greater fraction of subjects at higher rather than lower doses. These agents have a wide margin of safety; doses several times the currently recommended amounts have been safely given to subjects during the clinical trials. However, most studies have demonstrated that for benzodiazepines (and related agents such as imidothiaprines—e.g., zolpidem), side effects such as memory and gait disturbance increase proportionally with increases in dose (Abernethy, Greenblatt, & Shader, 1986; Greenblatt et al., 1989; Mendelson, 1992).

It may sometimes be appropriate to use doses of hypnotics above those recommended by the manufacturer. In some cases, in which criteria for TRI are met and there are no specific contraindications (e.g., past substance use, respiratory compromise), time-limited trials of doses as high as twice the reccommended levels may be used, after informed consent,

TABLE 17.2. ICSD Diagnoses That May Present with Insomnia Symptoms

I. Dyssomnias
  A. Intrinsic Sleep Disorders
      1. Psychophysiological Insomnia
      2. Sleep State Misperception
      3. Idiopathic Insomnia
      4. Narcolepsy
        . . .
      8. Obstructive Sleep Apnea Syndrome
      9. Central Sleep Apnea Syndrome
      10. Central Alveolar Hypoventilation Syndrome
      11. Periodic Limb Movement Disorder
      12. Restless Leg Syndrome
      13. Intrinsic Sleep Disorder NOS

  B. Extrinsic Sleep Disorders
      1. Inadequate Sleep Hygiene
      2. Environmental Sleep Disorder
      3. Altitude Insomnia
      4. Adjustment Sleep Disorder
      5. Insufficient Sleep Syndrome
      6. Limit-Setting Sleep Disorder
      7. Sleep-Onset Association Disorder
      8. Food Allergy Insomnia
      9. Nocturnal Eating (Drinking) Syndrome
      10. Hypnotic-Dependent Sleep Disorder
      11. Stimulant-Dependent Sleep Disorder
      12. Alcohol-Dependent Sleep Disorder
      13. Toxin-Induced Sleep Disorder
      14. Extrinsic Sleep Disorder NOS

  C. Circadian Rhythm Sleep Disorders
      1. Time Zone Change (Jet Lag) Syndrome
      2. Shift Work Sleep Disorder
      3. Irregular Sleep–Wake Pattern
      4. Delayed Sleep Phase Syndrome
      5. Advanced Sleep Phase Syndrome
      6. Non-24-Hour Sleep–Wake Disorder
      7. Circadian Rhythm Sleep Disorder NOS

II. Parasomnias
  A. Arousal Disorders
      1. Confusional Arousals
      2. Sleepwalking
      3. Sleep Terrors

  B. Sleep–Wake Transition Disorders
      1. Rhythmic Movement Disorder
      2. Sleep Starts
      3. Sleep Talking
      4. Nocturnal Leg Cramps

  C. Parasomnias Usually Associated with REM Sleep
      1. Nightmares
      2. Sleep Paralysis
      3. Impaired Sleep-Related Penile Erections
      4. Sleep-Related Painful Erections

TABLE 17.2. (cont.)

     5. REM Sleep-Related Sinus Arrest
     6. REM Sleep Behavior Disorder

  D. Other Parasomnias
     1. Sleep Bruxism
     2. Sleep Enuresis
     3. Sleep-Related Abnormal Swallowing Syndrome
     4. Nocturnal Paroxysmal Dystonia
       . . .
     6. Primary Snoring
     7. Infant Sleep Apnea
     8. Congenital Central Hypoventilation Syndrome
       . . .
     10. Benign Neonatal Sleep Myoclonus
     11. Other Parasomnia NOS

III. Sleep Disorders Associated with Medical/Psychiatric Disorders
  A. Associated with Mental Disorders
     1. Psychoses
     2. Mood Disorders
     3. Anxiety Disorders
     4. Panic Disorder
     5. Alcoholism

  B. Associated with Neurological Disorders
     1. Cerebral Degenerative Disorders
     2. Dementia
     3. Parkinsonism
     4. Fatal Familial Insomnia
     5. Sleep-Related Epilepsy
     6. Electrical Status Epilepticus of Sleep
     7. Sleep-Related Headaches

  C. Associated with Other Medical Disorders
     1. Sleeping Sickness
     2. Nocturnal Cardiac Ischemia
     3. Chronic Obstructive Pulmonary Disease
     4. Sleep-Related Asthma
     5. Sleep-Related Gastroesophageal Reflux
     6. Peptic Ulcer Disease
     7. Fibrositis Syndrome

IV. Proposed Sleep Disorders
     1. Short Sleeper
     2. Long Sleeper
     3. Subwakefulness Syndrome
     4. Fragmentary Myoclonus
     5. Sleep Hyperhidrosis
     6. Menstrual-Associated Sleep Disorder
     7. Pregnancy-Associated Sleep Disorder
     8. Terrifying Hypnagogic Hallucinations
     9. Sleep-Related Neurogenic Tachypnea
     10. Sleep-Related Laryngospasm
     11. Sleep Choking Syndrome

Note. NOS, not otherwise specified. Adapted from Diagnostic Classification Steering Committee (1990). Copyright 1990 by the American Sleep Disorders Association. Adapted by permission.

and under conditions of careful monitoring with clear targets to assess results.

Benzodiazepines and Related Agents. All benzodiazepines and related agents have sedative properties, although six are specifically marketed as hypnotics: flurazepam, temazepam, zolpidem, estazolam, quazepam, and triazolam. Many other benzodiazepines, such as clonazepam, lorazepam, and diazepam are, used clinically for management of insomnia and TRI. I focus here on selected problems of benzodiazepine treatment of insomnia relevant to TRI.

Benzodiazepines may depress the alerting mechanisms that terminate apneas. Thus, they must be used with care in patients with sleep apnea or obesity/hypoventilation ("Pickwickian syndrome"), after all of the alternatives have failed.

The long-term use of benzodiazepine hypnotics is a controversial topic. There is general agreement that it is best to seek alternatives to long-term use, and that treatment should be maintained with the lowest possible effective dose. If long-acting agents are used chronically, drug accumulation may occur and must be managed. Some investigators report that tolerance to the hypnotic effects of benzodiazepines develop over time, whereas others report that subjective and objective improvement in sleep can be demonstrated with lorazepam use for periods longer than 4 weeks (Church & Johnson, 1979; Gelenberg, 1992; Lamphere, Roeher, Zorick, Koshorek, & Roth, 1986; Mendels, 1994; Nino-Murcia, 1992; Scharf et al., 1994). My colleagues' and my clinical experience is that some patients with TRI can be safely and successfully managed with long-term benzodiazepine use. Over time, some of these patients may find that they need a drug only two or three nights per week. Careful record keeping and patient monitoring, to insure that dose escalation or performance problems from excessive daytime sedation do not arise, are important. It may also be useful to attempt to discontinue the drug gradually every year, to determine whether continued usage is still required. However, further systematic study of this area is required.

Antidepressants. All antidepressants tend to increase sleep continuity and are useful when lack of sleep maintenance is the chief complaint. The more sedating antidepressants (e.g., amitriptyline, doxepin) also immediately decrease sleep latency. Antidepressants can be helpful in the management of sleep disturbance in patients with depression, dysthymia, anxiety disorders, and personality disorders (Hohagen et al., 1994; Ware, 1983). Small doses (10–25 mg at bedtime) of agents such as amitriptyline or doxepin may relieve insomnia without causing unacceptable side effects. Larger doses may be called for if a patient has a partial response to low doses. Certainly, if major depression is present, effective treatment with antidepressants or other interventions is critical.

Trazodone is sedating but is no more effective for managing insomnia than are the tricyclics (Montgomery et al., 1983; Scharf et al., 1994). Although trazodone's lack of anticholinergic properties and lack of effects on the cardiac conduction system may prompt its use in older patients or those with cardiac arrhythmias, it has a relatively high propensity to cause orthostatic hypertension, which may make its use problematic in the elderly or debilitated.

Amitriptyline, in doses of 10–75 mg at bedtime, may be useful for management of adults with childhood-onset insomnia (Czeisler et al., 1981). Amitriptyline, nortriptyline, and doxepin (10–100 mg at bedtime) provide symptomatic and polysomnographic resolution of alpha–delta sleep, the type of insomnia often associated with fibromyalgia.

Stimulating antidepressants, such as imipramine, desipramine, protriptyline, fluoxetine, phenelzine, or tranylcypromine, may sometimes prolong sleep latency and cause insomnia. This can be managed with a shift from bedtime to morning dosing or with the addition of a benzodiazepine (e.g., lorazepam, 1 mg at bedtime). If the sleep disturbance remains intractable, switching to another agent may be necessary. Trazodone (50 mg at bedtime) may be safely and effectively used to manage insomnia induced by monoamine oxidase inhibitors (MAOIs) or selective serotonin reuptake inhibitors (SSRIs) (Nierenberg, Adler, Peselow, Zornberg, & Rosenthal, 1994; Nierenberg & Keck, 1989). However, despite their reputation as "stimulating," recent studies suggest that the SSRIs (e.g., fluoxetine) may be as likely to cause sedation as insomnia (Tollefson et al., 1994). The generally favorable side effect profile of the SSRIs may make them the treatment of choice for many mood and anxiety disorder patients, even in the presence of insomnia.

All antidepressants may induce sleep disturbance, including nocturnal myoclonus, sleepwalking, sleep talking, or nightmares. Effective management strategies may include lowering the dose of the antidepressant, adding a benzodiazepine (e.g., clonazepam, 0.5–2 mg at bedtime), or switching from bedtime to morning dosing. Sometimes switching among antidepressants may be necessary. Abrupt discontinuation of tricyclics or MAOIs may cause insomnia and nightmares. Gradual tapering of these agents is often necessary to minimize this adverse effect.

Use of Alternative Agents

Narcotics and Barbiturates. Several cases have been reported in which an opiate narcotic (hydromorphone) was used with apparent success to manage TRI (Hauri, 1987; Regestein, 1976, 1987; Regestein & Reich, 1983). It may be useful to consider barbiturates or opiates in cases of TRI where the patients can be carefully monitored over time and therefore treated safely. Since no controlled studies can be found to support or warn against this practice, it should be considered as a "last resort" and used only after appropriate consultation with drug abuse and sleep experts, as well as informed consent on the part of the patient.

Barbiturates (secobarbital, pentobarbital), methylprylon, glutethimide, and methaqualone have been used in the past as nypnotics, but have a lower margin of safety, greater propensity to cause dependence, and no advantage in effectiveness as compared to the benzodiazepines. These agents are rarely, if ever, used any more as hypnotics. Many patients appear to become tolerant of the hypnotic effects of these agents after regular use. The long-term use of these drugs may produce fragmentation of sleep, and in fact may worsen insomnia. If a patient taking one of these agents experiences recurrent sleep difficulties, it may be useful to taper the agent and consider alternate therapies.

Lithium. Lithium may be used alone or in combination with antidepressants and/or hypnotics for patients who have TRI secondary to underlying mood disorders, particularly bipolar disorders. Lithium has also been found to be useful in clinical practice as an adjunct to direct manipulation of sleep–wake times in patients with circadian rhythm abnormalities.

L-Tryptophan. L-Tryptophan in doses of 1–5 g at night was used to treat insomnia until the eosinophilia myalgia syndrome was linked to this agent several years ago. Although impurities in the production process appeared to produce the syndrome, rather than the L-tryptophan itself, this agent is still not back on the market in the United States.

Chloral Hydrate and Paraldehyde. The older agents chloral hydrate and paraldehyde have an objectionable taste and smell, but can be effective hypnotics in the short term. Their principal short-term indication is in the treatment of insomnia in patients undergoing alcohol detoxification, when benzodiazepine treatment is contraindicated. Chloral hydrate is rarely used as a maintenance agent, and in clinical practice, many patients appear to develop rapid tolerance to its therapeutic effects. However, for some patients its use one to three times per week may be useful, in doses of 500 to 1000 mg at bedtime, when other alternative interventions are unsuccessful.

Buspirone. Buspirone, a nonbenzodiazepine anxiolytic, does not seem to be useful as a hypnotic, and has little if any effect on sleep architecture.

Stimulants. In a few adult patients with symptoms of attention-deficit/hyperactivity disorder, use of stimulants such as methylphenidate (10–60 mg/day, taken during the day) may ameliorate insomnia. Very recent work suggests that clonidine (0.1 mg at bedtime) may help adult and pediatric patients with persistent insomnia secondary to methylphenidate use (Prince, Wilens, Spencer, Wozniak, & Biederman, 1994).

Antipsychotics. Antipsychotics may be useful for the treatment of insomnia in psychotic and delirious patients. For patients in a medical, surgical, or intensive care unit, dosing may begin with 0.5 mg/day of haloperidol (administered orally, intramuscularly, or intravenously), although larger doses are sometimes required (e.g., 1–10 mg/day). Some clinicians advocate the use of antipsychotic agents in patients with primitive character pathology who are prone to fragmentation. Small amounts of haloperidol or thiothixene (e.g., 0.5–2 mg at bedtime) may be useful when agitated ruminations interfere with sleep in these patients. However, the risk of tardive dyskinesia should limit the use of these agents for treatment of severe difficulties over a brief period of time.

CONCLUSION

This chapter proposes a definition of TRI and an approach to its evaluation and treatment, based on extrapolation from the literature and from clinical experience. Future research is necessary to better characterize the prevalence and phenomenology of refractory insomnia and to develop comprehensive therapeutic approaches to the treatment of these difficult conditions.

REFERENCES

Abernethy, D. R., Greenblatt, D. J., & Shader, R. I. (1986). Benzodiazepine hypnotic metabolism: Drug interactions and clinical indications. *Acta Psychiatrica Scandinavica, 332*(Suppl. 74), 32–38.

American Psychiatric Association. (1994). *Diagnostic and statistical manual of mental disorders* (4th ed.). Washington, DC: Author.

Balter, M. B., & Uhlenguth, E. (1992). New epidemiologic findings about insomnia and its treatment. *Journal of Clinical Psychiatry, 53*(12, Suppl.), 34–42.

Bootzin, R. R. (1977). Effects of self-control procedures for insomnia. In R. B. Stuart (Ed.), *Behavioral self-management strategies, techniques and outcome* (pp. 176–195). New York: Brunner/Mazel.

Bootzin, R. R., & Perlis, M. L. (1992). Nonpharmacologic treatments of insomnia. *Journal of Clinical Psychiatry, 53*(6, Suppl.), 37–41.

Brunner, D. P., Munch, M., Biederman, K., Huch, R., Huch, A., & Borbely, A. (1994). Changes in sleep and sleep electroencephalogram during pregnancy. *Sleep, 17*, 576–582.

Carskadon, M. A., Dement, W. C., Mitler, M. M., Guilleminault, C., Zarcone, V. P., & Spiegel, R. (1976). Self-reports versus sleep laboratory finding in 122 drug-free subjects with complaints of chronic insomnia. *American Journal of Psychiatry, 133*(12), 1382–1388.

Church, M. W., & Johnson, L. C. (1979). Mood and performance of poor sleepers during repeated use of flurazepam. *Psychopharmacology, 61*, 309–316.

Coleman, R. M., Roffwargh, P., Kennedy, S. J., Giulleminault, C., Cinque, J., Cohn, M., Karacan, I., Kupfer, D. J., Lemmi, H., Miles, L. E., Orr, W. C., Philips, E. R., Roth, T., Sassin, J. F., Schmidt, H. S., Weitzman, E. D., & Dement, W. C. (1982). Sleep–wake disorders based on a polysomnographic diagnosis: A national cooperative study. *Journal of the American Medical Association, 227*(7), 997–1003.

Czeisler, R. G., Coleman, R. M., Zimmerman, J. C., Moore-Ede, M. C., Dement, W. C., & Weitzman, E. D. (1981). Chronotherapy: Resetting the circadian clocks of patients with delayed sleep phase insomnia. *Sleep*, 4(1), 1–21.

Diagnostic Classification Steering Committee, American Sleep Disorders Association. (1990). *International classification of sleep disorders: Diagnostic and coding manual*. Rochester, MN: American Sleep Disorders Association.

Erman, M. K. (1987). Sleep disorders. *Psychiatric Clinics of North America*, 10(4), 525–541.

Frankel, R. L., Coursey, R. D., Buchbinder, R., & Snyder, F. (1976). Recorded and reported sleep in chronic primary insomnia. *Archives of General Psychiatry*, 33, 1615–1623.

Gelenberg, A. (1992). Introduction. The use of benzodiazepine hypnotics: A scientific examination of a clinical controversy. *Journal of Clinical Psychiatry*, 53(12, Suppl.), 3.

Gillin, J. C., & Byerly, W. F. (1990). The diagnosis and management of insomnia. *New England Journal of Medicine*, 322, 239.

Greenblatt, D. J., Abernathy, D. R., Divoll, M., Harmatz, J. S., & Shader, R. E. (1983). Pharmacokinetic properties of benzodiazepine hypnotics. *Journal of Clinical Psychiatry*, 3(2), 129–132.

Greenblatt, D. J., Harmatz, J. S., Engelhardt, N., & Shader, R. I. (1989). Pharmacokinetic determinants of dynamic differences among three benzodiazepine hypnotics. *Archives of General Psychiatry*, 46, 326–332.

Greenblatt, D. J., Harmatz, J. S., Zinny, M. A., & Shader, R. I. (1987). Effect of gradual withdrawal on the rebound sleep disorder after discontinuation of triazolam. *New England Journal of Medicine*, 317, 722–728.

Hauri, J. J. (1983). A cluster analysis of insomnia. *Sleep*, 6, 326–339.

Hauri, P. (1987). Editorial: Specific effects of sedative/hypnotic drugs in the treatment of incapacitating chronic insomnia. *American Journal of Medicine*, 83, 925–926.

Hauri, P. (1994). Primary insomnia. In T. Roth, M. H. Kryger, & W. C. Dement (Eds.), *Principles and practice of sleep medicine* (pp. 494–499). Philadelphia: W. B. Saunders.

Hauri, P., & Fisher, J. (1986). Persistent psychophysiologic (learned) insomnia. *Sleep*, 9(1), 38–53.

Hobson, J. A. (1983). *Sleep charting*. South Norwalk, CT: Medication.

Hohagen, F., Montero, R. F., Weiss, E., Lis, S., Schonbrunn, E., Dressing, H., Riemann, D., & Berger, M. (1994). Treatment of primary insomnia with trimipramine: An alternative to BZD hypnotics? *European Archives of Psychiatry and Clinical Neuroscience*, 244(2), 65–72.

Jonas, J. M., Coleman, B. S., Sheridan, A. Q., & Kalinske, R. W. (1992). Comparative clinical profiles of triazolam versus other shorter-acting hypnotics. *Journal of Clinical Psychiatry*, 53(12, Suppl.), 19–33.

Kramer, P. D. (1982). Insomnia: Importance of the differential diagnosis. *Psychosomatics*, 23, 129–137.

Lamphere, J., Roeher, T., Zorick, F., Koshorek, G., & Roth, T. (1986). Chronic hypnotic efficacy of estazolam. *Drugs in Experimental Clinical Research*, 12(8), 687–691.

Mellinger, G. D., Balter, M. B., & Uhlenhuth, E. H. (1985). Insomnia and its treatment. *Archives of General Psychiatry*, 42, 225–232.

Mendels, J. (1994). Evaluation of the safety and efficacy of quazepam for the treatment of insomnia in psychiatric outpatients. *Journal of Clinical Psychiatry, 55*(2), 60–65.

Mendelson, W. (1992). Clinical distinctions between long-acting and short-acting benzodiazepines. *Journal of Clinical Psychiatry, 53*(12, Suppl.), 4–7.

Monane, M. (1992). Insomnia in the elderly. *Journal of Clinical Psychiatry, 53*(6, Suppl.), 23–28.

Montgomery, I., Oswald, I., Morgan, K., & Adam, K. (1983). Trazodone enhances sleep and subjective quality but not in objective duration. *British Journal of Clinical Pharmacology, 16,* 139–144.

Moran, M. G., Thomson, T., & Nies, A. S. (1988). Sleep disorders in the elderly. *American Journal of Psychiatry, 145*(1), 1369–1378.

Moun, C. M., Culbert, J. P., & Schwartz, S. M. (1991). Non-pharmacological interventions for insomnia: A meta-analysis of treatment efficacy. *American Journal of Psychiatry, 151*(8), 1172–1180.

Nierenberg, A. A., Adler, H. A., Peselow, E., Zornberg, G., & Rosenthal, M. (1994). Trazodone for cannibis induced insomnia. *American Journal of Psychiatry, 151*(7), 1069–1072.

Nierenberg, A. A., & Keck, P. E. (1989). Management of monoamine oxidase inhibitor-associated insomnia with trazodone. *Journal of Clinical Psychopharmacology, 1,* 42–45.

Nino-Murcia, G. (1992). Diagnosis and treatment of insomnia and risks associated with lack of treatment. *Journal of Clinical Psychiatry, 53*(12, Suppl.), 43–49.

Prince, J., Wilens, T., Spencer, T., Wozniak, J., & Biederman, J. (1994). *Clonidine for ADHD-related sleep disturbance: A systematic review of 47 cases.* Paper presented at the Annual Meeting of the American Academy of Child and Adolescent Psychiatry, New York.

Prinz, P. N., Vitiello, M. V., Raskind, M. A., & Thorpy, M. J. (1990). Geriatrics: Sleep disorders and aging. *New England Journal of Medicine, 323,* 520.

Regestein, Q. R. (1976). Treating insomnia: A practical guide for managing chronic sleeplessness, circa 1975. *Comprehensive Psychiatry, 17*(4), 517–526.

Regestein, Q. R. (1987). Specific effects of sedative/hypnotic drugs in the treatment of incapacitating chronic insomnia. *American Journal of Medicine, 83,* 909–916.

Regestein, Q. R., & Reich, P. (1983). Incapacitating childhood-onset insomnia. *Comprehensive Psychiatry, 24*(3), 244–248.

Reite, M., Buysse, D., Reynolds, C., & Mendelson, W. (1995). The use of polysomnography in the evaluation of insomnia. *Sleep, 18*(1), 58–70.

Reynolds, C. F., Kupfer, D. J., Buysse, D. J., Coble, P. A., & Yeager, A. (1991). Subtyping DSM-III-R primary insomnia: A literature review by the DSM-IV work group on sleep disorders. *American Journal of Psychiatry, 148,* 423–438.

Reynolds, C. F., Kupfer, D. J., Hoch, C. C., & Sewitch, D. E. (1985a). Sleeping pills for the elderly: Are they ever justified? *Journal of Clinical Psychiatry, 46,* 9–12.

Reynolds, C. F., Kupfer, D. J., Taska, L. S., Hoch, C. C., Sewitch, D. E., & Spiker, D. G. (1985b). Sleep of healthy seniors: A revisit. *Sleep, 8,* 20–30.

Reynolds, C. F., Taska, L. S., & Sewitch, D. E. (1984). Persistent psychophysiologic insomnia: Preliminary research diagnostic criteria and EEG sleep data. *American Journal of Psychiatry, 141,* 804–805.

Rosekind, M. R. (1992). The epidemiology and occurrence of insomnia. *Journal of Clinical Psychiatry, 53*(6, Suppl.), 4–6.

Scharf, M. B., Roth, T., & Vogel, G. W. (1994). A multicenter placebo controlled study evaluating zolpidem in the treatment of chronic insomnia. *Journal of Clinical Psychiatry, 55*(5), 192–199.

Scharf, M. B., & Sachias, B. A. (1990). Sleep laboratory evaluation of the effects and efficacy of trazodone in depressed insomniac patients. *Journal of Clinical Psychiatry, 51*(9), 13–17.

Schweitzer, P. K., Koshorek, G., Muehlback, M. J., & Morris, D. D. (1991). Effects of estazolam and triazolam on transient insomnia associated with phase-shifted sleep. *Human Psychopharmacology, 6*(2), 99–107.

Spielman, A. J., Suskin, P., & Thorpy, M. J. (1987). Treatment of chronic insomnia by restriction of time in bed. *Sleep, 10,* 45–57.

Standards of Practice Committee, American Sleep Disorders Association. (1995). An American Sleep Disorders Association report: Practice parameters for the use of polysomnography in the evaluation of insomnia. *Sleep, 18*(1), 55–57.

Stepanski, E. J. (1994). Behavioral therapy for insomnia. In T. Roth, M. H. Kryger, & W. C. Dement (Eds.), *Principles and practice of sleep medicine.* Philadelphia: W. B. Saunders.

Tan, T. L., Kales, J. D., Kales, A., Martin, E. D., Mann, L. D., & Soldatos, C. R. (1987). Inpatient multidimensional management of treatment-resistant insomnia. *Psychosomatics, 28,* 266–272.

Tollefson, G. D., Greist, J. H., Jefferson, J. W., Heiligenstein, J. H., Saylor, M. E., Tollefson, S. L., & Koback, K. (1994). Is baseline agitation a relative contraindication for a selective serotonin reuptake inhibitor?: A comparative trial of fluoxetine versus imipramine. *Journal of Clinical Psychopharmacology, 14,* 385–391.

Walsh, J. K., Moss, K. L., & Sugarman, J. (1994). Insomnia in adult psychiatric disorders. In T. Roth, M. H. Kryger, & W. C. Dement (Eds.), *Principles and practice of sleep medicine* (pp. 500–508). Philadelphia: W. B. Saunders.

Ware, J. C. (1983). Tricyclic antidepressants in the treatment of insomnia. *Journal of Clinical Psychiatry, 44,* 25–28.

Weilburg, J. B. (1995). Approach to the patient with insomnia. In L. A. May, A. H. Goroll, & A. G. Mulley (Eds.), *Primary care medicine* (pp. 1062–1066). Philadelphia: J. B. Lippincott.

Weilburg, J. B., & Winkleman, J. (in press). Sleep disorders in general hospital patients. *Journal of Clinical Psychiatry.*

Weitzman, E. D., Czeisler, C. A., Coleman, R. M., Spielman, A. J., Zimmerman, J. C., & Dement, W. (1981). Delayed sleep phase syndrome. *Archives of General Psychiatry, 38,* 737–746.

Wooten, V. (1994). Medical causes of insomnia. In T. Roth, M. H. Kryger, W. C. Dement (Eds.), *Principles and practice of sleep medicine* (pp. 509–522). Philadelphia: W. B. Saunders.

Zorick, F. (1994). Overview of insomnia. In T. Roth, M. H. Kryger, & W. C. Dement (Eds.), *Principles and practice of sleep medicine* (pp. 483–486). Philadelphia: W. B. Saunders.

Zorick, F., Roth, T., Hartze, K., Piccone, P. M., & Stepanski, E. J. (1981). Evaluation and diagnosis of persistent insomnia. *American Journal of Psychiatry, 138*(6), 769–773.

V

TREATMENT-EMERGENT SIDE EFFECTS

18

Management of Antidepressant-Induced Side Effects

MARK H. POLLACK
JORDAN W. SMOLLER

Antidepressant agents have been the mainstay of pharmacologic treatment of patients suffering from mood and anxiety disorders over the past 30 years. The effectiveness of the tricyclic antidepressants (TCAs), selective serotonin reuptake inhibitors (SSRIs), monoamine oxidase inhibitors (MAOIs), and other antidepressants is well established; however, patients are often treated with suboptimal doses of antidepressants, either because of their own failure to adhere to the prescribed dosage regimen or because of their physicians' failure to prescribe adequate doses (Keller et al., 1982). The low-level pharmacotherapy may be explained in part by patients' and physicians' concern with the potential side effects of these medications. An examination of treatment of depression in the primary care setting by Katon et al. (1990) demonstrated that adequate pharmacotherapy was prescribed at relatively low rates in a group of depressed high utilizers of primary care. However, the likelihood of receiving adequate pharmacotherapy and remaining in treatment over time was correlated with the type of antidepressant medication prescribed: Patients receiving the better-tolerated antidepressants such as the secondary amine TCAs, (e.g., desipramine or nortriptyline), or newer antidepressants including the SSRIs, were more likely to remain in treatment than those receiving the older antidepressants, which have more side effects (e.g., amitriptyline). Simon, Von Korff, and Katon (1994), in a study of treatment of depression in a primary care setting, found that SSRI-treated patients were more likely to receive adequate levels of treatment, and patients for whom treatment was initiated with a TCA were likely over time to end up switching to an SSRI, presumably because of the SSRIs' greater tolerability.

Administration of adequate doses of antidepressants, both acutely and during maintenance treatment, is critical to achieving a sustained remission in depressed patients (Frank et al., 1990). The high rate of relapse associated with treatment discontinuation suggests that many depressed patients may require long-term treatment with antidepressants (Thase, 1990). Successful management of depression thus hinges in part on a patient's ability to tolerate full doses of antidepressants for extended periods of time. Critical to the effort to optimize outcome and facilitate administration of medication at adequate doses over time are the availability of better-tolerated antidepressants and the timely management of treatment-emergent adverse effects.

Management of antidepressant-induced side effects is critical to enhancing patient compliance. Compliance with a prescribed medication regimen diminishes as the incidence and severity of side effects increase (Christensen, 1978; Madden, 1973). The prescription of subtherapeutic doses of antidepressants, or rapid abandonment of treatment with one agent to switch to another in response to the emergence of side effects, can significantly prolong the period of untreated illness or promote relapse in patients responding to pharmacologic therapy. Many depressed patients who are labeled "treatment-resistant" or have residual symptoms after initial treatment respond to an increase in dosage (Fava et al., 1992). Attention to treatment-emergent adverse side effects may facilitate the dose increases necessary for successful treatment of refractory patients. Furthermore, a physician's concern about side effects and competence in responding to them enhance the therapeutic alliance with the patient and minimize premature abandonment of treatment.

PRINCIPLES OF SIDE EFFECT MANAGEMENT

A number of general principles apply to the treatment of all patients who may develop antidepressant-induced side effects:

1. Probable side effects should be anticipated with the patient. Some clinicians may avoid discussion of adverse effects, because of the belief that such discussion may produce side effects in suggestible patients. However, unanticipated side effects negatively alter the perceived value of medication and contribute to noncompliance (Becker & Maiman, 1975). Understandable explanations prevent a patient from becoming discouraged when side effects arise, and as predictions fulfilled may be paradoxically reassuring and increase the patient's confidence in the physician. Straightforward explanations about the mechanisms underlying side effects and potential management strategies may allay the patient's concerns and reduce

the sense of helplessness often engendered when side effects do emerge. It is helpful to follow discussion of potential side effects with an explanation of management interventions that will be used to minimize the patient's discomfort. For instance, when a clinician is initiating treatment with an SSRI, the following discussion may be useful:

> I'm starting you on this medication because I think it will be helpful for your condition. Most people tolerate the medication well. However, if you do have side effects they may include problems falling asleep, so we'll have you take the medication in the morning rather than at night. You may get an upset stomach, so take the pills after you eat breakfast and have some food in your stomach. If the stomach trouble persists, I can give you some other medication to help. You may feel a little bit more anxious for the first few days after starting the medication, so I'm going to have you start on a lower-than-usual dose to minimize that problem. In addition, some people experience difficulties with their sexual function while taking this medication. If this becomes a problem for you, there are a number of things we can do to try to counteract it.

Thus, the clinician has informed the patient of common potential side effects, but also informed him or her that various management strategies and "antidotes" are available to minimize possible distress.

2. Perhaps the most effective treatment strategy is prevention of side effects through appropriate drug selection. Many adverse side effects may be predicted from the neuropharmacologic profile of the medications, and may be minimized by judicious selection of appropriate agents. In general, the newer antidepressants—including the SSRIs (e.g., fluoxetine, sertraline, paroxetine, fluvoxamine), venlafaxine, and atypical antidepressants (e.g., bupropion, nefazadone)—are better tolerated than the older TCAs, with fewer side effects attributable to blockade of cholinergic, alpha-adrenergic, and histaminergic receptors. Among the TCAs, the secondary amines (e.g., desipramine and nortriptyline) generally have a more favorable side effect profile than the tertiary amines (e.g., imipramine, doxepin, and amitriptyline).

3. Whereas previous recommendations (Pollack & Rosenbaum, 1987) included an attempt to embark on a systematic, gradual effort to determine the lowest effective dose of medication as a means of reducing side effects, current evidence suggests that lowering the dose from that necessary to achieve acute remission increases the risk of relapse in depressed patients (Frank et al., 1990). Thus, attempts to manage side effects by dose reduction should in general be avoided, and other strategies should be adopted. However, elderly patients, children and adolescents, and those with organic brain syndromes may require and only tolerate lower doses of medication (Greenblatt, Sellers, & Shader, 1982).

4. Parallel to recommendations regarding the use of adjunctive treatment strategies for depressed patients who fail to respond to an antidepres-

sant trial (Fava et al., 1994), the most efficient treatment approach to emergent side effects often involves managing them with the judicious use of adjunctive agents, rather than precipitous discontinuation and switching to a different antidepressant. Rapid switching among antidepressants to decrease side effects may delay therapeutic response and result in relapse in responsive patients. In addition, as every antidepressant may have some side effects, "switching rather than fighting" may result in a new or similar set of difficulties while prolonging the duration of the patient's distress.

5. Adverse effects often diminish with time. Strategies to manage side effects can extend the period that the patient will tolerate treatment and "buy time" until adverse effects diminish spontaneously.

6. Many side effects traditionally associated with the use of antidepressant medication may be manifestations of the underlying disorder for which pharmacotherapy is being prescribed, and may improve with effective treatment. It is not always possible to distinguish medication-induced adverse effects from those secondary to mood or anxiety disorders, though symptoms that begin after initiation of treatment or get worse in a dose-dependent fashion are more likely to be medication-related. Though the association of some types of side effects with particular classes of agents may be unlikely because of their pharmacodynamic profile (e.g., the possibility of an SSRI's causing orthostatic hypotension), it is a truism that unanticipated adverse effects may occur with any agent; patients are rarely mollified by assurance that symptoms are "impossible" on their particular medication. Fortunately, some symptoms, regardless of etiology, will improve with appropriate management strategies.

In the remainder of this chapter, we review a number of the more commonly encountered adverse effects associated with administration of the antidepressants, and discuss interventions that improve a patient's comfort and compliance with treatment.

SEXUAL DYSFUNCTION

Sexual dysfunction associated with antidepressants is common, though often unrecognized, and is likely to be an occult reason why patients discontinue pharmacotherapy (Pollack, Reiter, & Hammerness, 1992). Patients may not report sexual difficulties because of embarrassment or confusion as to their cause; they may attribute their unwillingness to continue treatment to other adverse effects or difficulties. Clinicians should have a high index of suspicion for antidepressant-induced sexual difficulties, and, should query about sexual functioning both prior to treatment initiation and as part of the ongoing review of neurovegetative symptomatology at follow-up visits. Estimates vary as to the prevalence of sexual dysfunction attendant to antidepressants. Although package inserts tend to report an incidence in the range of 1–15% of treated patients, clinical experience and numerous reports suggest that the true prevalence is much higher (Herman et al., 1990; *Physicians' Desk Reference*, 1995). Harrison et al. (1986) reported that about one-third of TCA-treated patients and 40% of MAOI-treated patients experienced sexual dysfunction on medication; the prevalence of sexual dysfunction among SSRI-treated patients appears to be in this range. The incidence of its occurrence with the recently introduced agents nefazadone is reportedly low (Preskorn, 1995), an observation awaiting confirmation in further clinical experience. Among other available agents, bupropion appears to have relatively less propensity to cause sexual dysfunction (Gardner & Johnston, 1985).

The mechanism of action by which antidepressants affect sexual function is incompletely understood (Pollack et al., 1992). Normal sexual functioning is the result of a complex interaction of central and peripheral neurophysiologic functions, including sympathetic and parasympathetic autonomic activity, neurotransmitters (including serotonin, norepinephrine, acetylcholine, and dopamine), and hormones (including testosterone and estrogens); antidepressants may affect sexual function at a number of these levels (Segraves, 1989). Although erectile and ejaculatory disturbances may make sexual side effects more obvious in men, sexual dysfunction associated with antidepressant therapy is likely to occur with equal frequency in men and women (Gitlin, 1994).

Domains of sexual function that can be affected by antidepressants include (1) libido, (2) excitement (including erection in men and lubrication in women), (3) ejaculatory disturbance in men, and (4) orgasm in men and women.

Decreased Libido

Decreased libido as a side effect of antidepressant therapy may be difficult to distinguish from that related to the mood or anxiety disorder at which treatment is targeted. However, decreased libido that persists or worsens as the other psychiatric symptoms improve suggests the presence of a medication-induced adverse effect.

Impaired Erection

Difficulty in achieving or maintaining erection (and, rarely, penile anesthesia) may occur secondary to antidepressant administration (Mitchell & Popkin, 1983; Neill, 1991). Penile erection is primarily under parasympathetic control, and its disruption by antidepressants is presumably secondary to blockade at the cholinergic and perhaps alpha-adrenergic receptors (Pollack et al., 1992).

Priapism, a prolonged and painful engorgement of the penis, has been associated with the use of trazodone as well as a number of antipsychotics in frequencies of 1 per every 1000–10,000 men treated (Thompson, Ware, & Blashfield, 1990). It may occur secondary to the agent's $alpha_1$-adrenergic receptor blockade in the absence of anticholinergic activity, preventing detumescence of the engorged penis (Thompson et al., 1990). Priapism with trazodone usually occurs within the first 4 weeks of treatment (although it has occurred as late as 18 months after treatment initiation), and it can occur at any dose level (Warner, Peabody, Whiteford, & Hollister, 1987). The condition may occur without warning, although some patients may experience prodromal symptoms (unusual, painful, or frequent erections, or urination difficulties). Men taking trazodone should be warned about this potential side effect and instructed to discontinue medication immediately if any unusual erectile or urologic activity occurs. Priapism is a medical emergency necessitating evaluation by a urologist. It may respond to injection of alpha-adrenergic agonists such as metaraminol or to saline injection into the corpus cavernosa, promoting venoconstriction and detumescence; or to surgical interventions (Thompson et al., 1990)

Impaired Ejaculation

Ejaculation involves both parasympathetic and sympathetic activity (DeGroat & Booth, 1980). Retarded or delayed ejaculation, painful ejaculation, and anhedonic ejaculation (ejaculation without orgasm) (Pollack et al., 1992) have all been associated with antidepressant administration. The propensity of antidepressants to inhibit or delay ejaculation has been exploited therapeutically for the treatment of premature ejaculation (e.g., fluoxetine, 10–20 mg/day; sertraline, 50 mg/day; or paroxetine, 20–40 mg/day) (Waldinger, Hengeveld, & Zwinderman, 1994).

Orgasmic Dysfunction

Delayed orgasm or anorgasmia has been reported with the use of the TCAs, MAOIs, SSRIs, and atypical antidepressants (Gitlin, 1994). Orgasmic response is mediated in part by the inhibitory input of central serotonergic neurons and the excitatory effects of dopaminergic neurons (Pollack et al., 1992). Antidepressant-induced anorgasmia is presumed to be secondary to increased serotonergic activity. However, the effects of these agents on orgasmic function remain complex; spontaneous orgasms while yawning have been reported by patients on clomipramine (a serotonergic TCA) and fluoxetine (McLean, Forsythe, & Kapkin, 1983; Modell, 1989). Bupropion appears less likely to cause inhibited sexual function than other antidepressants (Gardner & Johnston, 1985), and we have found that an occasional patient experiences marked and even uncomfortable increases in libido associated with bupropion therapy.

Management of Sexual Dysfunction

There are relatively few systematic data available on the treatment of antidepressant-induced sexual dysfunction; however, a number of interventions have been found to be useful in clinical practice, case reports, and case series.

Yohimbine

Yohimbine is an alpha$_2$-adrenergic presynaptic inhibitor that increases norepinephrine and other catecholamines in the synapses. It has been demonstrated to be effective for male erectile impotence in controlled trials (Susset et al., 1989), and has been reported to increase libido and improve erectile and orgasmic functioning in patients treated with TCAs, SSRIs, and bupropion (Hollander & McCarley, 1992; Jacobsen, 1992; Pollack & Hammerness, 1993; Price & Grunhaus, 1990).

Yohimbine may cause increased anxiety and induce panic attacks in predisposed individuals; thus, treatment should be initiated at low doses, which should be titrated up slowly to minimize the development of anxiety. Dosing should start at 2.7 mg/day (one-half tablet) and should be increased every 2–3 days as tolerated by half a pill up to 5.4 mg (one pill) three times a day; occasional patients may require and benefit from doses of 30–45 mg/day (two or three pills three times a day). Patients may begin to respond a few days to a few weeks after initiation of treatment, and the trial should last at least a month to determine its effectiveness. Side effects of yohimbine may include increased anxiety, nausea, lightheadedness, and sweating. Because it acutely increases noradrenergic transmission, yohimbine should not be used in conjunction with MAOIs, in order to avoid a hypertensive reaction.

Some clinicians prescribe yohimbine and other adjunctive agents on an "as-needed" basis, 1–2 hours prior to intercourse. Although this schedule may be useful for some patients, we find that using yohimbine and other augmentation agents for sexual functioning on this basis may limit their effectiveness because patients are unable to "schedule" intercourse, find the decreased spontaneity off-putting, or experience increased performance anxiety when anticipating sexual activity after taking a medication. Thus, we generally prescribe yohimbine and the other adjunctive agents to be taken on a regular schedule.

Dopamine Agonists

Dopamine has a stimulatory effect on sexual arousal (Hyyppa, Falck, Aukia, & Rinne, 1975). A number of agents with dopaminergic properties have been used to treat decreased libido, as well as erectile, ejaculatory, and orgasmic dysfunction induced by antidepressants.

Amantadine (100 mg two or three times a day) was reported to reverse SSRI-induced decreased libido, erectile dysfunction, and anorgasmia (Balogh, Hendricks, & Kang, 1992). In our experience, pergolide initiated at 50 µg and titrated up by 100 µg (0.1 mg) every 2–3 days up to 2–5 mg/day in once- or twice-daily dosing may be used to treat antidepressant-induced sexual dysfunction, as well as being useful for treatment-refractory depressed patients (Bouckoms & Mangini, 1993). Bromocriptine, a potent dopaminergic agonist, may also be used to treat antidepressant-induced sexual dysfunction (2.5–10 mg/day in once- or twice-daily dosing), but is often poorly tolerated by patients because of gastrointestinal (GI) distress, sedation, and increased anxiety. Bupropion, an antidepressant with weak dopaminergic properties, has been used as an adjunct (75–100 mg once or twice a day) to reverse SSRI-induced sexual dysfunction in men and women (Labatte & Pollack, 1994). For some patients, a switch to monotherapy with bupropion may be useful (Walker et al., 1993), although many patients benefit from its use as an adjunct without the need for three-times-per-day dosing.

Cyproheptadine

Cyproheptadine is an agent with multiple properties, including antihistaminic and antiserotonergic effects. It has been reported to be helpful in reversing anorgasmia and libidinal, ejaculatory, and erectile dysfunction for patients on SSRIs, TCAs, and MAOIs (DeCastro, 1985; McCormick, Olin, & Brotman, 1990; Steele & Howell, 1986). Unfortunately, cyproheptadine can be difficult for some patients to tolerate because of sedation and significant weight gain. It should be initiated at a low dose (e.g., half a pill [2 mg] at bedtime) and titrated up to one to four pills (4–16 mg) per day, typically in once- or twice-a-day dosing. Some patients taking SSRIs have noted a loss of therapeutic antidepressant effect when they are placed on cyproheptadine; this presumably results from the antagonism of serotonergic effects (Feder, 1991).

Cholinergic Agonists

Cholinergic agents such as bethanechol (10–80 mg/day, given in twice-daily doses) or neostigmine (7.5–15 mg a half hour before sexual intercourse), have been reported helpful in enhancing libido (Kraupl-Taylor, 1972). However, clinical experience suggests that these agents are most likely to be effective for improving erectile potency and reversing ejaculatory retardation in men.

Other Agents

Buspirone (10–20 mg three times a day) has occasionally been helpful for reversing anorgasmia and other sexual dysfunction on serotonergic antidepressants. It may also be a useful adjunct for treatment-refractory depression in some cases (Bakish, 1991).

General Comments

There is no information from controlled studies demonstrating the relative response rates of these different interventions for antidepressant sexual dysfunction, which are summarized in Table 18.1. Our clinical experience has been that yohimbine, the dopaminergic agonists, and buspirone may be effective in as many as 40–50% of men and women for disturbances of libido, excitement, and orgasm, whereas the cholinergic agonists and cyproheptadine may be useful somewhat less frequently. In many cases, the sequential use of different adjunctive strategies may be necessary to find an effective agent for relief of antidepressant-associated sexual dysfunction; sometimes these adverse effects remit spontaneously over time

GASTROINTESTINAL DISTRESS

Patients receiving an antidepressant may experience significant GI distress, including dyspepsia, gas pain, nausea, bloating, diarrhea, and constipation. For most patients, the difficulties are time-limited, beginning during treatment initiation and remitting within a few days or weeks; however, some patients have persistent difficulties. Table 18.2 summarizes the intervention for the various forms of GI distress.

Nausea and Dyspepsia

Patients can often reduce dyspepsia or nausea by taking an antidepressant medication after meals or dividing up the daily dose rather than taking it once a day. Over-the-counter antacids may sometimes be helpful

TABLE 18.1. Agents Used in the Treatment of Antidepressant-Induced Sexual Dysfunction

Agent	Dose[a]
Yohimbine (Yocon)	5.4–16.2 mg b.i.d.–t.i.d.
Dopaminergic agonists	
Amantadine (Symmetrel)	100 mg t.i.d.–q.i.d.
Bupropion (Wellbutrin)	75–100 mg b.i.d.
Pergolide (Permax)	0.5–1.25 mg q.i.d.
Bromocriptine (Parlodel)	2.5–5.0 mg b.i.d.–q.i.d.
Buspirone (BuSpar)	10–20 mg t.i.d.
Cyproheptadine (Periactin)	4 mg q.d.–q.i.d.
Bethanechol (Urecholine)	10–20 mg q.d.–q.i.d.

[a]Abbreviations here and in Tables 18.2–18.3: q.d, every day; b.i.d., twice a day; t.i.d., three times a day; q.i.d., four times a day.

as well. A number of adjunctive agents have also proven useful for dyspepsia or nausea secondary to antidepressants:

1. The newer histamine (H_2) blockers, such as nizatidine (15–30 mg/day) famotidine (20–40 mg/day), or ranitidine (150 mg once or twice a day), may reduce nausea and dyspepsia secondary to SSRIs and other antidepressants. These agents have generally been well tolerated in clinical experience.

2. Cisapride (5 mg by mouth twice a day), a serotonin ($5\text{-}HT_3$) antagonist, has been reported to alleviate nausea induced by SSRIs (Bergeron & Blier, 1994).

3. Metoclopramide, an agent used to treat esophageal reflux and gastroparesis, has been used clinically to reduce antidepressant- and lithium-induced dyspepsia and nausea. Dosing is initiated at 5 mg/day and titrated up to 10–15 mg one to four times a day. Metoclopramide has dopamine-blocking properties, however, and may cause extrapyramidal symptoms and even tardive dyskinesia, so it should be used over the short term (4–12 weeks) and discontinued when possible.

Diarrhea

Among the antidepressants, the SSRIs may be more likely to cause diarrhea. For some patients this may remit after a few weeks of treatment, but for others it may persist. Management interventions that sometimes prove helpful include typical antidiarrheal agents, including diphenoxylate hydrochloride (5 mg two to four times a day); or over-the-counter remedies. Cypropheptadine (2–4 mg one or two times a day), an antihistamine with anti-serotonergic properties has also been useful for SSRI-induced diarrhea, as has use of Acidophilus culture (available in capsules) at a dose of 1 capsule/meal.

Constipation

Anticholinergic effects on the GI tract cause decreased intestinal motility, with consequent increased water absorption from the bowel and production of stool that is dry, hard, and difficult to pass. Constipation can be particularly uncomfortable or even dangerous for the elderly patient, in whom it may progress to severe obstipation with paralytic ileus and require emergent medical consultation.

Patients should be instructed to increase fluid intake as well as dietary bulk (i.e., vegetables, fruits, and whole grains). If other interventions are necessary, an over-the-counter bulk laxative (e.g., Metamucil, 1–2 tbsp. every morning) or other over-the-counter hydrophilic preparations (e.g., docussate sodium [Colace], 100 mg by mouth two to three times a day) may be used to soften the stool. Over-the-counter cathartic laxatives such as Milk of Magnesia (30 cc by mouth every day) can be used acutely or

TABLE 18.2. Strategies for the Treatment of Gastrointestinal Distress

Dyspepsia and nausea

Dose after meals

Over-the-counter antacids (e.g., Maalox, Mylanta)

H_2 blockers

Nizatidine (Axid), 15–30 mg q.d.

Famotidine (Pepcid), 20–40 mg q.d.

Ranitidine (Zantac), 150 mg q.d.–b.i.d.

Cisapride (Propulsid), 5 mg p.o. b.i.d.

Metoclopramide (Reglan), 10–15 mg q.d.–q.i.d.

Diarrhea

Diphenoxylate hydrochloride (Lomotil), 5 mg b.i.d.–q.i.d.

Cypropheptadine (Periactin), 2–4 mg q.d.–b.i.d.

Acidophilus (1 capsule/meal)

Loperamide (Imodium A-D), 2–4 mg b.i.d.–q.i.d.

Over-the-counter antidiarrheals (e.g., Kaopectate, Imodium A-D)

Constipation

Increase fluid intake and fiber

Over-the-counter laxatives

Metamucil, 1–2 tbsp. q. A.M.

Docussate sodium (Colace), 100 mg b.i.d.–t.i.d.

Milk of Magnesia, 30 cc q.d.

Bethanechol (Urecholine), 10–30 mg q.d.–t.i.d.

intermittently, but prolonged use may be ineffective and lead to intestinal dysmotility, exacerbating the constipation. Bethanechol (10–30 mg by mouth one to three times a day) has been used successfully in a number of patients to relieve antidepressant-induced constipation.

WEIGHT GAIN

For patients in whom significant weight loss is a symptom of depression, the weight gain associated with antidepressant use may be a welcome side effect in the short term. However, weight gain is a significant cause of treatment noncompliance, and may be the most common reason why patients on antidepressants (particularly the TCAs and MAOIs) discontinue treatment over time (Noyes, Garvey, Cook, & Samuelson, 1989). The mechanisms underlying antidepressant-induced weight gain are unknown, but have been hypothesized to include fluid retention, central nervous system (CNS) antihistaminic effects, changes in glucose metabolism, alterations in hypothalamic function, carbohydrate craving, and increased appetite associated with improved mood (Garland, Remick, & Zis, 1988). Clinically, the propensity of antidepressants to cause weight gain is correlated with their blockade of the histaminic receptors. Thus, older TCAs with more potency at the histamine receptors (e.g., amitriptyline, doxepin, and imipramine) are more likely to cause weight gain than the secondary amine TCAs (e.g., desipramine or nortriptyline) (Richelson, 1994). MAOIs may also cause significant weight gain over time, with phenelzine a greater offender than tranylcypromine (Rabkin, Quitkin, McGrath, Harrison, & Tricamo, 1985). Newer agents, such as the SSRIs, bupropion, venlafaxine, and nefazadone, have relatively small effects at the histamine receptors and generally little propensity to cause weight gain. Fluoxetine and the other SSRIs cause some minimal weight loss over the first 6 weeks of treatment, with patients who are markedly overweight losing somewhat more (e.g., 5–10 pounds) and those at normal weight experiencing little effect; patients do not continue to lose weight on the SSRIs during maintenance treatment (Cooper, 1988). Despite their lower propensity to cause weight gain, however, some patients clearly do gain weight on the SSRIs and other new agents.

No specific pharmacologic interventions have been found routinely helpful for treating antidepressant-induced weight gain. On occasion, the addition of anorectic agents (e.g., methylphenidate or fenfluramine) or thyroid hormones may have some short-term benefits in the treatment of obesity, although they have not been systematically studied for antidepressant-related weight gain (Hollingsworth, Amatruda, & Schei, 1970; Silverstone & Kyriakides, 1982). Thus, education and behavioral modifications are critical to reduce medication effects on weight gain. Before initiation of treatment with antidepressants, patients should be warned about the possibility of weight gain and instructed to minimize carbohydrate and fat intake (with low-calorie snacks to satisfy carbohydrate cravings if necessary). Patients who do gain weight need to be fastidious about their dietary intake and should attempt regular exercise commensurate with their age and health. The use of calorie-containing beverages such as sugared sodas to manage dry mouth should be proscribed.

Antidepressant-induced edema can be treated by elevation of the affected limb or administration of a diuretic such as hydrochlorothiazide (25–50 mg by mouth once or twice a day) (Pollack & Rosenbaum, 1987). Serum electrolytes, as well as levels of other medications such as lithium that might be affected by thiazide diuretics, should be monitored if this strategy is employed. Alternatively, a potassium-sparing diuretic such as amiloride (5–10 mg/day) may be used.

CENTRAL NERVOUS SYSTEM EFFECTS

We discuss a number of antidepressant-associated adverse CNS effects, including tremor; agitation and anxiety; fatigue and sedation; sleep disturbances; myoclonus; and paresthesias. In addition, we examine the purported association of antidepressants and increased suicidal ideation.

Tremor

High-frequency tremor is often seen with heterocyclic agents, SSRIs, and occasionally MAOIs, particularly tranylcypromine. Tremulousness may be caused or exacerbated by anxiety, and may respond to treatment with benzodiazepines, psychologic management, or other anxiolytic intervention. When antidepressant-induced tremor is worsened by caffeine intake, it may respond to a reduction in intake or a switch to decaffeinated beverages.

Antiparkinsonian agents (e.g., benztropine) are generally not as effective for antidepressant-induced tremors as they are for neuroleptic-induced tremor. Propranolol (10–20 one to three times a day) or atenolol (50–150 mg/day) may reduce tremor, as may low doses of benzodiazepines such as lorazepam (1.0–2.0 mg two to four times a day) or clonazepam (0.5–2.0 mg once or twice a day).

Increased Anxiety or Agitation

Although anxiety or agitation is most commonly reported as a concomitant of TCA therapy (Pohl, Yeragani, Balon, & Lycaki, 1988), initiation of most non-MAOI antidepressant therapy may be associated with increased anxiety, agitation, restlessness, and autonomic symptoms of arousal, particularly in patients with anxiety disorders or in those with anxious, agitated depression. In order to prevent premature abandonment of therapy, it is critical to anticipate the occurrence of these symptoms with predisposed individuals, reassure them that the symptoms are time-limited, and review steps that will be taken to minimize symptom impact. Patients at risk should initially be treated with low doses of the antidepressant (e.g., a "test dose" of 10–25 mg of imipramine or 5–10 mg of fluoxetine). Close to half of panic patients in one reported series discontinued fluoxetine when treatment was initiated at 20 mg/day (Gorman et al., 1987), whereas most responded positively to the drug when it was initiated at lower doses (Schneier et al., 1990). Once a patient is acclimated to the antidepressant within the first week or two of treatment, the dose may be titrated up to therapeutic levels. Some anxious or panic patients may benefit from the concurrent initiation of an antidepressant and a benzodiazepine, such as clonazepam (0.5 mg by mouth once or twice a day), lorazepam (0.5–1.0 mg/day, in once-daily to four-times-daily dosing), or alprazolam (0.5 mg four times a day). The benzodiazepine may sometimes be tapered and discontinued after 2–3 weeks, although many patients feel well on the combined treatment, are reluctant to discontinue the benzodiazepine and are appropriately maintained on the combination. Combined antidepressant and benzodiazepine treatment may diminish discomforting anxiety symptoms associated with antidepressant initiation and provide immediate relief of anxiety symptoms prior to the onset of therapeutic effect of the antidepressant. For some patients, restlessness on SSRIs may resemble neuroleptic-induced akathisia, with restlessness, pacing, purposeless movements, and anxiety (Lipinski, Mallya, Zimmerman, & Pope, 1989). This syndrome may respond to the addition of propranolol (20–40 mg two to four times a day) or clonazepam (0.5–2.0 mg once or twice a day).

Fatigue and Sedation

The TCAs vary in their propensity to cause sedation; the agents with greater antihistaminic and antiadrenergic properties (e.g., amitriptyline and doxepin) are the most sedating, and desipramine is among the least sedating. The non-TCA trazodone is also very sedating—a property that has been exploited therapeutically in its use as a soporific for patients on SSRIs and MAOIs (Nierenberg, Adler, Peselow, Zornberg, & Rosenthal, 1994). Although use of a sedating antidepressant may hasten sleep onset and improve sleep maintenance, many patients receiving these agents report morning "hangover" and daytime sedation; elderly patients may experience confusion, dizziness and ataxia if they get up at night to use the bathroom, and thus are at risk of serious injury from falls (Carr & Hobson, 1977).

Daytime fatigue and sluggishness or "poop-out" have been noted in some patients receiving MAOIs or SSRIs (Hoehn-Saric et al., 1991; Joffe, 1990; Teicher, Cohen, Baldessarini, & Cole, 1988). Patients can often distinguish this effect from the mood disturbance associated with depression. Sometimes this occurs after months of treatment in which a patient has experienced improved energy, and it may or may not be associated with nighttime insomnia. The mechanism of this effect is not clear. For patients in whom daytime sedation is associated with nighttime insomnia, the sleep disturbance may be corrected with the addition of a hypnotic (e.g., lorazepam, 1–2 mg at bedtime). For some patients, switching to nighttime dosing may relieve daytime sedation. Reduction in dose or a "drug holiday" of 2–4 weeks may also be helpful, although this may result in a relapse of the mood or anxiety disorder. For some patients, judicious use of caffeinated beverages during the day may reduce fatigue. For some patients on SSRIs, addition of low doses of stimulating antidepressants to the SSRIs (e.g., desipramine, 25–50 mg/day or bupropion 75–100 mg once or twice a day), with attention to TCA plasma levels because of SSRI inhibition of TCA hepatic metabolism, may be useful for fatigue as well as refractory depression (Weilburg, Rosenbaum, Meltzer-Brody, & Shustari, 1991). Addition of stimulants (e.g., methylphenidate, 10–40 mg/day; pemoline, 18.75–112.5 mg/day) may also be helpful. Other adjunctive strate-

TABLE 18.3. Strategies for the Treatment of Antidepressant-Induced Fatigue and Sedation

---

Correct sleep disturbance (e.g., bedtime hypnotic)

Bedtime dosing

Lower dose/"drug holiday"

Caffeine

Adding another antidepressant to an SSRI
  Desipramine (Norpramin), 25–50 mg/day
  Bupropion (75–100 mg once or twice a day)

Adding a stimulant to an SSRI
  Methylphenidate (Ritalin), 10–40 mg/day
  Dextroamphetamine (Dexedrine), 10–20 mg/day
  Pemoline (Cylert), 18.75–112.5 mg/day

Adding dopaminergic agonists to an SSRI or MAOI
  Amantadine (Symmetrel), 100 mg t.i.d.–q.i.d.
  Pergolide (Permax), 0.5–2.0 mg/day
  Bromocriptine, 1–10.0 mg/day

Thyroid supplementation of an SSRI or MAOI
  T_3, 25–50 mg/day

---

gies that have proven useful in clinical practice for fatigue associated with SSRIs or MAOIs include addition of dopaminergic agents (e.g., amantadine, 100 mg three to four times daily; pergolide, 0.5–2.0 mg/day; bromocriptine, 1–10 mg/day) or addition of thyroid hormone (e.g., T_3, 25–50 mg/day). Table 18.3 summarizes the strategies for treating fatigue and sedation.

Disturbed Sleep, Nightmares, and Hypnopompic Activity

Antidepressants may produce disturbed sleep, nightmares, and hypnogogic or hypnopompic activity (abnormal sensations, including hallucinations, while going to sleep or awakening). For TCA-treated patients, these effects may be secondary to medication-induced decreases in rapid-eye-movement sleep and increases in stage 3 and stage 4 sleep (Flemenbaum, 1976). Management strategies for these adverse effects include a change from bedtime to morning dosing, or divided dosing during the daytime. Provision of a benzodiazepine at bedtime may reduce sleep disturbance early in treatment and may be tapered off after onset of the therapeutic effect of the antidepressant. Adjunctive trazodone (50–300 mg at bedtime) has been successfully used to reduce insomnia associated with SSRIs, bupropion, and MAOIs, although the risk of priapism in men must be considered in the risk–benefit analysis (Nierenberg et al., 1994).

Although the SSRIs are typically considered activating, and more sedating agents are often used preferentially for depressed patients with sleep disturbance or agitation, systematic assessment suggests that the SSRIs are as effective as the TCAs for agitated depression and are generally better tolerated (Tollefson et al., 1994). In addition, SSRIs are actually as likely to produce sedation as insomnia (Cooper, 1988). The common strategy of initiating antidepressant treatment with a sedating agent such as amitriptyline or doxepin to treat depression-associated insomnia is often counterproductive because of sedation carryover during the day. The more sedating TCAs are also generally associated with a variety of adverse effects, including weight gain, orthostatic hypotension, and anticholinergic effects, all of which make achieving an adequate dose and maintaining long-term compliance difficult. Moreover, sedating antidepressants and benzodiazepines may decrease respiratory drive at night and promote increased sleep disturbance, particularly in patients with sleep apnea.

Attention to sleep hygiene and to bedtime stimulus control measures is often essential in managing insomnia. These measures include avoidance of caffeinated beverages, reduction in nighttime fluid intake to minimize nocturia, proper room ventilation and darkness, avoidance of daytime naps, and restriction of bedroom activities to sleep or sexual relations (Morin, Culbert, & Schwartz, 1994).

Myoclonus

Patients receiving antidepressants may complain of sudden jerking or twitching movements of their arms and legs; if this occurs at night, it may be severe enough to wake the patients up from sleep or disturb their bed partners. Myoclonus has been reported to occur in up to 40% of patients receiving imipramine; in 9%, it was severe enough to warrant treatment discontinuation (Garvey & Tollefson, 1987). The mechanism of this effect is unknown. Management strategies include changing from bedtime to daytime dosing or divided doses (for nocturnal myoclonus), or lowering the dose. In some cases, the addition of clonazepam (0.5–2.0 mg once or twice a day), trazodone (50–300 mg/day), cyproheptadine (4–16 mg/day), or valproate or carbamazepine at therapeutic levels may also be helpful.

Paresthesias

Numbness and tingling, or swollen, stiff, "pins-and-needles" feelings in the extremities, may occur in conjunction with use of MAOIs and other antidepressants. The paresthesias may be secondary to pyridoxine (vitamin B_6) deficiency induced by MAOI effects on the gastric absorption of this vitamin (Stewart, Harrison, Quitkin, & Liebowitz, 1984). They may respond to pyridoxine (50–150 mg at bedtime); however, excessive doses of vitamin B_6 may cause neuropathy. The addition of small doses of a benzodiazepine (e.g., clonazepam, 0.5–2.0 once or twice a day) may also be helpful.

Suicidal Ideation

Suicidal ideation has been reported as a rare adverse effect of antidepressant treatment (Damulji & Ferguson, 1988). Teicher, Glod, and Cole (1990) reported on a series of six severely depressed inpatients with complex presentations involving comorbid medical and psychiatric conditions, use of multiple medications, and histories of recurrent or refractory depression, who reportedly developed increased suicidal ideation after initiation of treatment with fluoxetine. This report sparked wide concern on the part of the mass media, patients, and professionals as to whether fluoxetine and other antidepressants cause suicidal ideation. Reviews of data from large numbers of patients in clinical trials (Dista Products Company, 1990) and clinical practice (Fava & Rosenbaum, 1991), suggested that increased suicidal ideation after initiation of antidepressant treatment is a very rare, idiosyncratic event and is not associated with any specific antidepressant, including fluoxetine. Most reports of "antidepressant-induced" suicidal ideation probably reflected untreated mood or other Axis I disorders, or were the products of unresolved Axis II pathology. For some patients, particularly those with poor impulse control or aggressiveness, markedly increased agitation and self-destructive impulses may be provoked by stimulating effects or akathisia associated with SSRI and other antidepressant therapy (Lipinski et al., 1989). Antidepressant-associated stimulation and dysphoria may be worsened if initial dosing is aggressively escalated in an attempt to achieve more comprehensive or rapid symptom relief. Antidepressant treatment may induce irritability, mood instability, and mania in patients with a bipolar diathesis, increasing their impulsivity and risk of self-harm. Treatment of these bipolar patients involves discontinuation of the antidepressant, and usually initiation of mood stabilizers.

In general, the risk of suicide attempts provoked by antidepressants can be reduced by effective treatment of the underlying disorder, initiation of treatment with low doses of antidepressants in the anxious or agitated patient, and recognition and treatment of akathisia and mania. The clinician needs to be sensitive to the presence of significant Axis II pathology and interpersonal difficulties, and to be available to patients who develop emergent symptomatology.

ANTICHOLINERGIC EFFECTS

The anticholinergic effects associated with blockade of the muscarinic cholinergic receptors include dry mouth, poor vision, urinary retention, constipation (discussed above in the section on GI distress), and confusion. Antidepressant agents vary widely in their effects at the muscarinic receptors (Richelson, 1994). The SSRIs, bupropion, trazodone, venlafaxine, and MAOIs are less anticholinergic than the secondary amines desipramine and nortriptyline, which are in turn less anticholinergic than the older tertiary amines such as amitriptyline, doxepin, and imipramine. Selection of agents with a low propensity to block the cholinergic receptors is the critical first step in minimizing anticholinergic effects. In addition, specific management strategies may be helpful for the different anticholinergic side effects.

Dry Mouth

Diminished parasympathetic stimulation resulting from muscarinic cholinergic blockade may decrease salivation; this effect can be exacerbated by anxiety or depression. Dry mouth associated with antidepressant therapy may persist over time, and its impact on the patient may vary, depending on its level of intensity and the patient's job and social activity. Persistent decreased salivation may be associated with the development of dental caries, stomatitis, and bad breath.

The patient should be encouraged to use sugarless gum and hard candies to stimulate salivary flow, but to avoid sugar-containing confections, as these may cause weight gain, dental cavities, and infection by sucrose-dependent organisms. Artificial saliva preparations, as well as toothpaste, ointments, and gums marketed specifically to treat xerostomia, may be helpful.

A 1% solution of pilocarpine (a cholinergic agonist indicated for the treatment of glaucoma) used as a mouth rinse three to four times a day will reverse cholinergic blockade and promote salivation (Bernstein, 1983). Patients may use this on an as-needed basis—for instance, when making oral presentations. The solution is prepared by mixing 4% pilocarpine solution and water in a 1:3 proportion.

A 10-mg tablet of bethanechol, a cholinergic agonist, dissolved sublingually may increase salivation (Bernstein, 1983). Bethanechol at a dose of 10–30 mg by mouth one to four times daily also promotes salivation. Dosing is started at low levels and titrated upward until dryness is relieved or adverse reactions to the bethanechol (e.g., abdominal cramping) develop. Other adverse reactions to bethanechol are those of cholinergic stimulation, including diarrhea, tremors, rhinorrhea, and tearing. These effects remit on decreasing or discontinuing the bethanechol. Doses of 10 mg three times a day appear to be safe and effective against a variety of anticholinergic side effects in elderly patients (Rosen, Pollock, Altieri, & Jonas, 1993).

Blurred Vision

Anticholinergic effects of antidepressants on the eyes are generally disturbances of near vision (presbyopia, "farsightedness") caused by pupillary dilation, sluggish reaction to light, and cycloplegia (paresis of the ciliary muscles acting on the lens). Blurred vision secondary to antidepressant therapy often remits within a few weeks after initiation of treatment.

However, for patients in whom visual disturbance persists or becomes markedly distressing, a number of interventions may be helpful.

A 1% solution of pilocarpine drops (one drop three times a day) may restore pupillary responsiveness and improve vision (Klein, Gittelman, Quitkin, & Rifkin, 1980). Bethanechol (10–30 mg one to three times a day) may also improve impaired vision (Bernstein, 1983). A change in prescriptive lenses may be helpful, if the patient is to be maintained on a stable dose of medication for a long period of time and tolerance to the adverse effect does not develop.

Those patients complaining of disturbances in distant vision (myopia, "nearsightedness") may be experiencing difficulties not referable to the antidepressant medication and should receive ophthalmologic evaluation.

Anticholinergic antidepressants may increase intraocular pressure in patients with both open-angle and (the less common form) narrow-angle glaucoma. Patients with narrow-angle glaucoma are at particular risk, because drainage of intraocular fluid may be precipitously compromised as a result of anticholinergic effects, and intraocular pressure may rise dramatically. Patients with a personal or family history of glaucoma, shallow interior chamber on ophthalmologic screening exam, presence of cataracts, farsightedness, history of eye pain, or tendency to see colored halos around lights are all at increased risk of anticholinergic-induced acute narrow-angle glaucoma and should receive ophthalmologic evaluation before initiation of treatment with TCAs. The newer agents lack significant anticholinergic effects and are generally less risky for the glaucoma patient; however, patients with glaucoma may receive anticholinergic antidepressants if the clinician manages their treatment in conjunction with an ophthalmologist, who can monitor and treat abnormal intraocular pressures.

Urinary Retention

Anticholinergic effects on the urinary bladder may cause urinary hesitation, dribbling, decreased flow, atonic bladder with stasis and secondary urinary tract infections, urinary retention, and even renal failure. Elderly patients and those with enlarged prostates or other outflow obstruction are at particular risk for developing these complications. MAOIs and newer agents, including trazodone, bupropion, and the SSRIs, may cause urinary hesitancy or retention in clinical practice, despite a lack of anticholinergic activity.

Clinical experience suggests that urinary hesitation without the presence of mechanical outflow obstruction (e.g., enlarged prostate) can be treated with bethanechol (10–30 mg three times daily), which stimulates contraction of the bladder (Everett, 1975). The use of this agent in patients with an enlarged prostate may be dangerous, however, because forceful contraction of the bladder against a fixed obstruction may damage the bladder. Severe urinary retention mandates discontinuation of the antidepressant and medical consultation. The use of agents with little effect at the muscarinic cholinergic receptors reduces the risk of urinary hesitation, as well as other anticholinergic adverse effects.

Central Anticholinergic Syndrome

The effects of excessive cholinergic blockade in the CNS may be manifested in delirium (including agitation, delusions, hallucinations, restlessness, myoclonic jerking, and choreoathetotic movements), which can occur with or without the presence of peripheral signs of anticholinergic excess (e.g., tachycardia, flushing, pupillary dilation, dry skin, decreased sweating, increased temperature, decreased bowel signs, and urinary retention). Patients may present in this state after accidental or purposeful overdose with TCAs, but delirium may also occur at lower (typically therapeutic) doses in elderly, brain-damaged, or child patients, all of whom may be particularly vulnerable to anticholinergic toxicity. Elderly patients taking multiple medications with anticholinergic effects who become confused or agitated after initiating treatment with TCAs should be suspected of suffering from anticholinergic toxicity, and the antidepressant should be discontinued. Selection of appropriate medication for the elderly should aim at minimizing the anticholinergic load in these individuals.

Central anticholinergic syndrome can be diagnosed and treated with physostigmine (a cholinesterase inhibitor that increases cholinergic transmission), given in one of two ways: 1–2 mg by slow-push intravenous administration (1 mg over 2 minutes) every 30 minutes, or 1–2 mg by intramuscular injection every hour. Physostigmine has a half-life of 1–2 hours, and the initial dose can be repeated in 20 minutes if there is no improvement. Residual agitation can be intramuscularly treated with a benzodiazepine such as lorazepam (0.5–2.0 mg by mouth or intravenously) every 30–60 minutes as needed. Administration of physostigmine should be titrated against the effects on mental status and vital signs (i.e., it should be administered at doses that maintain the pulse above 60 beats per minute). Physostigmine should be avoided in patients with unstable vital signs when possible; life support apparatus and cardiac monitoring equipment should be available when physostigmine is used, since cholinergic stimulation may cause bronchial constriction, hypotension, bradycardia, and abdominal cramping with nausea and vomiting. The adverse effects of physostigmine can be reversed with intravenous atropine (0.5 mg per 1 mg of physostigmine) (Rumach, 1973). Rapid intravenous administration of physostigmine may result in seizures, which can be treated with intravenous diazepam or lorazepam.

Physostigmine is relatively contraindicated in those patients with a history of respiratory distress, asthma, or cardiac conduction abnormality. Its use, especially in these patients, requires careful consideration of the benefits of rapidly reversing the adverse manifestations of continued anticholinergic toxicity, as opposed to the potential adverse consequences of the drug. For many patients, mentation may improve over time as the anticholinergic agent is discontinued, without the need for additional intervention; however, for some, anticholinergic-induced agitation and confusion may cause them to endanger themselves or others and may make overall care impossible until these symptoms are brought under control.

ORTHOSTATIC HYPOTENSION

Orthostatic hypotension is a common adverse effect of the MAOIs, TCAs, and trazodone, and is less commonly associated with treatment with the newer agents (the SSRIs, venlafaxine, bupropion, and perhaps nefazadone). For the non-MAOIs, orthostatic hypotension is presumably secondary to alpha$_1$-adrenergic receptor blockade (Richelson, 1994). Orthostatic hypotension associated with MAOI therapy may be attributable to the accumulation of "false transmitters" that displace catecholamines, or to increased catecholaminergic activation of inhibitory presynaptic alpha$_2$-adrenergic receptors (Baldessarini, 1985). The sensation of lightheadedness may be very distressing for some patients and occasionally dangerous, particularly in the elderly and in those with impaired ability to compensate for drops in blood pressure (e.g., patients receiving antihypertensive medications or those with cardiac disease) when associated with syncopal episodes.

Selection of an agent with a low propensity to block the alpha$_1$-adrenergic receptors (e.g., SSRIs, the other newer antidepressants, desipramine) may reduce the incidence of orthostasis (Richelson, 1994). Among the TCAs, nortriptyline has been reported to have a particularly low propensity to induce orthostatic blood pressure changes (Roose et al., 1981). Orthostasis during the day may sometimes be reduced by bedtime dosing or divided daytime dosing.

Thoughtful assessment may uncover factors that promote or exacerbate antidepressant-induced orthostasis, including a low-salt diet, restricted fluid intake, antihypertensive medications, hypothyroidism, hypoadrenalism, and dehydration. Modification or treatment of these factors may substantially reduce or eliminate hypotension associated with antidepressant treatment (Rabkin et al., 1985).

Patients should be warned about the potential for hypotension. Particularly during the first weeks of dosage adjustment, clinicians should advise patients to rise slowly from the prone position, dangling their feet from their beds or chairs for a full minute before attempting to stand, especially after long periods of lying down. In the event of experiencing lightheadedness on standing and walking, a patient should immediately sit in a chair or on the floor, to avoid a syncopal episode and head trauma or other injury. The use of foot boards and other exercises to strengthen calf muscles may prevent blood pooling in the legs; support hose or stockings and abdominal binders may be helpful as well (Kline, 1981).

Pharmacologic management of antidepressant-induced orthostasis may also be helpful for some patients. Triiodothyronine (T_3, 25–50 mg/day) or thyroxine (T_4, 0.1–0.2 mg/day may reduce antidepressant-induced orthostasis (Bernstein, 1983; Whybrow & Prange, 1981). Methylphenidate (from 10 mg to 30–40 mg/day) or dextroamphetamine (5–20 mg/day) may be useful for orthostasis, and these amphetamines normalized blood pressure in a series of patients treated with combined MAOI and TCA therapy. The stimulants were reported as therapeutic adjuncts to the MAOIs, and none of the patients in this series experienced a hypotensive reaction (Feighner, Herbstein, & Damlouji, 1985). Nonetheless, this combination may be best reserved for patients failing to respond to less aggressive interventions.

For patients on MAOIs, TCAs, or SSRIs, a cup of brewed coffee at the time of the day when symptoms are most pronounced or likely to occur can be helpful. We are not aware of patients on MAOIs experiencing hypertensive reactions as a result of using caffeinated beverages.

Fludrocortisone acetate, a potent mineralocorticoid, reliably alleviates antidepressant-induced hypotension by increasing intravascular sodium and fluid volume (Simonson, 1964). It is administered in doses of 0.1–0.25 mg two to four times a day, and is typically effective within 1–2 weeks of treatment initiation. Salt tablets (600–1800 mg twice a day) may also reduce symptoms of hypotension within a week of their initiation (Munjack, 1984). For some patients, salting their food more heavily or loosening up on salt restrictions may significantly improve feelings of lightheadedness. For most healthy patients, these interventions are safe and well tolerated; however, they may cause significant sodium and fluid retention in individuals with cardiac or renal impairment, and these patients should be carefully monitored for the development of hypertension, edema, congestive heart failure and hypokalemia.

Metoclopramide (10 mg by mouth three times a day) has been reported to reduce antidepressant-induced orthostasis (Patterson, 1987). Despite this drug's potential effectiveness, the risk of tardive dyskinesia because of dopamine blockade restricts its use to more refractory cases. Yohimbine (2.7–10.8 mg one to three times a day) has also been reported effective for maintaining blood pressure in antidepressant-treated patients (LeCrubier, Puech, & Des Lauriers, 1981) although its augmentation of catecholaminergic transmission may provoke hypertensive reactions in patients on MAOIs, and should be avoided in these individuals.

HYPERTENSIVE REACTIONS

Elevated blood pressure is not usually associated with administration of TCA, other heterocyclics, or SSRIs. The main clinical concern regarding hypertension has been the so-called "cheese reaction" in patients taking MAOIs who ingest tyramine (a pressor agent found in a variety of foodstuffs normally destroyed by the intestinal monoamine oxidase enzyme,

MAO-A) or sympathomimetic agents such as ephedrine or other vasoactive cold medications (Blackwell & Cantob, 1963; Harrison, McGrath, Stewart, & Quitkin, 1989; Rabkin, et al., 1985). Comprehensive lists of proscribed foods and medications are available for patient and clinician reference (Janciak, Davis, Preskorn, & Ayd, 1993).

The marked rise in blood pressure in patients on MAOIs may occur minutes to hours after the ingestion of tyramine or sympathomimetic drugs; it is characterized by severe occipital headache, flushing, palpitations, retroorbital pain, nausea, and/or sweating. The elevation of blood pressure may lead to intracerebral bleeding. There have also been a number of reports of spontaneous hypertensive crises without dietary indiscretions in patients taking MAOIs (Keck et al., 1989).

Although transient elevations in blood pressure have been reported with the addition of agents such as bupropion or venlafaxine, these generally do not appear to be clinically significant. The diastolic blood pressure increase with venlafaxine is usually not clinically relevant, and may be on the order of 2–7 mm Hg (Wyeth-Ayerst Laboratories, 1994); patients may occasionally experience greater increases, particularly at doses greater than 300 mg/day. Hypertensive patients should have their blood pressure monitored regularly while on venlafaxine.

Prevention is the most important management intervention for this potentially fatal adverse effect. Selective or reversible MAOIs that do not irreversibly or significantly affect MAO-A may one day be clinically available and clinically useful (Simpson & De Leon, 1989). However, for the present, ongoing patient education as to the importance of avoiding proscribed foods and drugs is essential. Patients should be given written material about dietary restrictions; this should be discussed with them prior to the initiation of treatment, and then periodically reviewed. Patients should be instructed to keep copies of these lists at their homes and offices and in their automobiles for ready reference. They should be cautioned about "cheating" on their diets and warned that failure to experience a hypertensive reaction after ingesting a proscribed substance does not predict future safety on repeat exposure.

Patients who develop characteristic signs and symptoms of a hypertensive reaction should be instructed to present themselves immediately to a medical office or emergency room. Patients should not lie down if they are feeling poorly and have reason to suspect a hypertensive reaction; lowering the head may increase central pressure because of the additional effects of gravity on the intravascular column of blood. For those with elevated blood pressure, the urine should be acidified with vitamin C tablets or by other means, and supportive measures for the respiratory, cardiovascular, and metabolic systems should be provided as necessary. Sodium nitroprusside or phentolamine can be used in the emergency room setting to reduce blood pressure.

Nifedipine, a calcium channel blocker with antihypertensive properties, has been used to reduce blood pressure quickly in patients experiencing a hypertensive reaction. A 10-mg capsule can be taken sublingually (the capsule should be crushed between the teeth, absorbed under the tongue, and then swallowed) every 30 minutes as needed. Responsible patients may carry 10-mg nifedipine tablets for sublingual use if they have ingested proscribed substances and develop headache or other symptoms of hypertensive reactions at some distance from a hospital. The patients may use the sublingual nifedipine every 30 minutes as necessary to control their blood pressure on the way to the hospital. Patients should be warned that the availability of this intervention should not encourage risk taking and that nifedipine is not a substitute for medical evaluation if symptoms develop; depending on the size and content of the meal, tyramine may be absorbed over a relatively long period of time, and may thus continue to elevate blood pressure.

DERMATOLOGIC EFFECTS

Cutaneous reactions to antidepressant medications are relatively common, occurring in 5–10% of patients (Warnock & Knesevich, 1988). They are most commonly erythematous maculopapular rashes, which tend to occur early in treatment, to be time-limited, and to remit spontaneously if antidepressant treatment is continued (Biederman, Gonzalez, Bronstein, De Monaco, & Wright, 1988). The decision about whether to continue the medication depends on the level of patient discomfort, evidence of systemic involvement, and history of therapeutic response to other agents. Dermatologic reactions that progress beyond a flat maculopapular rash or are associated with signs of systemic involvement (e.g., increased temperature, abnormalities in liver function tests, or elevated white blood cell count) may be indications of a generalized immune reaction and may necessitate immediate discontinuation of the medication. For patients with relatively localized maculopapular rashes, pruritus can be treated with an antihistamine such as terfenadine (60 mg twice daily or diphenhydramanine (25–50 mg one to three times daily), or with occasional administration of a topical steroid cream containing 1% hydrocortisone. If another antidepressant is substituted, it may be reasonable to use agents from a different class to minimize the possibility of cross-reactivity, although there are no systematic data suggesting the utility of this practice.

Occasionally, more severe dermatologic reactions (e.g., localized or generalized urticaria, erythema multiforme, or toxic epidural necrolysis) may occur. Recently, some patients on SSRIs and benzodiazepines such as clonazepam (Magro, Crowson, Hatta, & Duncan, 1993) have been reported to develop cutaneous erythematous plaques with atypical lymphoid infiltrates or pseudolymphomas. Dermatologic consultation is recommended, and although it is unclear whether these infiltrates may proceed to malignancies, it is most prudent to discontinue the offending agent immediately and consider alternative treatment strategies.

HAIR LOSS

Various antidepressants, as well as other psychotropic medications, may cause hair loss. The mechanism of action of this effect is unknown. Supplementation of trace minerals such as selenium may prevent hair loss in some patients receiving antidepressants; over-the-counter multivitamin formulations containing trace minerals have been clinically useful for this indication.

SWEATING

Excessive sweating is commonly associated with TCAs, but can occur with any antidepressant and may be extremely distressing for some patients. The mechanism is not clear, but it has been suggested that TCA-induced sweating may be mediated by an imbalance between alpha- and beta-adrenergic function (Butt, 1989; Leeman, 1990). Consistent with this hypothesis is a case report suggesting that the alpha$_1$-adrenergic antagonist terazosin (1–5 mg at bedtime) is effective in reducing TCA-induced sweating (Leeman, 1990). Clonidine (0.25 mg one to four times a day) may also be used to reduce sweating, with initiation of dosing at low levels (i.e., 0.1 mg/day) to minimize hypotensive effects (Kuritsky, Hering, Goldhammer, & Bechar, 1984). A solution of aluminum chloride hexahydrate (20% w./v.) in anhydrous alcohol, (Drysol), a potent antiperspirant, can be used to control excessive sweating localized to the axilla or palms (Yarrow, 1981). Simple measures such as daily showering or use of talcum powder may also provide some symptomatic relief.

CONCLUSIONS

The treatment of antidepressant-induced adverse effects is an important area of clinical concern, particularly as increasing evidence points to the need for long-term treatment of mood and anxiety disorders at full therapeutic levels in order to maximize outcome. Selection of well-tolerated agents and effective management of emergent adverse effects will improve patient compliance and permit acute and long-term treatment with optimal levels of pharmacotherapy.

REFERENCES

Bakish, D. (1991). Fluoxetine potentiation by buspirone: Three case histories. *Canadian Journal of Psychiatry, 36*, 749–750.

Baldessarini, R. (1985). *Chemotherapy in psychiatry: Principles and practice.* Cambridge, MA: Harvard University Press.

Balogh, S., Hendricks, S. E., & Kang, J. (1992). Treatment of fluoxetine-induced anorgasmia with amantadine [Letter]. *Journal of Clinical Psychiatry, 53,* 212–213.

Becker, J., & Maiman, L. (1975). Sociobehavioral determinants of compliance with health and medical care recommendations. *Medical Care, 13,* 10.

Bergeron, R., & Blier, P. (1994). Cisapride for treatment of nausea produced by selective serotonin reuptake inhibitors. *American Journal of Psychiatry, 151,* 1084–1086.

Bernstein, J. (1983). *Drug therapy in psychiatry.* Boston: John Wright.

Biederman, J., Gonzalez, E., Bronstein, B., De Monaco, H., & Wright, V. (1988). Desipramine and cutaneous reactions in pediatric outpatients. *Journal of Clinical Psychiatry, 49,* 178–183.

Blackwell, B., & Cantob, M. B. (1963). Hypertensive crisis due to monoamine oxidase inhibitors. *British Journal of Psychiatry, 113,* 349–365.

Bouckoms, A., & Mangini, L. (1993). Pergolide: An antidepressant adjuvant for mood disorders. *Psychopharmacology Bulletin, 29,* 207–211.

Butt, M. M. (1989). Managing antidepressant-induced sweating [Letter]. *Journal of Clinical Psychiatry, 50,* 146–147.

Carr, A. C., & Hobson, R. P. (1977). High serum concentration of antidepressants in elderly patients. *British Medical Journal, ii,* 1151.

Christensen, D. (1978). Drug taking compliance: A review and synthesis. *Health Services Research, 13,* 171–187.

Cooper, G. L. (1988). The safety of fluoxetine: An update. *British Journal of Psychiatry, 153*(3, Suppl.), 77–86.

Damulji, N. F., & Ferguson, J. M. (1988). Paradoxical worsening of depressive symptomatology caused by antidepressants. *Journal of Clinical Psychopharmacology, 8,* 347–349.

DeCastro, R. M. (1985). Reversal of MAOI-induced anorgasmia with cyproheptadine [Letter]. *American Journal of Psychiatry, 142,* 783.

DeGroat, W. C., & Booth, A. M. (1980). Physiology of male sexual function. *Annals of Internal Medicine, 92,* 329–331.

Dista Products Company. (1990). *Letter to doctors.* Indianapolis, IN: Eli Lilly & Company.

Everett, H. C. (1975). The use of bethanechol chloride with tricyclic antidepressants. *American Journal of Psychiatry, 132,* 1202–1204.

Fava, M., & Rosenbaum, J. F. (1991). Suicidality and fluoxetine: Is there a relationship? *Journal of Clinical Psychiatry, 52,* 108–111.

Fava, M., Rosenbaum, J. F., Cohen, L., Reiter, S., McCarthy, M., Steingard, R., & Clancy, K. (1992). High dose fluoxetine and the treatment of depressed patients not responsive to a standard dose of fluoxetine. *Journal of Affective Disorders, 25,* 229–234.

Fava, M., Rosenbaum, J. F., McGrath, P. J., Stewart, J. W., Amsterdam, J. D., & Quitkin, F. M. (1994). Lithium and tricyclic augmentation of fluoxetine treatment for resistant major depression: A double blind controlled study. *American Journal of Psychiatry, 151,* 1372–1374.

Feder, R. (1991). Reversal of antidepressant activity of fluoxetine by cyproheptadine in three patients. *Journal of Clinical Psychiatry, 52,* 163–164.

Feighner, J. P., Herbstein, J., & Damlouji, N. (1985). Combined MAOI, TCA and direct stimulant therapy of treatment resistant depression. *Journal of Clinical Psychiatry, 46,* 206–209.

Flemenbaum, A. (1976). Pavor nocturnus: A complication of single daily tricyclic or neuroleptic dosage. *American Journal of Psychiatry, 133*(5), 570–572.

Frank, E., Kupfer, D. J., Perel, J. M., Cornes, C., Jarret, D. B., Mallinger, A. G., Thase, M. E., McEachran, A. B., & Grochocinski, V. J. (1990). Three-year outcomes for maintenance therapies in recurrent depression. *Archives of General Psychiatry, 47*, 1093–1099.

Gardner, A. E., & Johnston, J. A. (1985). Bupropion: An antidepressant without sexual pathophysiological action. *Journal of Clinical Psychopharmacology, 5*, 24–29.

Garland, E. J., Remick, R. A., & Zis, A. P. (1988). Weight gain with antidepressants and lithium. *Journal of Clinical Psychopharmacology, 8*, 323–330.

Garvey, M. J., & Tollefson, G. D. (1987). Occurrence of myoclonus in patients treated with cyclic antidepressants. *Archives of General Psychiatry, 44*, 269–272.

Gitlin, M. J. (1994). Psychotropic medications and their effects on sexual function: Diagnosis, biology and treatment approaches. *Journal of Clinical Psychiatry, 55*, 406–413.

Gorman, J. M., Liebowitz, M. R., Fyer, A. J., Goetz, D. H., Campeas, R. B., Fyer, M. R., Davies, S. O., & Klein, D. F. (1987). An open trial of fluoxetine in the treatment of panic attacks. *Journal of Psychopharmacology, 7*, 329–332.

Greenblatt, D. J., Sellers, E. M., & Shader, R. I. (1982). Drug disposition in old age. *New England Journal of Medicine, 306*, 1081–1088.

Harrison, W. M., McGrath, P. J., Stewart, J. W., & Quitkin, F. M. (1989). Monoamine oxidase and hypertensive crisis: The role of OTC drugs. *Journal of Clinical Psychiatry, 52*, 64–65.

Harrison, W. M., Rabkin, J. G., Ehrlhardt, A. A., Stewart, J. W., McGrath, P. J., Ross, D., & Quitkin, F. M. (1986). Effects of antidepressant medications on sexual function: A controlled study. *Journal of Clinical Psychopharmacology, 6*, 144–149.

Herman, J. B., Brotman, A. W., Pollack, M. H., Falk, W. E., Biederman, J., & Rosenbaum, J. F. (1990). Treatment emergent sexual dysfunction with fluoxetine. *Journal of Clinical Psychiatry, 51*, 25–27.

Hoehn-Saric, R., Harris, G. J., Pearlson, J. D., Cox, C. S., Machlin, S. R., & Camargo, E. E. (1991). A fluoxetine-induced frontal lobe syndrome in an obsessive compulsive patient. *Journal of Clinical Psychiatry, 52*, 131–133.

Hollander, E., & McCarley, A. (1992). Yohimbine treatment of sexual side effects induced by serotonin reuptake blockers. *Journal of Clinical Psychiatry, 53*, 207–209.

Hollingsworth, O. R., Amatruda, T. T., & Schei, G. R. (1970). Quantitative and qualitative effects of L-triiodothyronine in massive obesity. *Metabolism, 19*, 934–945.

Hyyppa, M. T., Falck, S. C., Aukia, H., & Rinne, U. K. (1975). Neuroendocrine regulation of gonadotropin secretion and sexual motivation after L-tryptophan administration in man. In. M. Sandler & D. L. Gessa (Eds.), *Sexual behavior: Pharmacology and biochemistry.* New York: Raven Press.

Jacobsen, F. M. (1992). Fluoxetine-induced sexual dysfunction and an open trial of yohimbine. *Journal of Clinical Psychiatry, 53*, 119–122.

Janicak, P. G., Davis, J. M., Preskorn, S. H., & Ayd, F. J. (1993). *Principles and practice of pharmacotherapy.* Baltimore: Williams & Wilkins.

Joffe, R. T. (1990). Afternoon fatigue and somnolence associated with tranyl-cypromine treatment. *Journal of Clinical Psychiatry, 51*, 192–193.

Katon, W., Von Korff, M., Lin, E., Lipscomb, P., Russo, J., Wagner, E., & Polk, E. (1990). Distressed high utilizers of medical care: DSM-III-R diagnoses and treatment needs. *General Hospital Psychiatry, 12*, 355–362.

Keck, P. E., Vuckovic, A., Pope, H. G., Nierenberg, A., Gribble, G. W., & White, K. (1989). Acute cardiovascular response to monoamine oxidase inhibitors: A prospective assessment. *Journal of Clinical Psychopharmacology, 9*, 203–206.

Keller, M. B., Klerman, G. L., Lavori, P. W., Fawcett, J. A., Coryell, W., & Endicott, J. (1982). Treatment received by depressed patients. *Journal of the American Medical Association, 228*, 1848–1855.

Klein, D. F., Gittelman, R., Quitkin, F., & Rifkin, A. (1980). *Diagnostic and drug treatment of psychiatric disorders: Adults and children* (2nd ed.). Baltimore: Williams & Wilkins.

Kline, N. S. (1981). Eliminating hypotension with abdominal binders [Letter]. *American Journal of Psychiatry, 138*, 858.

Kraupl-Taylor, F. (1972). Loss of libido in depression. *British Medical Journal, i*, 305.

Kuritsky, A., Hering, R., Goldhammer, G., & Bechar, M. (1984). Clonidine treatment in paroxysmal localized hyperhidrosis. *Archives of Neurology, 41*, 1210–1211.

Labatte, L. H., & Pollack, M. H. (1994). Treatment of fluoxetine-induced sexual dysfunction with bupropion. *Annals of Clinical Psychiatry, 6*, 13–15.

LeCrubier, Y., Puech, A. J., & Des Lauriers, A. (1981). Favorable effects of yohimbine on clomipramine-induced orthostatic hypotension: A double blind study. *British Journal of Clinical Pharmacology, 12*, 90–93.

Leeman, C. P. (1990). Pathophysiology of tricyclic-induced sweating [Letter]. *Journal of Clinical Psychiatry, 51*, 258–259.

Lipinski, J. F., Mallya, G., Zimmerman, P., & Pope, H. G. (1989). Fluoxetine-induced akathisia: Clinical and theoretical implications. *Journal of Clinical Psychiatry, 50*, 339–342.

Madden, E. F. (1973). Evaluation of outpatient pharmacy counseling. *Journal of the American Pharmaceutical Association NS, 13*, 437.

Magro, C., Crowson, N., Hatta, T., & Duncan, L. M. (1993). A 47 year old woman with several large chronic scaling plaques. *Fitzpatrick's Journal of Clinical Dermatology, 11–12*, 24–28.

McCormick, S., Olin, J., & Brotman, A. W. (1990). Reversal of fluoxetine-induced anorgasmia by cyproheptadine in two patients. *Journal of Clinical Psychiatry, 51*, 383–384.

McLean, J. D., Forsythe, R. G., & Kapkin, I. A. (1983). Unusual side effects of clomipramine associated with yawning. *Canadian Journal of Psychiatry, 28*, 569–570.

Mitchell, J. E., & Popkin, M. K. (1983). Antidepressant drug therapy and sexual dysfunction in men: A review. *Journal of Clinical Psychopharmacology, 3*, 76–79.

Modell, J. G. (1989). Repeated observations of yawning, clitoral engorgement and orgasm associated with fluoxetine administration [Letter]. *Journal of Clinical Psychopharmacology, 9*, 63–65.

Morin, C. M., Culbert, J. P., & Schwartz, S. M. (1994). Nonpharmacologic interventions for insomnia: A meta-analysis of treatment efficacy. *American Journal of Psychiatry, 151*, 1172–1180.

Munjack, D. (1984). The treatment of phenelzine-induced hypotension with salt tablets: Case report. *Journal of Clinical Psychiatry, 45*, 89–90.

Neill, J. R. (1991). Penile anesthesia associated with fluoxetine [Letter]. *American Journal of Psychiatry, 148,* 1603.

Nierenberg, A. A., Adler, L. A., Peselow, E., Zornberg, G., & Rosenthal, M. (1994). Trazodone for antidepressant associated insomnia. *American Journal of Psychiatry, 151,* 1069–1072.

Noyes, R., Garvey, M. J., Cook, B. L., & Samuelson, L. (1989). Problems with tricyclic antidepressant use in patients with panic disorder or agoraphobia: Results of a naturalistic follow-up study. *Journal of Clinical Psychiatry, 50,* 163–169.

Patterson, J. F. (1987). Metoclopramide therapy of MAOI orthostatic hypotension [Letter]. *Journal of Clinical Psychopharmacology, 7,* 112–113.

Physicians' desk reference (48th ed.). (1995). Montvale, NJ: Medical Economics.

Pohl, R., Yeragani, V. K., Balon, R., & Lycaki, H. (1988). The jitteriness syndrome in panic disorder patients treated with antidepressants. *Journal of Clinical Psychiatry, 49,* 100–104.

Pollack, M. H., & Hammerness, P. G. (1993). Adjunctive yohimbine for treatment refractory depression. *Biological Psychiatry, 33,* 220–221.

Pollack, M. H., Reiter, S., & Hammerness, P. (1992). Genitourinary and sexual adverse effects of psychotropic medication. *The International Journal of Psychiatry in Medicine, 22,* 305–327.

Pollack, M. H., & Rosenbaum, J. F. (1987). Management of antidepressant-induced side effects: A practical guide for the clinician. *Journal of Clinical Psychiatry, 48,* 3–8.

Preshorn, S. H. (1995). Comparison of the tolerability of bupropion, fluoxetine, imipramine, nefaxodane, paroxetine, sertraline and venlafaxine. *Journal of Clinical Psychiatry, 56*(Suppl. 6), 12–21.

Price, J., & Grunhaus, I. J. (1990). Treatment of clomipramine-induced anorgasmia with yohimbine: A case report. *Journal of Clinical Psychiatry, 51,* 32–33.

Rabkin, J., Quitkin, F. M., McGrath, P., Harrison, W., & Tricamo, E. (1985). Adverse reactions to monoamine oxidase inhibitors: Part 2. Treatment correlates and clinical management. *Journal of Clinical Psychopharmacology, 5,* 2–9.

Richelson, E. (1994). The pharmacology of antidepressants at the synapse: Focus on newer compounds. *Journal of Clinical Psychiatry, 55*(Suppl. A), 34–39.

Roose, S. P., Glassman, A. H., Siris, S. G., Walsh, B. T., Bruno, R. L., & Wright, L. B. (1981). Comparison of imipramine and nortriptyline orthostatic hypotension: A meaningful difference. *Journal of Clinical Psychopharmacology, 1,* 316–319.

Rosen, J., Pollack, B. G., Altieri, L. P., & Jonas, E. A. (1993). Treatment of nortriptyline's side effects in elderly patients: A double blind study of bethanechol. *American Journal of Psychiatry, 150,* 1249–1251.

Rumach, B. H. (1973). Anticholinergic poisoning treatment with physostigmine. *Pediatrics, 52,* 449–451.

Schneier, F. R., Liebowitz, M. R., Davies, S. O., Fairbanks, J., Hollander, E., Campeas, R., & Klein, D. F. (1990). Fluoxetine in panic disorder. *Journal of Clinical Psychopharmacology, 10*(2), 119–121.

Segraves, T. (1989). Effects of psychotropic drugs on human erection and ejaculation. *Archives of General Psychiatry, 46,* 275–284.

Silverstone, E. T., & Kyriakides, M. (1982). Clinical pharmacology of appetite. In T. Silverstone (Ed.), *Drugs and appetite.* London: Academic Press.

Simon, G. E., Von Korff, M., & Katon, W. J. (1994). *Balancing cost and effectiveness of antidepressant drugs in primary care: A randomized trial.* Paper presented at the Eighth Annual NIMH International Research Conference on Mental Health Problems in the General Health Care Sector, McLean, VA.

Simonson, M. (1964). Controlling MAO inhibitor hypotension. *American Journal of Psychiatry, 121,* 1118–1119.

Simpson, G. M., & De Leon, J. (1989). Tyramine and new monoamine oxidase inhibitor drugs. *British Journal of Psychiatry, 155,* 32–37.

Steele, T. E., & Howell, E. F. (1986). Cyproheptadine for imipramine-induced anorgasmia [Letter]. *Journal of Clinical Psychopharmacology, 6,* 326–327.

Stewart, J. W., Harrison, W., Quitkin, F., & Liebowitz, M. R. (1984). Phenelzine-induced pyridoxine deficiency. *Journal of Clinical Psychopharmacology, 4,* 225–226.

Susset, J. G., Tessier, C. D., Wincze, J., Bansal, S., Malhotra, C., & Schwacha, M. G. (1989). Effect of yohimbine hydrochloride on erectile impotence: A double blind study. *Journal of Urology, 141,* 1360–1363.

Teicher, M. H., Cohen, B. M., Baldessarini, R. J., & Cole, J. O. (1988). Severe daytime somnolence in patients treated with an MAOI. *American Journal of Psychiatry, 145,* 1552–1556.

Teicher, M. H., Glod, C., & Cole, J. O. (1990). Emergence of intense suicidal preoccupation during fluoxetine treatment. *American Journal of Psychiatry, 147,* 207–210.

Thase, M. E. (1990). Relapse and recurrence in unipolar major depression: Short term and long term approaches. *Journal of Clinical Psychiatry, 51*(6, Suppl.), 51–57.

Thompson, J. W., Jr., Ware, M. R., & Blashfield, R. K. (1990). Psychotropic medication and priapism: A comprehensive review. *Journal of Clinical Psychiatry, 51,* 430–433.

Tollefson, G. D., Greist, J. H., Jefferson, J. W., Heiligenstein, J. H., Sayler, M. E., Tollefson, S. L., & Koback, K. (1994). Is baseline agitation a relative contraindication for a selective serotonin reuptake inhibitor?: A comparative trial of fluoxetine versus imipramine. *Journal of Clinical Psychopharmacology, 14,* 385–391.

Waldinger, M. D., Hengeveld, M. W., & Zwinderman, A. H. (1994). Paroxetine treatment of premature ejaculation: A double blind randomized placebo controlled study. *American Journal of Psychiatry, 151,* 1377–1379.

Walker, P. W., Cole, J. O., Gardner, E. A., Hughes, A. R., Johnston, J. A., Beatty, S. R., & Lineberry, C. G. (1993). Improvement in fluoxetine associated sexual dysfunction in patients switched to bupropion. *Journal of Clinical Psychiatry, 54,* 459–465.

Warner, M. D., Peabody, C. A., Whiteford, H. A., & Hollister, L. E. (1987). Trazodone and priapism. *Journal of Clinical Psychiatry, 48,* 244–245.

Warnock, J. K., & Knesevich, J. W. (1988). Adverse cutaneous reactions to antidepressants. *American Journal of Psychiatry, 145,* 425–430.

Weilburg, J. B., Rosenbaum, J. F., Meltzer-Brody, S., & Shustari, J. (1991). Tricyclic augmentation of fluoxetine. *Annals of Clinical Psychiatry, 3,* 209–213.

Whybrow, P. C., & Prange, A. G. (1981). A hypothesis of thyroid catecholamine receptor interaction. *Archives of General Psychiatry, 38,* 106–113.

Wyeth-Ayerst Laboratories (1994). *Effexor prescribing information.* Philadelphia: Author.

Yarrow, H. (1981). Treatment of axillary hyperhidrosis. *British Medical Journal, 282,* 150.

19

Acute and Chronic Adverse Effects of Neuroleptics

ALAN J. GELENBERG

For the past three decades, antipsychotic agents have been invaluable for alleviating symptoms of acute and chronic psychosis. At the same time, however, they have engendered a broad spectrum of unwanted effects on virtually all body systems, ranging in severity from annoying to potentially lethal. This chapter focuses on those side effects of neuroleptics that make patients want to stop treatment. The term "neuroleptic" refers to the tendency of antipsychotic agents to cause neurologic effects, most notably "extrapyramidal" reactions—that is, those affecting motor activities. (Table 19.1 lists some of the pharmacologic agents most commonly used in treating extrapyramidal reactions; their specific uses are discussed in greater detail below.) In this chapter, I use the terms "neuroleptic" and "antipsychotic drug" interchangeably. Since adverse drug effects are commonly cited as reasons for noncompliance with a treatment regimen, the chapter highlights diagnostic and treatment approaches that may alleviate such symptoms and foster greater patient acceptance of prescribed antipsychotic therapy. At the same time, the chapter addresses other treatment dilemmas and problems regarding this class of drugs.

DYSTONIC REACTIONS

Acute dystonic reactions, along with acute dyskinesias and oculogyric crises, typically occur early in the course of neuroleptic therapy or after a marked dosage increment (Gelenberg, 1991b). The muscle tightening and abnormal posturing of this syndrome are easily recognized if the drug-related precipitation is appreciated, although tetanus, seizures, and conversion reactions form part of the differential diagnosis. Males, young people, and patients taking high-potency neuroleptics are most likely to develop acute dystonic reactions.

Parenteral therapy provides the most rapid relief of acute dystonias. Commonly employed contraactive drugs include benztropine, diphenhydramine, and the benzodiazepines. After the acute dystonic reaction remits, the physician may provide an oral form of one of these contraactive agents. Alternatively, or in addition, the physician may wish to lower the dose of the antipsychotic agent or switch to one of lower potency.

Recent investigations have suggested that the prophylactic use of antiparkinsonian drugs can cut the rate of acute dystonic reactions by 50% or more (Gelenberg, 1987). Patients for whom this strategy may be most appropriate are those at greatest risk (i.e., young males on high-potency neuroleptics). Alternatively, the growing use of lower doses of antipsychotic drugs in the treatment of psychotic disorders may in itself obviate the need for such a prophylactic strategy. Whether or not the physician elects to prescribe a prophylactic antiparkinsonian drug, a patient being started on an antipsychotic agent should be warned about the possibility of an acute dystonic reaction, to diminish the intensity of what could otherwise be a frightening experience. Family members or other caretakers should be similarly forewarned.

AKATHISIA

Akathisia, an inner compulsion to be in restless motion, is a miserably uncomfortable symptom that frequently leads patients to resist or abandon neuroleptic treatment (Van Putten & Marder, 1987). More common (again) with higher-potency antipsychotic drugs, akathisia can at times be mistaken for the anxiety or agitation of an underlying psychiatric illness. A clue to its recognition, however, is the fact that an antipsychotic drug may recently have been initiated, changed, or increased in dose. In its more severe forms, akathisia can simulate or actually cause a worsening of psychosis, and thus can be an iatrogenic cause of treatment-resistant psychosis.

Like other types of extrapyramidal reactions to neuroleptics, akathisia can sometimes be managed by lowering the antipsychotic drug dose or by switching to a less potent agent. Thioridazine, in particular, is unlikely to cause extrapyramidal effects. Clozapine appears to cause few extrapyramidal effects, including akathisia.

Drugs that have been used (with variable rates of success) to alleviate akathisia include anticholinergic antiparkinsonian drugs (e.g., benztropine, trihexyphenidyl), sedating antihistamines (e.g., diphenhydramine),

TABLE 19.1. Agents Used in the Treatment of Neuroleptic-Induced Extrapyramidal Symptoms

Generic name	Trade name	Type of drug	Usual dose range (mg/day)	Injectable?
Amantadine	Symmetrel, etc.	Dopamine agonist	100–300	No
Benztropine	Cogentin, etc.	Antihistamine and anticholinergic	1–6	Yes
Biperiden	Akineton, etc.	Anticholinergic	2–6	Yes
Diphenhydramine	Benadryl, etc.	Antihistamine and anticholinergic	25–200	Yes
Lorazepam	Ativan, etc.	Benzodiazepine	0.5–8	Yes
Procyclidine	Kenadrin, etc.	Anticholinergic	6–20	No
Propranolol	Inderal, etc.	Beta-adrenergic blocker	20–160	No
Trihexyphenidyl	Artane, etc.	Anticholinergic	1–10	No

benzodiazepines, and more recently beta-adrenergic blockers (e.g., propranolol).

On broad average, the beta-adrenergic blockers have had a success rate of roughly 50% in alleviating the symptoms of akathisia. They certainly belong in our armamentarium against this troublesome side effect; however, because of their potential to cause some profound cardiorespiratory toxicity, they probably should be reserved for cases in which easier-to-use contraactive therapies (e.g., antiparkinsonian agents) have proved ineffective. Patients on other cardioactive substances, and those with some degree of heart block, heart failure, or other cardiac problems, should be managed in consultation with an internist when they are placed on beta-adrenergic blockers. Patients with bronchospastic conditions such as asthma should not receive these agents at all. Although a number of beta-adrenergic blockers have been tried and found successful in alleviating akathisia, the nonselective and oldest member of this group, propranolol, has been used most. I recommend initiating therapy with 10 mg by mouth and then assessing the symptomatic response, which should become apparent within a matter of minutes and peak within 1 hour. The dose can be titrated upward as necessary (rarely more than 40 mg at a time, although there should be no absolute ceiling dose), depending on therapeutic efficacy on the one hand, and such important side effects as hypotension and bradycardia on the other.

As with all adverse drug effects, a thorough discussion with the patient goes a long way toward alleviating secondary anxiety. In particular, the patient should be reassured that the hellish compulsion to move about is a reaction to the drug, rather than a worsening of the psychosis or a "punishment from God."

PARKINSONIAN SYNDROMES

A full description of Parkinson's syndrome as a neuroleptic reaction is beyond the scope of this chapter, but such a description can be found elsewhere (Gelenberg, 1984a). Parkinson's syndrome is characterized by three signs and symptoms: tremor, rigidity, and akinesia or bradykinesia. Bradykinesia or akinesia, a slowing or disinclination to move, is the feature of parkinsonism most commonly observed in neuroleptic-treated patients, and these signs are most likely to be associated with treatment noncompliance. Milder bradykinesia can make a patient feel listless, fatigued, apathetic, or depressed. On top of the other burdens of a major psychiatric disorder, the patient may find himself or herself lacking interest, energy, and pleasure. If misdiagnosed, this condition can be falsely attributed to a treatment-resistant depression in a psychotic patient.

In its more severe forms, akinesia can mimic catatonia, and patients become more psychotic as their bodies feel stiff and strange. For the clinician, the flattening of facial expressiveness, characteristic stance and posture, and attendant signs of parkinsonism will indicate the drug-related nature of this condition. The temporal relationship to the course of antipsychotic drug therapy should reaffirm this diagnosis.

Once again, lowering the antipsychotic drug dose may alleviate most or all parkinsonian symptoms and signs. Use of a lower-potency neuroleptic—in particular, thioridazine or clozapine—may also be an effective strategy. Anticholinergic antiparkinsonian drugs (e.g., benztropine) can often be helpful, although the physician should attend to unwanted anticholinergic effects, both peripheral (e.g., dry mouth, constipation, blurred vision) and central (from short-term memory difficulties all the way to a delirium).

When anticholinergic antiparkinsonian drugs are added to antipsychotic drugs that a patient is already taking, the patient's peripheral and central muscarinic blockade can climb to clinically troublesome levels. Among antipsychotic drugs, lower-potency drugs are more strongly anticholinergic, with thioridazine and clozapine the most anticholinergic of all. The elderly, and patients with certain medical conditions (e.g., glaucoma, prostatic hyperplasia), may be even more susceptible to these effects.

Amantadine, a dopamine agonist, is an antiparkinsonian drug that does not have anticholinergic effects. Some patients, however, experience unwanted stimulation and even worsening of psychosis on treatment with amantadine, and patients with decreased glomerular filtration (elevated serum creatinine) should be treated with lower doses and more cautious observation.

There is some evidence that between 62% and 96% of patients on maintenance treatment with antipsychotic drugs require long-term therapy with concomitant antiparkinsonian agents to avoid a recurrence of parkinsonian signs (Gelenberg, 1987). Alternatively, many astute clinicians find that the use of very low doses of antipsychotic agents for patients on maintenance therapy diminishes the need for such additional drug therapy.

TARDIVE DYSKINESIA

Tardive dyskinesia may afflict from 20% to 30% of neuroleptic-treated patients. Fortunately, most cases are mild; however, the relatively uncommon severe cases, particularly those involving dystonic posturing, can cause profound suffering and discomfort.

The dyskinesias themselves are less likely than other adverse reactions to foster noncompliance; in fact, many schizophrenic patients who develop tardive dyskinesia maintain that they are unaware of the movements. On the other hand, a physician's full disclosure of the risk of tardive dyskinesia, as part of an informed consent discussion with the patient, may serve as an excuse for noncompliance. Clinicians would be well advised, therefore, to consider the way in which they discuss the risk of tardive dyskinesia with patients. Patients can be reassured that our current understanding of the odds still favors their not developing this syndrome, and, more importantly, that most cases of tardive dyskinesia are mild and relatively untroubling. The physician can further reassure a patient that the two of them will work together to watch for early signs of this syndrome, and that at all times the physician will seek to use the lowest effective antipsychotic dose, which should further minimize the risk of the patient's developing tardive dyskinesia. Finally, when the physician has made a decision to recommend maintenance neuroleptic therapy, it stands to reason that the doctor has weighed the risks of the psychosis as being considerably greater than the probability and severity of dyskinesia—and this should be fully discussed with the patient and close relatives.

Unfortunately, at present there is no standard treatment for tardive dyskinesia. Fortunately, though, many patients can continue to take antipsychotic drugs without any marked worsening of the dyskinesias. The fortunate few who can discontinue antipsychotic drugs often find a gradual reversal of the syndrome.

Most schizophrenic patients will require ongoing maintenance treatment with an antipsychotic drug, to prevent the immediate reemergence of psychotic symptoms or an eventual relapse into an acute episode. For them, the best strategy is to find the lowest effective maintenance dose. With haloperidol, for example, many schizophrenic patients can be maintained on as little as 0.5–1.0 mg/day. With one of the two currently available decanoate esters of antipsychotic drugs (fluphenazine and haloperidol), as little as 0.25 cc injected at monthly intervals (or occasionally even less frequently) can maintain adequate symptom control. At times of stress, the clinician may wish to increase the dose of the antipsychotic drug for a brief period until the stress abates and the patient's symptoms again become quiescent.

For most patients, the abnormal involuntary movements of tardive dyskinesia are minimally troublesome, causing little pain or dysfunction. As mentioned above, continuing treatment with an antipsychotic drug is unlikely to make the movements worse, but it may decrease the likelihood of the movements' ever reversing.

Occasionally, dyskinesia can be severe and even disabling, and this is most likely when the movements are the sustained postures of tardive dystonia. One of the least hazardous approaches to symptom remission is the use of a benzodiazepine. Any benzodiazepine can be effective (e.g., diazepam, lorazepam, clonazepam), and the lowest effective dose should be employed; again, the physician must balance symptom alleviation against excessive sedation and incoordination.

A number of recent studies have suggested benefit from vitamin E at a dosage of 1200–1600 IU/day (Adler et al., 1993; Egan et al., 1992; Elkashef, Ruskin, Bacher, & Barrett, 1990; Lohr, Cadet, Lohr, Jeste, & Wyatt, 1987; Shriqui, Bradwejn, Annable, & Jones, 1992). In general, patients who have had tardive movement disorders for under 5 years show greater improvement than those who have had them for longer than 5 years. Patients with tardive dystonia, particularly those with blepharospasm, have sometimes been dramatically improved by treatment with botulinum toxin (Gelenberg, 1991a). Clozapine does not appear to engender tardive dyskinesia, and there is some evidence that it may actually produce improvement in dyskinetic and dystonic signs (Gelenberg, 1993a; Lieberman, Johns, Pollack, Borenstein, & Kane, 1991).

New antipsychotic drugs, termed "atypical" because they are less likely to produce extrapyramidal effects, are being introduced in the United States. The first has been risperidone. These drugs produce fewer of all types of extrapyramidal reactions. Whether they may cause tardive dyskinesia remains to be observed. Also unknown is whether they will have clozapine's ability to dampen dyskinetic and dystonic symptoms.

ANTICHOLINERGIC EFFECTS

By blocking the muscarinic acetylcholine receptor, antipsychotic agents produce a variety of peripheral and central anticholinergic effects (Gelenberg, 1984b). In the periphery, these parasympatholytic effects include dry mouth, problems of visual accommodation, constipation, and difficulty in initiating urination. Centrally, such atropine-like actions impair the ability to learn new information, and in the extreme may cause a full-blown delirium. Low-potency drugs have stronger anticholinergic effects than high-potency agents: Thioridazine appears to be the most strongly anticholinergic among the typical neuroleptics, and clozapine is even more so. By and large, antipsychotic drugs are less anticholinergic than antidepressants. Obviously, there is greater risk of anticholinergic toxicity if a patient is concomitantly taking another drug with similar effects, such as some antiparkinsonian agents, tricyclic antidepressants, or certain drugs used to treat allergies or upper respiratory infections (e.g., diphenhydramine).

Forewarning patients about common anticholinergic effects often improves compliance, as patients may be willing to tolerate effects that they know about in the hope of alleviating underlying psychiatric symptoms. Furthermore, some degree of tolerance develops to anticholinergic effects, leading to a diminution in intensity over time. When anticholinergic effects are particularly uncomfortable, the first treatment strategy to consider is to lower the anticholinergic burden by decreasing the dose of one or both drugs or by using a less anticholinergic agent. Reduction in dose is obviously contingent on the clinical need for the agent. Less anticholinergic among the antipsychotic drugs are the high-potency agents; among antiparkinsonian agents, the physician might consider amantadine.

The second best strategy for dealing with anticholinergic symptoms is the use of contraactive agents. For dry mouth, sugarless gum or sugarless lozenges may be helpful, and some patients periodically make use of a saliva substitute. Dry mouth and some of the other peripheral anticholinergic symptoms may at times be alleviated by such peripherally active parasympathomimetic agents as bethanechol or neostigmine; with these agents, however, there is the risk of such symptoms of cholinergic excess as abdominal cramps and diarrhea. Constipation may at times be alleviated by the use of over-the-counter bulk-forming agents and stool softeners; blurred vision may be improved by a change in corrective lenses.

OTHER ADVERSE EFFECTS
WITH IMPLICATIONS FOR COMPLIANCE

Patients taking one of the lower-potency antipsychotic drugs may experience photosensitivity, which can cause an exaggerated sunburn reaction. In times of potential high solar exposure, these patients should be encouraged to minimize time in the sun, particularly in the heat of the day, or to cover the skin as much as possible. Using a high-protection chemical screening agent is an alternative.

Weight gain troubles some patients. Lowering the dose of the drug, or switching to a higher-potency agent, may alleviate the appetite increase that underlies many such cases. In addition, patients can be encouraged to watch their caloric intake and to get more exercise. There is some evidence suggesting that molindone may promote less weight gain than other antipsychotic drugs (Gelenberg, 1993b). Confirmation of these observations, however, will require more systematic study.

A woman whose periods become scanty or stop altogether should have a gynecologic assessment and plasma prolactin assay. The psychiatrist may try to lower the dose of the antipsychotic drug if hyperprolactinemia appears to be the cause of amenorrhea (which may be associated also with galactorrhea). Coadministering bromocriptine can be discussed with an endocrinologist.

Both men and women sometimes experience diminished libido and delayed or absent orgasm when taking antipsychotic agents. Men occasionally report difficulty in achieving or maintaining erection, or retrograde ejaculation. Sometimes these problems are temporary; reassurance can go a long way. As in so many other adverse effects, lowering the dose of the antipsychotic drug may be helpful, or switching to a higher-potency agent may work. Contraactive strategies for the similar problem that exists with antidepressant drugs have included neostigmine, bethanechol, cyproheptadine, yohimbine, amantadine, and trazodone (Hopkins, 1992).

A woman of childbearing potential should be instructed to inform her physician before she tries to conceive a child, in order to allow for full discussion of the risks and potential benefits of drug therapy during pregnancy. As in most questions of drug therapy during pregnancy, there is a delicate balance of risks and unknown factors. Antipsychotic drugs have not been incriminated as teratogens, although we cannot rule out the possibility of a low-level association. There is concern about the possibility of what has been called "behavioral teratogenesis," in which exposure of the developing brain to a psychoactive drug may adversely affect central nervous system development. On the other side of the coin, an unchecked psychosis is not good for the health of the mother or of the developing fetus. A full discussion of these concerns can be found elsewhere (Cohen, Rosenbaum, & Heller, 1991).

SUMMARY AND CONCLUSIONS

Antipsychotic drugs cause a multitude of unwanted effects. This chapter has touched on those most likely to affect compliance adversely. In general, a full disclosure of common adverse effects before they occur can cement the therapeutic alliance and enlist the patient as an ally in a fight against the underlying pathology. A concerned clinician who takes the time to listen to a patient's complaints, and to uncover some that the patient may not freely volunteer at first, can head off potential noncompliance and further reassure the patient and family. Routine screening for adverse effects (e.g., an annual examination for tardive dyskinesia) further underscores this concern for the patient's safety, comfort, and well-being, and additionally strengthens the therapeutic bond. When problems do arise, the physician's concern and knowledge will foster a sense of a joint venture, rather than one of antagonism. Finally, the physician might consider a consultation—even one in the hallway or by telephone—the results of which should be shared with the patient (and sometimes family members). This emphasizes the physician's commitment to the best possible treatment for the patient.

REFERENCES

Adler, L., Peselow, E., Rotrosen, J., Duncan, E., Lee, M., Rosenthal, M., & Angrist, B. (1993). Vitamin E treatment of tardive dyskinesia. *Journal of Psychiatry, 150,* 1405–1407.

Cohen, L. S., Rosenbaum, J. F., & Heller, V. L. (1991). Psychotropic drug use in pregnancy. In A. J. Gelenberg, E. L. Bassuk, & S. C. Schoonover (Eds.), *The practitioner's guide to psychoactive drugs* (3rd ed., pp. 389–405). New York: Plenum Press.

Egan, M. F., Hyde, T. M., Albers, G. W., Elkashef, A. M., Alexander, R. C., Reeve, A., Blum, A., Saenz, R. E., & Wyatt, R. J. (1992). Treatment of tardive dyskinesia with vitamin E. *American Journal of Psychiatry, 149,* 773–777.

Elkashef, A. M., Ruskin, P. E., Bacher, N., & Barrett, D. (1990). Vitamin E in the treatment of tardive dyskinesia. *American Journal of Psychiatry, 147,* 505–506.

Gelenberg, A. J. (1984a). Extrapyramidal reactions to antipsychotic drugs. In T. Manschreck (Ed.), *Psychiatric medicine update* (pp. 177–193). New York: Elsevier/North-Holland.

Gelenberg, A. J. (1984b). Use and abuse of anticholinergic drugs in psychiatry. *Hillside Journal of Clinical Psychiatry, 6,* 148–155.

Gelenberg, A. J. (1987). Treating extrapyramidal reactions: Some current issues. *Journal of Clinical Psychiatry, 48*(9, Suppl.), 24–27.

Gelenberg, A. J. (1991a). Botulinum toxin for tardive dyskinesia. *Biological Therapies in Psychiatry Newsletter, 14,* 17.

Gelenberg, A. J. (1991b). Psychoses. In A. J. Gelenberg, E. L. Bassuk, & S. C. Schoonover (Eds.), *The practitioner's guide to psychoactive drugs* (3rd ed., pp. 125–178). New York: Plenum Press.

Gelenberg, A. J. (1993a). Clozapine and tardive dyskinesia. *Biological Therapies in Psychiatry Newsletter, 16,* 14–15.

Gelenberg, A. J. (1993b). Molindone and weight loss. *Biological Therapies in Psychiatry Newsletter, 16,* 27.

Hopkins, H. S. (1992). Antidotes for antidepressant-induced sexual dysfunction. *Biological Therapies in Psychiatry Newsletter, 15,* 33–36.

Lieberman, J., Johns, C., Pollack, S., Borenstein, M., & Kane, J. (1991). The effects of clozapine on tardive dyskinesia. *British Journal of Psychiatry, 158,* 503–510.

Lohr, J. B., Cadet, J. L., Lohr, M. A., Jeste, D. V., & Wyatt, R. J. (1987). Alphatocopherol in tardive dyskinesia. *Lancet, i,* 913–914.

Shriqui, C. L., Bradwejn, J., Annable, L., & Jones, B. D. (1992). Vitamin E in the treatment of tardive dyskinesia: A double-blind placebo controlled study. *American Journal of Psychiatry, 149,* 391–393.

Van Putten, T., & Marder, S. R. (1987). Behavioral toxicity of antipsychotic drugs. *Journal of Clinical Psychiatry, 48*(9, Suppl.), 13–19.

Index

Page numbers in italics refer to tables or figures.

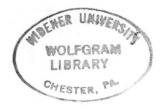